Critical Care Handbook of the Massachusetts General Hospital

Fourth Edition

Critical Care Handbook of the Massachusetts General Hospital

Fourth Edition

Massachusetts General Hospital
Harvard Medical School

Senior Editor
Luca M. Bigatello, M.D.

Associate Editors
Rae M. Allain, M.D.
Kenneth L. Haspel, M.D.
Judith Hellman, M.D.
Dean Hess, Ph.D., R.R.T.
Richard M. Pino, M.D., Ph.D.
Robert Sheridan, M.D.

 LIPPINCOTT WILLIAMS & WILKINS
A **Wolters Kluwer** Company
Philadelphia • Baltimore • New York • London
Buenos Aires • Hong Kong • Sydney • Tokyo

Acquisitions Editor : Brian Brown
Developmental Editor : Maria McAvey
Managing Editor : Franny Murphy
Project Manager : Fran Gunning
Manufacturing Manager : Ben Rivera
Marketing Manager : Angela Panetta
Design Coordinator : Terry Mallon
Production Services : TechBooks
Printer : R. R Donnelley-Crawfordsville

**WX
39
C934
2006**

© 2006 by Department of Anesthesia and Critical Care
Massachusetts General Hospital
Published by LIPPINCOTT WILLIAMS & WILKINS
530 Walnut Street
Philadelphia, PA 19106 USA
LWW.com

Printed in the USA.

Library of Congress Cataloging-in-Publication Data

Critical care handbook of the Massachusetts General Hospital / senior
    editor, Luca M. Bigatello; associate editors,
    Rae M. Allain ... [et al.]. —4th ed.
      p. ; cm.
    ISBN 0-7817-6244-8
    1. Critical care medicine—Handbooks, manuals, etc.   I. Bigatello,
Luca M.   II. Massachusetts General Hospital.
    [DNLM: 1. Critical Care—Handbooks.   2. Postoperative
Complications—Handbooks.   WX 39 C934 2006]
RC86.8C76 2006
616.02′8′09744—dc22

                                                              2005023753

To purchase additional copies of this book, call our customer service department at
(800) 638-3030 or fax orders to (301) 824-7390. International customers should call
(301) 714-2324.

Visit Lippincott Williams & Wilkins on the Internet: http://www.LWW.com.
Lippincott Williams & Wilkins customer service representatives are available from
8:30 am to 6:00 pm, EST.

                                          10 9 8 7 6 5 4 3 2 1

To Our Patients

Contents

I. Critical Care Principles

Appendices

Contributing Authors

Rae M. Allain, M.D. *Department of Anesthesia and Critical Care, Massachusetts General Hospital, Instructor in Anesthesia, Harvard Medical School*

Theodore A. Alston, M.D., Ph.D. *Department of Anesthesia and Critical Care, Massachusetts General Hospital, Assistant Professor of Anesthesia, Harvard Medical School*

Patricia R. Bachiller, M.D. *Department of Anesthesia and Critical Care, Massachusetts General Hospital, Clinical Resident in Anesthesia, Harvard Medical School*

Neeraj Badjatia, M.D. *Department of Neurology, Massachusetts General Hospital, Instructor in Neurology, Harvard Medical School*

Keith Baker, M.D., Ph.D. *Department of Anesthesia and Critical Care, Massachusetts General Hospital, Assistant Professor of Anesthesia, Harvard Medical School*

Hasan Bazari, M.D. *Department of Medicine, Massachusetts General Hospital, Assistant Professor of Medicine, Harvard Medical School*

William J. Benedetto, M.D. *Department of Anesthesia and Critical Care, Massachusetts General Hospital, Clinical Fellow in Critical Care, Harvard Medical School*

Sascha Beutler, M.D., Ph.D. *Department of Anesthesia and Critical Care, Massachusetts General Hospital, Clinical Fellow in Critical Care, Harvard Medical School*

Luca M. Bigatello, M.D. *Department of Anesthesia and Critical Care, Massachusetts General Hospital, Associate Professor of Anesthesia, Harvard Medical School*

Edward Bittner, M.D., Ph.D. *Department of Anesthesia and Critical Care, Massachusetts General Hospital, Instructor in Anesthesia, Harvard Medical School*

Sharon E. Brackett, RN, BS, CCRN *Staff Nurse, Surgical ICU, Department of Nursing, Massachusetts General Hospital*

Kathryn Ann Brush, RN, MS, CCRN *Clinical Nurse Specialist, Surgical ICU, Department of Nursing, Massachusetts General Hospital*

Roland Brusseau, M.D. *Department of Anesthesia and Critical Care, Massachusetts General Hospital, Clinical Fellow in Anesthesia, Harvard Medical School*

Andrew M. Cameron, M.D., Ph.D. *Department of Surgery, Liver Transplant Fellow, U.C.L.A. Medical Center*

Theresa Chang, M.D.   *Department of Anesthesia and Critical Care, Massachusetts General Hospital, Clinical Resident in Anesthesia, Harvard Medical School*

Kristopher R. Davignon, M.D.   *Department of Anesthesia and Critical Care, Massachusetts General Hospital, Instructor in Anesthesia, Harvard Medical School*

Kevin Dennehy, M.B., B.Ch.   *Department of Anesthesia and Critical Care, Massachusetts General Hospital, Assistant Professor of Anesthesia, Harvard Medical School*

Peter F. Dunn, M.D.   *Department of Anesthesia and Critical Care, Massachusetts General Hospital, Instructor in Anesthesia, Harvard Medical School*

Thomas W. Felbinger, M.D.   *Department of Anesthesiology, University of Hamburg Medical Center, Assistant Professor of Anesthesia, University of Hamburg*

Daniel F. Fisher, MS, RRT   *Respiratory Care Services, Massachusetts General Hospital*

Michael G. Fitzsimons, M.D.,   *Department of Anesthesia, Massachusetts General Hospital, Instructor in Anesthesia and Critical Care, Harvard Medical School*

Edward George, M.D., Ph.D.   *Department of Anesthesia and Critical Care, Massachusetts General Hospital, Instructor in Anesthesia, Harvard Medical School*

Fiona K. Gibbons, M.D.   *Department of Medicine, Pulmonary and Critical Care Division, Massachusetts General Hospital, Instructor in Medicine, Harvard Medical School*

Robert Goulet, M.S., R.R.T.   *Respiratory Care Services, Massachusetts General Hospital*

Loreta Grecu, M.D.   *Department of Anesthesia and Critical Care, Massachusetts General Hospital, Instructor in Anesthesia, Harvard Medical School*

David M. Greer, M.D., M.A.   *Department of Neurology, Massachusetts General Hospital, Assistant Professor of Neurology, Harvard Medical School*

Robert Hallisey, MS., Pharm, RPh   *Department of Pharmacy, Massachusetts General Hospital, Assistant Professor of Clinical Pharmacy, Massachusetts College of Pharmacy & Health Sciences*

Kenneth L. Haspel, M.D.   *Department of Surgical Critical Care, Lahey Clinic*

Judith Hellman, M.D. *Department of Anesthesia and Critical Care, and Department of Medicine, Massachusetts General Hospital, Assistant Professor of Anesthesia, Harvard Medical School*

James Helstrom, M.D. *Department of Anesthesia and Critical Care, Massachusetts General Hospital, Clinical Resident in Anesthesia, Harvard Medical School*

Dean R. Hess, Ph.D., RRT *Respiratory Care Services, Massachusetts General Hospital, Associate Professor of Anesthesia, Harvard Medical School*

Leigh R. Hochberg, M.D., Ph.D. *Department of Neurology, Massachusetts General Hospital, Instructor in Neurology, Harvard Medical School*

Brian L. Hoh, M.D. *Neurosurgical Service, Massachusetts General Hospital, Clinical Fellow in Surgery, Harvard Medical School*

William Hurford, M.D., FCCM *Professor and Chairman, Department of Anesthesia, University of Cincinnati College of Medicine*

Patrick G. Jackson, M.D. *Department of Surgery, Georgetown University Hospital, Assistant Professor of Surgery, Georgetown University School of Medicine*

Jason P. Jenkins, M.D. *Department of Anesthesia and Critical Care, Massachusetts General Hospital, Clinical Resident in Anesthesia, Harvard Medical School*

John C. Klick, M.D. *Department of Anesthesia and Surgery, Hartford Hospital, Instructor in Anesthesia and Surgery, University of Connecticut School of Medicine*

Jean Kwo, M.D. *Department of Anesthesia and Critical Care, Massachusetts General Hospital, Instructor in Anesthesia, Harvard Medical School*

Harish S. Lecamwasam, M.D., M.Sc. *Department of Anesthesia and Critical Care, Massachusetts General Hospital, Instructor in Anesthesia, Harvard Medical School*

Stephanie L. Lee, M.D., Ph.D. *Department of Medicine, Boston Medical Center, Associate Professor of Medicine, Boston University School of Medicine*

David T. Liu, M.D., Ph.D. *Department of Anesthesia and Critical Care, Massachusetts General Hospital, Clinical Fellow in Critical Care, Harvard Medical School*

Thomas E. MacGillivray, M.D., FACS *Department of Surgery, Massachusetts General Hospital, Instructor in Surgery, Harvard Medical School*

Bonnie T. Mackool, M.D., MSPH   *Department of Dermatology, Massachusetts General Hospital, Assistant Professor of Dermatology, Harvard Medical School*

Adrian A. Maung, M.D.   *Department of Surgery, Massachusetts General Hospital, Clinical Fellow in Surgery, Harvard Medical School*

Joseph Meltzer, M.D.   *Department of Anesthesia and Critical Care, Massachusetts General Hospital, Clinical Fellow in Critical Care, Harvard Medical School*

Frederic Michard, M.D., Ph.D.   *Critical Care Division, Lannelonggue Hospital, Paris France*

Richard J. Oeser, M.D.   *Department of Anesthesia and Critical Care, Massachusetts General Hospital, Clinical Resident in Anesthesia, Harvard Medical School*

Steven V. Panaro, M.D.   *Department of Anesthesia and Critical Care, Massachusetts General Hospital, Clinical Resident in Anesthesia, Harvard Medical School*

Shyam Parek, M.D.   *Department of Anesthesia and Critical Care, Massachusetts General Hospital, Clinical Resident in Anesthesia, Harvard Medical School*

Robert A. Peterfreund, M.D., Ph.D.   *Department of Anesthesia and Critical Care, Massachusetts General Hospital, Associate Professor of Anesthesia, Harvard Medical School*

Richard M. Pino, M.D., Ph.D.   *Department of Anesthesia and Critical Care, Massachusetts General Hospital, Assistant Professor of Anesthesia, Harvard Medical School*

Deborah A. Quinn, M.D.   *Department of Medicine, Pulmonary and Critical Care Division, Massachusetts General Hospital, Assistant Professor of Medicine, Harvard Medical School*

Stacey L. Remchuck, M.D.   *Department of Anesthesia and Critical Care, Massachusetts General Hospital, Clinical Fellow in Anesthesia, Harvard Medical School*

Ulrich Schmidt, M.D., Ph.D.   *Department of Anesthesia and Critical Care, Massachusetts General Hospital, Assistant Professor of Anesthesia, Harvard Medical School*

Lee H. Schwamm, M.D.   *Department of Neurology, Massachusetts General Hospital, Associate Professor of Neurology, Harvard Medical School*

Kenneth E. Shepherd, M.D. *Department of Anesthesia and Critical Care, Massachusetts General Hospital, Assistant Professor of Anesthesia, Harvard Medical School*

Robert Sheridan, M.D. *Division of Burns and Trauma, Shriners Hospital for Children and Massachusetts General Hospital, Associate Professor of Surgery, Harvard Medical School*

Jagmeet P. Singh, M.D., D.Phil *Department of Medicine, Massachusetts General Hospital, Instructor in Medicine, Harvard Medical School*

David J. Steele, M.D. *Department of Medicine, Renal Division, Massachusetts General Hospital, Instructor in Medicine, Harvard Medical School*

H. Thomas Stelfox, M.D., Ph.D. *Department of Anesthesia and Critical Care, Massachusetts General Hospital, Instructor in Anesthesia, Harvard Medical School*

B. Taylor Thompson, M.D. *Department of Medicine, Pulmonary and Critical Care Division, Massachusetts General Hospital, Associate Professor of Medicine, Harvard Medical School*

Catherine Valentine, M.D. *Department of Medicine, Infectious Disease Unit, Massachusetts General Hospital, Clinical and Research Fellow in Medicine, Harvard Medical School*

Lee V. Wesner, MD. *Department of Anesthesia and Critical Care, Massachusetts General Hospital, Instructor in Anesthesia, Harvard Medical School*

Preface

The *Critical Care Handbook of the Massachusetts General Hospital, Fourth Edition,* is a multi-disciplinary guide to the care of the critically ill patient. While individual intensive care units may focus their practice on selected patient populations—surgical, medical, cardiac units, etc.—the bases of critical illness are universal. We have strived to emphasize a physiological approach to critical care, equally valuable to trainees of various backgrounds such as medicine, anesthesia, and surgery, and to medical students, nurses, pharmacists and therapists interested in taking on the challenge of working in an intensive care unit. Accordingly, the authors are a heterogeneous group of individuals who have in common their expertise in the day-to-day care of critically ill patients and their dedication to academic medicine.

The *Handbook* is intended for the pocket of your scrubs or your work coat, as a valuable resource while you learn to work in an intensive care unit. As such, it covers classic topics like acute respiratory failure, hemodynamic monitoring, and sepsis, as well as selected subjects like endocrine imbalances and obstetric emergencies. We have also included chapters on the ethical issues of end of life, prophylaxis of complications, and evidence-based medicine. Of course, the *Handbook* is not the ultimate opinion in critical care, but a practical guide that will stimulate further learning from more extensive textbooks and current medical journals.

This edition of the *Handbook* has been completely rewritten, expanded, and reorganized. In addition, some source material from prior editions and from our companion handbook, *Clinical Anesthesia Procedures of the Massachusetts General Hospital,* has been included verbatim when appropriate. The integral contributions of editors and authors of these other handbooks are gratefully acknowledged; in particular, we appreciate the work of Dr. William E. Hurford, senior editor of the previous edition, who gave this publication a completely renewed substance.

We also wish to acknowledge the continuing guidance and leadership of Dr. Warren M. Zapol; the excellent editorial assistance of Mrs. Tracey Sughrue, and the enthusiastic support of the staff at Lippincott Williams & Wilkins.

Finally, we owe deep thanks to all the people who work in our intensive care units: doctors, nurses, therapists, technicians and aids; only through their dedication to teamwork, we can ever provide the best possible care to our patients.

Luca Bigatello

Critical Care Principles

1

Hemodynamic Monitoring. I

Sascha Beutler and Luca M. Bigatello

I. **The goal of hemodynamic monitoring** is to maintain adequate organ perfusion. In critically ill patients, hypoperfusion of vital organs may lead to multiple-organ-system dysfunction and death. The aim of this and the next chapter is to guide the clinician through the interpretation of hemodynamic data based on the application of circulatory physiology.

   A. **Organ perfusion** is determined by the difference between arterial and venous pressure divided by its resistance to flow:

   $$\text{Flow} = (P_{\text{arterial}} - P_{\text{venous}})/\text{Resistance}$$

   In the absence of a method for measuring the flow to individual organs, measuring the systemic arterial pressure is used as a substitute for estimating the adequacy of organ perfusion, assuming constant venous pressure and constant resistance.

   B. **The mean arterial pressure (MAP)** value provides the closest measure of perfusion pressure. A MAP of greater than 65 mm Hg is a reasonable target for most patients. At times (e.g., in chronic hypertension or spinal cord ischemia) higher levels are necessary. Under normal circumstances, organ blood flow is maintained within normal range by autoregulation. **Autoregulation** provides a constant blood flow through constriction or dilation of the afferent vessels during changes of arterial blood pressure. However, pathologic conditions such as chronic hypertension, trauma, and sepsis impair autoregulation significantly, and flow may become directly dependent on perfusion pressure (Fig. 1-1).

II. **Monitoring arterial blood pressure**

   A. **Noninvasive blood pressure (NIBP)** measurement involves occluding an artery by a pressurized cuff. Various techniques can be used:

      1. **Manual methods.** Although somewhat time consuming and prone to high individual variability, manual methods are still widely employed due to their ease of use and low cost. One manual technique involves the **auscultation** of the sounds (Korotkoff's sounds) generated by the turbulent flow of blood through a vessel previously occluded by a cuff (systolic pressure) and attending to the disappearance of these sounds (diastolic pressure). A second manual technique **(oscillometry)** involves watching a pressure gauge connected to the cuff as the cuff is slowly deflated to detect the systolic (first oscillations) and the diastolic blood pressure (disappearance of the oscillations).

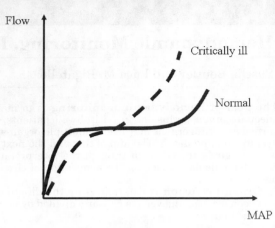

Flow

Critically ill

Normal

MAP

Fig. 1-1.   Autoregulation provides constant blood flow in healthy individuals over a wide range of blood pressure, but it may be impaired in critically ill patients, and flow may become dependent on perfusion pressure. MAP, mean arterial pressure.

2. **Automated noninvasive techniques** are becoming most common due to their obvious convenience. Most automated devices measure blood pressure by **oscillometry.** Typically, the cuff is inflated about 40 mm Hg above the previous systolic pressure (or about 170 mm Hg initially) and then incrementally deflated while sensing pressure oscillations in the cuff. The MAP correlates well with the lowest pressure at which maximum oscillations occur. The systolic and diastolic pressures are determined by algorithms, but generally correlate with the initial rise and final fall of oscillations about the maximum.
3. **Sources of error**
   a. **Cuff size.** The cuff should cover about two-thirds of the upper arm or thigh; that is, the width of the cuff should be 20% greater than the diameter of the limb. A cuff that is too narrow may produce falsely high measurements; a cuff that is too wide may produce falsely low values.
   b. **Movement.** Motion artifact increases the cycle time and is rejected by some instruments. Venous congestion may occur if the instrument is set to cycle too frequently; cycle times less than 2 minutes apart should be avoided for routine monitoring. Some instruments have a STAT mode, which cycles rapidly to give very frequent measurements but can compromise perfusion and result in nerve damage.
   c. **Arrhythmia.** In patients with arrhythmia, the actual value of blood pressure may not be recorded

during progressive cuff deflation because of the occasional lack of normal beats.

d. **Very low or very high blood pressure.** In these patients, it may be difficult for the instrument to sense the oscillations.

B. **Intraarterial blood pressure monitoring** is the gold standard of arterial blood pressure measurement. When correctly positioned and calibrated, the catheter-transducer-monitor system provides a highly accurate measurement of arterial blood pressure.

1. **Indications**

a. **Hemodynamic instability** is the most common indication for intraarterial blood pressure monitoring. As discussed previously, the presence of severe hypotension, hypertension, or a rapidly fluctuating blood pressure makes the noninvasive systems unreliable.

b. **Rigorous control of blood pressure** may be mandatory in some clinical situations, such as a leaking aortic aneurysm or a traumatic injury of the aorta, to decrease the likelihood of rupture.

c. **Frequent arterial blood sampling.** This indication has decreased in recent years because of the use of reliable respiratory monitoring with pulse oximetry and exhaled CO_2 analysis.

2. **Site of cannulation.** The radial artery at the wrist is the preferred site for an indwelling arterial catheter. The hand usually has good collateral blood supply through the ulnar artery, and the wrist constitutes an easy area for access and maintenance of the catheter. Acceptable alternative sites in adults include the femoral, axillary, brachial, and dorsalis pedis arteries. The choice of one of these sites depends on individual habits and on the patient's underlying medical condition. For example, the femoral artery may be considered in the septic hypotensive patient because the radial artery pressure may underestimate central pressure and lead to excessive vasopressor administration. On the other hand, in a patient with a history of previous aortic bypass surgery, the femoral site is contraindicated.

3. **Complications of arterial lines**

a. **Vascular complications** of clinical significance are rare, but can be devastating. Fastidious attention to the presence of adequate distal perfusion is of great importance. All sites are at risk for ischemic complications either because of their small caliber (radial and dorsalis pedis arteries), the lack of adequate collateral circulation (brachial and axillary arteries), or the frequent presence of atherosclerotic vascular disease (femoral and dorsalis pedis) arteries. The performance of Allen's test has poor predictive value for vascular complications.

    b. Infectious complications are rare, probably due to the high blood flow rate through and around the catheter. However, infection is possible, and arterial catheters should be treated like any other indwelling device, that is, using accurate sterile techniques and frequently inspecting the site for signs of inflammation and infection.

4. Function of the catheter-transducer-monitor system. The accuracy of intraarterial blood pressure measurement depends on the proper setup and function of the catheter-transducer-monitor system.

    a. Reference level. The level at which the arterial transducer should be referenced is not strictly codified—it should be at the level of interest. For example, in neurosurgical patients it may be at the height of the external meatus of the ear to reference the blood pressure to the intracranial circulation. In the majority of critically ill patients, the object of blood pressure monitoring is overall tissue perfusion, and the arterial pressure transducer is set at the level of the heart.

    b. Calibration. Clinicians should be familiar with the principles of calibration of a blood pressure monitoring system to be able to troubleshoot and resolve problems of catheter malfunction.

        (1) Static calibration. Given the high precision of the current monitors and disposable transducers, the calibration routine is often limited to the performance of the first step of the static calibration, that is, **zeroing.** The transducer is opened to air and the recorded pressure (the atmospheric pressure) is used by convention as the 0 mm Hg reference value. The second step of the static calibration entails the application of a higher level of pressure (e.g., 200 mm Hg) to assure accurate recordings over a clinically relevant pressure range. This **high calibration** is performed automatically by most current monitors.

        (2) Dynamic calibration. There are two components of a dynamic calibration of an oscillating system: the dampening and the resonance. **Dampening** indicates the tendency of an oscillating system to return to its resting state. With increased dampening, the pressure waveform appears flattened. Factors that increase dampening include loose connections, kinks, and large air bubbles. The ideal damping coefficient is 0.8 (with 1 corresponding to no damping). If properly set up, modern transducers have minimal dampening. Hence, if a trace looks flattened on the monitor screen, chances are that the reading is real, and that the blood pressure is dangerously low.

Resonance indicates the property of a system to vibrate (resonate) when hit by a certain force. When the systolic pressure "hits" the elastic arterial wall, this vibrates and, just like a musical fork, generates an infinite series of sine waves of increasing frequency and decreasing amplitude. The lowest frequency of the sine waves (fundamental frequency) is the heart rate, and the subsequent sine wave frequencies (harmonics) are its multiples. If the system resonates at a frequency lower than the 8th to the 10th harmonics (decreased resonant frequency), the pressure trace will appear "whipped" or "flinging," terms used to characterize traces with a higher systolic pressure and a more pronounced dicrotic notch. Excessive tubing length, multiple stopcocks, and inadequate debubbling of the system predispose to a decrease in its resonant frequency. The resonant frequency of a system can be tested with a **flush test,** consisting in applying to the transducer a pressure burst by flushing the system. If this maneuver is displayed on a strip chart recorder, the resonant frequency of the system can be calculated by measuring the distance between two subsequent peaks of the trace, as shown in Fig. 1-2.

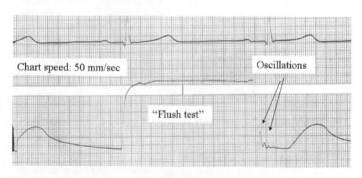

Fig. 1-2.   Flush test. The catheter–transducer system is pressurized by opening the flush ("square-wave sign") and then letting go of it. As the pressure rapidly returns to the patient's arterial pressure, the system "resonates." The resonance frequency is calculated by dividing the strip chart speed by the distance between two successive oscillations generated by the flush test. In this case, the distance is 2 to 3 mm, which holds a resonance frequency of 20 Hz. This is a common frequency of properly set up transducers, which will accurately reproduce most arterial traces at heart rates up to 120 beats/min.

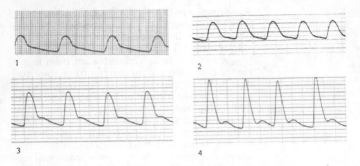

Fig. 1-3. Arterial blood pressure traces from different patients, all obtained with properly calibrated transducers. The first three traces are from radial artery catheters, the fourth trace is from a dorsalis pedis catheter.

   5. **Arterial blood pressure waveform on the monitor.** Current monitors' displays offer multiple options of blood pressure reading, including numeric values, cursors, and filters. In contrast to central venous pressures, the arterial blood pressure is only minimally affected by changes in intrathoracic pressure relative to its absolute value. Therefore, the numbers displayed on the monitor screen, which reflect an average over time (a few seconds) of each beat, are reasonably accurate for clinical purposes. Arterial pressure traces differ from individual to individual and from site to site (Fig. 1-3). For example, a pressure waveform recorded at the root of the aorta looks rounded, with a dicrotic notch located at the beginning of the descending portion of the curve. As arterial pressure is recorded more distally, the trace generally looks progressively more peaked, and the dicrotic notch migrates distally. Normal traces may look whipped and dampened, and the only way to assess the appropriateness of such a trace is to perform the dynamic calibration (see prior discussion).

III. **Physiologic approach to hypotension.** Hypotension is the most common reason for instituting invasive hemodynamic monitoring in critically ill surgical patients. A simple approach to the physiologic determinant of hypotension is shown in Fig. 1-4. Hypotension is due to either **low cardiac output** or **low vascular tone.** A low cardiac output can be due to a primary decrease in heart rate or to a decrease in **stroke volume** (cardiac output/heart rate). A decrease in stroke volume can be due to a decrease in **venous return** (volume depletion or, less frequently, obstruction to heart filling) or to **ventricular dysfunction.** Of course, several of these mechanisms may coexist, as it is often the case in critically ill patients who have been in the intensive care unit for days or weeks. As the complexity of a patient's presentation increases, it becomes increasingly difficult to discern

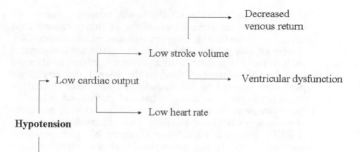

Fig. 1-4. Algorithm describing a physiologic approach to hypotension (see section III).

which mechanism is responsible for the circulatory failure—hypovolemia, ventricular dysfunction, or low vascular tone. This is why invasive hemodynamic monitoring is a common part of the management of critically ill patients, but also why invasive hemodynamic monitoring does not always provide the desired, clear-cut answer to our questions.

IV. **Physiology of central pressures monitoring.** We can use a central venous catheter to determine the central venous pressure **(CVP)** in the systemic circulation or a pulmonary artery **(PA)** catheter to determine, in addition to the CVP, the pulmonary artery pressure **(PAP)**, the pulmonary artery occlusion pressure **(PAOP)** in the pulmonary venous circulation, and the cardiac output **(CO)**. In either case, we measure an intravascular pressure that is intended to estimate a volume. In general, we assume that:

CVP ≅ Right ventricular end-diastolic volume (RVEDV)

PAOP ≅ Left ventricular end-diastolic volume (LVEDV)

However, variables in addition to the status of the intravascular volume of the systemic and pulmonary circulations can affect the measurement of central pressures. Therefore, these two basic assumptions do not hold true in many critically ill patients. There are four main physiologic conditions that may alter the foregoing relationships:

A. **Abnormal compliance of a cardiac chamber.** The relationship between pressure and volume (the *compliance*) of a cardiac chamber at end-diastole is not linear and is affected by pathologic conditions. For example, in a patient with concentric left ventricular hypertrophy secondary to chronic hypertension or aortic stenosis, the left ventricular compliance is decreased, and the measured pressure (the PAOP) tends to overestimate the desired volume (LVEDV).

B. **Increased intrathoracic pressure.** In the relationships CVP ≅ RVEDV and PAOP ≅ LVEDV the vascular pressures are intended to be **transmural** pressure, that is, the pressure inside the vessel minus the pressure outside. The transmural pressure is the pressure that actually distends the blood vessel and cardiac chamber. However, the pressure that we measure with a central catheter is the intravascular pressure, which is affected both by the volume of blood in the vessel and any other pressure applied to the outside of the vessel (intrathoracic pressure). Common causes of increased intrathoracic pressure in critically ill patients include positive-pressure ventilation, positive end-expiratory pressure (PEEP), intrinsic PEEP (see Chapter 3), and, possibly, increased abdominal pressure. In these situations, an increase in intravascular pressure may not reflect an increase in transmural pressure, and thus may not be a valid estimate of the intravascular volume. The effect of intrathoracic pressure changes on the measured vascular pressures (CVP, PAOP) is minimal at end-expiration, when it approaches atmospheric pressure. For this reason, central **pressures are read at end-expiration.** However, the alveolar pressure can be increased at end-expiration by **PEEP** or **intrinsic PEEP.** One can estimate the fraction of alveolar pressure that is transmitted to the pleural space based on the compliance of the lung and chest wall. Normally, these two values are nearly equal, and approximately half of the alveolar pressure is transmitted across the lung to the pleural space. Remembering to convert the units of measurement (cm H_2O for airway, mm Hg for vascular pressures), we find that 10 cm H_2O of PEEP will increase a CVP/PAOP by about 3 mm Hg (5 cm $H_2O \times 0.74$). When the compliance of the lung is significantly decreased (e.g., in acute respiratory distress syndrome), a smaller fraction of pressure is transmitted. When the compliance of the lung is increased (e.g., in chronic obstructive pulmonary disease) or the compliance of the chest wall is decreased (e.g., in abdominal distension), a larger fraction of the applied pressure is transmitted. We do not recommend discontinuing the applied PEEP to improve the accuracy of central pressure readings, for two reasons. First, PEEP discontinuation may cause lung derecruitment and hypoxemia; second, the pressure exerted on the blood vessel is real and has hemodynamic effects; hence, by discontinuing PEEP we create a situation that may be less relevant to the current patient's physiology.

C. **Valvular heart disease. Severe stenotic lesions** of the atrioventricular valves (tricuspid and mitral stenosis) limit the ability to estimate the pressure in the respective ventricle. In these valvular lesions, the pressure in the atria can be significantly higher than the pressure in the respective ventricles, which, with the progression of the lesion, tend to be underfilled. Therefore, pressure readings will overestimate ventricular volumes.

D. **Ventricular interdependence.** When the right ventricle (RV) is dilated from volume and pressure overload (from pulmonary hypertension or primary failure) the interventricular septum moves leftward and impinges onto the left ventricle (LV), decreasing its compliance. In these cases, an elevated PAOP is in part determined by the overload of the RV and may overestimate filling of the LV.

E. Despite the aforementioned sources of inaccuracy, measurement of central pressures with or without cardiac output measurement is widely used to diagnose the causes of hypotension and guide therapy. Clearly, the hemodynamic values have to be put in the patient's context and interpreted in the light of relevant clinical variables.

V. **Monitoring with a CVP catheter.** Standard central venous catheters permit monitoring the CVP without the capability of measuring the CO.

A. **Indications** of central venous cannulation include the following:

1. Measurement of right heart filling pressures as a guide to intravascular volume estimate and volume resuscitation.

2. Access for administration of drugs or parenteral nutrition into the central cannulation.

3. Intravenous access in patients with difficult peripheral access.

B. **Site of cannulation.** Techniques of central venous catheter insertion have been described extensively, and we refer to the *Clinical Anesthesia Procedures of the Massachusetts General Hospital*, for review and illustrations. The most common sites of cannulation are the internal jugular and the subclavian vein. The tip of the catheter should be positioned at the junction of the superior vena cava and the right atrium. It is controversial whether central pressure can be accurately measured through a femoral vein access, and we do not recommend it.

C. **Complications** of CVP catheter insertion and use include dysrhythmia, pneumothorax, pericardial tamponade, hydrothorax, air embolism and carotid or subclavian artery puncture, and infection. Transient **dysrhythmias** (premature atrial and ventricular contractions [PACs, PVCs]) occur frequently at the time of threading the guide wire, and resolve with retrieving it out of the right atrium. Occasionally, the tip of the catheter may either be placed or migrate into the right atrium or ventricle, causing recurrent arrhythmias. Placement of a CVP catheter constitutes a higher risk in the subclavian position because there the artery cannot be easily compressed; hence, subclavian cannulation should be avoided in patients at increased risk for bleeding.

D. **Waveform readings.** The zero reference point for venous pressures is at the fourth intercostal space on the midaxillary line, which corresponds to the position of the right and left atria when the patient is supine. The transducer is maintained at the same level with respect to the patient during sequential measurements. It should be noted that **changes in position may significantly affect the CVP,** even with correct leveling of the

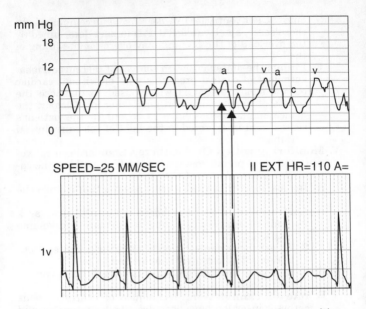

Fig. 1-5. The central venous pressure trace contains three positive deflections, which correspond to atrial contraction, (a) ventricular contraction in systole, (c) and right atrial filling (v) (see section **IV.D**). HR, heart rate. Shown here in relationship with the ECG tracing.

transducer. The CVP, like all central vascular pressures, is read at end-expiration, when the pleural pressure is close to zero (see section **IV.B**). The CVP value is considered normal in the order of 2 to 6 mm Hg. A CVP trace contains three positive deflections, the **a-, c-, and v-waves** (Fig. 1-5). These correspond respectively to atrial contraction, bulging of the tricuspid valve during isovolumic ventricular contraction, and right atrial filling against a closed tricuspid valve. The x-descent is thought to be caused by the downward displacement of the atrium during ventricular systole and the y-descent by tricuspid valve opening during diastole. The a-waves are absent in atrial fibrillation. Large a-waves (**cannon a-waves**) may occur when the atrium contracts against a closed valve, such as during atrioventricular dissociation. **Abnormally large v-waves** can be associated with tricuspid regurgitation; they begin immediately after the QRS complex and often incorporate the c-wave. Large v-waves are also observed during right ventricular failure and ischemia, constrictive pericarditis, or cardiac tamponade, due to the volume and/or pressure overload associated with these conditions.

E. **Interpretation.** Considering the number of variables that influence the measurement of the CVP in addition to the volume status of the systemic circulation, it is not surprising that it is frequently difficult to interpret CVP values. When the CVP is available as part of a monitoring system that can measure the CO, such as a PA catheter (see section **VI**) or a **PiCCO** monitor (Pulsion Medical, Munich, Germany; see Chapter 2), its value is significantly increased. We discuss the use of the combination of central pressures and CO values when we discuss this in reference to the PA catheter in section **VI**. When no measure of CO is available, the isolated value of CVP is less helpful, but can be improved by using the combined changes in CVP and MAP (as a surrogate of CO) in response to a volume challenge.

VI. Monitoring with a PA catheter permits measuring CVP, PAP, PAOP, and CO.

   A. Indications. The main indication for the placement of a PA catheter is the presence of **hemodynamic instability** (hypotension) of unclear physiologic etiology. Other indications include sampling of **mixed venous oxygen saturation** and **pacing capability.**

   B. Insertion. The internal jugular vein is used most commonly because of easy access from the head of the patient and the lower incidence of pneumothorax. Figure 1-6 shows the characteristic pressure waveforms seen as the pulmonary catheter is advanced through the successive structures of the heart. The PA catheter is first inserted to a depth of 20 cm, where the monitor should confirm a CVP waveform. The balloon is inflated with 1 to 1.5 ml of air, and the catheter is advanced until a right ventricular pressure waveform is seen. This should occur at a depth of about 30 to 35 cm. PVCs and, less often, bursts of ventricular tachycardia can occur at this time; the catheter should be advanced rapidly out of the RV into the PA, where the dysrhythmias generally cease. The catheter is then advanced slowly until a PAOP trace is obtained (generally at a depth of 50–55 cm). The PA trace should reappear with deflation of the balloon. If it does not, the catheter is withdrawn until the PA tracing reappears. **A high degree of caution must be applied to the transition from a PA to a PAOP** trace; sometimes, the change is not quite apparent, and the catheter may be advanced when it is already in the occlusion position, causing disastrous complications (PA rupture, see section **VI.C.2**). Such a situation occurs typically in the presence of a large *v*-wave on the PAOP trace (mitral regurgitation, congestive heart failure). Occasionally, the PA catheter may have to be placed under direct fluoroscopic guidance. Indications include the presence of a recently placed (generally 6 weeks) permanent pacemaker, the need for selective PA placement (e.g., following a right pneumonectomy), and the presence of significant structural abnormalities, such as severe right ventricular dilatation, and large intracardiac shunts.

   C. Complications include the following:
      1. PVCs, ventricular tachycardia, and **right-bundle-branch block.** Most of these occur during

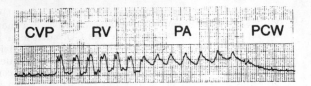

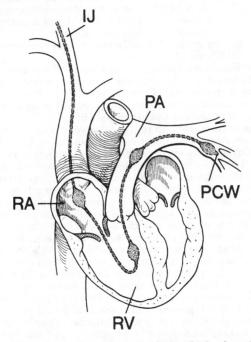

Fig. 1-6. Characteristic pressure waves seen during insertion of a pulmonary artery catheter. CVP, central venous pressure; IJ, internal jugular; RA, right atrium; RV, right ventricle; PA, pulmonary artery; PCW, pulmonary capillary wedge.

placement (see prior discussion) and are transient. However, in the presence of a left-bundle-branch block, the onset of a right-bundle-branch block will cause **complete heart block;** the catheter may not be able to float out of the right ventricle and the block may persist. Clinical judgment must be used prior to inserting a PA catheter in a patient with a left-bundle-branch block. Appropriate measures include setting up pacing capability, transcutaneous or transvenous, and aborting the procedure.

2. **PA rupture** is rare but has a high mortality. Factors predisposing to PA rupture include severe pulmonary

hypertension, the presence of a suture line, and, possibly, anticoagulation. However, given the lack of prospective data, all of these conditions are simply a reason to raise the level of caution, not to avoid placement or to be overconfident when these conditions are not present. The fundamental measure for avoiding PA rupture is using the appropriate technique. Balloon inflation should be slow, and stopped immediately when a PAOP tracing is obtained; the balloon should never be kept inflated for an extended period of time. The pulmonary artery pressure trace should be monitored at all times to rule out the migration into the occluded position. There is controversy as to whether the frequency of inflating the balloon for measurements correlates with the occurrence of rupture. Although somewhat counterintuitive, there is no evidence that the number of occlusions performed correlates with the incidence of rupture. Instead, one may argue that by not performing sufficient occlusions over time, the clinician is deprived of important information needed to guide optimal patient therapy. Hence, we tend to perform occlusion pressures as frequently as we record all other hemodynamic parameters.

3. **Pulmonary infarction** is another rare complication related mainly to poor technique. Although less devastating than a PA rupture, infarction is a serious complication and can be avoided by using proper technique.

4. PACs may occasionally form a **knot.** Fluoroscopic guidance may be needed to untangle and remove the catheter.

5. **Balloon rupture.** At no time should the balloon be filled with more than 1.5 ml of air.

6. **Complications at the site of insertion** are the same as described for CVP catheters in section **V.C.**

D. **Cardiac output/cardiac index.** Thermodilution CO is determined by injecting a fixed volume of cold (room temperature or lower) solution into the CVP port of the PAC. The cold tracer mixes with the blood as it passes through the right heart, and the temperature of the mixture is measured as it passes a thermistor near the tip of the PAC. The computation of the cardiac output uses a formula that must properly account for the volume and temperature of the injectate, the thermodynamic properties of blood, injectate solution, and catheter used, and the integral of the temperature–time curve.

1. **Interpretation** of CO usually is done in the setting of hypotension. Determining the CO allows diagnosis of a low-tone state [low systemic vascular resistance (SVR)], a low CO, or both. If the CO is low, a concurrent measurement of heart rate (HR) will help to determine whether the reason is related to the heart rate or ventricular performance (i.e., stroke volume = CO/HR). Instead of the cardiac output, the **cardiac**

index may be calculated by dividing CO by the body surface area (BSA). It may allow easier comparison between patients of different weights and heights.

2. **Accuracy and reliability**

a. **Serial** measurements are recommended for each cardiac output determination (generally three). Even then the cardiac output measurement can vary by as much as 10% without a change in the clinical condition of the patient.

b. **Respiration.** Cardiac output can vary over the respiratory cycle, depending on the mode of ventilation and baseline levels of venous return and cardiac performance. Accordingly, the timing of injection affects the measurement of a thermodilution CO measurement. If a consistent trend is desired, it is probably best to inject at a constant point in the respiratory cycle, usually at end-expiration. If an average over the respiratory cycle is desired, it is usual to take the mean of three measurements obtained at random times throughout the respiratory cycle.

c. **Low-output states** can affect the accuracy of the CO measurement, especially when room-temperature indicator solutions are injected. Iced injectate gives more accurate measurements.

d. **Tricuspid regurgitation** may produce both erroneously high and erroneously low readings. When the cold indicator fluid is recycled back and forth across the tricuspid valve, the thermodilution curve is prolonged and has a low amplitude, leading to erroneously high cardiac output measurements.

e. Intracardiac shunts **can also produce erroneous measurements because they create a difference between right and left ventricular outputs.**

E. **Pulmonary artery pressure and pulmonary artery occlusion pressure**

1. **Measurement.** For an accurate measurement of PAOP, the tip of the catheter should reside in a lung zone where pulmonary venous pressure is greater than alveolar pressure **(West zone III).** This is usually the case because the tip of the catheter has the tendency to float with the bloodstream when the balloon is inflated.

2. **Values.** The PAP is considered normal between 15 and 20 mm Hg systolic and 5 to 12 mm Hg diastolic pressure. The PAOP is intended to estimate the left atrial pressure (LAP). Because of the interposed lung, this estimate is delayed and dampened. The a- and c-waves typically are not very large. Consequently, the mean pressure at end-expiration reflects the left atrial pressure. The PAOP is considered normal between 5 and 12 mm Hg. The assumption that these central pressures reflect the volume in the pulmonary circulation may not be accurate. As highlighted in

the discussion of central pressure measurements, volume is only one parameter that influences the measurements; other variables (e.g., cardiac compliance, intrathoracic pressure, and ventricular interdependence) have to be kept in mind when interpreting the measured values.

   3. **Waveform PAP and PAOP.** The morphology of the PAP waveform is similar to that of the systemic arterial waveform, but is smaller and precedes it slightly. When the balloon at the tip of the catheter is inflated, the catheter occludes flow in the artery and the morphology of the waveform changes to more closely approximate that of the CVP: a-, c-, and v-waves as well as x- and y-descents.

   F. **Mixed venous oxygen saturation (Svo$_2$).** The oxygen saturation in the pulmonary artery (mixed venous) blood can be monitored continuously with a specialized PA catheter (oximetric PA catheter) or it can be measured *in vitro* with a blood sample obtained from the distal port of the catheter. Svo$_2$ rises with increases of perfusion above requirements and falls, with increasing oxygen extraction ratio, as perfusion becomes inadequate. Thus, a low Svo$_2$ may indicate either a decreased rate of oxygen delivery (anemia, low cardiac output) or an increased rate of oxygen consumption (see also Chapter 8).

   G. **PA catheters with pacing ports** provide specially positioned ports to pass temporary pacing wires, usually one port for atrial pacing and one port for ventricular pacing. Without pacing wires in place, these ports can also be used for drug infusions.

   H. **PA catheters and outcome.** Although it seems reasonable to believe that if hemodynamic data are interpreted correctly, they could benefit the care of unstable patients, such evidence is lacking. With the introduction of flow-directed balloon-tipped catheters in 1970, the PA catheter became accessible to many physicians and was soon adopted as a tool for guiding cardiovascular therapy in perioperative and critical care medicine. The effect of this technology on patient-centered outcomes was not initially tested in randomized trials. Since the mid 1990s several large outcome studies assessing the benefit of PA catheters have been conducted and have not shown clear evidence of such benefit. Although these results do not seem sufficiently strong to discourage the use of invasive hemodynamic monitoring, they underscore the importance of using appropriate indications for invasive monitoring and of correctly interpreting the data obtained.

VII. **Alternatives to central pressure monitoring.** The measurement of central vascular pressures (CVP, PAP, and PAOP) is a time-honored hemodynamic monitoring technique that may provide useful information for the management of unstable critically ill patients. However, it has significant limitations, as described earlier. Technological advances have provided alternative means of hemodynamic monitoring, often less invasive and possibly more accurate (see Chapter 2).

SELECTED REFERENCES

Guyton AC. Venous return. In: Dow P, Hamilton WF, eds. *Handbook of physiology. Section 2, Vol. 2: Circulation*. Washington, DC: American Physiological Society, 1963:1099–1133.

Hurford WE, Bailin MT, Davison JK, et al., eds. *Clinical anesthesia procedures of the Massachusetts General Hospital*, 6th ed. Baltimore: Lippincott Williams & Wilkins, 2002.

Jacobson E, Chorn R, O'Connor M. The role of the vasculature in regulating venous return and cardiac output: historical and graphical approach. *Can J Anaesth* 1997;44:849–867.

Kleinman B, Powell S, Kumar P, et al. The fast flush test measures the dynamic response of the entire blood pressure monitoring system. *Anesthesiology* 1992;77:1215–1220.

O'Quin R, Marini JJ. Pulmonary artery occlusion pressure: clinical physiology, measurement, and interpretation. *Am Rev Respir Dis* 1983;128:319–326.

Pinsky M. Pulmonary artery occlusion pressure. *Intensive Care Med* 2003;29:19–22.

Richard C, Warszawski J, Anguel N, et al. Early use of the pulmonary artery catheter and outcomes in patients with shock and acute respiratory distress syndrome: A randomized controlled trial. *JAMA* 2003;290:2713–2720.

Sandham JD, Hull RD, Brant RF, et al. A randomized, controlled trial of the use of pulmonary-artery catheters in high-risk surgical patients. *New Eng J Med* 2003;348:5–14.

Sharkey SW. Beyond the wedge: clinical physiology and the Swan-Ganz catheter. *Am J Med* 1987;83:111–122.

Slogoff S, Keats AS, Arlund C. On the safety of radial artery cannulation. *Anesthesiology* 1983;59:42–47.

Teboul JL, Pinsky MR, Mercat A, Anguel N, et al. Estimating cardiac filling pressure in mechanically ventilated patients with hyperinflation. *Crit Care Med* 2000;28:3631–3636.

Hemodynamic Monitoring. II

Edward Bittner and Frédéric Michard

Traditional pressure-based hemodynamic monitoring (see Chapter 1) is invasive and not always accurate. This chapter provides an overview of the hemodynamic parameters provided by less invasive methods and technologies, focusing on their clinical use.

I. **Analysis of arterial pressure respiratory variations during mechanical ventilation**
   A. **Mechanical ventilation** induces a complex series of changes in arterial pressure that can be reduced to a **rise during early insufflation followed by a decrease** that carries through during exhalation (Fig. 2-1).
      1. **The rise in arterial pressure** that occurs in the initial phase of insufflation is mainly due to pressuring blood out of the pulmonary capillaries toward the left side of the heart ("left ventricular preload" effect).
      2. **The decrease in arterial pressure** during late inspiration and onto exhalation is the consequence of a decreased right ventricular output during inspiration. Mechanical insufflation impedes right ventricular ejection by decreasing its filling and increasing its afterload. Changes in right ventricular output are turned into changes in left ventricular output after a phase lag of few beats because of the long blood pulmonary transit time.
      3. The decrease in arterial pressure in early exhalation is the major determinant of the respiratory variation in arterial pressure induced by mechanical ventilation.
   B. **Respiratory variation in arterial pressure, blood volume, and cardiac preload**
      1. The magnitude of the arterial pressure variation during the respiratory cycle is closely dependent on changes in **volume status:** It decreases with volume loading and increases with hypovolemia. It is also weakly and inversely correlated with the pulmonary artery occlusion pressure **(PAOP),** the left ventricular end-diastolic area measured by echocardiography (see section **V**), and the global end-diastolic volume **(GEDV)** measured by transpulmonary thermodilution (see section **II**).
      2. However, because the respiratory variation in arterial pressure is affected by other factors, such as cardiac performance, tidal volume, and respiratory compliance, it cannot be used as the sole

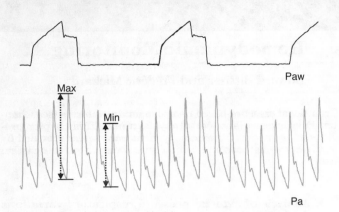

Fig. 2-1. Mechanical ventilation induces cyclic variation in systolic and pulse (systolic minus diastolic) pressure. Maximum values are observed at the end of mechanical insufflation and minimal values a few heart beats later, that is, during the expiratory period. The magnitude of the respiratory variation in arterial pressure mainly reflects the sensitivity of the heart to the cyclic changes in preload induced by mechanical insufflation. Paw, airway pressure; Pa, arterial pressure. From Michard F, et al. Am J Respir Crit Care Med, 2000;162:134–138, with permission.

parameter for assessing total blood volume or cardiac preload.

C. **The concept of fluid responsiveness**
1. The real clinical endpoint of fluid loading is not to normalize any index of cardiac preload, but to **increase the stroke volume and cardiac output.** Therefore, **predictors of fluid responsiveness** (i.e., a significant increase in cardiac output and stroke volume in response to fluid administration) may be more useful bedside endpoints than traditional estimates of preload such as the central venous pressure (CVP), PAOP, and GEDV.
2. In fully sedated and mechanically ventilated patients, the respiratory changes in stroke volume and arterial pressure reflect the sensitivity of the heart to changes in preload induced by mechanical insufflation and hence the sensitivity of the heart to a potential volume loading.
3. The arterial pressure variation induced by mechanical ventilation is an accurate predictor of the hemodynamic effects of a fluid challenge. Patients with a respiratory variation greater than 10% to 15% usually respond to a fluid challenge by a significant increase in stroke volume and cardiac output.
4. **Limitations**
   a. The respiratory variation in arterial pressure cannot be analyzed in patients with cardiac arrhythmias.

      b. The respiratory variation in arterial pressure is an accurate predictor of the hemodynamic effects of fluid therapy only in deeply sedated patients ventilated with standard ventilatory settings.

II. Transthoracic thermodilution

A. This method is based on the injection of a thermal (cold) indicator into a central vein and its detection in a systemic artery (transthoracic dilution), and is used by the PiCCO monitor (Pulsion Medical, Munich, Germany). Because critically ill patients are frequently instrumented with central venous lines, cardiorespiratory monitoring by the transthoracic thermodilution technique requires only the addition of a special thermistor-tipped arterial catheter. The mathematical analysis of the thermodilution curve allows the computation of **cardiac output, cardiac blood volume** (the **GEDV**), and an estimate of extravascular lung water, the extravascular thermal volume (see section **II.A.5**). The same arterial catheter is also used for blood pressure monitoring and blood sampling.

    1. Measurement of cardiac output. The cardiac output is calculated by the analysis of the thermodilution curve in a fashion similar to the way cardiac output is calculated with a PA catheter.

    2. Assessment of cardiac preload. From the analysis of the transthoracic thermodilution curve, the PiCCO monitor estimates the maximum volume of blood contained in the four heart chambers—the GEDV, an index of cardiac preload. Classic analysis of a thermodilution curve provides two parameters used to calculate the GEDV: the **mean transit time (MTt)** and the **exponential downslope time (DSt),** as illustrated in Fig. 2-2.

      a. The **MTt** is the time from injection of the cold bolus to the time of sampling; the product of the MTt and the cardiac output is primarily related to the total volume of distribution of the thermal indicator (intrathoracic thermal volume). This volume includes all intra- and extravascular volume in which the thermal indicator distributes, that is, heart and lungs.

      b. The **DSt** is the time of the downslope of the curve; the product of the DSt by the cardiac output is primarily affected by the volume of the largest mixing chamber that the bolus gets mixed into. In most individuals, the largest mixing chamber in this system is constituted by the lungs (pulmonary thermal volume), including both the pulmonary blood volume and the extravascular lung water.

      c. By subtracting the pulmonary thermal volume from the intrathoracic thermal volume, one is left with a volume that is in the chest but not in the lungs, that is, in the four chambers of the heart, the **GEDV.** A suggested normal GEDV is 600 to 800 ml/m^2, or 1,000 to 1,400 ml.

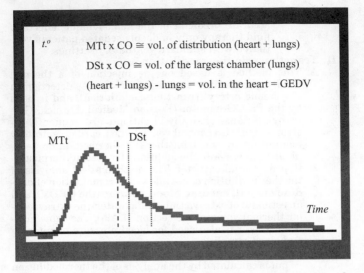

$$t^o \quad \text{MTt x CO} \cong \text{vol. of distribution (heart + lungs)}$$

$$\text{DSt x CO} \cong \text{vol. of the largest chamber (lungs)}$$

$$\text{(heart + lungs) - lungs = vol. in the heart = GEDV}$$

MTt   DSt

Time

Fig. 2-2.   Transpulmonary thermodilution curve; measurements and calculations. CO, cardiac output; Dst, downslope time; GEDV, global end-diastolic volume; MTt, mean transit time.

3. **Detection of fluid responsiveness**
   a. The arterial pressure variation, discussed in section **I,** is automatically calculated by the PiCCO over a period of a few seconds, and can be used as a predictor of fluid responsiveness in fully mechanically ventilated patients.
4. **Assessment of cardiac function**
   a. The ventricular ejection fraction **(EF),** although dependent on both myocardial function and afterload, is commonly used to assess ventricular function. The EF is calculated as the ratio of stroke volume to end-diastolic volume. Because transthoracic thermodilution provides the GEDV, an estimate of the volume of blood contained in the four heart chambers, the ratio of stroke volume to the GEDV has been proposed to assess the global function of the heart, or global ejection fraction **(GEF).**
   b. The GEF is low in case of right and/or left ventricular dysfunction. Patients with echocardiographic evidence of left ventricular systolic dysfunction have shown values of GEF below 18% to 20%.
5. **Estimate of pulmonary edema.** The PiCCO monitor also provides an index of pulmonary edema, the extravascular thermal volume. This index is derived from the estimate of the intrathoracic thermal volume (see section **II.A.2.a**) and the intrathoracic blood volume, based on its consistent linear correlation with the GEDV demonstrated in a study population of

critically ill patients. The difference between these two parameters should yield the volume of fluid in the thorax that is not intravascular, that is, edema fluid. The suggested normal value for the extravascular thermal volume seems to be below 7 to 10 ml/kg. The clinical usefulness of this parameter needs further validation in diverse populations of critically ill patients.

6. **Indications for transthoracic thermodilution**
   a. **Hemodynamic instability.** Transthoracic thermodilution is a less invasive alternative to the PA catheter for the physiologic assessment of patients with circulatory failure. The simultaneous assessment of cardiac output, cardiac preload (GEDV), and cardiac contractility/function (GEF) provides a useful combination of physiologic data. The arterial pressure variation analysis provides an additional assessment of volume status and volume responsiveness in patients who are on full mechanical ventilation.

7. **Limitations**
   a. Transpulmonary thermodilution does not provide a measurement of pulmonary artery (PA) pressure and PAOP. Therefore, it does not discriminate between right and left heart function, nor is it suitable for monitoring hemodynamically unstable patients with pulmonary hypertension.
   b. **Arterial access.** The thermistor-tipped arterial catheter has to be inserted in a large-caliber artery, usually the femoral or axillary artery.
   c. **Tricuspid and mitral regurgitation.** Because the thermal bolus is injected in the right side of the circulation and the thermal change is measured in the left side, it is possible that both tricuspid and mitral regurgitation may affect the measurement of cardiac output, GEDV, and GEF. This has not been systematically studied.
   d. **Atrial dilation and aortic aneurysms.** Significant anatomic changes in the size of the heart chambers and aorta may affect the GEDV and GEF independent of cardiac filling and function (see section **II.A.2**).

III. **Transpulmonary lithium dilution**
   A. This method is based on the injection of lithium chloride in a central or antecubital vein. Arterial blood is withdrawn from a standard arterial catheter through a lithium sensor, and cardiac output is derived from the lithium concentration–time curve. When the lithium-selective membrane is in contact with blood, the voltage across it is related to plasma lithium concentration. Blood flow through the sensor is obtained by a peristaltic pump. This method is used by the LiDCO monitor (LiDCO Ltd., London, UK).
      1. **Cardiac output measurement.** The cardiac output is calculated by the analysis of the dye-dilution curve

in a fashion similar to the way cardiac output is calculated with the PiCCO and the PA catheter.

2. **Detection of fluid responsiveness.** The LiDCO calculates the arterial pressure variation (see section **I**) in a similar fashion as the PiCCO (see section **II.A.3**). This feature can be used to assess fluid responsiveness.

3. **Advantages.** Transthoracic lithium dilution is similar in principle to transthoracic thermodilution, in that it provides accurate measurement of cardiac output without the need for right heart catheterization. The main advantage of the LiDCO is its lower level of invasiveness. The indicator, namely the lithium, can be injected through a large peripheral vein, such as an antecubital vein, and can be detected with a radial artery catheter.

4. **Limitations**

   a. In contrast to the transthoracic thermodilution method, the transthoracic lithium dilution technique does not provide any further analysis of the dilution curve and hence any information concerning cardiac preload, cardiac function, or extravascular thermal volume.

   b. Use of lithium chloride is contraindicated in patients undergoing treatment with lithium salts, in patients who weigh less than 40 kg (88 lb), and in patients who are in the first trimester of pregnancy.

IV. **Pulse contour analysis**

A. **Principles.** This method, used by both PiCCO and LiDCO monitors, is based on the beat-by-beat analysis of the systolic portion of the blood pressure trace to estimate the left ventricular stroke volume. The two monitors use different algorithms, which have not been directly compared. Both techniques require a calibration by an independent measure of stroke volume, that is, a manual injection of the respective indicator. Recalibration is suggested whenever a significant hemodynamic change is suspected to have occurred.

B. **Advantages**

1. **Continuous measurement of cardiac output,** obtained from direct measurement of heart rate and estimate of the stroke volume, may be useful in selected hemodynamically unstable patients, particularly patients in coronary care units, and following cardiac surgery.

2. **Calculation of stroke volume variation.** The stroke volume variation during full mechanical ventilation can serve the same function as the arterial pressure variation as described in sections **I.A, II.A.3,** and **III.A.2**. The stroke volume variation may be an equivalent or better predictor of fluid responsiveness than the arterial pressure variation.

C. **Limitations**

1. The main limitation of continuous cardiac output measurement through pulse contour analysis is that

it requires a calibration each time the mechanical properties of the arterial bed change. This includes changes in cardiac output, volume status, and vasoactive support. Unfortunately, these are often the situations when a clinician would like to be warned of a change in cardiac output.

2. The presence of arrhythmia or aortic valve regurgitation and the use of intraaortic counterpulsation may invalidate the algorithm used to calculate the stroke volume from the contour of the arterial blood pressure.

V. **Echocardiography**

A. Echocardiography has become an invaluable tool in the management of critically ill patients. It is essential that the intensivist be familiar with the strengths and limitations of echocardiography so as to be able to use it effectively in the intensive care unit (ICU). The intensivist must be able to communicate knowledgeably with both sonographers and cardiologists to ensure that clinically important information is obtained and that interpretation occurs in the appropriate clinical context.

1. **Two-dimensional echocardiography.** In clinical echocardiography, a mechanical vibrator (transducer) is placed in contact with the skin or the esophageal mucosa to create tissue vibrations—sound waves. These sound waves propagate and are subsequently reflected from various anatomic structures, including cardiac structures. The reflected sound waves travel back to the transducer, which uses the time delay for each reflected wave to create an image of the heart (Fig. 2-3).

2. **Doppler ultrasound** allows the display of blood flow and provides the ability to quantify the magnitude and direction of flow. It is based on the Doppler principle, which states that the motion of an object alters the frequency of a reflected ultrasound signal. This relationship between alteration in ultrasound frequency and blood flow velocity can be quantified using the Doppler equation (Fig. 2-4).

B. **Transthoracic versus transesophageal echocardiography**

1. **Transthoracic echocardiography (TTE)** can be considered the least invasive way of imaging cardiac structures. However, in many critically ill patients it results in suboptimal-quality images, particularly in patients who are morbidly obese, those who have multiple chest tubes or extensive dressings, and those who are receiving mechanical ventilation.

2. **Transesophageal echoradiography (TEE)** uses an ultrasound probe at the tip of an endoscope that is positioned in the esophagus or stomach. The proximity of the cardiac structures to the probe results in improved visualization.

C. **TEE versus the PA catheter**

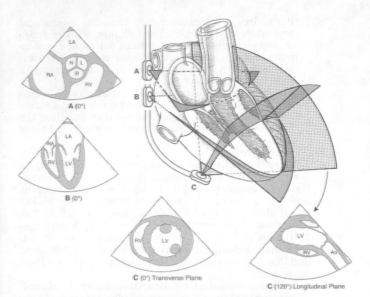

Fig. 2-3. Schematic representation of the views of the cardiac anatomy that can be obtained with the progressive advancement of the transesophageal echoradiography probe. A. Aortic valve. B. Long-axis four-chamber view. C. Short-axis view of the left ventricle. D. Left ventricle and its outflow tract. From Perrino AC, Reeves ST, eds. *A practical approach to transesophageal echocardiography.* Baltimore: Lippincott Williams & Wilkins 2003:272–285.

    1. **PA** catheterization is often used in critically ill patients to assess left ventricular preload and function. The PAOP is frequently used for assessing left ventricular preload. However, its values may be affected by factors other than ventricular preload and function, as discussed in Chapter 1. In contrast, TEE provides direct visualization of the left ventricle, providing direct estimates of left ventricular dimensions and function. In addition, TEE measurement of cardiac output has been shown to correlate well with thermodilution measurements.

    2. Several studies have compared the PA catheter and TEE in postoperative assessment. Echocardiography has consistently been shown to provide different and therapeutically important information beyond that provided by the PA catheter. However, echocardiography can be a time-consuming technique and therefore is probably more useful for hemodynamic diagnosis than for real-time hemodynamic monitoring.

D. Contraindications and complications of TEE

    1. TEE is an invasive procedure. Contraindications include the presence of significant esophageal or gastric pathology. Clinical judgment must be used in the

$$\Delta F = v\cos\theta \cdot \frac{2F_T}{c}$$

$$V = \frac{\Delta F}{\cos\theta} \cdot \frac{c}{2F_T}$$

Fig. 2-4. Calculating blood flow velocity; the Doppler equation. The Doppler equation calculates blood flow velocity based on two variables: the Doppler frequency shift (ΔF) and the cosine of the angle of incidence between the ultrasound beam and the blood flow. The Doppler frequency shift is measured by the electrocardiographic system, but $\cos\theta$ is unknown, and manual entry by the electrocardiographer is required for its estimation. V, blood flow velocity; F_T, transmitted signal frequency; F_R, reflected signal frequency; ΔF, difference between F_R and F_T; c, speed of sound in tissue; Δ, angle of incidence between the orientation of the ultrasound beam and that of the blood flow. From Perrino AC, Reeves ST, eds. *A practical approach to transesophageal echocardiography*. Baltimore: Lippincott Williams & Wilkins 2003:272–285.

presence of intermediate-severity conditions, such as small esophageal varices. In the general patient population (i.e., stable, ambulatory-setting patients) complications are rare, averaging 0.5% of all probe placements. Data specific to the ICU population are not available.

2. Placement of a TEE probe in an uncooperative patient can be associated with esophageal trauma, cardiovascular stress, dysrhythmias, and hypoxia. Bleeding can occur, particularly in the presence of coagulation abnormalities. Manipulation of the neck must be avoided in patients with cervical spine disease or injury. Emesis and aspiration are real concerns in nonfasting patients with an unprotected airway. The ICU is a safer setting for high-risk patients undergoing TEE because of the high level of monitoring and staffing and the ability to rapidly assure airway protection and hemodynamic control.

E. **Indications of echocardiography-Doppler**

1. Guidelines published by the American Heart Association, American College of Cardiology, and American Society of Echocardiography recommend echocardiography as a class I indication for **hemodynamic**

instability and for **suspected aortic dissection** in critically ill patients. In the following sections, we will refer mainly to TEE.

2. **Hypovolemia**
   a. Assessment of left ventricular chamber size (usually left ventricular end-diastolic area) by TEE has been shown to be a sensitive measure of left ventricular preload and hence of volume status.
   b. In deeply sedated and mechanically ventilated patients, the magnitude of the respiratory variation in aortic blood flow (Doppler) or in the vena cava diameter (two-dimensional echo) predicts the hemodynamic effects of a volume load (see also section **I**).

3. **Ventricular dysfunction.** TEE can provide a qualitative assessment of left ventricular chamber size and function. It can also estimate intracardiac filling pressures and hemodynamic indices such as stroke volume and cardiac output. The right ventricle is less easily accessible than the left ventricle by both TTE and TEE; however, an estimate of right ventricular function can be provided by the findings of right ventricular dilation, tricuspid regurgitation, abnormal septal wall motion, and decreased left ventricular chamber size.

4. **Valvular dysfunction.** TEE is invaluable in detecting significant valvular dysfunction. In addition to providing a diagnosis and establishing disease severity, TEE provides information as to its cause, for example, ventricular dysfunction, ruptured chordae, or leaflet perforation.

5. **Pericardial tamponade.** The initial step in diagnosing tamponade is to visualize pericardial fluid, which can be done easily with echocardiography in most patients. The most common sign of hemodynamically significant pericardial effusion is diastolic collapse of one or more (usually right-sided) cardiac chambers. Evidence of exaggerated alternation of left ventricular and right ventricular filling and output resulting from respiration is also a common finding.

6. **Pulmonary embolism.** Visualization of emboli within the main or right PA is very specific (but insensitive) for the diagnosis. The left PA is rarely seen because of the superimposed left main bronchus. The diagnosis is suggested when pulmonary emboli are suspected and there is evidence of acute right ventricular overload. Absence of these findings does not rule out the diagnosis.

7. **Endocarditis.** The hallmark of endocarditis is the presence of **vegetations,** which are attached to valves or areas of denuded endocardium. The size, mobility, location, and number of valves involved have prognostic information and are related to the likelihood of complications. TEE is the best test for

visualizing valvular vegetations, and has a 90% to 100% sensitivity.

8. **Aortic dissection.** TEE is becoming the standard modality for acute evaluation of suspected aortic dissection. The diagnosis requires visualization of an undulating intimal flap in at least two views. The sensitivity of TEE for thoracic aortic dissection is close to 100%. The ascending aorta and proximal arch are more difficult to visualize due to the position of the trachea and the left main bronchus. False-positive results may occur due to linear artifacts within the ascending aorta, which may simulate an intimal flap.

9. **Unexplained hypoxemia.** In patients with severe hypoxemia, TEE may be used to diagnose an intracardiac shunt. Right-to-left shunts can be demonstrated using color flow Doppler or agitated saline contrast.

10. **Myocardial infarction.** TEE can provide information regarding the extent of myocardial involvement and suspected complications. Mechanical complications such as acute valvular insufficiency, septal or free wall rupture, and ventricular pseudoaneurysm are readily diagnosed by TEE. One limitation of TEE is that the ventricular apex is not well visualized, and thus infarction, aneurysms, or thrombi may not be identified.

11. **Blunt chest trauma.** The most common abnormality following blunt chest trauma is **myocardial contusion.** Because of its proximity to the sternum, the right ventricle is the most vulnerable structure, although the left ventricle may also be injured. TEE findings include ventricular dilation and decreased systolic function. Assessment of valvular function is also important because lacerations of the annuli or chordal rupture can occur.

F. **Hand-held TTE**

1. Despite the multiple potential advantages of TTE and TEE over invasive pressure- based hemodynamic monitoring, current echocardiographic practice in ICU patients has significant shortcomings. Ideally, echocardiography in the ICU should be (a) easily available at all times, (b) read in real time, and (c) easily repeatable. This occurs very seldomly because very few ICU practices provide their own echocardiography service with 24-hour/d availability.

2. A possible alternative is to train intensivists to perform a simplified echocardiographic exam tailored to the specific needs of ICU patients. Similar approaches have been successful in anesthesia practice (mostly cardiac), where anesthesiologists have mastered the use of TEE for perioperative purposes, and in the emergency room, where physicians are trained in the use of TTE to diagnose/rule out a number of major injuries. Several academic institutions have

implemented this idea, using portable, hand-held ultrasound devices of the kind used to visualize central
venous blood vessels for catheterization, powered by
more sophisticated transducers designed specifically
for cardiac structures. Data on the effectiveness of this
approach on a large scale are not available.

VI. Esophageal Doppler monitoring

A. Technology. A Doppler probe measures flow in the descending aorta. The probe is the size of a nasogastric tube
and is placed like a nasogastric tube into the esophagus.
The basis for this technique is that blood flow through
the aorta is equal to the cross-sectional area of the descending aorta multiplied by the velocity of blood in the
aorta. This method is used by monitors such as the EDM
(Deltex Medical, Chichester, UK), the HemoSonic 100
(Arrow International, Reading, PA), and the CardioQ
(Deltex Medical, Chichester, UK). These monitors measure the blood flow velocity through the descending aorta
by using the Doppler principle (see section **V.A.2**) and
use different techniques to estimate its cross-sectional
area.

B. Advantages. The method is relatively noninvasive and
allows continuous monitoring of cardiac output. It also
provides the measurement of corrected **flow time** and
peak flow velocity, which have been proposed to assess cardiac preload and contractility, respectively. However, the accuracy of these measurements in critically
ill patients has not been tested in sizable controlled
studies.

C. Limitations

1. Esophageal Doppler monitoring estimates cardiac
   output based on blood flow in the descending aorta,
   which is only a portion of the total cardiac output.
   A correction factor is added that assumes that the
   ratio of flow distribution between the ascending and
   descending aorta remains constant over time.
2. Optimal probe position is crucial. To have a good ap-
   proximation of blood flow based on the Doppler equation, the ultrasound beam must be maintained within
   20 degrees of axial flow. The technique cannot be easily used in awake or moving patients.
3. The CardioQ and EDM systems use an estimation of
   aortic diameter from a nomogram to assess the cardiac output, whereas on the HemoSonic 100 the aortic diameter is measured by echocardiography (echo-
   Doppler probe).
4. Flow in the aorta is not always laminar. Turbulent
   aortic blood flow can be caused by tachycardia, anemia, and aortic valve disease and can alter velocity
   measurements.
5. Esophageal Doppler monitoring does not provide a
   validated assessment of cardiac preload and contractility.
6. Esophageal disease, severe coagulopathy, and patient
   agitation are contraindications.

7. Measurements of cardiac output by esophageal Doppler monitoring have been correlated well with both thermodilution and Fick methods; however, studies are limited.

VII. Indirect Fick method
A. Technology
1. **Fick's principle** is based on the conservation of mass. When applied to the lung, it states that the blood flow through the alveoli is equal to the uptake or the elimination of a gas divided by the difference in its concentration in the blood flowing in and out of the lungs. Traditionally, oxygen uptake ($\dot{V}O_2$) is used to calculate cardiac output with the Fick method:

$$\text{Cardiac output} = \dot{V}O_2/(CaO_2 - CvO_2)$$

where CaO_2 and CvO_2 are the arterial and mixed venous oxygen content, respectively.

2. Difficulty in measuring $\dot{V}O_2$ accurately and the sensitivity of the method to changes in hemoglobin concentration have led to substitution of O_2 with CO_2:

$$\text{Cardiac output} = \dot{V}CO_2/(CvCO_2 - CaCO_2)$$

where $\dot{V}CO_2$ is the CO_2 elimination and $CvCO_2$ and $CaCO_2$ are the mixed venous and arterial CO_2 content, respectively. The NICO monitor (Novametrix, Wallingford, CT) measures cardiac output noninvasively through the application of Fick's equation for CO_2. The $\dot{V}CO_2$ is measured at the airway with a flow and CO_2 sensor (volumetric capnometry; see Chapter 3). The $CaCO_2$ is obtained from arterial blood gases, or can be estimated from the end-tidal CO_2 ($EtCO_2$) concentration. The $CvCO_2$ is difficult to measure noninvasively, and the NICO monitor uses a **partial CO_2 rebreathing** technique to resolve the foregoing equation without measuring $CvCO_2$. The addition of a small rebreathing circuit at the airway causes an acute change in $PaCO_2$ and $\dot{V}CO_2$. The pulmonary blood flow calculation can thus be rewritten using the changes in each of the three terms involved, $\dot{V}CO_2$, $CvCO_2$, and $CaCO_2$. With the assumption that the $CvCO_2$ does not change significantly during the rebreathing period (due to the large CO_2 body stores), the $CvCO_2$ terms cancel out, and the pulmonary blood flow (also assumed not to change during rebreathing) is calculated from the changes in $\dot{V}CO_2$ and in $CaCO_2$. This technique gives a reasonable measurement of the cardiac output in normal individuals. However, the assumption that the pulmonary blood flow engaged in CO_2 exchange and the cardiac output are two similar values is no longer acceptable in the presence of acute respiratory failure. The NICO monitor provides an adjustment for the value of shunt, estimated noninvasively from the fraction of inspired oxygen and the arterial oxygen saturation by pulse oximetry.

B. Advantages. It is completely noninvasive.

C. Limitations

1. Its use is limited to intubated patients.
2. CO_2 rebreathing, albeit small, may not be well tolerated by patients with severe acute respiratory failure.
3. The relationships assumed are only valid when $PaCO_2$ is greater than 30 mm Hg.
4. Accuracy may be affected by nonsteady states.

SELECTED REFERENCES

Chaney JC, Derdak S. Minimally invasive hemodynamic monitoring for the intensivist: current and emerging technology. *Crit Care Med* 2002;30:2338–2345.

Cheitlin MD, Armstrong WF, Aurigemma GP, et al. ACC/AHA/ASE 2003 guideline update for the clinical application of echocardiography: summary article. *Circulation* 2003;108:1146–1462.

Combes A, Berneau JB, Luyt CE, et al. Estimation of left ventricular systolic function by single transpulmonary thermodilution. *Intensive Care Med* 2004;30:1377–1383.

Goedje O, Hoke K, Goetz AE, et al. Reliability of a new algorithm for continuous cardiac output determination by pulse-contour analysis during hemodynamic instability. *Crit Care Med* 2002;30:52–58.

Jaffe MB. Partial rebreathing cardiac output—operating principles of the NICO system. *J Clin Monitoring* 1999;15:387–401.

Jonas MM, Tanser SJ. Lithium dilution measurement of cardiac output and arterial pulse waveform analysis: an indicator dilution calibrated beat-by-beat system for continuous estimation of cardiac output. *Curr Opin Crit Care* 2002;8:257–261.

Lobato EB, Urdaneta F. TEE in the ICU. In: Perrino AC, Reeves ST, eds. *A practical approach to transesophageal echocardiography*. Baltimore: Lippincott Williams & Wilkins 2003:272–285.

Mahutte CK. Continuous cardiac output monitoring via thermal, Fick, Doppler, and pulse contour methods. In: Tobin MJ, ed. *Principles and practice of intensive care monitoring*. New York: McGraw-Hill, 1998:901–913.

Michard F, Alaya S, Zarka V, et al. Global end-diastolic volume as an indicator of cardiac preload in patients with septic shock. *Chest* 2003;124:1900–1908.

Michard F, Boussat S, Chemla D, et al. Relationship between respiratory changes in arterial pulse pressure and fluid responsiveness in septic patients with acute circulatory failure. *Am J Respir Crit Care Med* 2000;162:134–138.

Michard F, Perel A. Management of circulatory and respiratory failure using less invasive hemodynamic monitoring. In: Vincent JL, ed. *Yearbook of intensive care and emergency medicine*. Berlin: Springer, 2003:508–520.

Sakka SG, Ruhl CC, Pfeiffer UJ, et al. Assessment of cardiac preload and extravascular lung water by single transpulmonary thermodilution. *Intensive Care Med* 2000;26:180–187.

3

Respiratory Monitoring

Daniel Fisher and Dean Hess

I. **Monitoring** is a continuous, or nearly continuous, evaluation of the physiologic function of a patient in real time to guide management decisions, including when to make therapeutic interventions and assessment of those interventions. The decision to monitor, like any other clinical decision, should be based on clinical indications.
   A. **Safety.** Monitoring is often performed to assure patient safety. For example, pulse oximetry is used to detect hypoxemia and airway pressure is monitored to detect a mechanical ventilator disconnection. Although monitoring has improved safety, its impact on patient outcome in the intensive care unit (ICU) is less clear.
   B. **Assess interventions.** Invasive and noninvasive monitoring is commonly used in the ICU to assess patient response to clinical interventions. Titration of the inspired oxygen fraction (FiO_2) is commonly guided by pulse oximetry, the level of pressure support is guided by respiratory rate, and the inspiratory-to-expiratory ratio (I:E ratio) is guided by measurement of intrinsic positive end-expiratory pressure (auto-PEEP; see section **IV.B**).

II. **Gas exchange**
   A. **Arterial blood gases and pH.** Arterial blood gas analysis is often considered the gold standard for assessment of pulmonary gas exchange.
      1. **Arterial partial pressure of oxygen (PaO_2).** The normal arterial PaO_2 is 90 to 100 mm Hg breathing room air at sea level.
      2. **Decreased PaO_2 (hypoxemia)** occurs with pulmonary diseases resulting in shunt ($\dot{Q}_S/\dot{Q}_T$), ventilation-perfusion ($\dot{V}/\dot{Q}$) mismatch, hypoventilation, and diffusion defect. A low mixed venous PO_2 (e.g., decreased cardiac output) will magnify the effect of shunt on PaO_2. The PaO_2 is also decreased with decreased inspired oxygen (e.g., at high altitude).
      3. **Increased PaO_2 (hyperoxemia)** may occur when breathing supplemental oxygen. The PaO_2 also increases with hyperventilation.
      4. **Effect of FiO_2.** The PaO_2 should always be interpreted in relation to the level of supplemental oxygen. For example, a PaO_2 of 95 mm Hg breathing 100% oxygen is quite different from a PaO_2 of 95 mm Hg breathing air (21% oxygen).
      5. **Arterial partial pressure of CO_2 ($PaCO_2$).** The $PaCO_2$ reflects the balance between carbon dioxide production ($\dot{V}CO_2$) and alveolar ventilation ($\dot{V}_A$):

      $$PaCO_2 = \dot{V}CO_2/\dot{V}_A$$

      a. $Paco_2$ varies directly with carbon dioxide production and inversely with alveolar ventilation.

      b. $Paco_2$ is determined by alveolar ventilation and not minute ventilation per se.

      c. Minute ventilation affects $Paco_2$ only to the extent that it affects the alveolar ventilation.

  6. Arterial pH is determined by bicarbonate (HCO_3^-) concentration and $Paco_2$, as predicted by the **Henderson-Hasselbalch equation:**

$$pH = 6.1 + \log [HCO_3^- /(0.03 \times Paco_2)]$$

See Chapter 7 for a discussion of acid-base disorders.

B. Venous blood gases reflect tissue Pco_2 and Po_2.

  1. There is a large difference between Pao_2 and venous Po_2. Moreover, venous Po_2 is affected by oxygen delivery and oxygen consumption, whereas Pao_2 is affected by lung function. Thus, venous Po_2 should not be used as a surrogate for Pao_2.

  2. Normally, venous pH is slightly lower than arterial pH and venous Pco_2 is slightly higher than $Paco_2$. However, the difference between arterial and venous pH and Pco_2 is increased by hemodynamic instability. During cardiac arrest, for example, it has been shown that venous Pco_2 can be very high even when $Paco_2$ is low.

  3. When venous blood gases are used to assess acid-base balance, mixed venous or central venous samples are preferable to peripheral venous samples.

C. CO-oximetry. Spectrophotometric analysis of arterial blood is used to measure levels of oxyhemoglobin (oxygen saturation of hemoglobin), carboxyhemoglobin (carbon monoxide saturation of hemoglobin), and methemoglobin (amount of hemoglobin in the oxidized ferric form rather than the reduced ferrous form).

  1. Oxyhemoglobin (Hbo_2) measured by CO-oximetry is the gold standard for determination of oxygen saturation and is superior to other means of determining oxygen saturation, such as that calculated empirically by a blood gas analyzer or that measured by pulse oximetry. The normal Hbo_2 is about 97%.

  2. Carboxyhemoglobin ($Hbco$) levels should be performed whenever carbon monoxide inhalation is suspected. Endogenous carboxyhemoglobin levels are 1% to 2% and can be elevated in cigarette smokers and those living in polluted environments. Because carboxyhemoglobin does not transport oxygen, the Hbo_2 is effectively reduced by the $Hbco$ level.

  3. Methemoglobin. The iron in the hemoglobin molecule can be oxidized to the ferric form in the presence of a number of oxidizing agents, the most notable being nitrates. Because methemoglobin (metHb) does not transport oxygen, the Hbo_2 is effectively reduced by the metHb level.

D. **Continuous blood gas monitoring**
1. **Principles of operation.** Intraarterial blood gas systems use optical biosensors called fluorescent optodes. The optode consists of a miniaturized probe containing a fluorescent dye. Fluorescence is augmented with an increase in hydrogen ion concentration or PCO_2 and quenched with an increase in PO_2. Photosensors are used to quantify the signal for measurement of pH, PCO_2, and PO_2. Systems for continuous blood gas monitoring use a probe that passes through an arterial catheter and resides in the arterial lumen.
2. **Limitations.** The major limitations of these systems are cost of the system and the cost of labor needed to keep the sensors functioning for a prolonged period of time. Whether the benefits of continuous blood gas analysis outweigh the costs and technical constraints is not yet determined.
E. **Point-of-care blood gas monitoring** is performed near the site of patient care. Point-of-care analyzers are available to measure blood gases and pH. These analyzers can also make other measurements including electrolytes, glucose, lactate, urea nitrogen, hematocrit, and clotting studies (activated clotting times [ACT], prothrombin time [PT], and partial thromboplastin time [PTT]).
1. **Advantages.** Point-of-care analyzers are small and portable (some are hand held), they use very small blood volumes (several drops), and they provide rapid reporting of results (a few minutes). They are relatively easy to use (e.g., self-calibrating) and typically incorporate a disposable cartridge that contains the appropriate biosensors.
2. **Disadvantages.** The cost–benefit situation of these devices is unclear. Furthermore, appropriate documentation is necessary for compliance with the Clinical Laboratory Improvement Amendments of 1988 (CLIA'88) or Joint Commission on Accreditation of Healthcare Organizations (JCAHO) requirements. This involves two levels of quality-control checks at least twice daily. Instrument maintenance and quality control can be labor-intensive and confusing for those who are unfamiliar with these procedures. For example, the disposable cartridges are expensive and can require special handling and storage.
F. **Pulse oximetry**
1. **Principles of operation.** The pulse oximeter passes two wavelengths of light (e.g., 660 and 940 nm) from light-emitting diodes through a pulsating vascular bed to a photodetector. A variety of probes are available in disposable or reusable designs and include digital probes (finger or toe), ear probes, and nasal probes.
2. **Accuracy.** Pulse oximeters use empiric calibration curves developed from studies of healthy volunteers. The accuracy of pulse oximetry is $\pm 4\%$ to 5% at saturations of greater than 80% (and less at lower saturations). The implications of this accuracy relate

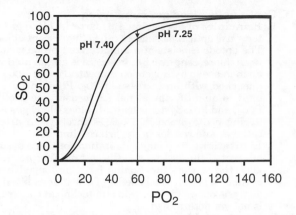

Fig. 3-1.   Oxyhemoglobin dissociation curve. Note that small changes in oxygen saturation relate to large changes in partial pressure of oxygen (Po_2) when the saturation is greater than 90%. Also note that the saturation can change without a change in Po_2 if there is a shift of the oxyhemoglobin dissociation curve.

to the oxyhemoglobin dissociation curve (Fig. 3-1). If the pulse oximeter displays an oxygen saturation (Spo_2) of 95%, the true saturation could be as low as 90% or as high as 100%. This range of Spo_2 translates to a Pao_2 range from as low as about 60 mm Hg to greater than 150 mm Hg.

3. **Limitations** of pulse oximetry should be recognized and understood by everyone who uses pulse oximetry data.

   a. **Saturation versus Po_2.** Due to the shape of the oxyhemoglobin dissociation curve, pulse oximetry is a poor indicator of hyperoxemia. It is also an insensitive indicator of hypoventilation. If the patient is breathing supplemental oxygen, significant hypoventilation can occur without Hbo_2 desaturation.

   b. **Differences between devices and probes.** Calibration curves vary from manufacturer to manufacturer. The output of the light-emitting diodes of pulse oximeters varies from probe to probe. For these reasons, the same pulse oximeter and probe should be used for each Spo_2 determination for a patient.

   c. **The penumbra effect** occurs when the pulse oximeter probe does not fit correctly and light is shunted from the light-emitting diodes directly to the photodetector.

   d. **Dyshemoglobinemia.** Pulse oximeters only use two wavelengths of light and therefore only evaluate two forms of hemoglobin: oxyhemoglobin and deoxyhemoglobin. **Carboxyhemoglobinemia** and **methemoglobinemia** result in significant inaccuracy of pulse oximetry. Carboxy-hemoglobinemia produces a SpO_2 greater than the true oxygen saturation and methemoglobine-mia causes the SpO_2 to move toward 85%. Fetal hemoglobin does not affect the accuracy of pulse oximetry.

  e. **Endogenous and exogenous dyes and pigments** such as intravascular dyes (particularly methylene blue) affect the accuracy of pulse oximetry. Nail polish can also affect the accuracy of pulse oximetry. Hyperbilirubinemia does not affect the accuracy of pulse oximetry.

  f. **Skin pigmentation.** The accuracy and performance of pulse oximetry are affected by deeply pigmented skin.

  g. **Perfusion.** Pulse oximetry becomes unreliable during conditions of low flow such as low cardiac output or severe peripheral vasoconstriction. An ear probe may be more reliable than a digital probe under these conditions. A dampened plethysmographic waveform suggests poor signal quality.

  h. **Anemia.** Although pulse oximetry is generally reliable over a wide range of hematocrit, it becomes less accurate under conditions of severe anemia.

  i. **Motion** of the oximeter probe can produce artifact and inaccurate pulse oximetry readings. Newer-generation oximeters incorporate noise-canceling algorithms to lessen the effect of motion on signal interpretation.

  j. **High-intensity ambient light,** which can affect pulse oximeter performance, can be corrected by shielding the probe.

  k. **Abnormal pulses.** Venous pulsations and a large dicrotic notch can affect the accuracy of pulse oximetry.

4. **Guidelines for use.** Although pulse oximetry improves the detection of desaturation, there is little evidence that its use improves outcome. In spite of this, pulse oximetry has become a standard of care in the ICU (particularly for mechanically ventilated patients). Pulse oximetry is useful for titrating supplemental oxygen in mechanically ventilated patients. A value of SpO_2 of greater than or equal to 92% reliably predicts a PaO_2 of greater than or equal to 60 mm Hg in white patients ($SpO_2 \geq 95\%$ in black patients). SpO_2 should be periodically confirmed by blood gas analysis.

G. **Capnometry** is the measurement of CO_2 at the airway and **capnography** is the display of a CO_2 waveform called the **capnogram** (Fig. 3-2). The PCO_2 measured at end-exhalation is called the **end-tidal PCO_2** ($PetCO_2$).

  1. **Principles of operation.** Quantitative capnometers measure CO_2 using the principles of infrared spectroscopy, Raman spectroscopy, or mass spectroscopy. Nonquantitative capnometers indicate CO_2 by a color

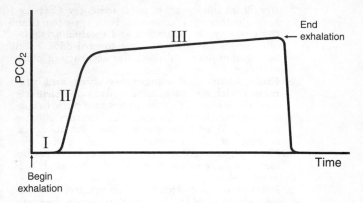

Fig. 3-2.   Normal capnogram. Phase I, anatomic dead space; phase II, transition from dead space to alveolar gas; phase III, alveolar plateau.

change of an indicator material. Mainstream capnometers place the measurement chamber directly on the airway, whereas sidestream capnometers aspirate gas through tubing to a measurement chamber in the capnometer.

2. The **$Petco_2$** represents alveolar Pco_2; it is determined by the rate at which CO_2 is added to the alveolus and the rate at which CO_2 is cleared from the alveolus. Thus, the $Petco_2$ is a function of the $\dot{V}/\dot{Q}$: with a normal $\dot{V}/\dot{Q}$, the $Petco_2$ approximates the $Paco_2$. With a high $\dot{V}/\dot{Q}$ (dead-space effect), the $Petco_2$ is lower than the $Paco_2$. With a low $\dot{V}/\dot{Q}$ (shunt effect), the $Petco_2$ approximates the mixed-venous Pco_2. The $Petco_2$ can be as low as the inspired Pco_2 (zero) or as high as the mixed venous Pco_2. Changes in $Petco_2$ can be due to changes in CO_2 production, CO_2 delivery to the lungs, or changes in alveolar ventilation.

3. **Abnormal capnogram.** The shape of the capnogram can be abnormal with obstructive lung diseases (Fig. 3-3).

4. **Limitations.** There is considerable intra- and interpatient variability in the relationship between $Paco_2$ and $Petco_2$. The $P(a\text{-}et)co_2$ is often too variable in critically ill patients to allow precise prediction of $Paco_2$ from $Petco_2$.

5. **Guidelines for clinical use.** The utility of $Petco_2$ to predict $Paco_2$ is limited in the ICU. Capnometry is useful for detecting esophageal intubation. $Petco_2$ monitoring to confirm tracheal intubation is generally regarded as a standard of care. Low-cost disposable devices are commercially available that produce a color change in the presence of exhaled CO_2.

6. **Volume-based capnometry** displays exhaled CO_2 as a function of exhaled tidal volume (Fig. 3-4). Note that

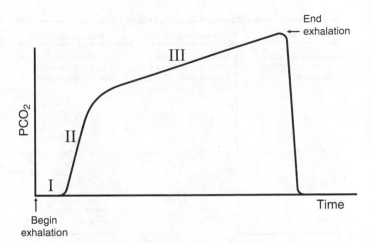

Fig. 3-3. An increased phase III occurs in the capnogram in patients with obstructive lung disease.

the area under the volume-based capnogram is the volume of CO_2 exhaled. Assuming steady-state conditions, this represents **carbon dioxide production** ($\dot{V}CO_2$). Because $\dot{V}CO_2$ is determined by metabolic rate, this can be used to estimate **resting energy expenditure** (REE): REE = $\dot{V}CO_2$ (L/min) × 5.52 kcal/L × 1,440 min/day (see also Chapter 9). Normal $\dot{V}CO_2$ is approximately 200 ml/min (2.6 ml/kg/min).

7. Using volume-based capnometry and a partial-rebreathing circuit allows measurement of **pulmonary capillary blood flow** using a modification

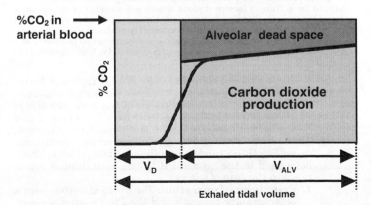

Fig. 3-4. The volume-based capnogram. Note that the area under the curve represents carbon dioxide elimination, which equals carbon dioxide production during steady-state conditions.

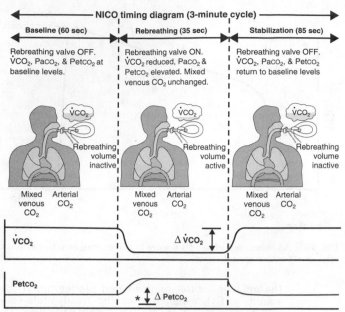

← —————— NICO timing diagram (3-minute cycle) —————— →

Baseline (60 sec)	Rebreathing (35 sec)	Stabilization (85 sec)

Rebreathing valve OFF. $\dot{V}CO_2$, $PaCO_2$, & $PetCO_2$ at baseline levels.

Rebreathing valve ON. $\dot{V}CO_2$ reduced, $PaCO_2$ & $PetCO_2$ elevated. Mixed venous CO_2 unchanged.

Rebreathing valve OFF. $\dot{V}CO_2$, $PaCO_2$, & $PetCO_2$ return to baseline levels

$\dot{V}CO_2$

Rebreathing volume inactive

$\dot{V}CO_2$

Rebreathing volume active

$\dot{V}CO_2$

Rebreathing volume inactive

Mixed venous CO_2 Arterial CO_2

Mixed venous CO_2 Arterial CO_2

Mixed venous CO_2 Arterial CO_2

$\dot{V}CO_2$ $\Delta \dot{V}CO_2$

$PetCO_2$ * $\Delta PetCO_2$

*3-5 mm Hg typical

Fig. 3-5. Use of the partial carbon dioxide rebreathing method to measure cardiac output using capnometry. Assuming that changes in Pulmonary capillary carbon dioxide content ($Cc'CO_2$) are proportional to changes in end-tidal CO_2 ($PetCO_2$), we can use the following equation to calculate pulmonary capillary blood flow (PCBF): $PCBF = \Delta \dot{V}CO_2/(S \times \Delta PetCO_2)$, where $\Delta \dot{V}CO_2$ is the change in CO_2 output and S is the slope of the CO_2 dissociation curve. Cardiac output is determined from PCBF and pulmonary shunt: $\dot{Q} = PCBF/(1 - \dot{Q}s/\dot{Q}t)$. Noninvasive estimation of pulmonary shunt ($\dot{Q}s/\dot{Q}t$) is adapted from Nunn's isoshunt plots, which are a series of continuous curves for the relationship between partial pressure of oxygen (PaO_2) and inspired oxygen (FiO_2) for different levels of shunt. PaO_2 is estimated using a pulse oximeter. $PaCO_2$, arterial partial pressure of CO_2. (NICO timing diagram courtesy of Novametrix, Wallingford, CT.)

of the Fick equation (Fig. 3-5). With corrections for intrapulmonary shunt, this allows noninvasive estimation of cardiac output. Studies of the accuracy of this method in critically ill patients have been mixed, and further validation in this patient population is needed.

H. Transcutaneous blood gas monitoring. Transcutaneous PO_2 ($PtcO_2$) and transcutaneous PcO_2 ($PtcCO_2$) have been used in the neonatal ICU, but with limited acceptance in the care of adults.

1. Principles of operation. The $PtcO_2$ electrode uses a polarographic principle and the $PtcCO_2$ used a Severinghaus electrode. To produce a $PtcO_2$ similar to PaO_2, the electrode is heated. The increase in PO_2 caused by heating roughly balances the decrease in PO_2 due to skin oxygen consumption and diffusion of oxygen across the skin. The $PtcCO_2$ is consistently greater than $PaCO_2$ and for this reason manufacturers incorporate a correction factor so that the displayed $PtcCO_2$ approximates $PaCO_2$.

2. **Limitations.** A number of factors limit the usefulness of transcutaneous monitoring in adults. The heated electrode can cause skin burns, and its position must be changed frequently to prevent burns. The transcutaneous PO_2 and PCO_2 are unreliable for 15 to 20 min after the electrode is placed. Compromised hemodynamics causes underestimation of PaO_2 and overestimation of $PaCO_2$. Given the technical and physiologic limitations of transcutaneous monitoring, it is rarely used in the adult ICU.

III. Lung Function
A. Indices of oxygenation
1. **Shunt fraction** is the gold standard index of oxygenation. It is calculated from the **shunt equation:**

$$\dot{Q}_S/\dot{Q}_T = (Cc'O_2 - CaO_2)/(Cc'O_2 - C\bar{v}O_2)$$

where $Cc'O_2$ is the pulmonary capillary oxygen content, CaO_2 is the arterial oxygen content, and $C\bar{v}O_2$ is the mixed venous oxygen content. Oxygen content is calculated from

$$CO_2 = (1.34 \times Hb \times HbO_2) + (0.003 \times PaO_2)$$

To calculate $Cc'O_2$, we assume the pulmonary capillary PO_2 is equal to the alveolar PO_2 and the pulmonary capillary hemoglobin is 100% saturated with oxygen. If measured when the patient is breathing 100% oxygen, the $\dot{Q}_S/\dot{Q}_T$ represents shunt (i.e., blood that flows from the right heart to the left heart without passing functional alveoli). If measured at FiO_2 less than 1.0, the $\dot{Q}_S/\dot{Q}_T$ represents shunt and $\dot{V}/\dot{Q}$ mismatch.

2. **PaO_2, $P(A-a)O_2$, PaO_2/PAO_2.** The **alveolar PO_2 (PAO_2)** is calculated from the **alveolar gas equation:**

$$PAO_2 = (FiO_2 \times EBP) - [PaCO_2 \times (FiO_2 + (1 - FiO_2)/R]$$

where EBP is the effective barometric pressure (barometric pressure minus water vapor pressure) and R is the respiratory quotient. For calculation of PAO_2, an R of 0.8 is commonly used. For FiO_2 greater than or equal to 0.6, the effect of R on the alveolar gas equation becomes

$$PAO_2 = (FiO_2 \times EBP) - (PaCO_2)$$

For FiO_2 less than 0.6, the alveolar gas equation becomes

$$PAO_2 = (FiO_2 \times EBP) - (1.2 \times PaCO_2)$$

An increased difference between PAO_2 and PaO_2, the **$P(A-a)O_2$ gradient,** can be due to shunt, $\dot{V}/\dot{Q}$ mismatch, or diffusion defect. The $P(A-a)O_2$ is normally equal to or less than 10 mm Hg breathing room air and equal to or less than 50 mm Hg breathing 100% oxygen. The ratio of the PaO_2 to PAO_2 **(PaO_2/PAO_2)** can also be calculated as an index of lung function and is normally greater than 0.75 at any FiO_2.

3. **PaO_2/FiO_2** is the easiest of the indices of oxygenation to calculate. The acute respiratory distress syndrome is associated with PaO_2/FiO_2 less than 200 and acute lung injury is associated with a ratio PaO_2/FiO_2 less than 300.

4. The **oxygenation index (OI)** is calculated from the FiO_2, mean airway pressure ($\bar{P}aw$), and PaO_2:

$$OI = (FiO_2 \times \bar{P}aw \times 100)/PaO_2$$

The OI is commonly calculated for critically ill neonates, but is seldom used in the care of critically ill adults.

B. **Indices of ventilation**

1. **Dead space** (V_D/V_T) is calculated from the **Bohr equation,** which measures the ratio of dead space to total ventilation:

$$V_D/V_T = (PaCO_2 - P\bar{E}CO_2)/PaCO_2$$

where $P\bar{E}CO_2$ is the mixed exhaled PCO_2. To determine $P\bar{E}CO_2$, exhaled gas is collected in a bag from the expiratory port of the ventilator and its CO_2 concentration is measured with a blood gas analyzer or capnometer. Alternatively, $P\bar{E}CO_2$ can be determined using volumetric capnometry (see section **II.F.6**):

$$P\bar{E}CO_2 = (\dot{V}CO_2 \times Pb)/\dot{V}_E$$

where Pb is barometric pressure. The normal V_D/V_T is 0.3 to 0.4.

IV. **Lung mechanics**

A. **Plateau pressure** (Pplat) is the mean peak alveolar pressure during mechanical ventilation.

1. **Measurement.** Pplat is measured by applying an end-inspiratory breath-hold for 0.5 to 2 seconds. During the breath-hold, pressure equilibrates throughout the system so that the pressure measured at the proximal airway approximates the peak alveolar pressure (Fig. 3-6). For valid measurement of Pplat, the patient must be relaxed and breathing in synchrony with the ventilator.

2. **An increased Pplat** indicates a greater risk of alveolar overdistention during mechanical ventilation. Many authorities recommend that Pplat be maintained at less than or equal to 30 cm H_2O in patients with acute respiratory failure. This assumes that chest wall compliance is normal. Higher plateau pressures may be necessary if chest wall compliance is decreased (e.g., abdominal distension).

B. **Auto-PEEP**

1. **Measurement.** Auto-PEEP is measured by applying an end-expiratory pause for 0.5 to 2 seconds (Fig. 3-7). The pressure measured at the end of this maneuver

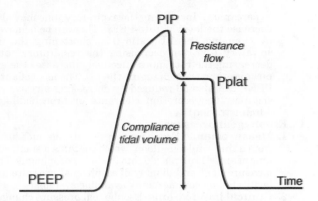

Fig. 3-6. Peak alveolar pressure (Pplat) is determined by applying an end-inspiratory breath-hold. The peak inspiratory pressure (PIP) – Pplat difference is determined by resistance and end-inspiratory flow, and the Pplat – positive end-expiratory pressure (PEEP) difference is determined by compliance and tidal volume.

that is in excess of the PEEP set on the ventilator represents the amount of auto-PEEP. For a valid measurement, the patient must be relaxed and breathing in synchrony with the ventilator—active breathing will invalidate the measurement. Measurement of auto-PEEP during active breathing requires the use of an esophageal balloon.

2. **Clinical implications.** Auto-PEEP is determined by the ventilator settings (tidal volume and expiratory time) and lung function (airways resistance and lung compliance). The level of auto-PEEP can be decreased by reducing the minute ventilation with a decrease in either tidal volume or respiratory rate (permissive

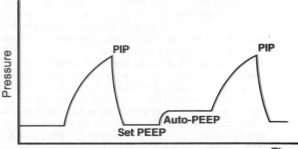

Fig. 3-7. Auto–positive end-expiratory pressure (auto-PEEP) is measured by applying an end-expiratory breath-hold. An increase in pressure above the level of PEEP set indicates the presence of auto-PEEP. PIP, peak inspiratory pressure.

hypercapnia). Increasing the expiratory time may also decrease the level of auto-PEEP. This can be achieved by changing the I:E ratio (i.e., shortening the inspiratory time) or decreasing the respiratory rate; decreasing the rate more effectively increases the expiratory time than changing the I:E. The level of auto-PEEP can also be reduced by decreasing airways resistance (i.e., secretion clearance or bronchodilator administration).

C. **Esophageal pressure**

1. **Measurement.** Esophageal pressure is measured from a thin-walled balloon, which contains a small volume of air (<1 ml) placed into the lower esophagus. The measurement and display of esophageal pressure are facilitated by commercially available systems.

2. **Clinical implications.** Esophageal pressure changes reflect changes in pleural pressure, but the absolute esophageal pressure does not reflect absolute pleural pressure. Changes in esophageal pressure can be used to assess respiratory effort and work of breathing during spontaneous breathing and patient triggered modes of ventilation, to assess chest wall compliance during full ventilatory support, and to assess auto-PEEP during spontaneous breathing and patient-triggered modes of ventilation. If exhalation is passive, the change in esophageal (i.e., pleural) pressure required to reverse flow at the proximal airway (i.e., trigger the ventilator) reflects the amount of auto-PEEP. Negative esophageal pressure changes that produce no flow at the airway indicate failed trigger efforts—in other words, the patient's inspiratory efforts are insufficient to overcome the level of auto-PEEP and trigger the ventilator (Fig. 3-8). Clinically, this is recognized as a patient respiratory rate (observed by inspecting chest wall movement) that is greater than the trigger rate on the ventilator.

D. **Gastric pressure**

1. Gastric pressure is measured by a balloon-tipped catheter similar to that used to measure esophageal pressure. It reflects changes in intraabdominal pressure. An alternative for measuring gastric pressure is measuring **bladder pressure.**

2. **Clinical implications.** During a spontaneous inspiratory effort, gastric pressure normally increases due to contraction of the diaphragm. A decrease in gastric pressure with spontaneous inspiratory effort is consistent with diaphragmatic paralysis (Fig. 3-9). A high baseline gastric pressure reflects elevated intraabdominal pressure, which may affect chest wall compliance and lung function.

E. **Compliance** (the inverse of elastance) is the change in volume (usually tidal volume) divided by the change in pressure required to produce that volume.

1. **Respiratory system, chest wall, and lung compliance**

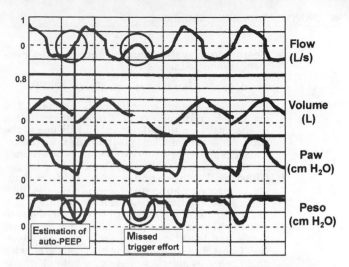

Fig. 3-8. Use of esophageal pressure to determine auto–positive end-expiratory pressure (auto-PEEP). The change in esophageal pressure required to trigger the ventilator is the level of auto-PEEP. Also note the presence of missed trigger efforts in which the inspiratory effort of the patient is not sufficient to overcome the amount of auto-PEEP. Paw, mean airway pressure; Peso, esophageal pressure.

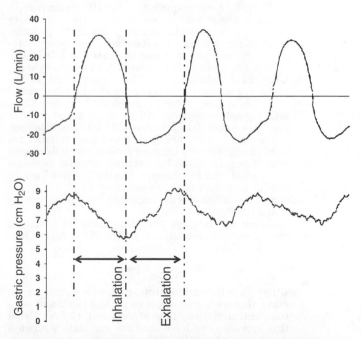

Fig. 3-9. Gastric pressure measurement in a patient with diaphragm paralysis. Note that the gastric pressure decreases during the inspiratory phase.

a. **Respiratory system compliance** is most commonly calculated in the ICU:

$$C = \Delta V/\Delta P = \text{tidal volume}/(\text{Pplat} - \text{PEEP})$$

Respiratory system compliance is normally 100 ml/cm H_2O and is reduced to 50 to 100 ml/cm H_2O in mechanically ventilated patients, likely due to the supine or semirecumbent position and microatelectasis. Respiratory system compliance is determined by the compliance of the chest wall and the lungs.

b. **Chest wall compliance** is calculated from changes in esophageal pressure (pleural pressure) during passive inflation. Chest wall compliance is normally 200 ml/cm H_2O and can be decreased due to abdominal distension, chest wall edema, chest wall burns, and thoracic deformities (e.g., kyphoscoliosis). Chest wall compliance is also decreased with an increase in muscle tone (e.g., a patient who is bucking the ventilator). Chest wall compliance is increased with flail chest and paralysis.

c. **Lung compliance** is calculated from changes in transpulmonary pressure. **Transpulmonary pressure** is the difference between alveolar pressure (Pplat) and pleural pressure (esophageal). Normal lung compliance is 100 ml/cm H_2O. Lung compliance is decreased with pulmonary edema (cardiogenic or noncardiogenic), pneumothorax, consolidation, atelectasis, pulmonary fibrosis, pneumonectomy, and mainstream intubation. Lung compliance is increased with emphysema.

2. **Clinical implications.** When compliance is decreased, a larger transpulmonary pressure is required to deliver a given tidal volume into the lungs. Thus, a decreased compliance will result in a higher Pplat and peak inspiratory pressure (PIP). To avoid dangerous levels of airway pressure, lower tidal volumes are used to ventilate the lungs of patients with decreased compliance. Deceased lung compliance also increases the work of breathing, decreasing the likelihood of successful weaning from the ventilator.

F. **Airways resistance** is determined by the driving pressure and the flow.

1. **Inspiratory airways resistance** can be estimated during volume ventilation from the PIP – Pplat difference and the end-inspiratory flow:

$$R_I = (\text{PIP} - \text{Pplat})/\dot{V}_I$$

where $\dot{V}_I$ is the end-inspiratory flow. A simple way to make this measurement is to set the ventilator for a constant inspiratory flow of 60 L/min (1 L/s). Using this approach, we have that the inspiratory airways resistance is the PIP – Pplat difference.

2. **Common causes** of increased airways resistance are bronchospasm and secretions. Resistance is also

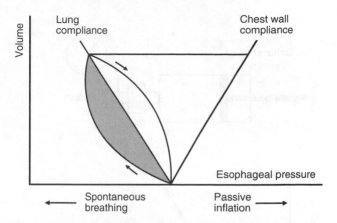

Fig. 3-10. Campbell diagram. The chest wall compliance curve is determined by plotting volume as a function of esophageal pressure during positive-pressure breathing with the chest wall relaxed. The lung compliance curve is determined from the point of zero flow at end-exhalation to the point of zero flow at end-inhalation during spontaneous breathing. Due to airways resistance, the esophageal pressure is more negative than predicted from the lung compliance curve. The areas indicated on the curve represent elastic work of breathing and resistive work of breathing. Note that a decreased chest wall compliance will shift that compliance curve to the right, thus increasing the elastic work of breathing. A decrease in lung compliance shifts that curve to the left, also increasing the work of breathing. An increased airways resistance causes a more negative esophageal pressure during spontaneous breathing, increasing the resistive work of breathing.

increased with a small–inner-diameter endotracheal tube. For intubated and mechanically ventilated patients, airways resistance should be less than 10 cm $H_2O/L/s$ at a flow of 1 L/s. Expiratory airways resistance is typically greater than inspiratory airways resistance.

G. **Work of breathing**
   1. **The Campbell diagram** (Fig. 3-10) is used to determine the work of breathing. The Campbell diagram includes the effects of chest wall compliance, lung compliance, and airway resistance on the work of breathing. Work of breathing is increased with decreased chest wall compliance, decreased lung compliance, or increased airways resistance.
   2. **Clinical implications.** Work of breathing requires special equipment and an esophageal balloon to quantify, and for that reason it is not frequently measured. Moreover, it is not clear that measuring work of breathing improves patient outcome. It may be useful for quantifying patient effort during mechanical ventilation, but this can often be achieved by simply observing the respiratory variation on a central venous pressure

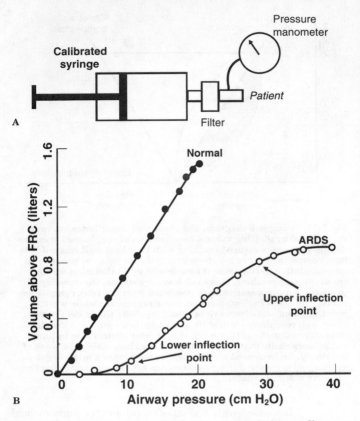

Fig. 3-11. A. Super-syringe set-up for measuring static compliance.
B. Inspiratory pressure–volume curve for a patient with normal lung
function and for a patient with acute respiratory distress syndrome
(ARDS). FRC, functional residual capacity.

tracing. Large inspiratory efforts produce large negative deflections of the central venous pressure trace
during inspiratory efforts. Increasing the level of ventilatory assistance should reduce these negative deflections.

H. The **static pressure–volume curve** measures the
pressure–volume relationship of the respiratory system.

1. **Measurement.** A calibrated syringe and pressure
manometer are used to determine the pressure–volume curve (Fig. 3-11A). The patient is preoxygenated
with 100% oxygen and the syringe is filled with oxygen. The patient is disconnected from the ventilator
and allowed to exhale to resting end-expiratory lung
volume (functional residual capacity). The syringe is

attached to the airway and the pressure is measured at 50- to 100-ml-step changes in volume from the syringe. Alternatively, the lungs can be slowly inflated while volume is plotted as a function of pressure (slow-flow technique).

2. **Lower and upper inflection points** can be determined from the pressure–volume curve (Fig. 3-11B). Some authors have suggested that the level of PEEP should be set above the lower inflection point to avoid alveolar collapse and Pplat should be set below the upper inflection point to avoid alveolar overdistention. However, the clinical benefits of this approach are not clear, and setting the ventilator using the pressure–volume curve is not currently recommended because there are important limitations to the clinical use of pressure–volume curves. Accurate measurements require heavy sedation (and often paralysis); it is unclear whether the inflation or deflation curve should be assessed; it can be difficult to precisely determine the inflection points; the respiratory system pressure–volume curve can be affected by both the lungs and the chest wall; and the pressure–volume curve models the lungs as a single compartment.

I. **Ventilator graphics,** typically scalar graphs of pressure, flow, and volume, can be displayed by many microprocessor-based ventilators. Flow–volume and pressure–volume graphics can also be displayed, but these are less useful. Dynamic pressure–volume loops typically reflect how the ventilator delivers flow and are of limited usefulness for detecting lower and upper inflection points.

1. **Airway pressure graphics** can be used to detect patient–ventilator dyssynchrony. An airway pressure waveform that varies from breath to breath indicates the presence of dyssynchrony (Fig. 3-12).

2. The **airway flow waveform** can be used to detect the presence of auto-PEEP (Fig. 3-13). Expiratory flow does not return to a zero baseline in the presence of auto-PEEP. Although the flow waveform is useful for detecting auto-PEEP, it does not quantitatively indicate the amount of auto-PEEP.

3. The **volume waveform** may be useful to detect the presence of an air leak (e.g., bronchopleural fistula). The difference between the inspiratory and expiratory tidal volumes indicates the volume of the leak (Fig. 3-14).

J. **Ventilator function**

1. **Alarms** are numerous on mechanical ventilators. The most important is the disconnect alarm.

a. A loss of airway pressure **(low-pressure alarm)** indicates a ventilator disconnect or a gross leak in the system. A **high-pressure alarm** indicates the presence of an elevated airway pressure. The high-pressure alarm also serves to cycle the ventilator to the expiratory phase to avoid injury due

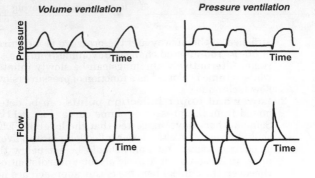

Fig. 3-12.   Patient–ventilator dyssynchrony. During volume-controlled ventilation, the pressure waveform varies from breath to breath. During pressure-controlled ventilation, the flow waveform varies from breath to breath.

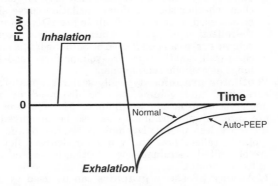

Fig. 3-13.   Flow waveform. The inspiratory flow is determined by the flow setting on the ventilator. Expiratory flow should return to zero. If the expiratory flow does not return to zero, auto–positive end-expiratory pressure is present. auto-PEEP, auto–positive end-expiratory pressure.

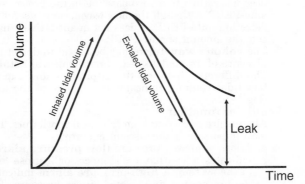

Fig. 3-14.   Volume waveform. If the exhaled volume does not equal the inhaled volume, a leak is present in the system.

overpressurization of the lungs. Appropriate setting of the high-pressure alarm is particularly important during volume ventilation. Common causes of a high-pressure alarm are obstruction of the ventilator circuit or the patient's airways (e.g., kinked ventilator circuit, kinked endotracheal tube, secretions, bronchospasm), a sudden decrease in lung compliance (pneumothorax, mainstream intubation, congestive heart failure), or patient–ventilator dyssynchrony ("bucking the ventilator").

b. **Exhaled tidal volume** should be monitored during volume ventilation to detect a leak. During pressure ventilation, the tidal volume should be monitored to detect changes in respiratory system compliance, resistance, auto-PEEP, or patient breathing efforts.

c. **FiO_2.** Although the blenders in mechanical ventilators are reliable, it is prudent to monitor FiO_2 in mechanically ventilated patients.

d. **Apnea.** With spontaneous breathing modes such as pressure support, there is risk of hypoventilation due to loss of respiratory drive. Current-generation ventilators initiate backup ventilatory support if the patient does not breathe during a preset period of time.

2. **Inspired gas conditioning.** Because the upper airway is bypassed, the inspired gas is warmed and humidified during mechanical ventilation. This has been traditionally accomplished using an active heated humidifier. Recently, there has been increased used of passive humidifiers (artificial noses) during mechanical ventilation.

a. **Airway temperature** is typically monitored during mechanical ventilation when active humidifiers are used. High temperatures should be monitored to avoid airway burns and low temperatures should be monitored to avoid delivery of inadequately humidified gas.

3. **Humidity** is not measured by current mechanical ventilators. The adequacy of delivered humidity can be assessed by observing the ventilator circuit near the patient for the presence of condensation. If the inspiratory circuit near the patient is dry, the delivered humidity is inadequate and steps should be taken to increase the level of humidification to avoid occlusion of the artificial airway with secretions. If an artificial nose is used, adequate humidification of the inspired gas is indicated by condensation within the proximal end of the endotracheal tube.

SELECTED REFERENCES

Banner MJ, Jaeger MJ, Kirby RR. Components of the work of breathing and implications for monitoring ventilator-dependent patients. *Crit Care Med* 1994;22:515–523.

Cardoso MM, Banner MJ, Melker RJ, et al. Portable devices used to detect endotracheal intubation during emergency situations: a review. *Crit Care Med* 1998;26:957–964.

Gehring H, Nornberger C, Matz H, et al. The effects of motion artifact and low perfusion on the performance of a new generation of pulse oximeters in volunteers undergoing hypoxemia. *Respir Care* 2002;47:48–60.

Hess DR. Capnometry. In: Tobin MJ, ed. *Principles and practice of intensive care monitoring*. New York: McGraw-Hill, 1998.

Hess D. Detection and monitoring of hypoxemia and oxygen therapy. *Respir Care* 2000;45:65–80.

Hess DR, Medoff MD, Fessler MB. Pulmonary mechanics and graphics during positive pressure ventilation. *Int Anesthesiol Clin* 1999;37(3):15–34.

Jubran A. Advances in respiratory monitoring during mechanical ventilation. *Chest* 1999;116:1416–1425.

Jubran A, Tobin MJ. Monitoring during mechanical ventilation. *Clin Chest Med* 1996;17:453–473.

Lucangelo U, Blanch L. Dead space. *Intensive Care Med* 2004;30:576–579.

Pilon CS, Leathley M, London R, et al. Practice guideline for arterial blood gas measurement in the intensive care unit decreases numbers and increases appropriateness of tests. *Crit Care Med* 1997;25:1308–1313.

Ranieri VM, Grasso S, Fiore T, et al. Auto-positive end-expiratory pressure and dynamic hyperinflation. *Clin Chest Med* 1996;17:379–394.

Shapiro BA. Point-of-care blood testing and cardiac output measurement in the intensive care unit. *New Horizons* 1999;7:244–252.

Yem JS, Tang Y, Turner MJ, et al. Sources of error in noninvasive pulmonary blood flow measurements by partial rebreathing: a computer model study. *Anesthesiology* 2003;98:881–887.

Airway Management

Peter F. Dunn, Robert L. Goulet,
and William E. Hurford

Endotracheal intubation is required to provide a patent airway
when patients are at risk for aspiration, when airway maintenance by mask is difficult, and for prolonged mechanical ventilation. This chapter discusses the evaluation of the airway,
techniques for endotracheal intubation, and management of the
chronically instrumented airway.

I. **Indications for endotracheal intubation**
   A. **Normal respiratory function** requires a patent
      airway, adequate respiratory drive, neuromuscular
      competence, intact thoracic anatomy, normal lung
      parenchyma, and the ability to cough, sigh, and defend
      against aspiration. Impairments in these parameters,
      singularly or in combination, may result in the need for
      endotracheal intubation and ventilatory support.
   B. **Endotracheal intubation**
      1. Provides relative protection against pulmonary
         aspiration.
      2. Maintains a patent conduit for respiratory gas
         exchange.
      3. Provides a means for coupling the lungs to mechan-
         ical ventilators.
      4. Establishes a route for clearance of secretions.
II. **Airway evaluation**
    A systematic evaluation of the need for tracheal intuba-
    tion is essential. The need for intubation can be immediate
    (e.g., cardiopulmonary arrest), emergent (e.g., impending
    respiratory failure), or urgent (e.g., decreased level of con-
    sciousness with inadequate airway control).
    A. **If cardiopulmonary resuscitation is underway,**
       bag-mask ventilation with 100% oxygen, followed by
       intubation, is required (see Chapter 14). Otherwise,
       perform a rapid evaluation to determine the need for
       intubation.
    B. **Apply oxygen by face mask.** The potential improve-
       ment in systemic oxygenation may allow more time to
       evaluate the patient and consider options.
    C. **Assess level of consciousness.** Obtundation, stupor,
       or coma may be of respiratory origin (e.g., hypoxemia or
       hypercapnia) or arise from metabolic, pharmacologic,
       and neurologic causes. Depressed consciousness can
       lead to airway obstruction, pulmonary aspiration, at-
       electasis, and pneumonia.
    D. **Integument. Cyanosis** is present when at least
       5 g/dl of deoxyhemoglobin is present. Thus, in anemia,

cyanosis may be absent despite a low oxygen saturation. With polycythemia, small decreases in oxygen saturation may manifest as cyanosis. Cold, diaphoretic skin suggests intense autonomic stress or circulatory failure.

E. **Respiration**
   1. Respiratory efforts should be noted, with particular attention to the rate and depth of thoracic movements. **Slow, deep respirations** (<10/min) suggest opioid effect or central nervous system (CNS) disorder. **Tachypnea** (>35/min) is a nonspecific finding that can be present with disorders that cause decreased respiratory system compliance [e.g., pulmonary edema, consolidation, acute respiratory distress syndrome (ARDS)] or increased respiratory load (e.g., increased dead space, fever). It is a common finding in pulmonary embolism and with respiratory muscle fatigue.
   2. **An absent gag reflex,** the inability to maintain an adequate airway in all head positions, or both indicates the need for intubation.
   3. **Evaluation for upper airway obstruction** includes visual (laryngeal tug, chest wall retraction, chest/abdomen discoordination), tactile (air flow felt by placing a hand in front of the patient's mouth and nose, position of trachea in the neck), and auscultory (stridor, absent breath sounds) indicators of either complete or partial obstruction. In the absence of coexisting processes (e.g., cervical spine injury), and depending on the etiology of obstruction (e.g., depressed mental status), obstruction may be relieved by extending the head at the atlanto-occiptal joint, performing a chin lift, jaw thrust, and/or inserting an oral or nasal airway prior to intubation (see later discussion).
   4. **Examine respiratory excursions** for symmetry, timing, and coordination. A pneumothorax, splinting, or large bronchial obstruction can cause side-to-side asymmetry. A long inspiratory time suggests upper airway or other extrathoracic obstruction; a prolonged expiratory time suggests intrathoracic obstruction, bronchospasm, or both. Discordant breathing efforts or the use of accessory muscles suggests respiratory muscle weakness or fatigue. Long inspiratory or expiratory pauses (e.g., Cheyne-Stokes or apneustic breathing) are caused by brainstem or metabolic abnormalities and depressant drugs.
   5. **Auscultate** the chest for presence of symmetric breath sounds, bronchospasm, rhonchi, or rales suggestive of secretions or pulmonary edema.
   6. **Pulse oximetry** aids in assessing the adequacy of oxygenation.
F. **The etiology of respiratory failure** usually is apparent. Readily reversible causes of respiratory failure may be addressed prior to intubation. Timely reversal of opioid- or benzodiazepine-induced respiratory

depression, residual pharmacologic neuromuscular blockade, pneumothorax, acute pulmonary edema, or mucous plugging of the airway may circumvent the need for intubation.

G. **Arterial blood gas** (ABG) tensions and pH may help to measure disease severity, document changes in condition over time, and assess the efficacy of interventions. The use of ABGs, however, should not substitute for clinical evaluation of the patient or delay needed interventions.

III. **Preparation for endotracheal intubation**

A. **A focused history and physical examination,** which may be obtained quickly while preparing the equipment needed for intubation (see later discussion), includes:

1. **Assessment of airway anatomy.** A receding mandible (micrognathia), small oropharynx, protruding, prominent upper incisors, and a short, muscular "bull" neck are associated with potentially difficult laryngoscopy and intubation. Temporomandibular joint or cervical spine immobility can make visualization of the glottis difficult. If these are recognized, alternative or additional intubation techniques may be employed (see section **V.A**).

2. **Allergies to Medications.**

3. **Assessment of aspiration risk,** including time since last gastric intake, trauma, recent vomiting, upper gastrointestinal (GI) bleeding, hemoptysis, bowel obstruction, history of esophageal reflux, morbid obesity, diabetes mellitus, and depressed mental status.

4. **Cardiovascular status** angina-ischemia, infarction, dysrhythmias, congestive heart failure, aneurysms, and hypertension.

5. **Neurologic status** increased intracranial pressure (ICP), ischemic symptoms, intracranial aneurysm and hemorrhage.

6. **Musculoskeletal status** neck and mandibular immobility or instability, neuromuscular disorders (especially recent cord denervation injuries, recent crush injuries, and burns).

7. **Coagulation status** platelet count, anticoagulation therapy, or coagulopathy (especially if a nasal intubation is anticipated).

8. **Past intubation problems** including history of periglottic or subglottic stenosis. The prior history is not entirely reliable because many other factors, such as airway edema, trauma, hemoptysis, and so on, may have intervened.

B. **Intubation method.** In an emergency, options are limited by the requirements for experience, expedience, and availability of specialized equipment. The most useful techniques are the following:

1. **Orotracheal intubation** is performed with direct laryngoscopy.

a. **Advantages** include ease and minimal equipment needs. It is the most familiar technique, allowing endotracheal tube (ETT) placement under direct vision.

b. **Disadvantages.** Adequate mandible and neck mobility are necessary to allow direct visualization. Topical, regional (block), or general anesthesia is often required.

2. **Nasotracheal intubation** may be performed as a blind procedure guided by breath sounds or under direct vision with laryngoscope or fiberoptic bronchoscope.

a. **Advantages.** Blind placement can be performed in a neutral head and neck position without general anesthesia or muscle paralysis. Nasotracheal intubation can be performed when the oral route is difficult or impossible (i.e., in a patient with limited mouth opening). A nasal tube also does not interfere with surgical repair of the mandible or oropharynx.

b. **Disadvantages.** It is more difficult to place the tube quickly. Spontaneous respiration must be present to guide the tube for blind placement. Placement by direct vision with the laryngoscope, with or without the Magill forceps, has the same disadvantages as the orotracheal intubation method. Tube diameter is limited by choanal size. Severe nasal hemorrhage, which can be life threatening, can occur. Transient bacteremia commonly occurs during the intubation. Once placed, a nasally placed tube tends to soften and kink in the nasopharynx, which can increase airway resistance and makes passage of a suction catheter more difficult. Nasal intubation is relatively contraindicated in the presence of suspected nasopharyngeal injury, nasal polyps, basilar skull fracture, epistaxis, coagulopathy, planned systemic anticoagulation or thrombolysis (i.e., the patient with an acute myocardial infarction), or immunocompromise. Sinusitis and otitis occur frequently with nasal intubation.

3. **Fiberoptic laryngoscopes** consist of glass fibers that are bound together to make a flexible unit (the insertion tube) for the transmission of light and images. Flexible fiberoptic laryngoscopy may be performed orally or nasally.

a. **Advantages.** They are very useful with distorted anatomy or in patients requiring maximal head-neck stability (i.e., unstable neck fractures).

b. **Disadvantages.** More skill is required than with other techniques. Fiberoptic intubation is not the technique of choice for emergency intubation of apneic patients. In patients with upper airway bleeding or vomiting, visualizing hypopharyngeal anatomy is difficult because of the limited capacity to clear secretions with the suction channel of the fiberscope.

4. **The laryngeal mask airway (LMA)** can be an important adjunct for establishing an emergency airway, especially in patients in whom mask ventilation is difficult or impossible and traditional endotracheal intubation has been unsuccessful.

   a. **Advantages.** The LMA is a fast and reliable method of establishing an airway when other methods have failed. Endotracheal intubation subsequently can be accomplished by placing an ETT through the lumen of the LMA with or without the assistance of a fiberoptic bronchoscope.

   b. **Disadvantages.** The LMA does not protect the airway against aspiration of gastric contents. The LMA may not be tolerated by an awake or agitated patient.

5. **Airway support devices** such as oral or nasopharyngeal airways do not prevent aspiration or guarantee continued airway patency. At best, they are temporary measures.

IV. **Techniques for airway management**

A. **Make thorough preparations for intubation prior to the initial attempt.** Time to establish the best possible intubating conditions usually is well spent. Equipment required for intubation is listed in Table 4-1.

   1. **Essential equipment** includes a Yankauer-tipped suction, a laryngoscope with an appropriate blade (usually Macintosh 3 or Miller 2 for adults and Miller 1 for small children), and an appropriately sized ETT with a stylet inserted and the cuff checked by briefly inflating it with approximately 10 ml of air.

   2. **Check that suction is available and functioning** in the form of a Yankauer or "tonsil tip" suction device.

   3. **The appropriate size** for the endotracheal tube depends on the patient's age, body habitus, and indication for intubation. A 7.0-mm endotracheal tube is a reasonable choice for most women and an 8.0-mm endotracheal tube for most men. Suggested pediatric tube sizes are listed in Table 4-2. The absence of air leaking past the ETT during positive-pressure ventilation with the cuff down indicates too tight a fit at the laryngeal or tracheal level. For an emergent intubation, a tube 0.5 mm smaller than usual will facilitate intubation.

   4. **Position the patient**

      a. In the supine position, the pharyngeal and laryngeal axes of the patients are offset, making a good view of the glottis extremely difficult during direct laryngoscopy (Fig. 4-1). Positioning the patient in the so-called "sniffing" position, with the occiput elevated by folded blankets and the head in extension, aligns the oral, pharyngeal, and

**Table 4-1. Suggested contents
of an emergency intubation kit**

Equipment	Drugs
Intravenous catheters (14–22 gauge)	Atropine
Laryngoscope blades:	*cis*-Atracurium
Macintosh 2, 3, 4; Miller 0, 1, 2, 3	
Endotracheal tubes (3–8 mm inner diameter)	Ephedrine
12-ml Syringes	Epinephrine
Magill forceps	Esmolol
Colorimetric end-tidal CO_2 detectors	Ethyl aminobenzoate (Hurricaine) spray
Nasal airways	Etomidate
Oral airways	Glycopyrrolate
Tape	Labetalol
Yankauer suction catheters	Lidocaine (1% and 4%)
Tube changers	Lidocaine ointment
Guide wires	Midazolam
Cotton-tipped swabs	Naloxone (Narcan)
Nasogastric tubes	Oxymetazoline (Afrin) spray
Jet ventilator	Pancuronium
	Phenylephrine
	Phenylephrine/lidocaine spray
	Propofol
	Propranolol
	Saline
	Succinylcholine
	Surgilube
	Viscous lidocaine

laryngeal axes so that the pathway from the lips to the glottis is nearly a straight line.

  b. Move the bed away from the wall and remove the headboard to allow access to the patient's head. If the headboard is fixed, or for patients in unusual locations or traction, move the patient diagonally in the bed to afford access to the patient and airway. Adjust the height of the bed so that the patient's head is at your mid-chest level.

  c. The trauma patient presents special challenges. All patients with multiple trauma, head, or facial injury must be presumed to have a cervical spine injury until excluded by a full evaluation. In such patients, excessive motion of the spine may produce or exacerbate a spinal cord injury. During airway manipulations, an assistant should stabilize the head and neck in a neutral position by maintaining in-line cervical traction. Note that the greatest cervical displacement appears to occur during bag and mask ventilation,

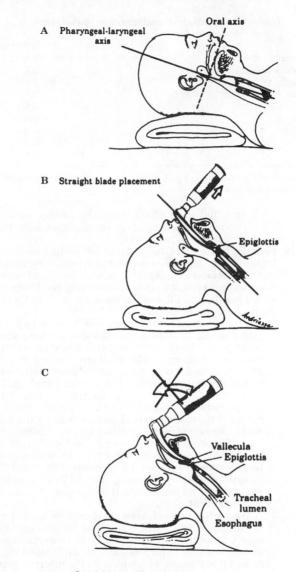

Fig. 4-1. A. The "sniffing position" aligns the oral, pharyngeal, and laryngeal axes for visualization of the glottis during laryngoscopy. B. The handle of the laryngoscope should be lifted in the direction of the long axis of the handle to view the glottis. C. The laryngoscope should not be used as a lever, to prevent damage to teeth or the alveolar ridge.

Table 4-2. Pediatric endotracheal tube sizes

Age	Size (mm)
Premature infant	2.5
Term infant	3.0
1–4 mo	3.5
4 mo–1 yr	4.0
1.5–2.0 yr	4.5
2.5–3.5 yr	5.0
4–6 yr	5.5
7–9 yr	6.0–7.0

Tube size should be adjusted to give airway leak pressures less than 25 cm H_2O; all tubes uncuffed.

and that orotracheal intubation causes no more cervical displacement or neurologic sequelae than nasotracheal intubation.

B. **Ventilation** should be assisted (or maintained) and 100% oxygen administered by mask and self-inflating bag (e.g., Ambu or Laerdahl) as soon as the airway is clear. In the obtunded patient, the airway can be opened with a gentle chin lift and the mask applied tightly over the patient's nose and mouth.

1. **An oropharyngeal airway (OPA)** may facilitate establishing a patent airway in the obtunded patient when proper head positioning and chin lift/jaw thrust alone are ineffective. The adult sizes are 80, 90, and 100 mm (Guedel sizes 3, 4, and 5, respectively), which reflect the length from the flange to the distal tip. The size can be estimated by measuring the OPA from the ear lobe to the corner of the patient's lips. The device is normally inserted backward along the hard palate and rotated into position as it approaches the posterior wall of the pharynx. Improperly placed, the OPA may obstruct the airway by pushing the tongue posteriorly or by pressing the epiglottis against the glottic opening. The OPA may induce vomiting or laryngospasm in an awake or semiconscious patient.

2. **A nasopharyngeal airway** should be considered as an adjunct to mask ventilation in patients with intact oropharyngeal reflexes or in those in whom mouth opening is impossible. The adult sizes range from 6.0 to 9.0 mm, which indicate the internal diameter of the tube. The tube should be well lubricated and gently inserted through the naris, along the floor of the nasal cavity (parallel to the hard palate), until the flange rests against the outer naris. **Coagulopathy** is a relative contraindication to its use, as is the presence of a basilar skull fracture (especially involving the ethmoid bone). Although the risk is less than with an OPA, vomiting and laryngospasm may still occur in some patients.

C. **An intravenous line** should be freely running and its adequacy demonstrated prior to laryngoscopy. In cases of cardiac arrest, in which the administration of sedatives and paralytic agents is unnecessary, intubation may precede the establishment of adequate intravenous access; the endotracheal tube can be used as an alternative route of drug administration (see Chapter 14).

D. **Monitoring during intubation** should include continuous electrocardiography (ECG), pulse oximetry, and frequent measurements of blood pressure.

E. **Orotracheal intubation**

1. **The laryngoscope** is composed of a handle, which usually contains batteries for the light source, and a laryngoscope blade, which usually contains a light bulb in the distal one-third of the blade. The Macintosh and Miller blades are most commonly used.

a. **The Macintosh blade** is curved, and the tip is inserted into the vallecula (the space between the base of the tongue and the pharyngeal surface of the epiglottis) (Fig. 4-2). Pressure against

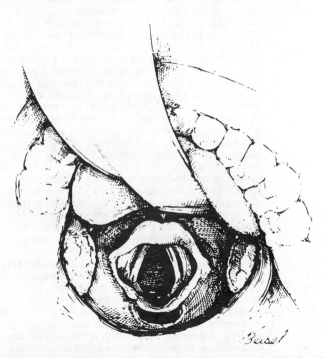

Fig. 4-2. View of the glottis by direct laryngoscopy with a Macintosh blade. Notice that the tip of the blade has been placed in the vallecula (the tip of the Miller blade is placed under the epiglottis, lifting it to view the glottis).

the hyoepiglottic ligament elevates the epiglottis to expose the larynx. The Macintosh blade provides a good view of the oro- and hypopharynx, thus allowing more room for ETT passage with diminished epiglottic trauma. Size ranges vary from No. 1 to No. 4, with most adults requiring a Macintosh No. 3 blade.

   b. The Miller blade is straight, and it is passed so that the tip lies beneath the laryngeal surface of the epiglottis. The epiglottis is then lifted to expose the vocal cords. The Miller blade allows better exposure of the glottic opening but provides a smaller passageway through the oro- and hypopharynx. Sizes range from No. 0 to No. 3, with most adults requiring a Miller No. 2 or No. 3 blade.

2. **A malleable stylet** inserted through the ETT (without extending past the tip) can be used to provide a 40- to 80-degree anterior bend 2 to 3 inches from the tip of the ETT ("hockey stick" configuration). This will allow passage of the tube along the posterior aspect of the epiglottis, facilitating intubation under difficult circumstances.

3. **Laryngoscopy.** Hold the laryngoscope in your left hand close to the junction of the blade and the handle. Open the patient's mouth with your right hand by applying a scissoring motion with your thumb and index finger on the patient's upper and lower premolars or gums. Insert the laryngoscope into the right side of the patient's mouth, taking care to avoid the teeth and pinching the lips between the blade and teeth. If using a Macintosh blade, insert it without resistance along the curve of the anterior pharynx. Once the blade is inserted, sweep the blade to the midline, utilizing the large flange of the blade to push the tongue out of the way. The epiglottis and vallecula will be visualized. Advance the blade into the vallecula and lift the handle in a direction parallel to its long axis to expose the vocal cords and laryngeal structures. If using a Miller blade, the tip of the blade is placed past the vallecula and is used to compress and elevate the epiglottis on lifting the handle. The laryngoscope blade should never be used as a lever with the upper teeth or maxilla as the fulcrum because damage to the maxillary incisors or gingiva may result.

4. **If the cords cannot be visualized**

   a. Secondary to vomitus or foreign material, suctioning or manual extraction is required.

   b. Due to an anterior position of the larynx, apply pressure to the thyroid or cricoid cartilages or change to a straight blade.

   c. Increase head flexion.

   d. Remove the laryngoscope and ventilate the patient with bag and mask. **Do not permit**

hypoxemia during a prolonged laryngoscopy in a patient who can be ventilated by mask.

5. **To insert the endotracheal tube,** hold it in your right hand as one would hold a pencil and advance it through the oral cavity from the right corner of the mouth and then through the vocal cords. Place the proximal end of the endotracheal tube cuff just below the vocal cords, remove the stylet, if used, and note the markings on the tube in relation to the patient's incisors or lips. In the average adult, the proper depth of insertion is approximately 21 cm for women, measured at the upper incisors, and 23 cm for men. Inflate the cuff just to the point of obtaining a seal in the presence of 20 to 30 cm H_2O positive airway pressure.

6. **Esophageal intubation remains one of the most common mistakes in airway management associated with a fatal outcome.** No single technique for verifying endotracheal placement is foolproof.

   a. **Verification of proper endotracheal tube position** usually includes the persistent detection of carbon dioxide (CO_2) in end-tidal samples of exhaled gas and auscultation over the stomach and both lung fields.

   b. **The measurement of the CO_2 concentration** in exhaled gas has become a standard for verifying tracheal placement of an endotracheal tube. In the absence of a capnometer, disposable colorimetric CO_2 detectors can be used to confirm the presence of carbon dioxide. This technique is not foolproof; carbon dioxide will not be present if pulmonary circulation is absent (i.e., in a dead patient or in the absence of adequate chest compressions during cardiopulmonary circulation).

   c. Small concentrations of carbon dioxide may be detected after an esophageal intubation, especially if bag and mask ventilation has insufflated previously exhaled air into the stomach. With an esophageal intubation, the amount of CO_2 detected in exhaled gas should decrease with repetitive breaths. With an endotracheal intubation, the end-tidal CO_2 concentration should be stable during repetitive exhalations. If it is not, additional confirmation is necessary.

7. **Physical signs and symptoms** of an endotracheal intubation include observation of the tube passing through the vocal cords, observation of chest and abdominal movement with ventilation, auscultation of breath sounds over both the right and left chest as well as the abdomen, palpation of the abdomen, and palpation of the trachea as the tube is passed. The exhaled tidal volume also may be measured

and is reduced with an esophageal intubation. Water vapor may be observed to fill the endotracheal tube on expiration and disappear on inspiration after proper placement. Other techniques for confirming endotracheal tube placement include fiberoptic endoscopy, the use of a self-inflating bulb (the esophageal detector) or an airflow whistle on the proximal end of the endotracheal tube, and chest radiography. Although any or all of these tests may be performed, one must acknowledge that any single test lacks adequate predictive value to reliably exclude an esophageal intubation.

8. **In the absence of direct visualization** of the endotracheal tube passing between the vocal cords, a very high index of suspicion of incorrect tube placement must be maintained for the first several minutes following intubation. Only after adequate oxygenation and ventilation appears certain (i.e., after several minutes) it is safe to leave the patient under the care of others.

9. **If the tube position is uncertain** despite these maneuvers, or the patient is deteriorating without a readily explained cause (e.g., pneumothorax), **remove the tube** and reinstitute bag and mask ventilation prior to another intubation attempt. If the patient regurgitates through an ETT placed in the esophagus, some advocate leaving the esophageal tube in place to act as a conduit for vomitus. This is acceptable only if the tube does not interfere with repeat visualization of the cords.

10. **If the tube has been advanced too far,** the right mainstem bronchus may be selectively intubated, resulting in absence of breath sounds over the left lung field and the right apex. Listening for breath sounds high in each axilla may decrease the chances of being misled by transmitted breath sounds from the opposite lung. Pull the tube back, with the cuff deflated, while ventilating and auscultating the left lung field until left-sided breath sounds are heard.

11. **When the ETT is in good position,** securely fasten it with tape, preferably to taut skin overlying bony structures. Note the depth of the tube at the incisors or gums in the patient's chart along with a description of the procedure.

12. **Obtain a chest radiograph** following intubation to confirm tube position and bilateral lung expansion. The distal end of the tube should rest within the mid-trachea, which is approximately 5 cm above the carina in the adult.

F. **Nasotracheal intubation**
   1. **Nasal mucosal vasoconstriction and anesthesia** are achieved with a solution of 0.25% phenylephrine–3% lidocaine or 2% lidocaine with 1:200,000 epinephrine using cotton-tipped swabs.

Even during general anesthesia, vasoconstriction with a topical solution such as oxymetazoline (Afrin) is advisable.

2. **Common endotracheal tube size** is 6.0 to 6.5 mm for women and 7.0 to 7.5 mm for men. Insertion to a depth of 26 cm in women, measured at the naris, and 28 cm in men usually results in proper position.

3. **General preparations** are as described for orotracheal intubation.

4. **Nasal passage** of the tube. Generously lubricate the nares and tube. Initially probe the nasopharynx with a well-lubricated nasal airway to establish which naris has greater patency. If both nares are patent, the right naris is preferred because the bevel of most ETTs, when introduced through the right naris, faces the flat nasal septum, reducing damage to the turbinates. Advance the tube in a direction that is perpendicular to the face and parallel to the hard palate. Inexperienced operators often tend to direct the tube cephalad, which tends to damage the turbinates. As the tube is passed into the nasopharynx, it may impact against the posterior nasopharyngeal wall. Retract the tube slightly, extend the patient's neck, and readvance. Forcible advancement of the tube at this point risks tearing the mucosa and creating a false passage. After passage through the naris into the pharynx, advance the tube through the glottic opening.

5. **Tracheal insertion** can be accomplished by several methods:

   a. **A Magill forceps** can be used to guide the tube into the trachea while direct laryngoscopy is performed. The laryngoscopic technique is the same as that used for oral intubation. The forceps is used to direct the tip of the endotracheal tube anteriorly and through the glottis. Grasp the tube with the forceps proximal to the endotracheal tube cuff. This reduces the chance of damaging the endotracheal tube cuff during insertion and permits the distal end of the tube to be inserted through the glottic opening. An assistant should advance the tube under the direction of the laryngoscopist.

   b. **Blind techniques** require a spontaneously breathing patient. While listening for breath sounds at the proximal end of the tube, advance the ETT during inspiration. A cough followed by a deep inhalation, condensate forming in the tube during exhalation, and loss of voice suggest tracheal entry. Sudden loss of breath sounds suggests passage into the esophagus, vallecula, or piriform recess:

      (1) **Extending the neck or providing cricoid pressure** may help direct the tube away from the esophagus.

(2) **Anterior flexion** directs the tube away from the vallecula.

(3) **Tilting the head** (not rotation) toward the side of the tube insertion and rotating the tube toward the midline directs the tube away from the piriform recess.

(4) **Inflating the cuff** of the ETT may help lift it off the posterior wall of the pharynx and direct the tube through the cords in a patient with an anterior larynx. In this instance, the cuff is deflated as the tube passes between the cords.

c. The **Endotrol** tracheal tube (Mallinckrodt, Inc., Glens Falls, NY) has a cord running up the concave side from the proximal end to the tip of the tube. Pulling on a ring attached to the proximal end of the cord flexes the tube anteriorly, which may direct the tip toward the glottis. It is sometimes useful for blind nasal intubation, especially when the neck cannot be manipulated.

d. **A fiberoptic bronchoscope** can be used to direct the ETT into the trachea (see later discussion).

G. **Fiberoptic intubation** can be used for both nasal and oral endotracheal intubation and should be considered as a first option in an anticipated difficult airway rather than as a last resort. Fiberoptic intubation should be considered for patients with known or suspected cervical spine pathology, head and neck tumors, morbid obesity, or a history of difficult ventilation or intubation. Facility with a fiberoptic bronchoscope should be obtained on mannequins and elective intubations prior to attempting emergency fiberoptic intubation.

1. **Standard equipment** for oral or nasal fiberoptic intubation includes a sterile fiberoptic scope with light source, an oral bite block or Ovassapian airway, topical anesthetics and vasoconstrictors, and suction.

2. **Technique.** To perform a fiberoptic intubation, place an endotracheal tube over a lubricated fiberoptic scope, attach suction tubing to the suction port, and grasp the control lever with one hand and use the other hand to advance and maneuver the insertion tube. An oral Ovassapian airway is helpful and well tolerated for oral laryngoscopy. Administration of an anticholinergic may help dry secretions that may obscure the view. After the administration of topical or general anesthesia, flex the tip of the insertion tube scope anteriorly and position it within the hypopharynx. Advance the scope toward the epiglottis. To avoid entering the piriform fossa, keep the insertion tube of the fiberoptic scope in the midline as it is advanced. If the view becomes impaired, retract the scope until the view clears, or remove it and clean the lens, and then reinsert it in the midline. As the tip of the scope slides beneath the epiglottis, the vocal cords will be seen. Advance the scope with

the tip in a neutral position until tracheal rings are noted. Then, stabilize the scope and advance the endotracheal tube over the insertion tube and into the trachea. Sometimes the tip of the endotracheal tube becomes caught against the arytenoids during advancement. If there is resistance, turning the endotracheal tube 90 degrees counterclockwise will allow passage through the vocal cords.

3. **Nasal intubation** can be performed similarly. Anesthetize and vasoconstrict the nasal mucosa, as discussed previously. With the ETT loaded on the scope, pass the scope under direct vision through the nasopharynx and into the trachea. Tongue retraction is usually not needed, but may occasionally be helpful. Maintain the scope's position in the trachea while an assistant passes the ETT over the scope and through the nose.

4. **An alternate technique** involves passage of the nasotracheal tube into the oropharynx as in blind nasal intubation. Lubricate the scope, pass it through the ETT, and guide the tube's passage through the cords and position within the trachea under direct vision.

H. **The LMA** has assumed an important role in airway management in the operating room and as an emergency airway adjunct in other locations.

1. LMAs come in both pediatric and adult sizes (Table 4-3). The most common adult sizes are No. 3 and No. 4.

2. The LMA may be easily placed with minimal experience (Fig. 4-3) and an airway established in most patients. The most common causes of failure include the folding of the LMA cuff back on itself in the oropharynx and the folding of the epiglottis down over the larynx by the tip of the LMA. These can be overcome by keeping the cuff pressed against the hard palate

Table 4-3. **Laryngeal mask airway sizes**

Patient Age/Size	LMA Size	Cuff Volume (ml)	ETT Size (ID)
Neonates/infants to 5 kg	1	4 ml	3.5 mm
Infants 5–10 kg	1.5	7 ml	4.0 mm
Infants/children 10–20 kg	2.0	10 ml	4.5 mm
Children 20–30 kg	2.5	14 ml	5.0 mm
Children 30 kg to small adults	3.0	20 ml	6.0 cuffed
Average adults	4.0	30 ml	6.0 cuffed
Large adults	5.0	40 ml	7.0 cuffed

LMA, laryngeal mask airway; ETT, endotracheal tube; ID, inner diameter.

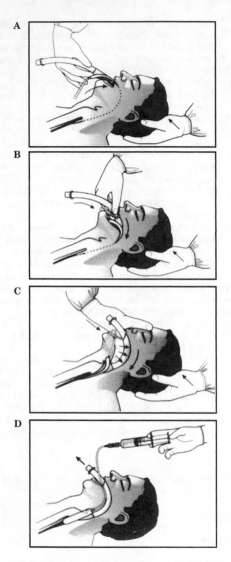

Fig. 4-3.   A. With the head extended and the neck flexed, carefully flatten the laryngeal mask airway (LMA) tip against the hard palate. B. The index finger pushes the LMA in a cranial direction following the contours of hard and soft palate. C. Maintaining pressure with the finger on the tube in the cranial direction, advance the mask until definite resistance is felt at the base of the hypopharynx. D. Inflation without holding the tube allows the mask to seat itself optimally. (From Brain AIJ, Denman WT, Goudsouzian N. *Laryngeal mask airway instruction manual.* San Diego, CA: Gensia, 1996. With permission).

during insertion and using the correct size of LMA. The LMA should not be placed in patients with intact upper airway reflexes.

3. The LMA does not protect against the possibility of gastric aspiration and is not suitable for long-term mechanical ventilation. An ETT may be placed through the lumen of the LMA, either blindly or with the aid of a fiberscope. The **Fasttrach LMA** is specially designed to permit subsequent endotracheal intubation through the LMA. The LMA also may be used as a temporary airway until a tracheostomy can be performed.

I. **Other specialized techniques for endotracheal intubation** include **retrograde wire-guided intubation,** use of a **light-wand stylet,** and **tactile intubation.**

J. **Cricothyrotomy** is performed as an emergency procedure when ventilation via mask or LMA is impossible and endotracheal intubation is unsuccessful.

1. **Technique.** Localize the cricothyroid notch (Fig. 4-4). Incise the skin and superficial subcutaneous

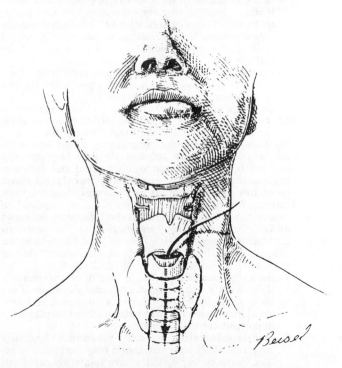

Fig. 4-4.   The cricothyroid membrane is the entry point of an artificial airway during cricothyrotomy.

tissues and pierce the cricothyroid membrane. Expand the membrane opening bluntly or with a scalpel and pass a small tracheostomy tube (No. 4 through No. 6) or a cut ETT (6.0 or 6.5 mm inner diameter [ID]) into the trachea.

2. **A needle cricothyrotomy** can be used to provide life-saving transtracheal jet oxygenation while other means are explored to secure the airway. A 14-gauge intravenous catheter attached to a syringe is used to puncture the cricothyroid membrane. Tracheal placement is confirmed by aspirating air from the catheter. The needle is removed and air again aspirated from the catheter. Firmly maintaining the catheter in position, attach it by tubing to a jet ventilator or, if this is unavailable, to a wall oxygen flowmeter opened to its maximal setting. By cyclically interrupting the flow of oxygen, gas flow is delivered at a 1:2 ratio of inspiration to expiration (1 second on; 2 seconds off). The chest should be observed to rise and fall with each jet.

3. **Complications.** The flow from the wall at 50 psi can exceed 500 ml/s. Inadequate time for expiration can result in high airway pressures and barotrauma, leading to poor venous return and pneumothorax. Other complications of this technique are subcutaneous and mediastinal emphysema, tracheal mucosal trauma, bleeding, and misplacement of the catheter.

K. **Emergency tracheostomy** entails significant time and risk of bleeding, which usually precludes its use as an emergency airway technique.

V. **Pharmacologic aids to intubation** include **neuromuscular blocking drugs (NMBDs),** sedatives, narcotics, and general and local anesthetics (see Chapter 6).

A. **NMBDs** induce complete respiratory arrest and abolish protective airway reflexes. Because laryngoscopy and intubation can be extremely painful and distressing, **patients who are chemically paralyzed must be either spontaneously or pharmacologically sedated.** When pharmacologic paralysis is required to secure the airway, patient survival depends on rapid and skillful laryngoscopy and intubation. Neuromuscular blocking drugs are slow in onset, and for that reason are quite dangerous for the patient who cannot tolerate even a few seconds of depressed ventilation.

1. **Succinylcholine** (1.0–1.5 mg/kg intravenously [IV]), with its rapid onset and brief duration of action, is the NMBD of choice for emergent endotracheal intubation in many patients. See Chapter 6 for important contraindications.

2. **Nondepolarizing muscle relaxants** typically have relatively slow onsets and long durations of action. Some newer NMBDs have relatively rapid onsets (e.g., rocuronium) and brief durations of action (e.g., mivacurium). These agents may also be useful

for intubation in selected patients. See Chapter 6 for additional details concerning the use of these agents.

3. **When rapid airway control is needed and succinylcholine is contraindicated,** large doses of *cis*-atracurium (>0.2 mg/kg IV) or **rocuronium** (1.2 mg/kg IV) can be used to decrease the onset of neuromuscular blockade from 1 to 1.5 minutes. Both drugs have relatively prolonged durations of action.

4. **All patients requiring emergent airway management are at risk for aspiration of gastric contents.** Thus, when paralysis is chosen, the intubation should follow a **"rapid sequence."** Administer the neuromuscular blocking agent immediately after rendering the patient rapidly unconscious with a drug such as propofol, etomidate, or ketamine. Apply cricoid pressure **(the Sellick maneuver)** with the onset of unconsciousness. To minimize gastric insufflation and the risk of regurgitation, under ideal circumstances, avoid positive-pressure ventilation until the airway is secured by an endotracheal tube. If the intubation is not immediately successful, positive-pressure ventilation may be administered via bag and mask with maintenance of cricoid pressure or via a laryngeal mask airway.

B. **Sedative-hypnotics, analgesics, and amnestics** are used during airway manipulation primarily to blunt autonomic responses and to obtund consciousness, pain, and recall (see Chapter 6).

C. **Benzodiazepines,** especially **midazolam** and **diazepam,** are frequently employed for IV sedation and amnesia during endotracheal intubation. Onset is rapid (60–90 seconds), and duration is brief (20–60 minutes) following single-dose administration (see Chapter 5). Cardiovascular side effects are minimal. For sedation, incremental doses of midazolam 0.5 to 1.0 mg IV or diazepam 2 mg IV may be repeated until the desired effect is achieved. The dose for induction of anesthesia 0.1 to 0.2 mg/kg IV for midazolam and 0.3 to 0.5 mg/kg for diazepam.

D. **Opioids. Fentanyl** and **morphine** are commonly employed for analgesia, sedation, and cough suppression during endotracheal intubation. Intravenous fentanyl has a rapid onset (1 minute) and in usual doses (50–500 μg) has a brief duration of action. Intravenous morphine (2–10 mg) has a longer peak onset time (5–10 minutes) and a longer duration of action (1–3 hours) (see Chapter 5 for additional details). The newer opioids **alfentanil, sufentanil,** and **remifentanil** offer more rapid onset times (30–60 seconds) and shorter durations with conventional doses than fentanyl, but are rarely indicated for endotracheal intubation.

E. β**-adrenergic blocking drugs** such as **esmolol** (10–20 mg IV in the adult) may blunt the cardiovascular response to laryngoscopy and intubation. Doses should be titrated to effect.

F. **Lidocaine** (1.0–1.5 mg/kg IV) may augment anesthesia and blunt the hemodynamic response to intubation. Lidocaine must be administered several minutes prior to laryngoscopy to be maximally effective.

G. **Oropharyngeal topical anesthesia** can be provided with viscous lidocaine, aerosol anesthetic sprays, or inhalation of aerosolized lidocaine. Topical anesthesia with unmetered aerosol sprays poses a risk of overdose and toxicity.

H. Glossopharyngeal **nerve blocks,** superior laryngeal nerve blocks, and translaryngeal ("transtracheal") blocks are occasionally useful in selected patients. In general, these blocks diminish the ability to guard against aspiration. Nerve blocks are relatively contraindicated in patients with coagulopathy.

VI. **Special intubating situations**

A. **A difficult intubation** is defined as the inability to place an ETT after three attempts by an experienced laryngoscopist. Unfortunately, no single clinical exam is able to predict accurately those patients who will have difficult laryngoscopies.

1. The **American Society of Anesthesiologists (ASA) Difficult Airway Algorithm** (Fig. 4-5) outlines protocols to be used when a difficult airway is encountered. Although the algorithm was designed initially to aid the decision-making process when a difficult airway is encountered in the operating room, it is also useful for emergent airway situations in other locations such as the intensive care unit.

   a. For a patient with a recognized difficult airway and spontaneous respirations, the choices for establishing a secure airway include awake direct laryngoscopy, fiberoptic laryngoscopy, blind nasal intubation, or an elective surgical airway.

   b. When intubation attempts have failed and spontaneous or assisted ventilation is absent, quick action is required to establish oxygenation and ventilation by other means. The ASA Difficult Airway Algorithm mentions three temporary means for delivering oxygen and eliminating carbon dioxide: the laryngeal mask airway, the Combitube, and transtracheal jet ventilation via cricothyrotomy.

2. **Backup personnel** should be called if a difficult intubation is anticipated (e.g., in patients with severe facial injuries, airway burns, or unstable cervical spine injuries).

3. The use of the LMA should be considered when mask ventilation is inadequate and endotracheal intubation has failed.

4. A **surgical airway** should be considered if intubation has failed and the airway cannot be maintained with bag and mask or LMA. A surgical cricothyrotomy should be performed by personnel with

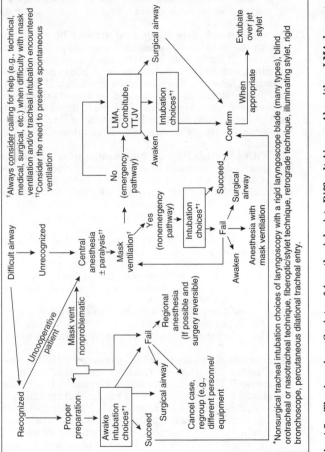

Fig. 4-5. The American Society of Anesthesiologists Difficult Airway Algorithm. LMA, laryngeal mask airway; TTJV, transtracheal jet ventilation.

*Nonsurgical tracheal intubation choices of laryngoscopy with a rigid laryngoscope blade (many types), blind orotracheal or nasotracheal technique, fiberoptic/stylet technique, retrograde technique, illuminating stylet, rigid bronchoscope, percutaneous dilational tracheal entry.

training in the technique. In the absence of a physician specifically trained in cricothyrotomy, a **needle or catheter percutaneous cricothyrotomy** should be considered when bag and mask or LMA ventilation and attempts at intubation have been unsuccessful. It should be noted that serious complications are common with this technique when performed under emergency conditions, including bleeding and subcutaneous emphysema that may make a subsequent surgical cricothyrotomy impossible.

B. **A full stomach, vomiting, and airway bleeding** increase the hazards of pulmonary aspiration during intubation. If intubation is anticipated, oral and gastric feedings should be discontinued for 8 hours prior to intubation; however, this is seldom practical. If present, the nasogastric (NG) tube should be placed on suction. The elective placement of an NG tube to drain the stomach prior to intubation may be effective for liquid gastric contents, but its presence is not a guarantee of an empty stomach.

1. **With obtundation or neuromuscular incompetence,** the presence of oral foreign matter requires immediate oral intubation with laryngoscopic visualization. Suction with a Yankauer tip should be available. During intubation, estimate severity of aspiration and determine the pH of the suctioned material.

2. **In the conscious patient,** awake intubation is generally preferred unless contraindicated by cardiovascular or neurologic problems. Topical local anesthesia makes the procedure more comfortable, although its use decreases protective airway reflexes, increasing the risk of aspiration.

3. **A "rapid-sequence" intubation** (see prior discussion) is performed if general anesthesia is required. The technique is similar to a rapid-sequence induction.

4. **Increased intracranial pressure (ICP)** (see Chapter 11). Pain or tracheal stimulation can increase ICP, even in comatose individuals. Intubation should be accomplished with minimal stimulation in any patient at risk for increased ICP. Adjuncts to consider include local anesthetic blocks, general anesthesia, including barbiturates, etomidate, or opioids, intravenous lidocaine, and the use of neuromuscular blockade to facilitate intubation.

C. **Myocardial ischemia or recent infarction** demands that heart rate and blood pressure be maintained within a narrow range. Hypertension (or hypotension) and tachycardia can exacerbate myocardial ischemia. Pharmacologic adjuncts to consider during endotracheal intubation include deep opioid anesthesia, local anesthetic blockade of airway reflexes, and the use of adequate β-adrenergic blockade. A pharmacologic method of treating hypotension (e.g., phenylephrine) and hypertension (e.g., nitroglycerine) should be immediately available.

D. **Neck injury** with potentially unstable cervical vertebrae presents the risk of precipitating or aggravating spinal cord damage during intubation. The head, neck, and thorax should be maintained in a neutral position **(inline stabilization).** Oral intubation is preferred during emergent situations. During intubation, a second individual should provide light in-line traction to maintain the head and neck in a neutral position. Flexion and anterior head motion pose the greatest risks for cord injury. Extension is less of a hazard but should be minimized. If the intubation is difficult or the pharyngeal and vocal cord anatomy is not easily visualized, an awake fiberoptic intubation (oral or nasal), intubation through an LMA (with or without fiberoptic assistance), or proceeding to cricothyrotomy in more emergent situations is prudent.

E. **Oropharyngeal and facial trauma.** The nasal route is relatively contraindicated if there is a possibility of cranial vault disruption, because of the potential for tubes and catheters to penetrate the brain. Once the airway is secured, a fiberoptic nasal intubation can be performed electively, if needed, to facilitate operative repair. In the case of a massively disrupted face, a cricothyrotomy or tracheostomy may be preferable.

F. **Emergency neonatal and pediatric intubations** (see Chapter 39). Children generally are less cooperative than adults, making certain techniques (e.g., awake fiberoptic intubation) difficult. Hypoxemia occurs more rapidly during apnea in children than in adults. In addition, the tracheal cartilage in prepubertal individuals is not fully developed, predisposing them to tracheal malacia and stenosis. Cuffed ETTs are usually avoided because the cuff material requires a smaller tube size in already narrow airways and because of the risk of tracheal damage from mucosal ischemia due to compression by the inflated cuff. Tubes placed in pediatric patients should have a leak of air regurgitating back around the tube into the pharynx with positive-pressure ventilation. A leak at less than 25 cm H_2O of positive airway pressure is optimal. A greater leak makes ventilation more difficult, and a lesser leak is likely to cause tracheal edema on extubation and to increase the risk of tracheal damage.

G. **Immunocompromised patients** require intubation with a technique that will minimize tracheal contamination. Aspiration is disastrous in this population, and nasal intubation should be avoided because of the risks of sinusitis and bacteremia. Perform intubation under direct vision, with care taken to keep the ETT as sterile as possible prior to passage through the cords.

VII. **Endotracheal and tracheostomy tubes**
A. **Tube materials**

1. **Polyvinyl chloride (PVC)** tubes are disposable, flexible, and transparent; they are the current standard tube. Siliconized PVC tracheostomy tubes are pliable and more easily conform to a patient's airway.

2. **Silicone** tubes are softer than PVC but are more likely to kink.

3. **Armored or anode** tubes have metal-coil–reinforced bodies with a rubber, silicone, or PVC coating. They are less likely to kink than PVC but are more flexible, usually requiring a stylet for placement.

B. **Cuff designs**

1. **High-pressure, low-compliance** cuffs have a small surface area of contact with the trachea and can produce tracheal damage more easily than low-pressure cuffs. High-pressure cuffs can be found on certain specialty tubes. Some low-pressure cuffs (such as those found on double-lumen endobronchial tubes) may generate high pressures if overinflated.

2. **Low-pressure, high-compliance** cuffs are found on standard disposable ETTs. They present a high surface area for tracheal contact at relatively low cuff pressures, preserving tracheal mucosal blood flow.

3. **Foam-filled** cuffs, as seen on **Kamen-Wilkinson** tubes or **Bivona** tubes, are sometimes used in patients with tracheal dilatation or in patients who require high cuff pressures to attain a seal (Fig. 4-6). The cuff is deflated for insertion, then left open to atmosphere and allowed to inflate passively within the trachea. A minimal cuff volume is required to ensure acceptable lateral wall pressures. Air and moisture are periodically aspirated from the cuff. If the cuff requires additional air to create a seal, the tube takes on the characteristics of the standard high-compliance tube.

4. **Lanz** cuffs have a balloon-within-a-shield pilot valve system to buffer the cuff pressure. The pilot system has a thick plastic guard surrounding a highly compliant inner balloon that distends at pressures above 28 cm H_2O, relieving high tracheal cuff pressure. The tracheal cuff is similar to the standard low-pressure, high-compliance cuffs found on other disposable tubes. Creating a seal at high airway pressures can be difficult.

C. **Tracheostomy tube designs.** Many tracheostomy tubes are available (see Fig. 4-7). Representative tubes include the following:

1. **Portex DIC (disposable inner cannula).** The body of the DIC tube has a uniform radius of curvature, designed to accept a thin-walled, nonpliable inner cannula. With the inner cannula inserted, the inner diameter of the tube is reduced by 1 mm. This tube is available in fenestrated and nonfenestrated, cuffed and uncuffed versions.

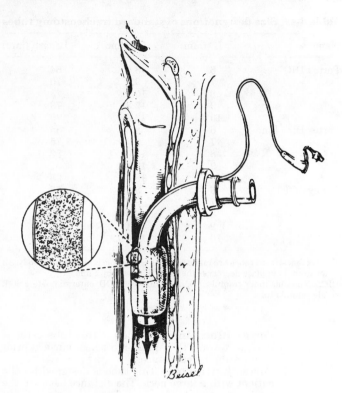

Fig. 4-6. Kamen-Wilkinson tube (Fome-Cuf, Bivona Medical Technologies, Gary, IN).

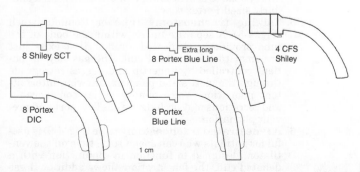

Fig. 4-7. Tracheostomy tube designs.

Table 4-4. Size designations of standard tracheostomy tubes

Name	ID (mm)	OD (mm)	Length (mm)
Portex DIC[a]	6	8.2	64
	7	9.6	70
	8	10.9	73
	9	12.3	79
	10	13.7	79
Portex Blue Line	6	8.3	55
	7	9.7	75
	8	11.0	82
	9	12.4	87
	10	13.8	98
Shiley SCT	6	8.3	67
	7	9.6	80
	8	10.9	89
	9	12.1	99
	10	13.3	105

[a]Portex fenestrated tubes are made from the disposable inner cannula body. An inner cannula in place decreases the inner diameter by 1 mm.
DIC, disposable inner cannula; ID, inner diameter; OD, outer diameter; SCT, single-cannula tube.

2. **Portex Blue Line.** The body of this tube extends straight toward the anterior tracheal surface prior to initiating its curvature.
3. **Portex Extra Long.** This tube is designed for the patient with a large neck. The distance between the tracheostomy tube flange and the initiation of curvature is longer than in the standard tracheostomy tube.
4. **Shiley SCT (single-cannula tube).** This tube is longer in vertical dimension (see Table 4-4) and has a larger-volume cuff than a Portex tube of equivalent internal diameter. The larger cuff usually allows the Shiley tube to seal at lower cuff pressure than a similarly sized Portex tube.
5. **Talking tracheostomy tube** or Communitrach (Fig. 4-8). A separate lumen within the body of the tube provides a dedicated air flow that exits just proximal to the tracheal cuff. The gas flow is patient controlled by fingertip and passes retrograde through the glottis and pharynx, allowing intermittent phonation. Voice quality varies considerably, and secretions may occlude the gas flow port and prevent phonation.
6. **A fenestrated tracheostomy tube** (Fig. 4-9) is useful for patients who can spend some time off the ventilator. Designed to function in conjunction with a deflated cuff, the fenestration allows additional gas flow through the lumen of the tube to the pharynx. In conjunction with a one-way speaking valve (such

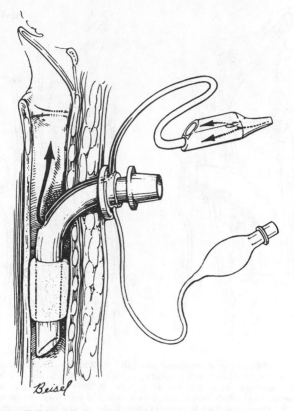

Fig. 4-8. Talking tracheostomy tube.

as the Passy-Muir valve), excellent phonation is possible. A removable inner cannula blocks this fenestration and is used when the patient is receiving mechanical ventilation. An uncuffed fenestrated tube can be used for selected patients who do not require the tracheostomy to facilitate mechanical ventilation or protect the airway. Occlusion of the fenestration with secretions or by tissue of the tracheal wall due to tube malposition is a common problem. The size and pattern of fenestrations vary among tubes (Fig. 4-10).

7. **Sizes** of tracheostomy tubes vary depending on the manufacturer and style of tube (Table 4-4).

VIII. **Maintenance of endotracheal and tracheostomy tubes**
A. **General care**
1. **Suctioning.** The pharynx and trachea of intubated patients may require suctioning to clear secretions.
2. **Cuff pressures** should be kept less than 30 cm H_2O and monitored routinely. Increased occlusion

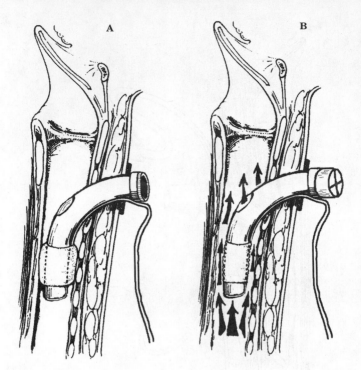

Fig. 4-9. Fenestrated tracheostomy tube. A. With the cuff inflated and the long, hollow inner cannula in place, function is similar to that of the standard cuffed tracheostomy tube. B. With the inner cannula removed, the cuff deflated, and the occluder or one way speaking valve in place, gas flow is routed through the glottis and pharynx.

pressures may suggest the need for a larger tube or a similarly sized tube with a larger cuff.

3. **Securing the tube.** Tape or a tube holder should be reapplied as needed. For an oral tube, avoid excessive pressure on the lips. Patients with **nasotracheal tubes** should be periodically assessed for sinusitis, otitis media, and necrosis of the nares.

B. **Common endotracheal and tracheostomy tube problems**

1. **Cuff leaks** are usually evident as audible pharyngeal gas flow diverted anteriorly around the cuff during positive-pressure ventilation. A large leak may prompt urgent reintubation with a new tube. Usually, however, addition of a small volume of air to the cuff recreates a seal. Causes of persistent cuff leaks include:

a. **Supraglottic cuff position.** A cuff that holds air but does not seal the airway may be within or above the vocal cords. Cuff position can be evaluated by chest radiograph or laryngoscopic

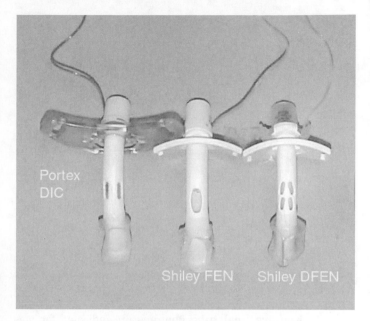

Fig. 4-10. Fenestration patterns.

examination. Deflate the cuff; advance the tube, and reconfirm intratracheal placement.

    b. Damaged cuff system. A cuff unable to hold any air is likely to require immediate replacement. Slow cuff leaks allow time for further evaluation. Small leaks can occur from the pilot valve or balloon, the cuff, or the cuff–tube interface.

    c. Tracheal dilation as a cause of persistent cuff leaks often can be diagnosed with the aid of a chest radiograph. The tissue–air interface at an inflated cuff is visible radiographically as a widened trachea. A larger tube or one with a larger cuff volume may be required. Alternatively, a foam cuff tube (e.g., Kamen-Wilkinson or Bivona) may be tried.

  2. Airway obstruction is an emergency forewarned by the high-pressure-limit alarm during volume ventilation or by low-volume alarms during pressure ventilation. Quickly evaluate the airway. A kinked tube may allow manual ventilation, but not allow a suction catheter to pass. Manipulation of the head and neck may temporarily increase flow through a kinked tube. Inability to manually ventilate requires immediate tube replacement.

  3. Malpositioned tracheostomy tubes (Fig. 4-11) can damage the tracheal mucosa, impede airflow, or predispose a patient to inadvertent decannulation.

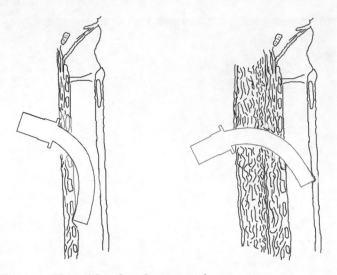

Fig. 4-11.   Malpositioned tracheostomy tubes.

C. **Endotracheal tube changes** are indicated for mechanical tube failure or changing tube size or position (e.g., nasal to oral). Common techniques for tube changes include the following:

1. **Direct laryngoscopy**

2. **Bronchoscopic change.** With a new ETT loaded onto the fiberscope, the fiberscope is advanced to the cords. After the pharynx and supperglottic areas are suctioned, an assistant deflates the cuff on the indwelling ETT and the fiberscope is advanced through the cords and into the trachea. While the endoscopist maintains intratracheal visualization of the fiberscope position, the assistant slowly withdraws the old ETT, and the new ETT is advanced over the fiberscope into the trachea. This technique is particularly useful in patients in whom direct laryngoscopy is contraindicated or technically difficult.

3. **Specially designed long, malleable stylets (tube changers)** can be used to perform tube changes blindly or under direct vision. Pass the stylet through the existing ETT and remove the tube, being careful not to dislodge the stylet. Then slip a new ETT into the trachea over the stylet. Many tube changers have a lumen for oxygen administration or, if necessary, jet ventilation.

4. **When changing nasal tubes,** change to an oral tube as an intermediate step rather than attempt placement of bilateral nasal tubes.

IX. **Tracheostomy** may be performed as an open surgical procedure or as a percutaneous, bedside procedure. The

bedside percutaneous procedure is a safe procedure that is gaining in popularity because it reduces the risk of transporting critically ill patients to the operating room, the cost of operating room resources, and the delay in scheduling encountered with today's busy operating room schedules.

A. **Advantages** of tracheostomy over translaryngeal intubation include the following:
   1. Improved patient comfort.
   2. Decreased risk of laryngeal dysfunction and/or damage.
   3. Improved oral hygiene.
   4. Improved ability to communicate, including the ability to phonate when the cuff can be deflated.
B. **Disadvantages** of tracheostomy include the following:
   1. Possibility of tracheal stenosis at the stoma site.
   2. Stomal infection, which may secondarily infect nearby open skin areas and vascular catheters.
   3. Erosion of neighboring vascular tissue can lead to hemorrhage.
   4. Operative complications.
   5. Scarring and granulation tissue at the stoma site.
C. **Deciding the appropriate time** for conversion from ETT to tracheostomy is a controversial issue. It is generally accepted, but not proved, that incidence and severity of glottic damage are related to duration of intubation. In clinical practice, elective tracheostomy is considered after 3 weeks of translaryngeal intubation.
D. **Replacement of tracheostomy tubes**
   1. **Changing a fresh tracheostomy tube.** The tract for the tracheostomy tube can be extremely difficult to cannulate in the initial postoperative period. If a tracheostomy change is required before the stoma is 7 to 10 days old, the tube should be changed over a malleable stylet and provisions for immediate orotracheal intubation should be immediately available in case the tract is lost. It is preferable for the surgeon who performed the tracheostomy to be present because exploration of the tract may be necessary.
   2. **Tracheostomy tube changes.** Proper cleanliness, function, and mobility of the appliance should be assessed regularly and the appliance changed as needed.
      a. Be prepared to perform an orotracheal intubation, if necessary.
      b. Administer 100% oxygen.
      c. Clean the tracheostomy site and suction the patient.
      d. Check the new tube and test for cuff integrity. Insert the obturator through the lumen of the new tube to provide a smooth surface at the tip of the tracheostomy tube.
      e. Deflate the cuff and remove the existing tube. Expect some resistance to decannulation as the

deflated cuff is pulled past the anterior tracheal wall.

f. Visualize the stoma tract and insert the new tube. Inflate the cuff and be prepared to manually ventilate with 100% oxygen.

g. Evaluate for proper intratracheal placement, as for any endotracheal tube (see section **IV.E**).

E. **Airway bleeding.** Suctioning of blood from the airway requires prompt evaluation.

1. Commonly, this bleeding represents **mucosal erosion** from the repeated trauma of suctioning. Fiberoptic bronchoscopy is the most direct means of assessment. If the source is not obvious, pull the tube back with the bronchoscope in place to view the trachea underlying the cuff. If, after examination, the etiology of the persistent bleeding is in doubt, obtain a repeat examination by an otorhinolaryngologist. If bleeding is not significant, a period of healing without irritation is warranted. Alternatively, a tracheostomy tube or ETT can be placed distal to the area of erosion until healing occurs.

2. With tracheostomy, the risk of erosion into the mediastinal blood vessels exists. If this occurs, the patient can **exsanguinate.** If bleeding continues and is of sufficient quantity, there is a risk of clotting within the ETT and airway obstruction. Emergent orotracheal intubation and surgical exploration may be necessary.

F. **Decannulation** is considered once indications for airway support are no longer present. The patient should have adequate oxygenation and ventilation and be able to clear secretions and protect the lungs from aspiration.

1. **Vocal cord dysfunction and aspiration** can occur due to prolonged intubation. Such dysfunction may spontaneously resolve within several weeks following extubation.

a. **Continued presence of a tracheostomy tube** can increase the chance of aspiration by mechanical interference with coordinated swallowing. Decreasing this potential problem may involve inserting a smaller uncuffed tracheostomy tube (such as a No. 4 Shiley) to decrease the mechanical stresses due to movement of the tracheostomy tube during swallowing. The smaller tube will maintain stomal patency and allow suctioning of the airway.

b. **A nasogastric tube** can contribute to decreased coordination during swallowing.

c. **Protecting such patients from aspiration** may involve:

(1) **Tracheostomy.** A cuffed tracheostomy tube can be used to prevent gross aspiration until cord function improves.

(2) **Extubation,** prohibiting oral intake, with enteral or parenteral feeding until the patient is no longer at risk. An enteral feeding tube should be located in the duodenum to decrease the chance of reflux and aspiration.

d. **Consultation with a speech and swallowing therapist** is appropriate. Coordination of swallowing can be assessed by fiberoptic visualization or, radiographically, by a modified barium swallow. Patient education and training can reduce the risks of aspiration and improve swallowing.

2. The following airway appliances may be considered as the patient progresses toward decannulation:

a. **Fenestrated tracheostomy tubes** allow breathing either through the tracheostomy or through the natural airway. The patient can speak normally when the inner cannula is removed, the cuff is down, and the opening of the tube is either occluded or fitted with a one-way speaking valve. A fenestrated tube provides no protection against aspiration when configured in this manner.

b. **A small cuffless tracheostomy tube,** such as the No. 4 Shiley CFS (Fig. 4-7), is often the last airway appliance used prior to decannulation. Most often, it serves as a safety device and as a conduit for suction. Resistance to airflow around such tubes, even when the tube is capped, is seldom clinically significant.

SELECTED REFERENCES

Benumof JL. The LMA and the ASA Difficult Airway Algorithm. *Anesthesiology* 1996;84:686–689.

Benumof JL, Dagg R, Benumof R. Critical hemoglobin desaturation will occur before return to an unparalyzed state following 1 mg/kg intravenous succinylcholine. *Anesthesiology* 1997;87:979–982.

Benumof JL, Scheller MS. The importance of transtracheal jet ventilation in the management of the difficult airway. *Anesthesiology* 1989;71:769–778.

Bishop MJ, Weymuller EA Jr, Fink BR. Laryngeal effects of prolonged intubation. *Anesth Analg* 1984;63:335–342.

Brain AIJ, Denman WT, Goudsouzian N. *Laryngeal mask airway instruction manual.* San Diego, CA: Gensia, 1996:21–25.

Cousins MJ, Bridenbaugh PO. *Neural blockade in clinical anesthesia and management of pain,* 2nd ed. Philadelphia: Lippincott, 1988:533–576.

Deutschman CS, Wilton P, Sinow J, et al. Paranasal sinusitis associated with nasotracheal intubation: a frequently unrecognized and treatable source of sepsis. *Crit Care Med* 1986;14:111–114.

Dorsch JA, Dorsch SE. Endotracheal tubes. In: *Understanding anesthesia equipment,* 3rd ed. Baltimore: Williams & Wilkins, 1994:439–541.

El-Gaqnzouri AR, McCarthy RJ, Tuman KJ, et al. Preoperative airway assessment: predictive value of a multivariate risk index. *Anesth Analg* 1996;82:1197–1204.

Eubanks DH, Bone RC. *Airway management, comprehensive respiratory care: a learning system,* 2nd ed. St. Louis, IL: Mosby, 1990.

Fluck RR Jr, Hess DR, Branson RD. Airway and suction equipment. In: Branson RD, Hess DR, Chatburn RL, eds. *Respiratory care equipment.* Philadelphia: Lippincott, 1995:116–144.

Hauswald M, Sklar DP, Tandberg D, et al. Cervical spine movement during airway management: cinefluoroscopic appraisal in human cadavers. *Am J Emerg Med* 1991;9:535–538.

Hurford WE. Nasotracheal intubation. *Respir Care* 1999;44:643–649.

Hurford WE. Orotracheal intubation outside the operating room: anatomic considerations and techniques. *Respir Care* 1999;44:615–629.

McKourt KC, Salomela L, Miraklew RK, et al. Comparison of rocuronium and suxamethonium for use during rapid induction of anaesthesia. *Anaesthesia* 1998;53:867–871.

Mehta S, Mickiewicz M. Pressure in large volume, low pressure cuffs: its significance, measurement, and regulation. *Intensive Care* 1986;31:199–201.

Ovassapian A, Randel GI. The role of the fiberscope in the critically ill patient. *Crit Care Clin* 1995;11:29–51.

Roberts JT. *Clinical management of the airway.* Philadelphia: Saunders, 1994.

Velmahos GC, Gomez H, Boicey CM, et al. Bedside percutaneous tracheostomy: prospective evaluation of the current technique in 100 patients. *World J Surg* 2000;24:1109–1115.

Weis FR, Hatton MN. Intubation by use of the light wand: experience in 253 patients. *J Oral Maxillofac Surg* 1989;47:577–580.

Whited RE. A prospective study of laryngotracheal sequelae in long term intubation. *Laryngoscope* 1984;94:367–377.

Wilson DJ. Airway appliances and management. In: Kacmarek RM, Stoller JK, eds. *Current respiratory care.* Philadelphia: BC Decker, 1988:80–89.

Wilson RS. Tracheostomy and tracheal reconstruction. In: Kaplan JA, ed. *Thoracic anesthesia.* New York: Churchill Livingstone, 1991:441–461.

5

Mechanical Ventilation

Fiona K. Gibbons and Dean R. Hess

I. **Mechanical ventilation** provides artificial support of gas exchange.
   A. **Indications:**
      1. **Hypoventilation**
         a. **Arterial pH** rather than arterial partial pressure of carbon dioxide ($PaCO_2$) should be evaluated for treatment of hypoventilation. Chronic compensated hypercapnia usually is a stable condition that does not require mechanical ventilatory support.
         b. **Hypoventilation resulting in an arterial pH of less than 7.30** often is considered an indication for mechanical ventilation, but patient fatigue and associated morbidity must be considered and may prompt initiation of mechanical ventilation at a higher or lower pH.
      2. **Hypoxemia**
         a. **Supplemental oxygen** should be administered to all hypoxemic patients, regardless of diagnosis (e.g., appropriate oxygen therapy should not be withheld from hypercapneic patients with chronic obstructive pulmonary disease [COPD]).
         b. Patients with **hypoxemic respiratory failure** due to atelectasis and/or pulmonary edema may benefit from **continuous positive airway pressure (CPAP)** administered by face mask.
         c. **Endotracheal intubation and mechanical ventilation** should be considered for severe hypoxemia (arterial oxygen saturation by pulse oximetry [SpO_2] <90% at a fraction of inspired oxygen [FiO_2] equal to 1.0) unresponsive to more conservative measures.
      3. **Respiratory fatigue**
         a. **Excessive work of breathing** (e.g., tachypnea, dyspnea, use of accessory muscles, nasal flaring, diaphoresis, tachycardia) may be an indication for mechanical ventilation before abnormalities of gas exchange occur.
      4. **Airway protection**
         a. Mechanical ventilation may be initiated in patients who require endotracheal intubation for airway protection, even in the absence of respiratory abnormalities (e.g., decreased mental status or increased aspiration risk).
         b. **The presence of an artificial airway** is not an absolute indication for mechanical ventilation.

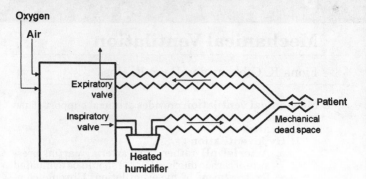

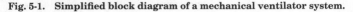

Fig. 5-1. Simplified block diagram of a mechanical ventilator system.

For example, many long-term tracheostomy patients do not require mechanical ventilation.

B. Goals of mechanical ventilation
   1. Provide adequate oxygenation.
   2. Provide adequate alveolar ventilation (Pa_{CO_2}).
   3. Promote patient–ventilator synchrony.
   4. Apply positive end-expiratory pressure (PEEP) to maintain alveolar recruitment.
   5. Avoid alveolar overdistension.
   6. Avoid auto-PEEP.
   7. Use the lowest possible Fi_{O_2}.

II. The ventilator system (Fig. 5-1)
   A. The ventilator is powered by gas pressure and electricity. Gas pressure provides the energy required to inflate the lungs.
      1. Gas flow is controlled by **inspiratory and expiratory valves.** The electronics (microprocessor) of the ventilator controls these valves so that gas flow is determined per the ventilator settings.
         a. An inspiratory valve controls flow and/or pressure during the inspiratory phase. The expiratory valve is closed during the inspiratory phase.
         b. The expiratory valve controls PEEP. The inspiratory valve is closed during the expiratory phase.
   B. The ventilator circuit delivers flow between the ventilator and the patient.
      1. Due to gas compression and the elasticity of the circuit, part of the gas volume delivered from the ventilator is not received by the patient. This **compression volume** is typically about 3 to 4 ml/cm H_2O. Some ventilators compensate for this; others do not.
      2. The volume of the circuit through which the patient rebreathes is **mechanical dead space.** Mechanical dead space should be less than 50 ml. When low tidal volumes are used (e.g., lung-protective ventilation strategies), the mechanical dead space should be as low as practically possible.

C. Gas conditioning
  1. **Filters** may be placed in the inspiratory and expiratory limbs of the circuit.
  2. **The inspired gas** is actively or passively humidified.
     a. **Active humidifiers** pass the inspired gas over a heated water chamber for humidification. Some active humidifiers are used with a **heated circuit** to decrease condensate within the circuit.
     b. **Passive humidifiers** (artificial noses or heat and moisture exchangers) are inserted between the ventilator circuit and the patient. They trap heat and humidity in the exhaled gas and return that on the subsequent inspiration. Passive humidification is satisfactory for many patients, but it is less effective than active humidification, increases the resistance to inspiration and expiration, and increases mechanical dead space.
     c. The presence of **water droplets** in the inspiratory circuit near the patient (or in the proximal endotracheal tube if a passive humidifier is used) suggests that the inspired gas is adequately humidified.

D. Delivery of inhaled medications during mechanical ventilation
  1. Inhaled medications can be delivered by **metered-dose inhaler** or **nebulizer** during mechanical ventilation. Dry-powder inhalers cannot be adapted to the ventilator circuit.
  2. A variety of factors influence aerosol delivery during mechanical ventilation (Fig. 5-2).

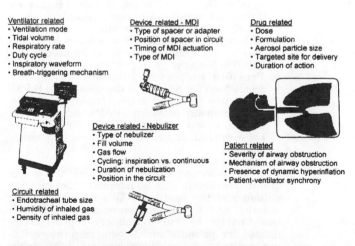

Ventilator related
• Ventilation mode
• Tidal volume
• Respiratory rate
• Duty cycle
• Inspiratory waveform
• Breath-triggering mechanism

Device related - MDI
• Type of spacer or adapter
• Position of spacer in circuit
• Timing of MDI actuation
• Type of MDI

Drug related
• Dose
• Formulation
• Aerosol particle size
• Targeted site for delivery
• Duration of action

Device related - Nebulizer
• Type of nebulizer
• Fill volume
• Gas flow
• Cycling: inspiration vs. continuous
• Duration of nebulization
• Position in the circuit

Patient related
• Severity of airway obstruction
• Mechanism of airway obstruction
• Presence of dynamic hyperinflation
• Patient-ventilator synchrony

Circuit related
• Endotracheal tube size
• Humidity of inhaled gas
• Density of inhaled gas

Fig. 5-2. **Factors affecting aerosol delivery during mechanical ventilation.** MDI, metered-dose inhaler. (From Dhand R. Basic techniques for aerosol delivery during mechanical ventilation. *Respir Care* 2004;49:611–622. With permission.)

3. With careful attention to technique, either inhalers or nebulizers can be used effectively during mechanical ventilation.

III. Classification of mechanical ventilation

A. Negative- versus positive-pressure ventilation:

1. The **iron lung** and **chest cuirass** create negative pressure around the thorax during the inspiratory phase. Although useful for some patients with neuromuscular disease requiring long-term ventilation, these devices are almost never used in the intensive care unit (ICU).

2. **Positive-pressure ventilation** applies pressure to the airway during the inspiratory phase. Positive-pressure mechanical ventilation is used almost exclusively in the ICU.

3. **Exhalation** occurs passively with both positive-pressure ventilation and negative-pressure ventilation.

B. Invasive versus noninvasive ventilation

1. **Invasive ventilation** is delivered through an endotracheal tube (orotracheal or nasotracheal) or a tracheostomy tube.

2. Although mechanical ventilation through an artificial airway remains the standard in the most acutely ill patients, **noninvasive positive-pressure ventilation (NPPV)** can be used successfully in some patients with rapidly reversible conditions, such as an exacerbation of COPD. There are many patients, however, in whom NPPV is not appropriate (Table 5-1).

   a. Noninvasive ventilation can be applied with a nasal or an oronasal mask. Oronasal masks are preferred in acutely ill dyspneic patients, in whom mouth leak is often problematic.

   b. Although bilevel or BiPAP ventilators are available for NPPV, any ventilator can be used to provide this therapy.

   c. **Pressure support ventilation** is most commonly used for NPPV. For the bilevel and BiPAP ventilators, this is achieved by setting inspiratory positive airway pressure (**IPAP**) and expiratory positive airway pressure (**EPAP**). The difference between IPAP and EPAP is the level of pressure support.

C. Full versus partial ventilation

1. **Full ventilatory support** provides the entire minute ventilation with no interaction between the patient and the ventilator. This usually requires sedation and sometimes neuromuscular blockade (see Chapter 6). Full ventilatory support is indicated for patients with severe respiratory failure, patients who are hemodynamically unstable, patients with complex acute injuries while they are being stabilized, and all patients receiving paralysis.

**Table 5-1. Patient selection for
noninvasive positive-pressure ventilation**

Diagnosis

- COPD exacerbation: high-level evidence supports NPPV use
- Hypoxemic respiratory failure: NPPV may be useful in patients developing respiratory failure who are immunocompromised, post solid-organ transplantation, and post lung resection surgery
- Post extubation: NPPV may be useful to allow early extubation in selected patients, but is not useful in patients who develop respiratory failure following planned extubation.
- Acute cardiogenic pulmonary edema: either CPAP or NPPV may be useful, NPPV may be more useful if the patient is hypercarbic

Indications

- Respiratory distress with dyspnea, use of accessory muscles, abdominal paradox
- pH <7.35 with $Paco_2$ >45 mm Hg
- Respiratory rate >25/min

Relative contraindications

- Respiratory arrest
- Unstable cardiovascular status
- Uncooperative patient
- Facial, esophageal, or gastric surgery
- Craniofacial trauma or burns
- High aspiration risk
- Unable to protect airway
- Anatomic lesion of upper airway
- Extreme anxiety
- Massive obesity
- Copious secretions

COPD, chronic obstructive pulmonary disease; CPAP, continuous positive airway pressure; NPPV, noninvasive positive-pressure ventilation.

2. **Partial ventilatory support** provides a variable portion of the minute ventilation, with the remainder provided by the patient's inspiratory effort. The patient–ventilator interaction is important during partial ventilatory support.
   a. Partial ventilatory support is indicated for patients with moderately acute respiratory failure or patients who are recovering from respiratory failure (e.g., during ventilator discontinuation).
      (1) **Advantages** of partial ventilatory support include avoidance of muscle atrophy during long periods of mechanical ventilation, preservation of the ventilatory drive and breathing pattern, decreased requirement for sedation and neuromuscular blockade, a better hemodynamic response to positive-pressure

Table 5-2. Volume-controlled versus pressure-controlled ventilation

	Pressure-Controlled Ventilation	Volume-Controlled Ventilation
Tidal volume	Variable	Set
Peak inspiratory pressure	Limited by pressure control setting	Variable
Plateau pressure	Limited by pressure control setting	Variable
Inspiratory flow	Descending ramp; variable	Set; constant or descending ramp
Inspiratory time	Set directly	Set (flow and volume settings)
Respiratory rate	Minimum set (patient can trigger)	Minimum set (patient can trigger)

ventilation, and better ventilation of dependent lung regions.

    (2) **Disadvantages** of partial ventilatory support include a high work of breathing for the patient and difficulty achieving adequate gas exchange.

IV. **Phase variables**

    A. The **trigger variable** starts inspiration.

       1. The trigger variable is time when the ventilator initiates the breath.

       2. When the patient initiates the breath, the ventilator detects either a pressure change (**pressure trigger**) or a flow change (**flow trigger**).

       3. The **trigger sensitivity** is set to prevent excessive patient effort but avoid autotriggering. Pressure sensitivity is commonly set at 0.5 to 2 cm H_2O, and flow triggering is set at 2 to 3 L/min.

       4. Both pressure triggering and flow triggering are equally effective when sensitivity is optimized and closely monitored.

    B. The **control variable** remains constant throughout inspiration, regardless of impedance. Most common are volume control and pressure control (Table 5-2).

       1. **Volume control.** The term volume control is commonly used, although the ventilator actually controls flow (the time derivative of volume).

          a. With volume-controlled ventilation, **tidal volume delivery is constant** regardless of changes in airways resistance or respiratory system compliance.

          b. A decrease in respiratory system compliance or an increase in airways resistance results in an increased peak airway pressure during volume-controlled ventilation.

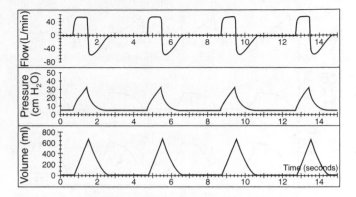

Fig. 5-3. Constant-flow volume ventilation.

    c. With volume-controlled ventilation, the **inspiratory flow is fixed** regardless of patient effort. This unvarying flow may induce patient–ventilator dyssynchrony in patients making vigorous inspiratory efforts.

       (1) Inspiratory flow patterns during volume-controlled ventilation include **constant flow** (rectangular wave) (Fig. 5-3), **descending-ramp flow** (Fig. 5-4), and flow approximating a sine wave.

       (2) Use of the constant-flow waveform results in a higher peak pressure, which is largely borne by the airways and not the alveoli.

       (3) Use of a descending-ramp waveform results in maximal flow early in the breath when lung volume is minimal. This reduces peak pressures but decreases expiratory time, which

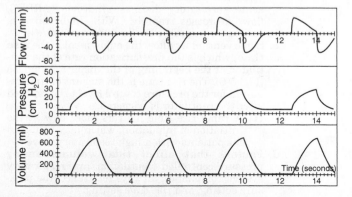

Fig. 5-4. Descending-ramp volume ventilation.

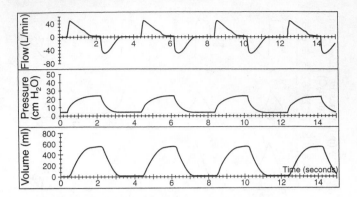

Fig. 5-5.   Pressure-controlled ventilation.

may increase the risk of auto-PEEP and hemodynamic compromise.

d. The **inspiratory time** during volume-controlled ventilation is determined by the inspiratory flow, inspiratory flow pattern, and tidal volume.

e. Volume-controlled ventilation is preferred when a minimum assured minute ventilation is desirable (e.g., avoidance of hypercarbia in patients with intracranial hypertension).

2. **Pressure-controlled ventilation**

a. With pressure-controlled ventilation (Fig. 5-5), **the pressure applied to the airway is constant** regardless of the airways resistance or respiratory system compliance.

b. **The inspiratory flow** during pressure-controlled ventilation is descending and is determined by the pressure control setting, airways resistance, and respiratory system compliance. With low respiratory system compliance [e.g., acute respiratory distress syndrome (ARDS)], flow decreases rapidly. With high airways resistance (e.g., COPD), flow decreases slowly.

c. Some ventilators allow the adjustment of the **rise time,** which is the pressurization rate of the ventilator at the beginning of the inspiratory phase (Fig. 5-6). The rise time is the amount of time required for the pressure control level to be reached after the ventilator is triggered.

   (1) A rapid rise time delivers more flow at the initiation of inhalation, which may be useful for patients with a high respiratory drive.

d. **Factors that affect tidal volume** during pressure-controlled ventilation are respiratory system compliance, airways resistance, the pressure setting, and rise time setting.

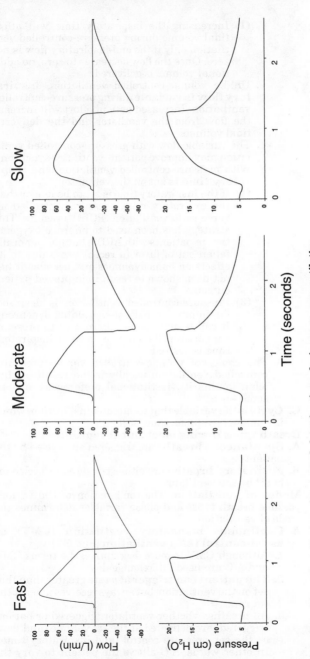

Fig. 5-6. Examples of fast, moderate, and slow rise times during pressure ventilation.

      (1) Increasing the inspiratory time will affect tidal volume during pressure-controlled ventilation only if the end-inspiratory flow is not zero. Once the flow decreases to zero, no additional volume is delivered.

  e. Unlike volume-controlled ventilation, **inspiratory flow is variable** during pressure-controlled ventilation. Increased patient effort will increase the flow from the ventilator and the delivered tidal volume.

  f. The variable flow with pressure-controlled ventilation may improve patient–ventilator synchrony.

  g. With pressure-controlled ventilation, **the inspiratory time is set** on the ventilator.

      (1) If the inspiratory time is set to be longer than the expiratory time, pressure-controlled inverse ratio ventilation (PCIRV) results. This strategy has been used to improve oxygenation in patients with ARDS, but has generally fallen out of favor in recent years due to its effects on hemodynamics and because it has not been shown to result in improved patient outcome.

      (2) Pressure-controlled ventilation is desirable for improving patient–ventilator synchrony. It can be used as an alternative to pressure support ventilation when a fixed inspiratory time is desired.

  3. The choice of volume-controlled versus pressure-controlled ventilation usually is the result of clinician familiarity, institutional preferences, or personal bias.

C. Cycle is the variable that terminates inspiration, which is commonly volume, time, or flow.

V. Breath types during mechanical ventilation

  A. Spontaneous breaths are triggered and cycled by the patient.

  B. Mandatory breaths are either triggered or cycled (or both) by the ventilator.

VI. Modes of ventilation. The combination of the various possible breath types and phase variables determines the mode of ventilation.

  A. Continuous mandatory ventilation (CMV) or assist-control (A/C) ventilation (Fig. 5-7)

    1. Although CMV is more descriptive, the terms CMV and A/C are used interchangeably.

    2. The patient can trigger at a rate greater than that set on the ventilation, but always receives at least the set rate.

    3. All breaths, whether ventilator triggered or patient triggered, are delivered at the set volume (and flow) or the set pressure control (and inspiratory time). In other words, A/C allows the patient to vary the respiratory rate, but not the breath delivery after the ventilator is triggered.

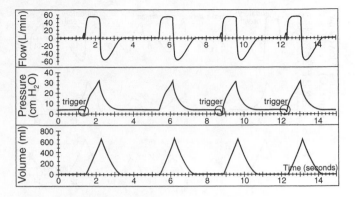

Fig. 5-7. Continuous mandatory ventilation (assist-control ventilation).

    4. Triggering at a rapid rate may result in hyperventilation, hypotension, and dynamic hyperinflation.
- **B. Synchronized intermittent mandatory ventilation (SIMV)** (Fig. 5-8)
  - **1.** With SIMV, the patient receives the mandatory set tidal volume (and flow) or the set pressure control (and inspiratory time) at the rate set on the ventilator.
  - **2.** The mandatory breaths are synchronized with patient effort.
  - **3.** Between the mandatory breaths, the patient may breathe spontaneously.
  - **4.** The spontaneous breaths may be pressure supported (Fig. 5-9).
  - **5.** The patient's inspiratory efforts may be as great during the mandatory breaths as the spontaneous breaths. Thus, it is a myth that SIMV rests the

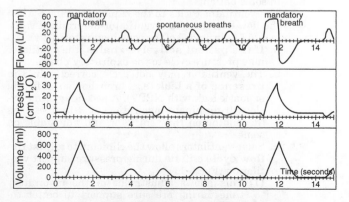

Fig. 5-8. Synchronized intermittent mandatory ventilation.

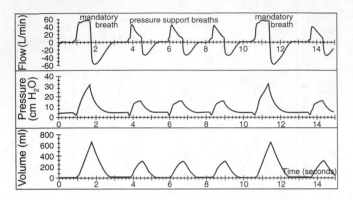

Fig. 5-9. Synchronized intermittent mandatory ventilation with pressure support.

patient during the mandatory breaths and works the patient during the spontaneous breaths.

6. The different breath types during SIMV may induce patient–ventilator dyssynchrony.
7. Note that the CMV and SIMV become synonymous if the patient is not triggering the ventilator (e.g., with neuromuscular blockade).

C. **Pressure support ventilation (PSV)** (Fig. 5-10)
1. **The patient's inspiratory effort** is assisted by the ventilator at a preset pressure with PSV. All breaths are spontaneous breath types.
   a. A pressure **rise time** can be set during pressure support ventilation, similar to pressure control ventilation.
2. The ventilator delivers breaths only in response to patient effort. Thus, appropriate apnea alarms must be set on the ventilator. The lack of a backup rate may result in apnea and sleep-disordered breathing in some patients.
3. The ventilator cycles to the expiratory phase when the flow decreases to a ventilator-determined value (e.g., 5 L/min or 25% of the peak inspiratory flow).
   a. **If the patient actively exhales,** the ventilator may pressure cycle to the expiratory phase.
   b. The ventilator may not cycle correctly **in the presence of a leak** (e.g., bronchopleural fistula or mask leak with NPPV). A secondary time cycle will terminate inspiration at 3 to 5 seconds (depending on the ventilator and adjustable on some).
   c. Some ventilators allow the clinician to **adjust the flow cycle** criteria during pressure support ventilation (Fig. 5-11).
      (1) This allows adjustment of the inspiratory time during pressure support to better coincide with the patient's neural inspiration

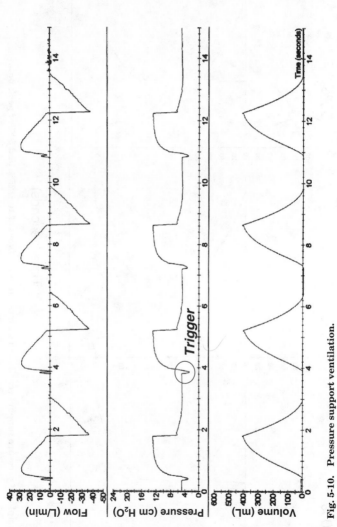

Fig. 5-10. Pressure support ventilation.

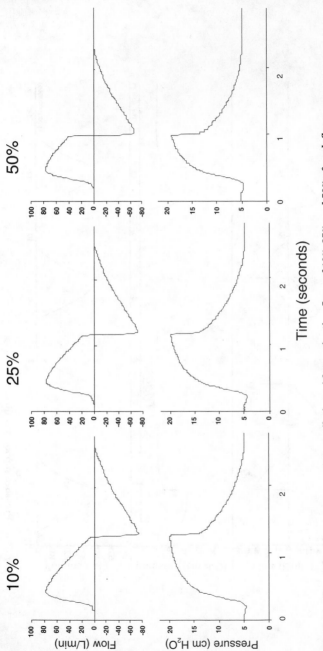

Fig. 5-11. Examples of pressure support ventilation with termination flows of 10%, 25%, and 50% of peak flow.

(thus avoiding active exhalation or double triggering).

(2) If the ventilator is set to cycle at a greater percentage of peak flow, the inspiratory time is decreased. Conversely, if the ventilator is set to cycle at a lower percentage of the peak flow, the inspiratory time is increased.

(3) As a general rule, a higher flow cycle is necessary for obstructive lung disease and a lower flow cycle is necessary for restrictive lung disease (e.g., patients recovering from acute lung injury).

4. The tidal volume, inspiratory flow, inspiratory time, and respiratory rate may vary from breath to breath with PSV.

5. **Tidal volume** is determined by the level of pressure support, rise time, lung mechanics, and the inspiratory effort of the patient.

D. **Continuous positive airway pressure (CPAP)**

1. With CPAP, the ventilator provides no inspiratory assistance.

2. Strictly speaking, CPAP applies a positive pressure to the airway. Current ventilators, however, allow the patient to breath spontaneously without applying positive pressure to the airway (CPAP = 0).

3. Modern ventilators offer little resistance to breathing and do not significantly increase the patient's work of breathing. This is particularly true with flow triggering.

4. CPAP can be applied to an endotracheal tube (invasive) or to a face mask (noninvasive).

E. **Dual-control modes.** Although the ventilator is capable of controlling only pressure or volume at any given time, recently developed modes allow the ventilator to combine features of pressure control (variable flow) and volume control (constant tidal volume).

1. **Volume support (VS).** This mode alters the level of pressure support on a breath-to-breath basis to maintain a clinician-selected tidal volume. The maximum pressure change from breath to breath is less than 3 cm H_2O and can range from 0 cm H_2O above PEEP to 5 cm H_2O below the high-pressure alarm setting.

2. **Pressure-regulated volume control (PRVC), and AutoFlow and VCt.** This mode (PRVC on the Servo ventilator, AutoFlow on the Draeger ventilator and VCt on the Puritan Bennet 840 ventilator) is a form of pressure-limited, time-cycled ventilation (i.e., pressure controlled) that uses tidal volume as a feedback control for continuously adjusting the pressure limit. The pressure limit will increase or decrease at less than 3 cm H_2O per breath in an attempt to deliver the desired tidal volume. The pressure limit will fluctuate between 0 cm H_2O above the PEEP level to 5 cm H_2O below the high-pressure alarm setting.

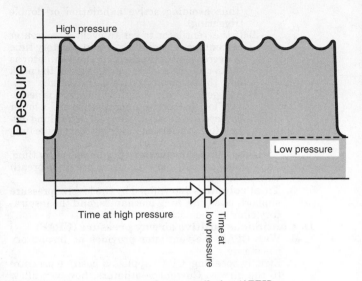

Fig. 5-12. Airway pressure release ventilation (APRV).

3. The clinical utility of VS, PRVC, AutoFlow, and VCt is yet to be determined.
   a. If the patient makes a vigorous inspiratory effort, the tidal volume may exceed the desired tidal volume, which could result in overdistention lung injury.
   b. If the patient makes vigorous inspiratory efforts that cause the volume to exceed the target, the ventilator will take away support. This may increase the patient's work of breathing.
   c. If the lungs become stiffer, the ventilator will increase the pressure, which could result in overdistention lung injury.
F. **Airway pressure release ventilation** (APRV) produces alveolar ventilation as an adjunct to CPAP (Fig. 5-12).
   1. Airway pressure is transiently released to a lower level, after which it is quickly restored to reinflate the lungs. The duration of the high-pressure level is greater than the duration of the low-pressure level.
   2. Minute ventilation is determined by lung compliance, airways resistance, the magnitude of the pressure release, the duration of the pressure release, and the magnitude of the patient's spontaneous breathing efforts.
   3. Oxygenation is determined by the high-pressure setting. Spontaneous breathing by the patient may also provide recruitment of dependent lung regions.

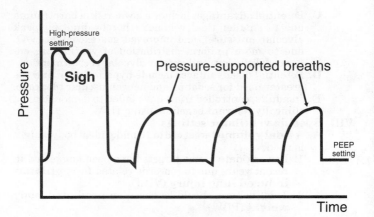

Fig. 5-13. BiLevel or PCV+ used with pressure support ventilation to produce a sigh. PEEP, positive end-expiratory pressure.

4. Because the patient is allowed to breathe spontaneously at both levels of CPAP, the need for sedation may be decreased.
5. The role of APRV in patient outcomes is yet to be determined.
6. A modification of APRV is PCV+ or BiLevel mode. APRV and PCV+ are available on the Drager Evita 4, and BiLevel is available on the Puritan-Bennett 840.
   a. Without spontaneous breathing, PCV+ is similar to PCV, and APRV is similar to Pressure controlled inverse ratio ventilation (PCIRV).
   b. PCV+ or BiLevel can be used to provide **sighs** during PSV or CPAP.
      (1) Several periods (two to four per minute) of elevated airway pressure (20–40 cm H_2O) are used periodically (1–3 seconds at the higher pressure level) (Fig. 5-13).
      (2) The patient can breathe spontaneously at the higher pressure.
      (3) This strategy may be useful in spontaneously breathing patients prone to atelectasis.
G. The choice of the mode of ventilation depends on the capability of the ventilator, the experience and preference of the clinician, and, most important, the needs of the patient. Rather than relying on a single "best" mode of ventilation, one should determine the mode that is most appropriate for each individual situation.

VII. **High-frequency ventilation (HFV)**
   A. With HFV, the patient is ventilated with higher-than-normal rates (i.e., >60/min) and smaller tidal volumes (<5 mL/kg).
   B. With HFV, gas exchange occurs as a result of bulk gas flow and diffusion.

C. Potential advantages include a lower risk of barotrauma due to smaller tidal volumes (thereby limiting peak alveolar pressure), and improved gas exchange ($\dot{V}/\dot{Q}$) due to more uniform distribution of ventilation, enhanced diffusion, and greater alveolar recruitment.

D. Potential disadvantages include hyperinflation and the greater need for sedation and neuromuscular blockade.

E. In adults, controlled trials have failed to demonstrate a clinically relevant benefit to using HFV.

VIII. **Specific ventilator settings**

A. **A tidal volume** target of 6 to 10 ml/kg ideal body weight is used.

1. Lower tidal volume targets have been suggested in recent years due to concerns related to **ventilator-induced lung injury (VILI).**

2. Tidal volume should be based on **predicted body weight** (PBW):

male patients: $PBW = 50 + 2.3 \times [\text{height (inches)} - 60]$

female patients: $PBW = 45.5 + 2.3 \times [\text{height (inches)} - 60]$

3. Use a tidal volume of 6 ml/kg for patients with **ARDS and acute lung injury (ALI).**

4. Use a tidal volume of 6 to 8 ml/kg with **obstructive lung disease.**

5. Use a tidal volume of 8 to 10 ml/kg with **neuromuscular disease** or **postoperative ventilatory support.**

6. **Monitor the plateau pressure** and consider tidal volume reduction if the plateau pressure is greater than 30 cm H_2O.

a. Because lung injury is a function of transalveolar pressure, a higher plateau pressure may be acceptable if chest wall compliance is decreased.

B. **Respiratory rate**

1. The respiratory rate and tidal volume determine **minute ventilation.**

2. Set the rate at 15 to 25/min to achieve a minute ventilation of 7 to 10 L/min.

a. With low tidal volumes and a low pH, a higher respiratory rate may be necessary.

b. A lower respiratory rate may be necessary to avoid air trapping and dynamic hyperinflation.

3. Adjust the rate to achieve the desired pH and Pa_{CO_2}.

4. Avoid high respiratory rates that produce air trapping.

5. **A high-minute-ventilation** (>10 L/min) requirement is due to an increased carbon dioxide production or a high dead space.

C. **Inspiratory:expiratory (I:E) ratio**

1. **Inspiratory time** is determined by flow, tidal volume, and flow pattern during volume-controlled ventilation. Inspiratory time is set directly with pressure control ventilation.

2. **Expiratory time** is determined by the inspiratory time and respiratory rate.
3. The expiratory time generally should be longer than the inspiratory time (e.g., I:E of 1:2).
4. **The expiratory time should be lengthened** (e.g., higher inspiratory flow, lower tidal volume, lower respiratory rate) if the blood pressure drops in response to positive-pressure ventilation or if auto-PEEP is present. If air trapping is significant and accompanied by an acute drop in blood pressure, the patient may be temporarily disconnected from the ventilator (about 30 seconds), then reconnected.
5. **Longer inspiratory times** increase mean airway pressure and may improve arterial partial pressure of oxygen (PaO_2) in some patients.
   a. There is little role for an inverse I:E (i.e., inspiratory time longer than expiratory time).
   b. When long inspiratory times are used, hemodynamics and auto-PEEP must be closely monitored.

D. **Oxygen concentration (FiO_2)**
1. Initiate mechanical ventilation with an FiO_2 of 1.0.
2. Titrate the FiO_2 using pulse oximetry.
3. Inability to reduce the FiO_2 to less than 0.60 indicates the presence of shunt (intrapulmonary or intracardiac).

E. **Positive end-expiratory pressure**
1. **The use of PEEP may increase oxygenation** in lung diseases characterized by alveolar collapse. Positive end-expiratory pressure maintains alveolar recruitment, increases the functional respiratory capacity, decreases intrapulmonary shunt, and may improve lung compliance.
   a. Because lung volumes are typically decreased with acute respiratory failure, it is reasonable to use a PEEP of at least 5 cm H_2O with the initiation of mechanical ventilation for most patients.
   b. **Maintaining alveolar recruitment** in disease processes like ARDS may decrease the likelihood of ventilator-associated lung injury.
   c. Although higher levels of PEEP often increase PaO_2, evidence has not shown that higher levels of PEEP (compared to modest levels of PEEP) decrease mortality.
2. A number of methods have been used to titrate the best level of PEEP.
   a. PEEP can be titrated to a desired level of oxygenation, such as the level of PEEP that allows the FiO_2 to be decreased to 0.6 without hemodynamic compromise.
   b. PEEP can be set 2 to 3 cm H_2O above the lower inflexion point of the pressure–volume curve. However, this is difficult to measure reliably in critically ill patients, and its role in the determination

of appropriate PEEP setting remains to be determined.

c. In patients with COPD, PEEP may be used to counter balance auto-PEEP and improve the ability to trigger the ventilator.

d. In patients with left ventricular failure, PEEP may improve cardiac performance by decreasing venous return and left ventricular afterload.

3. **Adverse effects of PEEP**

a. PEEP may **decrease cardiac output.** Hemodynamics should be monitored during PEEP titration.

b. High levels of PEEP may result in **alveolar overdistention** during the inspiratory phase. It may be necessary to decrease the tidal volume with high PEEP.

c. PEEP may **worsen oxygenation with unilateral lung disease** because it results in a redistribution of pulmonary blood flow from overdistended lung units to the unventilated lung units. PEEP may worsen oxygenation with cardiac shunt (e.g., patient foramen ovale).

IX. **Complications of mechanical ventilation**

A. **Ventilator-induced lung injury**

1. **Overdistension injury** occurs if the lung parenchyma is subjected to an abnormally high transpulmonary pressure.

a. Overdistension injury produces inflammation and increased alveolar-capillary membrane permeability.

b. Tidal volume should be limited (e.g., 6 ml/kg in patients with ARDS) to decrease the risk of overdistention lung injury.

c. The results of a recent multicenter trial (the ARDSNet trial) suggest that plateau pressure be maintained at less than or equal to 30 cm H_2O to prevent overdistension injury.

d. A priority should be given to use of the lowest tidal volume *and* plateau pressure possible to minimize the risk of lung injury during mechanical ventilation.

e. Because the risk of overdistension lung injury is related to transpulmonary pressure, higher plateau pressures may be acceptable if chest wall compliance is reduced (e.g., abdominal distention, chest wall burns, chest wall edema, obesity).

2. **Derecruitment injury**

a. PEEP levels that are not high enough to maintain alveolar recruitment may result in alveolar opening and closing with each respiratory cycle. This may result in inflammation and increased alveolar-capillary membrane permeability.

b. This injury may be avoided by use of appropriate levels of PEEP with ARDS: often 10 to 15 cm H_2O, and sometimes 15 to 20 cm H_2O.

3. **Oxygen toxicity**
    a. High concentrations of oxygen for long periods may cause lung damage and may promote atelectasis.
    b. Although it is prudent to reduce the FiO_2 provided that arterial oxygenation is adequate (SpO_2 >90% in most patients; some patients tolerate lower SpO_2), the precise role of oxygen toxicity in patients with acute lung injury is unclear.
    c. Appropriate levels of inspired oxygen should never be withheld for fear of oxygen toxicity.

B. **Patient–ventilator dyssynchrony**
  1. **Trigger dyssynchrony** refers to the inability of the patient to trigger the ventilator.
      a. Trigger dyssynchrony may be due to an **insensitive trigger setting** on the ventilator. This is corrected by adjusting the trigger sensitivity.
      b. An alternative approach to triggering may be tried, such as flow triggering instead of pressure triggering.
      c. A common cause of trigger dyssynchrony is the presence **of auto-PEEP** (see Chapter 3). If auto-PEEP is present, the patient must generate enough inspiratory effort to overcome the auto-PEEP before triggering can occur. Techniques for decreasing the level of auto-PEEP should be employed (e.g., administer bronchodilators, increase expiratory time). In patients with expiratory flow limitation (e.g., COPD), increasing the set PEEP on the ventilator may counterbalance the auto-PEEP and improve trigger synchrony.
  2. **Flow dyssynchrony**
      a. During volume ventilation, the ventilator flow is fixed and may not meet the patient's inspiratory flow demands. The inspiratory pressure waveform will demonstrate a characteristic scalloped pattern.
      b. Flow dyssynchrony may be improved during volume ventilation by increasing the inspiratory flow or changing the inspiratory flow pattern.
      c. Changing volume control to pressure control or pressure support, in which flows are variable, may be helpful.
  3. **Cycle dyssynchrony** occurs when the patient's expiratory effort begins before or after the end of the inspiratory phase set on the ventilator. Cycle dyssynchrony occurs during volume-controlled or pressure-controlled ventilation if the inspiratory time is inappropriately short or long. This is corrected by adjusting the inspiratory time.
      a. If the inspiratory flow rate is too low or the inspiratory time setting is too short, the patient may double trigger the ventilator. If the inspiratory flow rate is too high or the inspiratory time setting is too long, the patient may actively exhale.

    b. With high airways resistance and high lung compliance (e.g., COPD), a prolonged time may be required during pressure support ventilation for the inspiratory flow to decrease to the flow cycle criteria set in the ventilator. The patient may actively exhale to terminate the inspiratory phase.

      (1) This problem may be corrected by using pressure control rather than pressure support setting.

        (a) The inspiratory time is set so that inspiratory flow does not reach zero.

      (2) Some ventilators allow the clinician to adjust the termination flow during pressure support to improve synchrony.

      (3) Sometimes this problem improves with the use of a lower pressure support setting.

      (4) The problem may improve with the use of more aggressive attempts to reduce airways resistance (bronchodilators, secretion clearance).

C. Auto-PEEP

  1. Auto-PEEP is the result of gas trapping (dynamic hyperinflation) due to insufficient expiratory time and/or increased expiratory airflow resistance. The pressure exerted by this trapped gas is called auto-PEEP.

  2. The increase in alveolar pressure due to auto-PEEP may adversely affect hemodynamics.

  3. The presence of auto-PEEP can produce trigger dyssynchrony as discussed previously.

  4. Detection of auto-PEEP (see Chapter 3):

    a. Some ventilators allow auto-PEEP to be measured directly.

    b. In spontaneously breathing patients, auto-PEEP can be measured using an **esophageal balloon.**

    c. The **patient's breathing pattern** can be observed. If exhalation is still occurring when the next breath is delivered, auto-PEEP is present.

    d. Inspiratory efforts **that do not trigger the ventilator** suggest the presence of auto-PEEP.

    e. If flow graphics is available on the ventilator, it can be observed that **expiratory flow** does not return to zero before the subsequent breath is delivered.

  5. Factors affecting auto-PEEP

    a. Physiologic factors. A high airways resistance or high respiratory system compliance increases the likelihood of auto-PEEP.

    b. Ventilator factors. A high tidal volume, high respiratory rate, or prolonged inspiratory time will increase the likelihood of auto-PEEP.

Reducing the minute ventilation decreases the likelihood of auto-PEEP.

D. Barotrauma
1. **Alveolar rupture** during positive-pressure ventilation may lead to air extravasation through the bronchovascular sheath into the pulmonary interstitium, mediastinum, pericardium, peritoneum, pleural space, and subcutaneous tissue.
2. Sudden hemodynamic instability or sudden increase in peak inspiratory pressure in a mechanically ventilated patient should raise the suspicion of a **tension pneumothorax.**

E. Hemodynamic perturbations
1. Positive-pressure ventilation increases intrathoracic pressure and **decreases venous return.** Right ventricular filling is limited by the reduced venous return.
2. When alveolar pressure exceeds pulmonary venous pressure, pulmonary blood flow is affected by alveolar pressure rather than left atrial pressure, producing an **increase in pulmonary vascular resistance.** Consequently, right ventricular afterload increases and right ventricular ejection fraction falls.
3. **Left ventricular filling is limited** by reduced right ventricular output and decreased left ventricular diastolic compliance.
4. Increased right ventricular size affects left ventricular performance by shifting the interventricular septum to the left.
5. **Intravascular volume replacement** counteracts the negative hemodynamic effects of PEEP.
6. Increased intrathoracic pressure may **improve left ventricular ejection fraction and stroke volume.** This beneficial effect may be significant in patients with poor ventricular function.

F. Nosocomial pneumonia
1. Mechanically ventilated patients are at risk for ventilator-associated pneumonia.
2. Ventilator-associated pneumonia is most often related to aspiration of secretions around the cuff of the endotracheal tube.
   a. Because the source of ventilator-associated pneumonia is usually not the ventilator per se, the tubing and humidifier on the ventilator do not need to be changed at regular intervals.
   b. Continuous aspiration of subglottic secretions has been shown to decrease the incidence of ventilator-associated pneumonia.
   c. Semirecumbent position (elevation of the head of the bed by 30 degrees) has been shown to decrease the risk of ventilator-associated pneumonia.
   d. The use of NPPV decreases the risk of ventilator-associated pneumonia.

SELECTED REFERENCES

Branson RD, Johannigman JA. What is the evidence base for the newer ventilation modes? *Respir Care* 2004;49:742–760.

Brower RG, Lanken PN, MacIntyre N, et al. Higher versus lower positive end-expiratory pressures in patients with the acute respiratory distress syndrome. *N Engl J Med* 2004;351:327–336.

Chatburn RL. Computer control of mechanical ventilation. *Respir Care* 2004;49:507–517.

Chatburn RL, Primiano FP Jr. A new system for understanding modes of mechanical ventilation. *Respir Care* 2001;46:604–621.

Dhand R. Basic techniques for aerosol delivery during mechanical ventilation. *Respir Care* 2004;49:611–622.

Hall JB, Schmidt GA, Wood LD, eds. *Principles of critical care.* New York: McGraw-Hill, 1998.

Hess DR. The evidence for noninvasive positive-pressure ventilation in the care of patients in acute respiratory failure: a systematic review of the literature. *Respir Care* 2004;49:810–829.

Hess D, Kacmarek RM. *Essentials of mechanical ventilation.* 2nd ed. New York: McGraw-Hill, 2002.

Kallet RH. Evidence-based management of acute lung injury and acute respiratory distress syndrome. *Respir Care* 2004;49:793–809.

NIH/NHLBI ARDS Network. Ventilation with lower tidal volumes as compared with traditional tidal volumes for acute lung injury and the acute respiratory distress syndrome. *N Engl J Med* 2000;342:1301–1308.

Analgesia, Sedation, and Neuromuscular Blockade

James Helstrom and Ulrich Schmidt

The discomfort of a patient in the intensive care unit (ICU) can be due to multiple factors. Pain can arise from the physical burdens imposed by severe disease, operative wounds, traumatic injuries, and indwelling tubes and catheters. Near-continuous stimulation from personnel and equipment can quickly disrupt normal circadian rhythms and promote anxiety and delirium. Careful delineation of the individual contributions that pain, anxiety, and delirium make to patient behavior is crucial to a treatment strategy that maximizes patient comfort while enhancing clinical goals. Although overlaps exist with regard to the clinical effects of drug classes, a thorough understanding of the indications and adverse effects of the individual drug classes is essential because effective treatment demands that drugs be targeted only toward the specific condition for which they have been shown to be most effective.

Surveys of ICU survivors acknowledge poor control of agitation and pain. Pain increases sympathetic nervous system activation and raises circulating catecholamine levels. The hypermetabolic response to critical illness is worsened by pain and results in impaired wound healing, increased oxygen demand, hypercoagulability, and immunosuppression that may contribute to poor patient outcomes. Pain can alter breathing patterns and mechanics, and may contribute to the retention of pulmonary secretions and atelectasis, resulting in hypoxemia and infection. In addition, pain and agitation may have long-term psychological effects, and excessive use of sedatives and analgesics may have unintended effects including longer ventilation and ICU stay.

I. Pain and analgesia

A. **Pain assessment** by self-reporting is the preferred means of determining the adequacy of pain control. Pain can either be communicated directly or with the aid of simple tools such as the Visual Analog Scale (VAS) or a numeric rating system. However, assessment of analgesic needs through direct patient interaction is often difficult for patients supported by mechanical ventilation, patients who have altered levels of consciousness, and patients who have severe illness. In the absence of direct patient feedback, nurses and family members may be recruited to make surrogate assessments regarding patient comfort.

   1. The **VAS** consists of a 10-cm line bounded by extremes of pain such as "no pain" and "pain that could not be more severe" and represents a continuum on which patients place their current pain level. The VAS has been

tested for validity and reliability in many non-ICU populations and is regarded as the standard analgesic assessment tool. Effective use of the VAS demands directed motor activity and the ability to comprehend and follow complex directions.

2. The **numeric rating system** is an assessment tool similar to the VAS but uses discrete integers to quantify pain intensity, in distinction to the analogue scale. The rating scale (typically from 0 to 10) can be administered verbally or in writing, and requires minimal motor coordination. It has been independently validated and correlates well with the VAS in cardiac surgical patients.

3. The **faces scale** (happy to frowning to grimacing) does not require verbal ability and has been used traditionally as a self-reporting tool for adults and children.

B. **Treatment of pain**

1. **Nonpharmacologic** approaches for analgesia should initially be optimized to lessen analgesic and sedation requirements. Proper positioning of patients with respect to injuries or sites of procedure/surgical incisions, eliminating sites of catheter- or line-related irritation, and appropriate positioning of the endotracheal tube in mechanically ventilated patients can profoundly impact patient comfort.

2. **Regional analgesia**

   a. **Epidural analgesia** is the regional pain management technique that is appropriate for ICU patients even though prospective studies have not shown an overall outcome benefit. Known benefits include excellent pain control, facilitation of pulmonary toilet secondary to analgesia, and an increased postoperative activity level. A combination of a local anesthetic and opioid as the epidural infusion will provide synergistic pain relief necessitating lower cumulative doses of the individual component medications. Common **complications** associated with epidural placement are the result of local anesthetic actions: **hypotension** secondary to sympathetic blockade and paresis/paralysis of the lower extremities due to central inhibition of motor neurons. Hypovolemia, myocardial dysfunction, and other causes of low-tone states must always be considered before accepting the epidural as a cause for hypotension. Similarly, an epidural abscess and hematoma, although rare events, must be ruled out in the ICU patient who has difficulty moving lower extremities. Respiratory depression secondary to the systematic absorption of epidural opiates may occur and can be corrected by reducing or eliminating the narcotic in the epidural solution. The administration of naloxone is occasionally required.

   b. **Intercostal and paravertebral analgesia.** Paravertebral block or catheter placement can provide adequate postoperative pain control following procedures involving the thorax, upper abdomen, or flank. Catheters (or intermittent injections) are placed immediately lateral to the thoracic spine and medial to the parietal pleura. Adverse events are rare, and hypotension and urinary retention are reported to be less than that associated with epidural analgesia. Intercostal analgesia is invariably associated with intermittent nerve block. Intercostal injections can provide effective analgesia for 6 to 24 hours depending on the choice of local anesthetic; these blocks are performed in the same plane as paravertebral injections but more laterally and are a viable alternative for pain associated with rib fractures.

   c. **Anticoagulation and regional analgesia.** Deep vein thrombosis and therapeutic anticoagulation can impact both the placement and removal of epidural catheters. Epidural catheters can be safely placed and removed for patients on subcutaneous heparin and after holding heparin infusions for 4 hours. In contrast, catheters should not be manipulated within 12 hours of low-molecular-weight heparin administration. The IIb/IIIa platelet inhibitors have long half-lives that necessitate epidural removal prior to starting these drugs in the postoperative period.

C. Drugs used for pain control
  1. Nonnarcotic analgesics
    a. Acetaminophen. Acetaminophen is an analgesic and antipyretic, providing relief from mild to moderate pain. As an adjunct to opioid-based therapy, acetaminophen can provided improved pain control relative to higher doses of opioid alone. It should not be used for patients with hepatic insufficiency.

    b. Nonsteroidal antiinflammatory drugs (NSAIDs). NSAIDs provide analgesia through nonselective inhibition of cyclooxygenase, an enzyme responsible for prostaglandin synthesis in the arachadonic acid cascade. Reduction in prostaglandin production is nonspecific, and reductions in proinflammatory mediators are complemented by decreases in gastric prostaglandins PGI_2 and PGE_2, and renal afferent PGX, resulting in an increased risk of gastrointestinal bleeding, renal failure, and platelet dysfunction. NSAID use has been found to decrease opioid requirements postoperatively, although the precise role of NSAIDs in the ICU has not been systematically studied.

  2. Opioid agonists (Table 6-1) produce analgesia by interacting with μ and κ receptors, whereas side effects are mediated by interactions at additional receptor types. Comparative trials of opioids are lacking in ICU patients, and specific agents are chosen based on

Table 6-1.   Common opioids used in the intensive care unit

Drug	Adult Dose[a] (mg)	Duration of Action (h)	Approximate Conversion Factor	Metabolism	Comments
Codeine/ acetaminophen (Tylenol 3)	30/300	4		Hepatic to morphine	Limit is based on maximal acetaminophen dose of 4 g/d
Parenteral	—		0.08		
Oral	15–60		0.05		
Fentanyl	0.050– 0.10	0.5–2	80	Hepatic	Rapid IV injection can result in skeletal muscle and chest wall rigidity
Parenteral			80		
Transdermal patch	—	4		Hepatic; eliminated in urine, principally as glucuronide conjugates	25, 50, 75, or 100 μg/h Pediatric use not well established
Hydromorphone (Dilaudid)					
Parenteral	1–4		4		
Oral	1–4		1.33		
Meperidine (Demerol)		3–4		Hepatic; normeperidine (active metabolite) is dependent on renal function and can accumulate with high doses or in patients with decreased renal function	Use caution in patients with hepatic or renal failure seizure disorders or receiving high doses; normeperidine (a CNS stimulant) can accumulate and precipitate twitching, tremor, or seizures; MAO inhibitors, fluoxetine, and other serotonin-uptake inhibitors, greatly potentiate the effects of meperidine
Parenteral	50–150		0.1		

					Comments
Methadone (Dolophine)		4–12 h, increases to 22–48 h with repeated doses			Phenytoin, pentazocine, and rifampin can increase the metabolism of methadone and may precipitate withdrawal; increased toxicity: CNS depressants, phenothiazines, tricyclic antidepressants, and MAO inhibitors can potentiate the adverse effects of methadone
Parenteral	2–10		1.0		
Oral	2–10		0.7		
Morphine		4–5		In the liver via glucuronide conjugation; excreted unchanged in urine	Histamine release; can cause hypotension in patients with acute myocardial infarction
Parenteral	5–10		1.0		
Oral[b]	10–30		0.33		
Oxycodone/ acetaminophen (Percocet)		6		Hepatic	Limit is based on maximal acetaminophen dose of 4 g/d
Oral	5/325		0.33		

IV, Intravenous; CNS, central nervous system; MAO, monoamine oxidase.

Published tables vary widely in suggested equianalgesic doses. Titration to clinical responses is always necessary. Recommended doses do not apply to patients with hepatic or renal insufficiency or other conditions affecting drug metabolism and kinetics.

[a]These doses (oral, intravenous) are recommended starting doses for acute pain. Optimal doses for each patient are determined by titration, and the maximal dose is limited by adverse effects. Any oral or parenteral analgesic may be converted into its intramuscular morphine equivalent by multiplying the dose by the conversion factor.

[b]Controversy exists concerning actual conversion factor (3:1 ratio).

pharmacology and adverse effect profile. In the ICU, opiate infusions are often used for sedation of intubated patients in addition to analgesia. **Patient-controlled analgesia (PCA)** provides quality analgesia, less sedation, reduced opioid consumption, and diminished complications, including respiratory depression. It is useful for postoperative patients of short duration in the ICU. Side effects can include alterations in mental status, respiratory depression, hypotension, and inhibition of gastrointestinal motility. Daily awakening from analgesia and sedation allowed more effective analgesia titration, a lower cumulative morphine dose, and shorter duration of mechanical ventilation and ICU care.

a. **Morphine** is the standard narcotic against which other narcotics are compared. The peak onset of action is 10 to 30 minutes after parenteral administration, with persistence for 4 to 5 hours. Morphine-6-glucoronide is an active metabolite that can accumulate in renal disease.

b. **Fentanyl** is 100-fold more potent than morphine, with an almost immediate onset of action and a duration of 30 to 60 minutes. With increased time of infusions, the analgesic effect is diminished secondary to redistribution in fat. Clinically significant histamine release rarely occurs with fentanyl.

c. **Hydromorphone** is five- to sevenfold more potent than morphine, with an onset time of 15 minutes and a duration of analgesia of approximately 4 to 6 hours. The metabolites of hydromorphone are inactive, and the drug is not associated with significant histamine release.

d. **Meperidine** is six to eightfold less potent than morphine. Because its active metabolite, normeperidine, has a long half-life, lowers the seizure threshold, and accumulates with renal insufficiency, meperidine is seldom used in the ICU.

e. **Methadone**, when administered parenterally, is approximately equipotent with morphine, whereas oral administration is approximately one-half as potent. It has a duration of 15 to 40 hours. An additional property is the antagonism of N-methyl-D-aspartate receptors. We have observed analgesia with methadone when equipotent doses of hydromorphone and morphine have failed. The enteral dose is efficacious when a patient has an enteral feeding tube, a large opiate requirement, and will be transitioned to a step-down unit or a hospital floor bed.

f. **Acetaminophen (APAP) with oxycodone or codeine** is an oral analgesic that is useful when parenteral narcotics are no longer needed. As with parenteral narcotics, respiratory depression and sedation, especially in the elderly, is possible. The maximum doses of both drugs are based on the acetaminophen content, which should not exceed 4 g/d. APAP with oxycodone (Percocet) is available in formulations of 2.5, 5, 7.5, and 10 mg of narcotic combined with 325, 500, or 650 mg of APAP, and can be given every 6 hours. APAP with codeine (Tylenol with codeine) has 30 or 60 mg of codeine and 300 mg of APAP, and can be administered every 4 hours.

3. **Ketamine** is a rapid-acting drug, structurally related to phencyclidine, that produces an anesthetic state characterized by profound analgesia, normal pharyngeal-laryngeal reflexes, normal or slightly enhanced skeletal muscle tone, and cardiovascular and respiratory stimulation. It has been associated with hallucinations that can be effectively blocked with benzodiazepine administration. Ketamine is useful for procedures associated with painful stimulation such as debridement and dressing changes in burn patients.

II. **Sedation**

A. Numerous scales have been developed to describe patient behavior and aid the clinician in communicating sedation goals. Although there is no gold standard for use in the ICU, applying various scales to protocol-driven intervention plans has been shown to be of clinical benefit.

1. The **Ramsay Sedation Scale** scores six levels of agitation (Table 6-2). Although it is the most commonly used reference scale in the literature, the individual categories are not mutually exclusive, which makes it somewhat difficult to use clinically.

2. **The Richmond Agitation–Sedation Scale (RASS)** (Table 6-3) is advantageous because it describes a spectrum of sedation from unarousable to combative with appropriate descriptions for more accurate assessments.

3. The **Bispectral Index (BIS)** is a noninvasive measure of brain function that uses a proprietary algorithm to assess sedation level. The BIS attaches to the patient's forehead and provides a continuous reading using a scale of 0 to 100, with 100 representing normal wakefulness, less than 60 associated with deep

Table 6-2.   Ramsay Sedation Scale

Level	Response
1	Anxious, agitated, restless
2	Cooperative, oriented, tranquil
3	Responds to commands only
4	Asleep, brisk response to stimulus
5	Asleep, sluggish response to stimulus
6	Unarousable

From Ramsay MA, Savege TM, Simpson BR, et al. Controlled sedation with alphaxalone-alphadolone. *Br Med J* 1974;2:656–659. With permission.

Table 6-3. Richmond Agitation–Sedation Scale

Score	Term	Description
+4	Combative	Overtly combative or violent; immediate danger to staff
+3	Very agitated	Pulls on or removes tube(s) or catheter(s) or has aggressive behavior toward staff
+2	Agitated	Frequent nonpurposeful movement or patient–ventilator dyssynchrony
+1	Restless	Anxious or apprehensive but movements not aggressive or vigorous
0	Alert and calm	
−1	Drowsy	Not fully alert, but has sustained (>10 seconds) awakening, with eye contact, to voice
−2	Light sedation	Briefly (<10 seconds) awakens with eye contact to voice
−3	Moderate sedation	Any movement (but no eye contact) to voice
−4	Deep sedation	No response to voice, but any movement to physical stimulation
−5	Unarousable	No response to voice or physical stimulation

Procedure

1. Observe patient. Is patient alert and calm (score 0)?
   Does patient have behavior that is consistent with restlessness or agitation (score +1 to +4 using the criteria listed in last column)?
2. If patient is not alert, in a loud speaking voice, state the patient's name and direct the patient to open his or her eyes and look at the speaker. Repeat once if necessary. Can prompt the patient to continue looking at the speaker.
   Patient has eye opening and eye contact, which is sustained for more >10 seconds (score −1).
   Patient has eye opening and eye contact, but this is not sustained for 10 seconds (score −2).
   Patient has any movement in response to voice, excluding eye contact (score −3).
3. If the patient does not respond to voice, physically stimulate the patient by shaking the shoulder and then rubbing the sternum if there is no response to shaking of the shoulder.
   Patient has any movement to physical stimulation (score −4).
   Patient has no response to voice or physical stimulation (score −5).

From Sessler CN, Gosnell MS, Grap MJ, et al. The Richmond Agitation–Sedation Scale. Validity and reliability in adult intensive care unit patients. *Am J Respir Crit Care Med* 2002;166:1338–1344. With permission.

Table 6-4. Common benzodiazepines used in the intensive care unit

Drug	Adult Dose (Range)	Half-Life (h)	Active Metabolites
Alprazolam (Xanax)	0.75–4 mg/d	12–15	None
Diazepam (Valium)	6–40 mg/d	20–50	N-desmethyldiazepam N-methyloxazepam (temaxepam) Oxazepam
Lorazepam (Ativan)	2–6 mg/d	10–20	None
Midazolam (Versed)	2.5–30 mg/d	1–4	Alpha-hydroxymidazolam
Oxazepam (Serax)	30–120 mg/d	3–6	None

sedation, and less than 40 an indication of a deep hypnotic state. Although it has had some utility in the operating room, only a few studies have examined its usefulness for the critically ill patient.

B. **Drugs used for sedation.** In the presence of even an optimal ICU environment, many patients will require some treatment for anxiety, agitation, or delirium. As noted, the goal should be to use the minimum amount of medication necessary to (a) provide an acceptable patient experience, (b) significantly reduce the potential for injury, and (c) allow for appropriate therapy.

1. **Benzodiazepines** (Table 6-4) are sedatives that potentiate the actions of γ-aminobutyric acid (GABA) on inhibitory receptors throughout the neuroaxis. Benzodiazepines have no analgesic properties and are routinely used with analgesics. Benzodiazepines are metabolized by several different hepatic microsomal enzyme systems. Because active metabolites are generated that are biotransformed more slowly than the parent compound, the duration of action of many benzodiazepines bears little relationship to the elimination half-life of the administered drug. All benzodiazepines are lipophilic and can accumulate with prolonged infusions. Paradoxical agitation has been observed with small doses of benzodiazepines and is most likely a disinhibition phenomenon found most in individuals with neurologic deficits or underlying cognitive dysfunction. Long-term benzodiazepine infusions should be discontinued gradually because abrupt cessation can precipitate withdrawal syndromes.

a. **Midazolam** has a rapid onset of action but a rapidly developing tolerance. Accumulation of midazolam has been reported in ICU patients receiving prolonged infusions and for patients who are morbidly obese. Significant inhibition of metabolism can occur with concomitant administration of inhibitors of cytochrome 3A4 such as macrolide antibiotics, diltiazem, and propofol.

b. Lorazepam is the most commonly used ICU sedative, with a duration of action of 8 to 15 hours and no active metabolites. In addition to sedation, it is administered to prevent symptoms of withdrawal from ethanol and for the acute treatment of grand mal seizures. The propylene and polyethylene glycol diluents of this drug have been shown to precipitate an anion gap acidosis and reversible acute tubular necrosis with prolonged administration. Dosing regimens vary, but invariably begin with 1 to 2 mg administered every 4 to 8 hours. Lorazepam is available in parenteral and oral forms.

c. Diazepam is a rapidly acting benzodiazepine with several long-acting metabolites. The long half-lives of diazepam (40 hrs) and its active metabolic nordiazepam (70 hrs), diminish the utility of diazepam for short to medium courses of sedation.

2. Propofol is a nonanalgesic sedative and hypnotic induction agent for general anesthesia. Additional beneficial effects include bronchodilation; seizure suppression; antiemesis; and decreased intracranial pressure via a dose-dependent decrease in cerebral blood flow and cerebral metabolic oxygen demand. For intubated patients, the drug is administered by intravenous infusion titrated to effect. The most common side effects are respiratory depression and hypotension related to systemic vasodilation. Although propofol is considered a drug with a short duration of action, sedation in critically ill patients may persist sometimes for days following the cessation of a prolonged infusion. Because the drug is formulated in a lipid emulsion, long-term use can be associated with hypertriglyceridemia. There is increasing evidence for a **"propofol infusion syndrome"** characterized by a lactic acid metabolic acidosis, profound myocardial depression, rhabdomyolysis, and renal failure in association with the use of large quantities of propofol. The precise etiology is unknown but is hypothesized to be the result of the alteration of free fatty acid metabolism when triggered by exogenous steroid and catecholamine administration.

3. Opioids (Table 6-1) are the first line of therapy when pain is suspected as the primary cause of agitation. Despite possessing modest sedating effects, opiates do not diminish awareness and will not produce amnesia.

4. α2-Agonists activate sympathetic interneurons in the central nervous system and serve as a negative feedback mechanism to downregulate the sympathetic response. **Clonidine** is the prototypical α2-agonist. In addition to its use as an antihypertensive, it can ameliorate withdrawal syndromes in the ICU. The starting dose is 0.1 mg daily, which can be advanced to 0.3 mg by either enteral or cutaneous patch routes. Sudden discontinuation can precipitate rebound hypertension. **Dexmedetomidine** is a more selective intravenous α2-agonist and is approved as a short-term sedative (<24 hours). It provides anxiolysis and sedation without respiratory depression. A loading dose of 1 μg/kg is given over 10 minutes followed by infusion at 0.2 to 0.8 μg/kg/h.

III. **Agitation, anxiety, and delirium**

    A. These can be the result of metabolic derangements, neurologic abnormalities, infection and discomfort associated with invasive monitors and tubes, and near-constant stimuli. **Agitation** is excessive motor activity that is the result of internal discomfort. **Anxiety** is an unpleasant alteration of mood with intact cognition. **Delirium**, in contrast, is marked by cognitive dysfunction with an unpleasant alteration of mood. In addition to being unpleasant for the patient and family, these behaviors may have adverse consequences including self-extubation, removal of arterial and venous catheters, increased systemic myocardial oxygen consumption, and failure to participate in therapeutic interventions. ICU delirium has been recently shown to be an independent predictor of increase in 6-month mortality and hospital stay. Although pharmacologic therapies are the mainstay of treatment and the subject of recent consensus guidelines, the identification and correction of the etiologies responsible for the mental status changes is of first importance. The **differential diagnosis** of agitation and delirium should be done aggressively with drug screening, treatment of pain, laboratory tests, and radiographic imaging to rule out serious and potential life-threatening causes.

    B. **Agitation** has multifactorial causes from the interaction of medical, environmental, and patient-related factors.

        1. **Pain.** Inadequate analgesia is a frequent cause of agitation in critically ill patients. Although most commonly considered in the postoperative period, pain control is an important component of comprehensive care in many medical patients including those with pancreatitis, rheumatologic conditions, and decubiti.

        2. **Therapeutic drugs** such as sodium nitroprusside can cause confusion when used for a few days in an elderly patient.

        3. **Metabolic abnormalities:** hypoxemia, hypercarbia, CNS hypoperfusion, uremia, hepatic encephalopathy, and hypoglycemia.

        4. **Infection and fever.**

        5. **Neurologic events:** hemorrhage, infection, or embolic phenomena (including thrombi and air).

        6. **Environmental factors:** continuous noise and ambient light, frequent vital sign measurements, lack of mobility, suboptimal room temperature, and sleep deprivation.

7. **Withdrawal syndromes** related to recreational drugs, alcohol, and nicotine use.

C. **Delirium** is a global disorder of cognition and attention that may occur in 80% of critically ill patients and is frequently unrecognized. It manifests as a reduced level of consciousness, abnormal psychomotor activity (both increased and decreased), and disturbed sleep–wake cycle. Thinking is disorganized and incoherent; the ability to distinguish imagery and dreams from facts is impaired, and delusions or visual or auditory hallucinations can frequently occur.

1. **Etiologic factors.** Etiologic factors for delirium closely parallel those for agitation including primary intracranial disease, systemic diseases secondarily affecting the brain (toxic-metabolic encephalopathy), exogenous toxic agents including physician-prescribed medications, addiction/withdrawal syndromes, and preexisting history of psychosis. Toxic-metabolic delirium is especially common in the elderly, and these individuals are prone to delirium triggered by medications with anticholinergic properties.

2. **Treatment** of delirium is with antipsychotic agents that do not have respiratory depressant properties. These drugs are associated with a dose-dependent increased in the QT interval, resulting in an increased risk of ventricular dysrhythmias, especially torsades de pointes. The effects are worsened when they are administered with the multitude of other drugs that will prolong the QT interval. It is prudent to obtain an electrocardiogram at baseline and to daily measure the QTc to assure that it is neither increasing rapidly nor is greater than 500 msec. There should be a constant survey for the presence of neuroleptic malignant syndrome (see Chapter 13), which is possible with these drugs.

a. **Haloperidol** is useful for the management of ICU-related delirium. The initial starting dose is 1 mg intravenously (IV). Adequate sedation will occur in about 1 hour. If the treatment of delirium is inadequate, each successive dose should be doubled as needed based on the treatment effect and QTc. Because the elimination half-life is 13 to 35 hours, whereas the peak serum level of each dose is within 20 minutes, oversedation of patients, especially the elderly, may occur. Therefore, it is useful to have a target total dose in mind (e.g., 20 mg) and stop administering the drug once this dose is reached. The maintenance dose ranges from 1 to 2 mg IV every 4 to 8 hours. Extrapyramidal side effects are infrequent with IV haloperidol but may be difficult to distinguish from agitation.

b. **Quetiapine (Seroquel)** is an orally available, atypical antipsychotic agent structurally related to **olanzapine** and **clozapine.** The recommended initial dose of quetiapine is 25 mg twice daily, with incremental increases up to 300 to 400 mg daily. Peak serum concentrations are reached within 1.5 hours of administration. Quetiapine is extensively metabolized by the liver microsomal enzyme system, and dosage adjustments must be made for patients with liver dysfunction as well as elderly patients; no adjustments are necessary in renal failure.

IV. Neuromuscular blockade (NMB)

A. **NMB** is currently used in about 10% of ICU populations to facilitate endotracheal intubation and mechanical ventilation, control intracranial pressure (ICP), for procedures, and to decrease tension of the abdominal wall.

1. **Mechanical ventilation.** Despite adequate sedation and analgesia, NMB may be needed so the patient can tolerate mechanical ventilation and gas exchange can be improved through eliminating dysynchrous breathing, instituting inverse-ratio ventilation, and increasing chest wall compliance.

2. **Endotracheal intubation** can be facilitated in the ICU with NMB. Caution should be exercised with the use of succinylcholine (see section **IV.C.1**).

3. **Elevated intracranial pressure (ICP)** can increase the morbidity associated with neurologic injury. Administration of NMB has been demonstrated to prevent rises in ICP associated with tracheobronchial suctioning.

4. **Procedures/diagnostic studies** such as tracheostomy, percutaneous endoscopic gastrostomy (PEG), bronchoscopy, and placement of central venous access may be expedited with the use of NMB.

B. **Complications of NMB** include awareness, delay in diagnoses, and prolonged muscular weakness.

1. **Awareness.** Monitoring the level of awareness and sedation in ICU patients is difficult because the typical signs of agitation and pain are lost and clinicians must depend on autonomic signs of inappropriate sedation, which can be blocked by medication. The use of the Bispectral Index may at least provide some objective indication that a patient is adequately sedated during NMB, although data to conclusively support this are absent.

2. **Prolonged weakness** may result from the use of neuromuscular blockers in concert with the cumulative effects of inflammatory disease, critical illness neuropathy, critical illness myopathy, deconditioning, and corticosteroids (see Chapter 30).

3. **Physical examination** of a patient under neuromuscular blockade is limited and may delay the diagnoses of new-onset neurologic abnormalities (e.g., inability to detect focal neurologic changes) and abdominal processes (absence of guarding).

C. **Neuromuscular blocking agents**

1. **Succinylcholine** is primarily used to facilitate endotracheal intubation. It is contraindicated in patients

with denervation and crush injuries, burns, and immobility/deconditioning because of the risk of hyperkalemia secondary to the activation of postjunctional receptors. One cannot underestimate the risk in giving succinylcholine to patients who have been in the ICU for prolonged periods. Hyperkalemic cardiac arrests have occurred following the administration of succinylcholine to patients who have received the drug uneventfully only a short time previously.

2. **Cisatracurium** is a benzylisoquinoline that is useful for critically ill patients because it is metabolized by Hofmann elimination, which is independent of organ function. A useful starting dose is 0.15 mg/kg followed by an infusion titrated to effect.

3. **Vecuronium and pancuronium** are steroidal drugs that have been implicated in muscular weakness more than the benzylisoquinolines. These drugs are metabolized in the liver to metabolites with neuromuscular blocking properties that are eliminated by the kidney. Their action is prolonged with renal insufficiency. Infusions of pancuronium may result in profound paralysis secondary to a "channel block" of the acetylcholine receptor. The initial bolus dose is 0.1 mg/kg for vecuronium and 1 mg/kg for pancuronium.

D. **Monitoring** of neuromuscular blockade is via the response of the adductor pollicis muscle to simulation of the ulnar nerve with a train-of-four pattern. Unfamiliarity of the nursing staff with the technique, improperly placed electrodes, cold extremities, neuropathy, and edema will contribute to inaccurate assessments. The response of the orbicularis oculi to facial nerve stimulation may be useful in edematous patients.

E. **Reversal** of NMB with neostigmine/glycopyrrolate or edrophonium/atropine is preferable to spontaneous recovery for patients in the immediate postoperative period. Partial paralysis in an awaking patient is associated with anxiety, hypertension, tachycardia, and insufficient respiratory efforts.

SELECTED REFERENCES

Eli EW, Shintani A, Truman B, et al. Delirium as a predictor of mortality in mechanically ventilated patients in the intensive care unit. *JAMA* 2004;291:1753–1762.

Frazer GL, Prato BS, Riker RR, et al. Frequency, severity, and treatment of agitation in young versus elderly patients in the ICU. *Pharmacotherapy* 2000;20:75–82.

Jacobi J, Fraser GL, Coursin DB, et al. Clinical practice guidelines for the sustained use of sedatives and analgesics in the critically ill adult. *Crit Care Med* 2002;30:119–141.

Kress JP, Pohlman AS, O'Connor MF, et al. Daily interruption of sedative infusions in critically ill patients undergoing mechanical ventilation. *N Engl J Med* 2000;342:1471–1477.

Larsson L, Xiaopeng L, Edstrom L, et al. Acute quadriplegia and loss of muscle myosin in patients treated with non-depolarizing neuromuscular blocking agents and corticosteroids: mechanisms at the cellular and molecular levels. *Crit Care Med* 2000;28:34–45.

Ramsay MA, Savege TM, Simpson BR, et al. Controlled sedation with alphaxalone-alphadolone. *Br Med J* 1974;2:656–659.

Segredo V, Caldwell JE, Mathhay MA, et al. Persistent paralysis in critically ill patients after long-term administration of vecuronium. *N Engl J Med* 1992;327:524–528.

Sessler CN, Gosnell MS, Grap MJ, et al. The Richmond Agitation-Sedation Scale. Validity and reliability in adult intensive care unit patients. *Am J Respir Crit Care Med* 2002;166:1338–1344.

Simmons LE, Riker RR, Prato BS, et al. Assessing sedation during intensive care unit mechanical ventilation with the Bispectral Index and the Sedation-Agitation Scale. *Crit Care Med* 1999;27:1499–1504.

Venn RM, Grounds RM. Comparison between dexmedetomidine and propofol for sedation in the intensive care unit: patient and clinician perceptions. *Br J Anaesth* 2001;87:684–690.

Fluids, Electrolytes, and Acid-Base Status

David T. Liu and David Steele

Optimal management of fluids, electrolytes, and acid-base status in critically ill patients requires a general understanding of their normal composition and regulation. Disease processes, trauma, and surgery can all affect the manner by which the body controls its fluid balance and electrolytes.

I. **Fluid compartments.** There are multiple fluid compartments in the body, separated by semipermeable membranes and structures.
   A. **The total body water (TBW)** ranges from 50% to 70% of the body mass and is determined by lean body mass, gender, and age (Table 7-1). There is an inverse relationship between TBW and percentage body fat due to the low water content of adipose tissues.
   B. **Compartments of TBW**
      1. The **intracellular** compartment is approximately 66% of TBW (approximately 40% of body mass).
      2. The **extracellular** compartment is approximately 34% of TBW (approximately 20% of body mass), and can be further divided:
         a. The **intravascular** compartment is comprised of plasma, and is approximately 5% of total body mass.
         b. The **extravascular** compartment is comprised of lymph, interstitial fluid, bone fluid, fluids of the various body cavities, and mucosal/secretory fluids. The extravascular compartment represents approximately 15% of total body mass.
   C. **Ionic composition of the fluid compartments.** Various physiologic terms describe the concentrations of ions in a solution:
      1. **Molarity:** moles of solute per liter of solution.
      2. **Molality:** moles of solute per kilogram of solvent.
      3. **Osmolarity:** osmoles per liter of solution. The number of osmoles is determined by multiplying the number of moles of solute by the number of freely dissociated particles from one molecule of solute. For example, 1 mole of NaCl will yield 2 osmoles (Osm) in solution.
      4. **Osmolality:** osmoles per kilogram of solvent.
      5. **Electrical equivalence:** moles of ionized substance multiplied by its valence. For example, **1 mole of calcium is equal to 2 equivalents in solution.** For a calcium solution to be electrically neutral, it has to combine with 2 moles of opposite charge, such as chloride.

Table 7-1. Total body water as a percentage of body weight (%)

	Male	Female
Thin	65	55
Average	60	50
Obese	55	45
Neonate		75–80
First year		65–75
Ages 1–10 years		60–65
Ages 10 years to adult		50–60

6. Electrolytes in physiology are generally described in terms of milliequivalents per liter (mEq/L). The fluids of each compartment are electrically neutral. Average concentrations of each electrolyte in various compartments are given in Table 7-2.

   a. Serum osmolality (S_{osm}) can be estimated using the equation

   $$S_{osm}(mOsm/kg\ H_2O) =$$
   $$(2 \times [Na] + ([BUN]/2.8) + ([glucose]/18)$$

   with blood urea nitrogen (BUN) and glucose concentration expressed in mg/dl and sodium concentration expressed in mEq/L. In general, this estimate is within 10% of measured osmolality.

   b. In the setting of unequal distribution of nonpermeable proteins between compartments, the **Gibbs-Donnan effect** allows for unequal concentrations of small diffusible ions between the compartments.

Table 7-2. Fluid electrolyte composition of body compartments

		Plasma (mEq/L)	Interstitial (mEq/L H_2O)	Intracellular[a] (mEq/L H_2O)
Cations	Na	142	145	10
	K	4	4	159
	Ca	5	5	<1
	Mg	2	2	40
Anions	Cl	104	117	3
	HCO_3	24	27	7
	Proteins	16	<0.1	45
	Others	9	9	154

[a]Intracellular electrolytes are difficult to measure and most of the measurements are from myocytes, which might or might not be applicable to other cell types.

D. Movement of water in the body

1. Water is generally readily permeable through cell membranes and moves freely throughout the different fluid compartments. Movement of water is largely determined by **osmotic pressure** and **hydrostatic pressure.** The osmotic pressure is dependent on the number of osmotically active molecules in the solution and is much greater than hydrostatic pressure. In normal states, all fluid compartments are essentially iso-osmolar. Water diffuses down an osmotic gradient to keep the extracellular and intracellular milieu iso-osmolar.

2. The movement of water between extracellular interstitial and intravascular compartments is described by **Starling's equation:**

$$Q_f = K_f \left[(P_c - P_i) - \sigma(\pi_c - \pi_i) \right]$$

where Q_f is the fluid flux across the capillary membrane, K_f is a constant, P_c and P_i are the hydrostatic pressures in the capillary and the interstitium, respectively, σ is the *reflection coefficient* (see later discussion), and π_c and π_i are the colloid osmotic pressures in the capillary and interstitium, respectively.

   a. Large, negatively charged intravascular proteins to which vascular membranes are impermeable are responsible for the osmotic pressure gradient between intravascular and interstitial compartments. This component of osmotic pressure, known as the **oncotic pressure** or **colloid osmotic pressure,** contributes a small amount to the total osmotic pressure of the fluids. The positive ions that are associated with the negatively charged proteins also contribute to the osmotic pressure. **Albumin** is the predominant type of protein responsible for the oncotic pressure, accounting for approximately two-thirds of the total oncotic pressure. Cells do not contribute to the oncotic pressure.

   b. The **reflection coefficient** σ describes the permeability of a substance through a specific capillary membrane. Its value ranges from 0 (completely permeable) to 1 (impermeable), and varies in different disease states; it is approximately 0.7 in healthy tissues.

   c. **Basic dynamics at the capillary.** Fluids exit the capillary at the arteriolar end, where the hydrostatic pressure is greater than the oncotic pressure. This increases the oncotic pressure of the plasma. As the plasma flows down the capillary, the hydrostatic pressure dissipates. Toward the venous end of the capillary, fluid is reabsorbed because the oncotic pressure is greater than the hydrostatic pressure. Perturbations in this balance can lead to increased interstitial fluid. **Edema** occurs when the rate of interstitial fluid accumulation is greater than the rate of removal of interstitial fluids by the lymphatic system.

II. **Fluid deficits and replacement therapy**

A. **Fluid volume deficits** and appropriate fluid therapy are dependent on the source and type of fluid loss. Because all membranes are permeable to water, fluid deficits in one compartment will affect all other compartments. Fluid losses can be broadly classified based on the initial source of loss. Fluid losses also lead to electrolyte abnormalities.

1. **Intracellular fluid (ICF) compartment** deficits arise from **free water loss.**

   a. **Sources of free water loss** include
      (1) **Insensible losses** through skin and respiratory tract.
      (2) **Renal losses** secondary to inability to recollect water, such as in neurogenic or nephrogenic diabetes insipidus (see section **III.C**).

   b. With free water loss, intracellular and extracellular volumes both decrease in proportion to their volumes in the body; therefore, two-thirds of the loss will be intracellular. Similarly, **free water replacement** will be distributed in proportion to their volumes in the body, and only one-third of the administered free water will end up in the extracellular space.

   c. Therapy includes replacement of water with either **hypotonic saline** (5% dextrose in water with 0.45% sodium chloride solution) or **free water** (5% dextrose in water). Electrolytes (especially sodium) must be monitored with therapy.

2. **Extracellular fluid (ECF) compartment** deficit

   a. In general, ECF losses are isotonic. Losses may occur in each compartment, and fluid losses from one are rapidly reflected in others.

   b. Clinical manifestations include the following:
      (1) From 3% to 5%: dry mucous membranes and oliguria
      (2) From 6% to 10%: tachycardia and orthostatic hypotension
      (3) From 11% to 15%: hypotension
      (4) Greater than 20%: anuria and circulatory collapse

   c. **Causes of ECF losses** include **blood loss, vomiting, diarrhea,** and **distributional changes.**
      (1) **Distributional change** of ECF volume is due to the transudation of isotonic fluids from a functional interstitial fluid compartment to a nonfunctional compartment. This results in intravascular volume depletion. Examples include tissue injury from surgery or trauma ("third spacing"), burn injuries, ascites

Table 7-3. Composition of crystalloid solutions

	Na	Cl	K	Ca	Buffer	Dextrose	pH	Osmolarity
D5W	0	0	0	0	0	5	4.5	252
D5 0.45% NaCl	77	77	0	0	0	5	4.0	406
0.9% NaCl	154	154	0	0	0	0	5.0	308
7.5% NaCl	1283	1283	0	0	0	0	5.0	2567
Lactated Ringer's	130	109	4	3	28[a]	0	6.5	273

Na, Cl, K, Ca, and buffer concentrations are in mEq/L; dextrose is g/100 ml.
D5W, 5% dextrose in water; D5 0.45% NaCl, 5% dextrose in water with 0.45% sodium chloride solution.
[a]Lactate.

> formation, fluid accumulation inside an obstructed bowel, and pleural effusions.
>
> **(2) Replacement** of ECF volume loss usually requires isotonic salt solutions. Volumes required to replace ECF deficits can vary considerably among patients based on the inciting event and comorbid processes.

3. Intravascular fluid (plasma volume) deficit

   a. Intravascular volume deficits will lead to interstitial fluid depletion as the two compartments equilibrate.

   b. Manifestations include the following:

   (1) From 15% to 30% of intravascular volume: sinus tachycardia while supine.

   (2) Greater than 30% loss of intravascular volume: decreased arterial blood pressure, decreased central venous pressures.

B. Fluid replacement therapy

   1. Crystalloid solutions (Table 7-3)

   a. Maintenance fluids are used to replace constitutive losses of fluids and electrolytes.

   (1) Insensible water losses include normal losses by skin and lungs, and total approximately 600 to 800 ml/d. **Sensible losses** of water include losses from the kidney and gastrointestinal (GI) tract. The obligate minimal urine output is 0.3 ml/kg/h and the average urine output is 1 ml/kg/h in an average 70-kg person (approximately 1,700 ml/d).

   (2) Electrolytes. Daily loss of sodium is approximately 1 to 2 mEq/kg. Daily loss of chloride and potassium is approximately 1 to 1.5 mEq/kg. A total of 1 mEq/kg of each electrolyte should be replaced each day.

   (3) Glucose supplement as a caloric source should range from 100 to 200 mg/kg/h. However, glucose should not be a routine part of replacement fluids in critically ill patients because of the potential metabolic and neurologic imbalances caused by its rapid administration. Enteral or parenteral nutrition provides the needed dietary glucose (see Chapter 9).

(4) General guidelines for hourly maintenance fluid replacement based on body weight
  i. 0 to 10 kg: 4 ml/kg/h
  ii. 11 to 20 kg: 40 ml + 2 ml/kg/h for each kg above 10 kg
  iii. >20 kg: 60 ml + 1 ml/kg/h for each kg above 20 kg

(5) Maintenance fluid composition. In general, **hypotonic maintenance fluids** are used to replace insensible losses. Additional losses from other sources are often present in critically ill patients (e.g., through drains, fistulas, etc.) and require **isotonic fluid repletion.**

b. For **ECF repletion,** isotonic solutions are used.

(1) Because electrolytes are permeable through capillary membranes, crystalloids will rapidly redistribute from the intravascular compartment throughout the entire ECF, in the normal distribution of 75% extravascular to 25% intravascular.

(2) 0.9% sodium chloride (normal saline) contains sodium and chloride (both 154 mEq/L) and has an osmolarity of 308 mOsm/L and a pH of 5.0. Thus, normal saline is hypertonic and more acidic than plasma. Normal saline has a high chloride content and can cause hyperchloremic acidosis.

(3) Lactated Ringer's solution (LR) contains sodium (130 mEq/L), potassium (4 mEq/L), calcium (3 mEq/L), chloride (109 mEq/L), and lactate (28 mEq/L). LR has an osmolarity of 272.5 mOsm/L and a pH of 6.5. LR is slightly hypotonic. It does not cause hyperchloremia.

c. Isotonic crystalloid solutions can be used to replace volume deficits from **blood loss.** Replacement volumes of 2 to 5 ml of isotonic solution are infused per 1 ml of blood loss.

2. Colloid Solutions (Table 7-4). Colloid solutions are most commonly used for intravascular volume expansion. Unlike crystalloid solutions, the colloid elements do not freely cross intact capillary membranes and therefore do not redistribute as readily into the entire ECF compartment. In general, it takes two to six times less colloid solutions than crystalloid solutions to achieve the same level of intravascular volume expansion.

a. Albumin is a natural blood colloid and the most abundant plasma protein. Albumin infusions can maintain plasma oncotic pressure and hence may

Table 7-4. Physiologic and chemical characteristics of colloid solutions

Fluid	Weight–Average Molecular Weight (kd)	Oncotic Pressure (mm Hg)	Serum Half-Life (h)
5% Albumin	69	20	16
25% Albumin	69	70	16
6% Hetastarch	450	30	2–17

be more effective than crystalloid in expanding intravascular volume. However, the use of albumin as a means of expanding intravascular volume has been shown to have an equivalent effect as crystalloids on the outcome of critically ill patients. **5%** (5 g/dl) and **25%** (25 g/dl) **albumin** solutions are commercially available. They are prepared in isotonic saline, with the 25% albumin preparation in small volumes (called "salt-poor" due to the relatively lower salt load). The oncotic pressure of 5% albumin is similar to that of plasma. Twenty-five percent albumin has a higher oncotic pressure, and can expand plasma volume by four to five times of infused volume. Twenty-five percent albumin is reserved for mobilizing edema fluid, although the efficacy of this therapy is not proven.

   b. Hetastarch is a high-molecular-weight synthetic colloid (hydroxyethyl starch, branched glucose polymers). Hetastarch is available in the United States as 6% solution in normal saline **(Hespan)** and in LR **(Hextend).** The oncotic pressure of these preparations is approximately 30 mm Hg. The increased plasma oncotic pressures after infusion can last for 2 days. Side effects include elevation in serum amylase, anaphylactoid reactions, and coagulopathy. Use of hetastarch in coagulopathic states is controversial, but to decrease the risk of possible coagulopathy, it is recommended that the maximum dose be 20 ml/kg/d.

  3. Transfusions of blood and blood components are important for maintaining the oxygen-carrying capacity of blood and for coagulation. A detailed discussion of transfusions as a part of fluid management can be found in Chapter 10.

III. Electrolytes and electrolyte abnormalities: sodium

  A. The normal range of serum (plasma) sodium concentration is 136 to 145 mEq/L. Abnormalities in serum sodium suggest abnormalities in both water and sodium balance. The adult requirement for sodium ranges from **1 to 2 mEq/kg/d.** The requirement is higher in infants. The kidneys of healthy individuals precisely control sodium balance by excreting the exact amount of intake (range 0.25 to 6+ mEq/kg/d). This process is modulated by neurohumoral systems, including the renin-angiotensin-aldosterone system, atrial natriuretic peptide, antidiuretic hormone, parathyroid hormone (PTH), and the sympathetic nervous system.

B. **Hyponatremia** is defined by a serum sodium of less than 136 mEq/L. Severe hyponatremia can cause central nervous system (CNS) and cardiac abnormalities, such as seizures and dysrhythmias. Hyponatremia can be classified based on concomitant plasma tonicity.

1. **Isotonic hyponatremia** (approximately 290 mOsm/kg H_2O) occurs when there are elevated levels of other ECF constituents such as protein and lipids. This form of hyponatremia is also known as **pseudohyponatremia** and is an artifact of measurement due to lipid and protein displacement of volume for a given volume of plasma. Therapy for this hyponatremia is not required.

2. **Hypertonic hyponatremia** is due to the movement of intracellular water into the extracellular fluid compartment under the influence of **osmotically active substances** (e.g., glucose, mannitol) with consequent dilution of ECF sodium. A common example of hypertonic hyponatremia is seen with **hyperglycemia**, which can decrease serum sodium concentration by approximately 1.6 mEq/L for each 100 mg/dl of blood glucose. Removal of the osmotically active etiologic substance and restoration of volume are goals of therapy.

3. **Hypotonic hyponatremia** is the most common form of hyponatremia. This true type of hyponatremia is due to higher TBW relative to total body sodium. Hypotonic hyponatremia is further classified based on the extracellular fluid volume status (hypovolemic, hypervolemic, and isovolemic). In all three scenarios, the extracellular compartment volume status does not always correlate with the intravascular or effective arterial volume status.

a. **Hypovolemic hypotonic hyponatremia** can result from renal or nonrenal sources. In either case, water and salt are lost, but the loss of sodium is larger than the loss of water.

(1) Renal causes include the use of diuretics (particularly thiazide diuretics), mineral corticoid deficiency, hypothyroidism, and, rarely, renal salt-wasting nephropathy, cerebral salt wasting, and certain types of renal tubular acidosis.

(2) Nonrenal causes include fluid losses from the GI tract and intravascular volume depletion via third spacing.

(3) Renal and nonrenal causes can be distinguished by urine electrolytes. A urine sodium of greater than 20 mEq/L suggests a renal

source, whereas a urine sodium of less than 10 mEq/L suggests a nonrenal etiology.

(4) **The goal of therapy is to replace extracellular volume with isotonic sodium solutions** and to allow for appropriate renal free water excretion.

b. **Hypervolemic hypotonic hyponatremia** is associated with congestive heart failure (CHF), renal failure, and cirrhosis.

(1) Mechanism: in these disease processes, the effective *arterial* intravascular volume is low even if the *total* intravascular volume is normal or increased. The activation of the renin-angiotensin-aldosterone system and the sympathetic nervous system, and the release of antidiuretic hormone (ADH) lead to oliguria and salt retension. The result is expansion of ECF volume.

(2) Manifestations include edema, elevated jugular venous pressures, pleural effusions, and ascites.

(3) The goal of therapy is to control the primary disease process. Fluid and salt restriction and the use of proximal and loop diuretics may also be appropriate.

c. **Isovolemic hypotonic hyponatremia**

(1) Causes: syndrome of inappropriate ADH secretion (SIADH), psychogenic polydypsia, medications (e.g., opiates, oxytocin, carbamazepine, chemotherapeutics, nonsteroidal antiinflammatory agents), physiologic nonosmotic stimulus for ADH release (e.g., nausea, anxiety, pain), hypothyroidism, and adrenal insufficiency.

(2) Despite an absence of volume deficit or osmotic stimuli, ADH is increased, which causes an increase in free water retention.

(3) Therapy depends on the primary cause and the clinical presentation. In general, treatment involves water restriction. In some cases, **demeclocycline** is used to induce a nephrogenic diabetes insipidus to balance the effect of the excess ADH secretion.

d. **General guidelines for managing hypotonic hyponatremia.** Normal saline should be used for patients who are hypovolemic or who have hyponatremia induced by diuretic use. If the patient is euvolemic, treatment will vary depending on presentation. Often, euvolemic patients are best treated with water restriction. Hypervolemic patients are treated with diuretics along with free water restriction.

e. **Urgent intervention is required** in patients with symptomatic hyponatremia (nausea, vomiting, lethargy, altered level of consciousness, and seizures). The sodium deficit can be calculated from

$$\text{Sodium deficit} = \text{TBW} \times (140 - [\text{Na}]_{serum})$$

The rate of correction of the serum sodium is important and must be tailored to the individual patient. Both delayed and rapid correction can be associated with neurologic injury. Controlled correction can generally be achieved with **hypertonic saline** (3% NaCl) in euvolemic patients and with infusion of normal saline in hypovolemic patients. The rate of infusion should result in a correction of serum sodium of 1 to 2 mEq/L per hour for the first 24 hours or until serum sodium reaches a level of 120 mEq/L and then be reduced to a correction rate of 0.5 to 1 mEq/L per hour.

C. **Hypernatremia** is defined by serum sodium of greater than 145 mEq/L. Hypernatremia is also a description of total body sodium content relative to total body water and can exist in hypovolemic, euvolemic, and hypervolemic states. In all cases, the serum is hypertonic. Clinical manifestations of hypernatremia include tremulousness, irritability, spasticity, confusion, seizures, and coma. Symptoms are more likely to occur when the rate of change is rapid. When the change is gradual and chronic, cells in the central nervous system will increase the cellular osmolality, thereby preventing cellular water loss and dehydration. This process starts approximately 4 hours after the onset and stabilizes in 4 to 7 days. This change in CNS cellular osmolality is an important concept when considering therapy.

1. **Hypovolemic hypernatremia**
   a. Caused by the loss of hypotonic fluids through extrarenal (e.g., excessive sweating and osmotic diarrhea) or renal (e.g., osmotic diuresis and drug-induced) sources. There is loss of water and salt, with a greater proportion of water loss, which results in a decrease in the ECF volume and the effective arterial intravascular volume.
   b. It is recommended that isotonic saline be used for initial volume repletion, followed by hypotonic crystalloid solutions, such as 0.45% normal saline.

2. **Euvolemic hypernatremia**
   a. Caused by the loss of free water through extrarenal (e.g., excessive insensible loss through skin or respiration) or renal (e.g., diabetes insipidus) sources.
   b. Measuring urine osmolality (Uosm) is important. Extrarenal processes cause a high Uosm (>800 mOsm/kg H_2O), whereas renal processes cause a low Uosm (approximately 100 mOsm/kg H_2O).
   c. In most cases of hypernatremia from free water loss, the intravascular and extracellular fluid **volumes appear normal.**
   d. Therapy involves replacement of free water.

e. **Central** and **nephrogenic diabetes insipidus (DI;** see also Chapter 27) are among the renal causes of euvolemic hypernatremia. Evaluation of Uosm and the response to ADH may help to determine the site of the lesion.

(1) **Central (neurogenic) DI** can be caused by pituitary damage from tumor, trauma, surgery, granulomatous disease, and idiopathic causes. Central DI is treated with desmopressin (intranasal, 5–10 μg daily or twice daily).

(2) **Nephrogenic DI** can be caused by severe hypokalemia with renal tubular injury, hypercalcemia, chronic renal failure, interstitial kidney disease, and drugs (e.g., lithium, amphotericin, demeclocycline). Therapy includes correcting the primary cause if feasible, and possibly free water repletion.

3. **Hypervolemic hypernatremia** is caused by addition of excess sodium and usually results from the infusion or intake of solutions with high sodium concentration. The acute salt load leads to intracellular dehydration with extracellular fluid expansion, which can cause edema or CHF. The goal of therapy is to remove the excess sodium; this can be accomplished by using non–medullary gradient disrupting diuretics (e.g., thiazides).

4. **Free water deficit** and correction of hypernatremia

$$\text{Free water deficit} = \text{TBW} \times \{1 - (140/[\text{Na}])\}$$

The correction of hypernatremia should occur at approximately 1 mEq/L/h. Roughly one-half of the calculated water deficit is administered during the first 24 hours and the rest over the following 1 to 2 days. Aggressive correction is dangerous, especially in chronic hypernatremia, where rapid correction can cause cerebral edema. Rapid correction is reasonable if the hypernatremia is acute (<12 hours). Neurologic status should be carefully monitored while correcting hypernatremia, and the rate of correction should be decreased if there is any change in neurologic function.

IV. **Electrolyte abnormalities: potassium**

A. In an average adult, the total body potassium is approximately 40 to 50 mEq/kg. Most of the potassium is in the intracellular fluid compartment. In general, intake and excretion of potassium are matched. **Average daily intake is approximately 1 to 1.5 mEq/kg.** Although the serum potassium is used as a marker for total body potassium, potassium can have dynamic transcellular redistribution depending on the acid-base status, tonicity, and levels of insulin and catecholamines. The **ECG** is useful in diagnosing true potassium imbalance because the level of polarization of an excitable cell and the ability for repolarization are determined by the extracellular and intracellular potassium concentrations.

B. **Hypokalemia:** serum potassium concentration of less than 3.5 mEq/L. A general rule is that a 1 mEq/L decrease in serum potassium represents approximately a total body potassium deficit of 200 to 350 mEq.

1. **Causes** of hypokalemia
   a. Transcellular redistribution:
      (1) **Alkalemia** (a 0.1 to 0.7 mEq/L change per 0.1-unit change in pH).
      (2) Increased circulating **catecholamines.**
      (3) Increased **insulin.**
   b. Renal-associated causes:
      (1) Depletion of total body potassium from excessive renal excretion due to diuretics and osmotic diuresis.
      (2) Hypomagnesemia.
      (3) Hyperaldosteronism.
      (4) Renal artery stenosis.
      (5) Renal tubular acidosis.
      (6) High-dose penicillins.
   c. Acute leukemias.
   d. Excessive GI losses:
      (1) Secretory diarrhea, villous adenoma.
      (2) Emesis.
   e. Dietary deficiency.
   f. Lithium toxicity.
   g. Hypothermia.

2. **Manifestations** of hypokalemia include myalgias, cramps, weakness, paralysis, rhabdomyolysis, urinary retention, ileus, and orthostatic hypotension. **Electrocardiogram (ECG) manifestations,** in order of progression of worsening hypokalemia, are decreased T-wave amplitude, prolonged QT interval, U wave, dragging of ST segment, and increased QRS duration. **Arrhythmias** are also common, including atrial fibrillation, premature ventricular beats, supraventricular tachycardia, junctional tachycardia, and Mobitz type I second-degree atrioventricular block (Wenckebach).

3. **Therapy** of hypokalemia. **Intravenous potassium replacement** is appropriate in patients who have severe hypokalemia or who cannot take oral preparations. The rate of replacement should be governed by the clinical signs. The recommended maximal rate of infusion is 0.5 to 0.7 mEq/kg/h, with continuous ECG monitoring. Oral potassium preparations include immediate-release and slow-release preparations. Serum potassium levels should be monitored carefully during repletion. Potassium-sparing diuretics are sometimes used to treat renal losses of potassium. **Hypomagnesemia** should be corrected prior to potassium repletion (see section **V.C**).

C. **Hyperkalemia:** serum potassium of greater than 5.5 mEq/L.

1. **Causes** of hyperkalemia
   a. Hemolysis of sample.
   b. Leukocytosis (white blood cell count >50,000/mm^3).
   c. Thrombocytosis (platelet count >1,000,000/mm^3).
   d. Transcellular redistribution:
      (1) Acidemia.
      (2) Insulin deficiency.
      (3) Drugs (digitalis, β-blockers, succinylcholine).
   e. Malignant hyperthermia.
   f. Cell necrosis (rhabdomyolysis, hemolysis, burns).
   g. Increased intake via replacement therapy and transfusions.
   h. Decreased renal potassium secretion
      (1) Renal failure.
      (2) Hypoaldosteronism.
      (3) Diminished distal renal tubule sodium.
      (4) Drugs, including heparin, angiotensin-converting-enzyme inhibitors, and potassium-sparing diuretics (spironolactone, amiloride, triamterene).
2. **Manifestations** of hyperkalemia include muscle weakness and cardiac conduction disturbances. **ECG changes** include atrial and ventricular ectopy (serum potassium between 6 and 7 mEq/L), decreased QT, and peaked T waves. Worsening hyperkalemia will lead to loss of P waves, widening of the QRS complex, and eventual merging of the widened QRS complex with the T wave, leading to ventricular fibrillation.
3. **Therapy** for hyperkalemia is emergent for any level of hyperkalemia with ECG changes, and particularly when the serum potassium concentration is greater than 6.5 mEq/L. Continuous ECG monitoring is recommended.
   a. **Calcium chloride** or **calcium gluconate** should be given to stabilize the cellular membrane and to decrease excitability of the cells. Calcium does not have an effect on the extracellular potassium. The duration of calcium therapy is approximately 60 minutes, so repeat dosing may be necessary.
   b. Emergency measures to shift extracellular potassium intracellularly and thereby restore the polarized state of the cell include the use of **sodium bicarbonate** and **insulin with glucose** (1 U of intravenous [IV] insulin for 2 g of dextrose).
   c. Total body potassium can be reduced by using loop diuretics (e.g., **furosemide**) or exchange resins such as sodium polystyrene sulfonate (**kayexalate** either orally [PO] or rectally; time for effect orally is 120 minutes and rectally is 60 minutes).
   d. **Hemodialysis** should be initiated if hyperkalemia is not controlled adequately with these measures.
V. **Electrolyte abnormalities: calcium, phosphorus, and magnesium**

A. Calcium acts as a key signaling element for many cellular functions and is the most abundant electrolyte in the body (see also Chapter 27). Most of the calcium is stored in bone. The intestine and kidney play crucial roles in maintaining calcium balance. After entry, calcium equilibrates into exchangeable pools in blood, bone, and soft tissues. In the extracellular fluid, calcium is ionized (approximately 50%), bound to protein (approximately 40%), or chelated by anions (approximately 10%). The non–protein-bound calcium is filtered in the glomerulus, with 98% reabsorbed. The ionized form is the physiologically active form. The intracellular concentration of calcium is approximately 1,000-fold lower than the extracellular calcium. Normal values of total serum calcium range from 8.5 to 10.5 mg/dl (4.5 – 5.5 mEq/L). However, because calcium is bound to protein (approximately 40%), the appropriate range of total serum calcium that can provide for adequate ionized calcium is dependent on the total serum calcium and the amount of serum protein (with the predominant protein species being albumin). The **ionized calcium** provides a better functional assessment, with normal values ranging from 4 to 5 mg/ dL (2.1 – 2.6 mEq/L or 1.05 – 1.3 mmol/L). Ionized calcium can be affected by the pH of the serum, with acidemia leading to higher ionized calcium and alkalemia to lower ionized calcium. Modulators of calcium homeostasis include PTH and 1,25 vitamin D, which increase calcium levels, and calcitonin, which decreases calcium levels.

1. **Hypercalcemia:** defined as total serum calcium of greater than 10.5 mg/dL or ionized calcium of greater than 5.0 mg/dL (2.6 mEq/L or 1.29 mmol/L).

   a. **Causes** of hypercalcemia (see also Chapter 27)
      (1) Primary hyperparathyroidism.
      (2) Immobilization.
      (3) Malignancy:
          i. Direct bone invasion.
          ii. Paraneoplastic syndromes.
      (4) Granulomatous diseases (tuberculosis, sarcoidosis), secondary to increased 1,25 vitamin D production by the granulomatous tissue.
      (5) Thyrotoxicosis.
      (6) Primary bone reabsorption/formation abnormalities (Paget's disease).
      (7) Adrenal insufficiency.
      (8) Pheochromocytoma.
      (9) Milk-alkali syndrome, caused by daily high intake of calcium (>5 g/d) and alkali.
      (10) Drugs (thiazides, vitamin D, lithium, estrogens).

   b. **Diagnosis**
      (1) PTH levels: low in malignancy-associated hypercalcemia, high in primary, secondary, and tertiary hyperparathyroidism.
      (2) 1,25 Vitamin D levels: elevated in granulomatous disease.

   (3) Parathyroid hormone–related protein: ele-
        vated in malignancy-associated hypercalcemia
        (breast, lung, thyroid, renal cells).
   (4) Serum protein electrophoresis: monoclonal
        band associated with myeloma.
   (5) Thyroid-stimulating hormone (TSH).
   (6) Chest radiographs to evaluate for malignancy
        and granulomatous disease.
   c. Manifestations of hypercalcemia include GI symp-
        toms (vomiting, nausea, constipation, cramps),
        arthralgias, weakness, bone pain, lethargy, change
        in mental status, and, in severe cases, shock and
        coma. Hypercalcemia can also cause hyperten-
        sion and arrhythmias. ECG abnormalities include
        shortened QT interval, increased PR and QRS
        intervals, T-wave flattening, and atrioventricular
        block. Polyuria and dehydration also occur due to
        an inability of the kidneys to concentrate urine.
   d. Treatment should be initiated if neurologic symp-
        toms are present, total serum calcium is greater
        than 12 to 13 mg/dL, and the calcium/phosphate
        product is greater than 75. Primary treatment
        should be directed at correcting the underling
        cause.
   (1) Immediate therapy is **hydration** with normal
        saline to restore volume status and decrease
        serum calcium concentration by dilution.
   (2) After establishing euvolemia, normal saline
        should be used in combination with a loop di-
        uretic, with the goal of generating a **urine out-
        put** of 3 to 5 ml/kg/h. For example, for severe
        hypercalcemia, 2 to 3 L of normal saline can be
        given over 3 to 6 hours along with 20 to 40 mg
        of IV **furosemide** every 2 to 4 hours.
   (3) Other electrolytes should be carefully moni-
        tored and repleted as indicated.
   (4) Hemodialysis should be considered if rehy-
        dration and diuretic therapy is ineffective or
        if the patient cannot tolerate such therapies
        (e.g., in patients with renal failure or CHF).
   (5) In addition to rehydration, osteoclast in-
        hibitors such as **pamidronate** (60–90 g IV
        over 4 hours, one dose every 7 days), **calci-
        tonin** (4 IU/kg IV every 12 hours for four
        doses), and **plicamycin** (25 μg/kg IV over 4 to
        6 hours for 3 to 4 days) may be useful. **Gluco-
        corticoids** may be useful if the hypercalcemia
        is secondary to certain types of malignancies
        (e.g., lymphoma), sarcoidosis, or vitamin D in-
        toxication. **Calcium-channel blockers,** such
        as verapamil, can also be used to treat the car-
        diotoxic effects of hypercalcemia.
2. Hypocalcemia: defined as ionized calcium of less
    than 4 mg/dL (0.96 mmol/L).
    a. Causes of hypocalcemia (see also Chapter 27).

(1) **Sequestration of calcium:** can be caused by hyperphosphatemia (from renal failure), pancreatitis, intravascular citrate (from packed red blood cells), ethylenediaminetetraacetic acid (EDTA) administration, and alkalemia.

(2) **PTH deficiency:** can be caused by surgical excision of parathyroid gland, autoimmune parathyroid disease, amyloid infiltration of parathyroid gland, severe hypermagnesemia, hypomagnesemia, human immunodeficiency virus (HIV) infection, and hemachromatosis.

(3) **PTH resistance:** due to congenital abnormality or secondary to hypomagnesemia.

(4) **Vitamin D deficiency:** caused by malabsorption or poor nutritional intake, liver disease, anticonvulsants (phenytoin), inadequate sunlight, and renal failure.

(5) **Inappropriate calcium deposition:** can be due to formation of complex with phosphorus in hyperphosphatemic states (rhabdomyolysis); calcium deposition in the setting of acute pancreatitis; bone deposition in hungry bone syndrome post-parathyroidectomy.

(6) **Sepsis** and **toxic shock syndrome.**

b. **Manifestations** of hypocalcemia include generalized excitable membrane irritability leading to paresthesias and progressing to tetany and seizures. The classic physical exam findings include **Trousseau's sign** (spasm of the upper extremity muscles that causes flexion of the wrist and thumb with the extension of the fingers; can be elicited by occluding the circulation to the arm) and **Chvostek's sign** (contraction of ipsilateral facial muscles elicited by tapping over the facial nerve at the jaw). ECG changes include prolonged QT and heart block.

c. **Diagnosis**

(1) Confirm true hypocalcemia by checking ionized calcium and pH.

(2) Rule out hypomagnesemia.

(3) Check PTH level; if it is low or normal, hypoparathyroidism may be involved; if it is high, check serum phosphorus level. A low phosphorus level is indicative of pancreatitis or vitamin D deficiency, whereas a high phosphorus level suggests rhabdomyolysis and renal failure.

d. **Therapy** of hypocalcemia: infusion of calcium at 4 mg/kg of elemental calcium with either **10% calcium gluconate** (93 mg of calcium/10 ml) or **10% calcium chloride** (272 mg of calcium/10 ml). A bolus should be followed by an infusion because the bolus will increase the ionized form of calcium for 1 to 2 hours. Patients on digoxin may require ECG monitoring. To avoid precipitation of calcium salts, **IV calcium solutions should not be mixed**

with IV bicarbonate solutions. Calcium chloride is caustic to peripheral veins and should be given via central venous access if possible. Suspected vitamin D or PTH deficiency is treated with calcitriol ($0.25\ \mu g$ up to $1.5\ \mu g$ PO once a day). Oral calcium repletion with at least 1 g of elemental calcium a day should be given together with vitamin D therapy.

B. **Phosphorus** exists mainly as a free ion in the body. Phosphorus equilibrates in various tissues and bone pools. Approximately 0.8 to 1 g of phosphorus is excreted in the urine per day. Phosphorus excretion is affected by PTH (which inhibits proximal and distal nephron phosphorus reabsorption), vitamin D, high–dietary-phosphorus intake, cortisol, and growth hormone.

1. **Hypophosphatemia** occurs in approximately 10% to 15% of hospitalized patients.

   a. **Causes**
      (1) **GI:** malnutrition, malabsorption, vitamin D deficiency, diarrhea, and use of aluminum-containing antacids.
      (2) **Renal losses:** primary hyperparathyroidism, post renal transplantation, ECF expansion, use of diuretics (acetazolamide), Fanconi's syndrome, post obstructive diuresis, post acute tubular necrosis (ATN), and glycosuria/diabetic ketoacidosis (DKA).
      (3) **Redistribution:** alkalosis, post alcohol withdrawal, parenteral hyperalimentation, burns, and continuous venovenous hemofiltration.

   b. **Clinical symptoms** usually occur when phosphorus is less than 1.0 mg%.
      (1) Neurologic: metabolic encephalopathy.
      (2) Muscular: myopathy, respiratory failure, cardiomyopathy.
      (3) Hematologic: hemolysis, white blood cell dysfunction.

   c. **Diagnosis**
      (1) Urinary phosphorus less than 100 mg/d implies GI losses.
      (2) Urinary phosphorus greater than 100 mg/d suggests renal wasting.
      (3) Elevated serum calcium suggests hyperparathyroidism.
      (4) Elevated PTH suggests primary or secondary hyperparathyroidism or vitamin D–resistant rickets.

   d. **Treatment**
      (1) Increase oral intake to 1,000 mg/d.
      (2) Give 450 mg of elemental phosphorus per 1,000 kcal of hyperalimentation.
      (3) Dose of IV phosphorus should not exceed 2 mg/kg (0.15 mmol/kg) of elemental phosphorus.

2. **Hyperphosphatemia**
   a. **Causes**

(1) **Renal:** decreased glomerular filtration rate (GFR), increased tubular reabsorption, hypoparathyroidism and pseudohypoparathyroidism, acromegaly, thyrotoxicosis.

(2) **Endogenous:** tumor lysis, rhabdomyolysis.

(3) **Exogenous:** vitamin D administration, phosphate enemas.

b. **Clinical symptoms** are related to hypocalcemia due to calcium phosphate deposition and decreased renal production of 1,25 vitamin D.

c. **Treatment**

(1) Use of phosphate binders to reduce GI absorption.

(2) Volume expansion and dextrose 10% in water with insulin may reduce acutely elevated phosphorus levels.

(3) Use of hemodialysis and peritoneal dialysis.

C. **Magnesium:** Serum magnesium is maintained between 1.8 and 2.3 mg/dL (1.7–2.1 mEq/L); 15% is protein bound.

1. **Hypermagnesemia** is rare in patients with normal renal function unless large amounts of magnesium are given.

a. **Causes**

(1) Acute and chronic renal failure.

(2) Magnesium administration: $MgSO_4$ for toxemia of pregnancy, magnesium-containing antacids and laxatives.

b. **Signs and symptoms**

(1) Cardiac dysrhythmias.

(2) Decreased neuromuscular transmission.

(3) CNS dysfunction: confusion, lethargy.

(4) Hypotension.

(5) Respiratory depression.

(6) Death at higher levels.

c. **Treatment**

(1) Adverse effects of hypermagnesemia are antagonized by IV calcium.

(2) Hemodialysis to remove magnesium in renal failure.

2. **Hypomagnesemia** is defined as serum magnesium below 1.8 mg/dL.

a. **Causes**

(1) GI:

i. Decreased intake (chronic alcoholism).

ii. Starvation.

iii. Magnesium-free enteral feedings.

iv. Decreased GI intake due to nasogastric suction and malabsorption.

(2) Increased renal losses:

i. Diuretic therapy.

ii. Post obstructive diuresis.

iii. Recovery (polyuric phase) from ATN.

iv. DKA.

v. Hypercalcemia.

          vi. Primary hyperaldosteronism.

          vii. Barter's syndrome.

          viii. Aminoglycoside, cisplatin, and cyclosporine nephrotoxicity.

    (3) Manifestations

        (a) Hypomagnesemia causes hypokalemia and hypocalcemia; hypokalemia is the result of excess urine losses, which can only be corrected with magnesium repletion.

        (b) ECG changes mimic hypokalemia.

        (c) Digoxin toxicity is magnified by hypomagnesemia.

        (d) Neuromuscular fasciculations with Chvostek's and Trousseau's sign may be present.

    (4) Treatment for hypomagnesemia should be initiated when ECG changes and/or tetany are present.

        (a) IV: with $MgSO_4$, 6 g in 1 L of 5% dextrose in water over 6 hours.

        (b) PO: with magnesium oxide, 250 to 500 mg four times a day.

VI. Standard approach to acid-base physiology. The normal extracellular hydrogen ion (H^+) concentration is 40 nEq/L (one-millionth the milliequivalent-per-liter concentrations of sodium, potassium, and chloride). Maintenance of acid-base homeostasis depends on the presence of buffers. The standard approach to acid-base balance is based on the bicarbonate buffer system:

$$H^+ + HCO_3^- \Leftrightarrow H_2CO_3 \Leftrightarrow H_2O + CO_2$$

Although other buffers are present in the plasma (e.g., H^+ + Protein$^-$ ⇔ HProtein and other fixed acids), the bicarbonate buffer is the most significant because the acid and the conjugate base can be regulated by the lungs and kidneys, respectively. The H_2CO_3 species is in equilibrium with dissolved CO_2; therefore, the **Henderson-Hasselbalch equation** to describe weak acids and its conjugate base is as follows:

$$pH = 6.1 + \log \{[HCO_3^-]/(0.03 \times Paco_2)\}$$

where $Paco_2$ is the arterial partial pressure of carbon dioxide. Because pH = –log[H], the equation can be rearranged to

$$[H^+] = 24 \times (Paco_2/[HCO_3^-])$$

and used to calculate the bicarbonate for a specific $Paco_2$ at a specific pH. The hydrogen ion concentration can be quickly estimated when the pH is near 7.4 by adding or subtracting 10 nEq/L per change in 0.1-pH units from 40 nEq/L. Although buffers maintain acid-base homeostasis in the short term, compensatory changes in CO_2 and bicarbonate are responsible for continued maintenance of pH. Basic aspects of simple acid-base disorders and compensatory changes are included in Table 7-5, and the

Table 7-5. Simple acid-base disorders and compensatory changes

Disorder	Mechanism	Primary Disturbance	Compensation	Compensatory Change
Metabolic acidosis, pH <7.37	H^+ retention or production; HCO_3^- loss	↓ HCO_3^- from 24 mEq/L	↓ $PaCO_2$	$\Delta PaCO_2 = 1.2 \times \Delta HCO_3^-$
Metabolic alkalosis, pH >7.43	HCO_3^- retention or production; H^+ loss	↑ HCO_3^- from 24 mEq/L	↑ $PaCO_2$	$\Delta HCO_3^- = 0.7 \times \Delta PaCO_2$
Respiratory acidosis, pH <7.37	$PaCO_2$ retention	↑ $PaCO_2$ from 40 mm Hg	↑ HCO_3^-	Acute: $\Delta HCO_3^- = 0.1 \times \Delta PaCO_2$; $\Delta pH = 0.08/10$ mm Hg $\Delta PaCO_2$ Chronic: $\Delta HCO_3^- = 0.4 \times \Delta PaCO_2$; $\Delta pH = 0.03/10$ mm Hg $\Delta PaCO_2$
Respiratory alkalosis, pH >7.43	Excessive $PaCO_2$ reduction	↓ $PaCO_2$ from 40 mm Hg	↓ HCO_3^-	Acute: $\Delta HCO_3^- = 0.2 \times \Delta PaCO_2$; $\Delta pH = 0.08/10$ mm Hg $\Delta PaCO_2$ Chronic: $\Delta HCO_3^- = 0.5 \times \Delta PaCO_2$; $\Delta pH = 0.03/10$ mm Hg $\Delta PaCO_2$

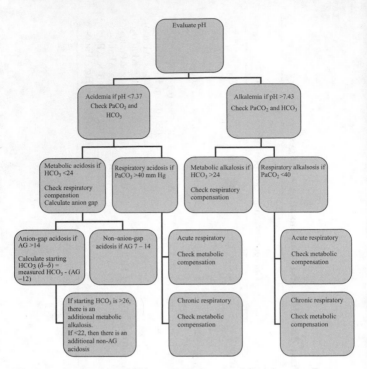

Fig. 7-1. **Approach to acid-base disturbances.** AG, anion gap; $Paco_2$, arterial partial pressure of carbon dioxide.

approach to an acid-base disturbance is shown in Fig. 7-1. In general, the pH, $Paco_2$, and bicarbonate are used to determine the primary disorder. The adequacy of compensation is then determined (see Table 7-5). If there is inadequate compensation, then there is likely to be a mixed acid-base disturbance.

A. Metabolic acidosis causes a primary decrease in serum bicarbonate due to one of three mechanisms: (a) a strong acid is generated either by endogenous production or by exogenous intake/administration and is buffered by bicarbonate; (b) bicarbonate is lost from the GI tract or is underproduced or lost by the kidney; and (c) there is ECF dilution due to high-dose administration of non–bicarbonate-containing IV fluids (large infusions of normal saline). Metabolic acidoses are classified as anion-gap and non–anion-gap types (Table 7-6).

    1. Anion-gap metabolic acidosis: The anion gap is based on the presence of unmeasured anions and is calculated as $Na - (Cl^- + HCO_3^-)$, with normal values between 7 and 14 mEq/L. **Albumin** is the largest constituent of the unmeasured anions. If albumin is low, the presence of other unmeasured anions, such as

Table 7-6. Classification of metabolic acidoses

Anion-gap metabolic acidosis
Endogenous
  Diabetic ketoacidosis; severe ketoacidosis (alcohol, starvation);
    uremia; lactate
Exogenous
  Toxins
    Ethylene glycol, methanol, salicylate

Non–anion-gap metabolic acidosis
Gastrointestinal losses
  Diarrhea; pancreatic, biliary, and enterocutaneous fistulas;
    ostomies
  Ureterosigmoidostomy
Infusion and ingestion of chloride-containing salts: total
  parenteral nutrition; cholestyramine
Renal tubular acidosis (RTA)
  Distal RTA
  Proximal RTA
  Type IV RTA
Metabolic acidosis of renal failure

---

lactic acid, will be falsely low based on the calculated anion gap. If the albumin concentration is less than 4 g/dl, the normal anion-gap range should be corrected by subtracting 2.5 mEq/L for every 1 g/dl of albumin below 4 g/dl.

  a. **Lactic acidosis** occurs when there is inadequate tissue O_2 delivery.
      (1) **Causes:** septic, cardiogenic, and hypovolemic shock, seizures.
      (2) **Treatment.** The primary goal is to restore tissue perfusion. Bicarbonate therapy may not be effective because it produces only a transient rise in pH and causes increased local CO_2 production, which may exacerbate intracellular acidemia. Bicarbonate therapy may also reduce endogenous hepatic lactate utilization. However, in severe acidemia small amounts of sodium bicarbonate are often infused to maintain arterial pH above 7.20.

  b. **Diabetic keto-acidosis** (DKA; see Chapter 27). Insulin deficiency and glucagon excess lead to hepatic production of ketoacids. Administration of insulin stops ketoacid production. DKA is treated with IV infusion of insulin and saline to replace fluid losses from the glycosuria-driven osmotic diuresis. Again, small amounts of bicarbonate are often infused intravenously to maintain arterial pH above 7.20.

  c. **Starvation ketosis.** Ketones are present in serum and urine. Treatment includes refeeding and correction of associated metabolic and electrolyte abnormalities such as hypophosphatemia and hypokalemia.

d. **Alcoholic ketoacidosis.** This condition is caused by chronic alcoholism and binge drinking. Serum alcohol and lactate levels are increased. Treatment should include saline, glucose with 100 mg of thiamine, and IV phosphorus.

e. **Salicylate intoxication** (see Chapter 31). Manifestations include respiratory alkalosis secondary to stimulation of the respiratory center and metabolic acidosis secondary to interference with oxidative metabolism.

f. **Ethylene glycol ingestion** (see Chapter 31). Ingestion of this toxin, a component of automobile antifreeze, causes renal failure. Patients present with an anion and osmolar gap and calcium oxalate crystals in the urine.

g. **Methanol ingestion** (see Chapter 31). This produces an acidosis with an elevated anion gap and osmolar gap.

2. **Non–anion-gap metabolic acidosis.** The **urine anion gap (UAG)** is a useful tool in the differential diagnosis of non–anion-gap acidosis:

$$UAG = (Na_{urine} + K_{urine}) - Cl_{urine}$$

UAG is negative if the cause of the acidosis is nonrenal (e.g., GI losses) and the unaccounted-for cation in the urine is NH_4^+. UAG is positive if the cause of the acidosis is renal in origin.

a. **Nonrenal non–anion-gap acidosis**

(1) **Metabolic acidosis associated with GI losses.** Bicarbonate wastage and consequent non–anion-gap metabolic acidosis are frequently seen with diarrhea, ileus, enterocutaneous fistulae, ostomies, laxative abuse, and villous adenoma of the rectum. Therapy includes bicarbonate replacement. In patients with volume contraction and avid renal sodium retention, decreased distal renal sodium delivery may impair the ability of the distal nephron to excrete hydrogen ions. Thus, volume repletion is also crucial.

(2) **Ureterosigmoidostomy.** The diversion of urine through intestinal segments can cause a non–anion-gap metabolic acidosis, hypokalemia, and occasionally hypocalcemia and hypomagnesemia. Given the frequency of these abnormalities when urine is diverted into the sigmoid colon, urinary diversions are now preferentially done with ileal conduits (which has a lower frequency of causing hyperchloremic acidosis).

b. **Renal tubular acidosis (RTA)**

(1) **Type 1 RTA**

   i. **Mechanisms:** direct impairment of apical membrane H^+/ATPase and decreased ability to excrete protons distally; increased permeability of the apical membrane or tight intercellular junctions to protons allowing hydrogen ions backdiffusion; or decreased Na absorption in principal cells, which may result in a reduction in luminal electronegativity and impede hydrogen ions excretion in adjacent intercalated cells.
   ii. **Diagnosis:** positive UAG, urine pH greater than 5.5, percentage filtered bicarbonate excreted less than 10, low serum potassium, and possible nephrocalcinosis and nephrolithiasis.
   iii. **Therapy:** bicarbonate replacement (1–2 mEq/kg/24 h) and potassium supplements.
(2) **Type 2 (proximal) RTA**
   i. **Mechanism:** impaired **proximal bicarbonate** reabsorption with transient bicarbonate loss in urine.
   ii. **Diagnosis:** UAG is an unreliable measure due to the presence of additional anion (bicarbonate) in the urine, urine pH less than 5.5, percentage filtered bicarbonate greater than 15, low serum potassium. If it is associated with a generalized tubular absorption disorder, urine phosphate, amino acids, and glucose are present (Fanconi's syndrome).
   iii. **Therapy:** high doses of bicarbonate (10–25 mEq/kg/24 h), aggressive potassium supplementation, and calcium and vitamin D supplementation.
(3) **Hyperkalemic (type IV) RTA**
   i. **Mechanisms:** selective aldosterone deficiency (common in patients with type 1 and type 2 diabetic nephropathy) and hyporeninemic hypoaldosteronism. This RTA is frequently encountered in patients with tubulointerstitial disease with mild to moderate renal insufficiency.
   ii. **Diagnosis:** positive UAG, urine pH less than 5.5, percentage filtered bicarbonate less than 10, high serum potassium.
   iii. **Therapy:** exchange resins (kayexalate) for hyperkalemia (which will also enhance ammonium excretion and hence acid secretion), and loop diuretics.
(4) **Renal failure**
   i. **Mechanism of generating acidosis.** With nephron loss, net acid excretion is maintained by increased ammonium production per functioning nephron; however,

when GFR falls below 30 to 40 ml/min, ammonium production falls below the level required to excrete the daily acid load. The retained acid (hydrogen ions) is buffered in the ECF by bicarbonate and in the tissues by cells and bone, and bicarbonate levels fall concomitantly.

    ii. **Therapy.** Oral sodium bicarbonate (650 mg PO twice to three times daily; 30–45 mEq bicarbonate) to maintain a serum bicarbonate level of greater than 20 mEq/L may be appropriate to reduce the adverse effects of prolonged acidosis (muscle wasting and bone demineralization).

B. Metabolic alkalosis

  1. Causes

    a. GI losses. There are proton losses from the upper GI tract due to nasogastric suctioning and vomiting.

    b. Diuretics. These cause a contraction alkalosis and chloride and potassium wasting, which disturb normal renal handling of protons and bicarbonate. **Contraction alkalosis** refers to the reduction in ECF volume around a fixed quantity of bicarbonate as is seen when diuretics cause ECF depletion by the excretion of bicarbonate-free urine.

    c. Hyperaldosteronism generates a metabolic alkalosis by increasing distal hydrogen ions excretion.

    d. Other

      (1) Post hypercapneic alkalosis.

      (2) Hypokalemia by cellular translocation of protons.

      (3) Bicarbonate or citrate administration.

  2. Metabolic alkalosis may be characterized based on urine chloride concentrations and responsiveness to chloride infusion (either as NaCl or as KCl).

    a. Chloride-unresponsive metabolic alkaloses are due to endogenous overproduction of aldosterone or mineralocorticoid derivatives.

    b. Chloride-responsive metabolic alkaloses are reversible with chloride repletion, and a number of factors play a role in the maintenance of an established chloride-responsive metabolic alkalosis:

      (1) Effective circulating volume depletion.

      (2) Chloride depletion and a low urine chloride.

      (3) Potassium depletion.

C. Respiratory acidosis is a primary increase in $PaCO_2$ due to inadequate excretion of CO_2. Increased CO_2 results in increased carbonic acid production that is buffered by tissue buffers. Renal compensation results in a net increase in bicarbonate production. Full compensation usually takes more than 24 hours.

D. Respiratory alkalosis is a primary decrease in $PaCO_2$ that usually results from alveolar hyperventilation. The alkalemia is buffered with intracellular protons. Renal compensation over a period of days causes a net excretion of bicarbonate. Clinical manifestations are perioral parasthesia, muscle cramps and hyperreflexia, seizures, and cardiac arrhythmias.

E. **Mixed acid-base disorders.** In contrast to emergency room and operating room patients (who generally start out with a normal acid-base status), critically ill patients frequently develop multiple acid-base abnormalities over time, of different and coexisting etiologies. The diagnosis of mixed acid-base disturbances highlights the need for a systematic approach to the analysis of acid-base disorders. Historical information should be sought, including drug and toxin exposure and the use of medications, such as diuretics, that may affect acid-base homeostasis. The presence of underlying disease of major organ systems such as cardiac, pulmonary, hepatic, or renal disease should be considered. The presence of diarrhea and the use of parenteral nutrition are examples of other relevant information. Laboratory data should include electrolytes, BUN and creatinine, urine electrolytes, the anion gap, and arterial blood gas. Whereas the ratios of pH, $PaCO_2$ and bicarbonate vary in a fixed way in simple acid-base disorders (see Table 7-5), these ratios do not behave according to these properties in mixed acid-base disturbances. The following general rules must be considered.

1. **Overcompensation does not occur** in primary disorders. Therefore if the change in ratio of $PaCO_2$ to bicarbonate or of bicarbonate to $PaCO_2$ is out of the ranges outlined in Table 7-5, a mixed acid-base disorder is present.

2. **A low** bicarbonate is due to either a primary acidosis or respiratory alkalosis. A bicarbonate of less than 15 mEq/L is usually due to a metabolic acidosis.

3. **An elevated bicarbonate** is due either to metabolic alkalosis or respiratory acidosis. A bicarbonate of greater than 40 mEq/L is usually due to a metabolic alkalosis.

4. **Severe acidemia can result from a combination** of metabolic and respiratory acidosis in which $PaCO_2$ and bicarbonate may not be markedly abnormal, but the pH may be very low.

5. **In mixed metabolic acidosis and respiratory alkalosis,** bicarbonate and $PaCO_2$ are both reduced, and the $PaCO_2$ will be lower than predicted based on the expected respiratory compensation for metabolic acidosis.

6. **Mixed metabolic acidosis and alkalosis** primarily affects bicarbonate; pH, and bicarbonate may be high, low, or normal; an elevated anion gap suggests an underlying anion-gap acidosis; vomiting is a frequent component of this mixed disorder.

7. **Combined metabolic alkalosis and respiratory acidosis** occurs with a high bicarbonate and $PaCO_2$.

The elevation in bicarbonate will be greater than predicted for primary compensation of a respiratory acidosis. This disorder is frequently seen in patients with a combination of pulmonary and cardiac disease who are on diuretics.

8. **Mixed metabolic and respiratory alkalosis causes a severe alkalemia;** a mixed disorder of this type is noted when a respiratory alkalosis is not accompanied by an appropriate decrease in bicarbonate or metabolic alkalosis is not accompanied by an appropriate increase in $PaCO_2$; mechanical ventilation and diuretic use often underlie this disorder.

9. **A triple acid-base disorder** with metabolic acidosis and alkalosis and either respiratory acidosis or alkalosis can be seen in alcoholic or diabetic patients who present with lactic acidosis or ketoacidosis, vomiting, and respiratory alkalosis due to sepsis or cirrhosis.

VII. **Physicochemical systems approach to acid-base physiology**

A. Although changes in bicarbonate can be used as an indicator of nonrespiratory acid-base disturbance, changes in bicarbonate are not primary, but instead result from the cumulative effects of multiple processes, both metabolic and respiratory. Therefore, the standard approach to acid-base analysis requires the calculation of compensation, the anion gap, subsequent manipulation of the anion gap in states of low or high weak acids, and starting bicarbonate $(\Delta - \Delta)$ calculations to reveal all the acid-base disturbances found in the system. However, an alternative method is to first define the system, all its components, and the interactions of the components. The components that can be primarily and individually affected are independent variables, and the components of the system that are changed due to changes in the independent variables are the dependent variables. The **Stewart physicochemical model** for acid-base physiology dissects and describes mathematically the determinants of acid-base balance in aqueous solutions. The system is based on three independent variables, (a) the **strong ion difference (SID)**, (b) the **total weak acids (A_{tot}),** and (c) the **$PaCO_2$,** and the constraints set by the law of mass action (in the form of equilibrium constants), the law of mass conservation, and maintenance of electroneutrality in solution. Other changes in the system, including changes in hydrogen ions and bicarbonate, are the result of changes in one or more of the independent variables.

1. **SID.** Strong ions are from compounds that can fully dissociate with an equilibrium dissociation constants K greater than 10^{-4} (acids) or less than 10^{-12} (bases) in solution. The SID is the difference between the sum of concentrations of all strong cations and all strong anions: $SID = [Na] + [K] + [Ca] + [Mg] - [Cl] - [other strong anions]$. In normal conditions, other strong anions do not exist, and the contributions of Ca and Mg

are minimal; therefore, SID is [Na] + [K] − [Cl] and is approximately equal to 40 mEq/L.

    2. A_{tot}. Weak acids are compounds that are partially dissociated at body pH, with equilibrium dissociation constants between 10^{-4} and 10^{-12}. These include proteins (albumin being the predominant species in plasma), sulfates, and phosphates.

    3. $Paco_2$. Dissolved plasma CO_2 is regulated by ventilation.

B. With the system defined, one can evaluate the independent variables to determine the type of acid-base disturbance present. The following rules apply.

    1. Metabolic alkalosis

        a. Low A_{tot}: secondary to low albumin from nephrotic syndrome and cirrhosis.

        b. High SID: from chloride loss secondary to vomiting, villous adenoma, or increased Na from hyperaldosteronism, Barters syndrome, and Na load from total parenteral nutrition.

    2. Metabolic acidosis

        a. Low SID due to increased chloride or decreased sodium.

        b. High A_{tot} due to increases in albumin or phosphates.

    3. With **metabolic acidosis,** one can calculate the **strong ion gap (SIG),** which is the difference between the apparent strong ion difference ($SID_a = [Na^+] + [K^+] − [Cl^-]$) and the effective strong ion difference ($SID_e = [HCO_3^-] + [A^-]$, where $[A^-] = 2.8 \times$ [albumin (in g/dl)] + $0.6 \times$ [phosphorus (in mg/dl)]. If SIG is greater than 0 mEq/L, then there are elevated unaccounted-for anions accounting for the acidosis (e.g., lactic acid, ketones, formate, methanol, and salicylates); if SIG is zero, then the acidosis is due to Cl^- retention (secondary to RTA, rapid saline infusion, and anion exchange resins).

    4. Respiratory disturbances are similarly described by the traditional method, which relies on the independent variable $Paco_2$.

C. The Stewart model is controversial. Proponents feel that complex acid-base disorders are easier to understand, explain, and rationalize using the Stewart model and that the Stewart model is mathematically valid. Detractors suggest the model adds little clinically and increases complexity.

SELECTED REFERENCES

Adrogue HJ, Madias NE. Management of life-threatening acid-base disorders. First of two parts. *N Engl J Med* 1998;338(1):26–34.

Adrogue HJ, Madias NE. Management of life-threatening acid-base disorders. Second of two parts. *N Engl J Med* 1998;338(2):107–111.

Adrogue HJ, Madias NE. Hypernatremia. *N Engl J Med* 2000;342: 1493–1499.

Adrogue HJ, Madias NE. Hyponatremia. *N Engl J Med* 2000;342: 1581–1589.

Choi PT, Yip G, Quinonez LG, et al. Crystalloids vs. colloids in fluid resuscitation: a systematic review. *Crit Care Med* 1999;27:200–210.

Fencl V, Leith DE. Stewart's quantitative acid-base chemistry: applications in biology and medicine. *Respir Physiol* 1993;91:1–16.

Finfer S, Bellomo R, Boyce N, et al. A comparison of albumin and saline for fluid resuscitation in the intensive care unit. *N Engl J Med* 2004;350:2247–2256.

Greenberg A, Cheung AK, National Kidney Foundation. *Primer on kidney diseases,* 2nd ed. San Diego, CA: Academic Press, 1998.

Jones NL. A quantitative physicochemical approach to acid-base physiology. *Clin Biochem* 1990;23:189–195.

Maxwell MH, Kleeman CR, Narins RG. *Maxwell & Kleeman's Clinical disorders of fluid and electrolyte metabolism,* 5th ed. New York, McGraw-Hill, 1994.

Rose BD, Rennke HG. *Renal pathophysiology: the essentials*. Baltimore: Williams & Wilkins, 1994.

Tinker JH, Morgan GE, Longnecker DE. *Principles and practice of anesthesiology,* 2nd ed. St. Louis, MO: Mosby, 1998.

8

Hemodynamic Management

Stacey Remchuk, Keith Baker,
and Luca Bigatello

I. **Management** of patients who are hemodynamically unstable requires treatment in the intensive care unit (ICU), where they can receive appropriate monitoring and resuscitative measures. The goal of hemodynamic management is to preserve end-organ perfusion and function. Lack of appropriate therapy will lead to tissue hypoperfusion, cellular damage, multiple-organ-system dysfunction, and death. The correct understanding of hemodynamic monitoring is key to optimal hemodynamic management.

II. **Hypotension and shock** is a syndrome of decreased tissue perfusion resulting in cellular damage. Initially, neurohumoral compensatory mechanisms help to maintain perfusion to vital organs. If appropriate supportive treatment is not promptly instituted, these compensatory mechanisms are overwhelmed and progressive tissue ischemia leads to organ failure. Clinical signs of end-organ hypoperfusion include oliguria/anuria, mental status changes, and acidemia. Shock is classified on the basis of its cause and characteristic hemodynamic pattern.

A. **Types of shock**

1. **Hypovolemic shock** is caused by an acute volume loss equal to or greater than 20% to 25% of the circulating blood volume. Causes of hypovolemic shock include hemorrhage, and sequestration of fluid within the body, such as in bowel obstruction. Hypovolemic shock is characterized by decreased blood pressure (BP), decreased cardiac output (CO), decreased central venous pressure (CVP), and decreased pulmonary artery pressure (PAP).

2. **Cardiogenic shock** is caused by primary failure of the heart to generate an adequate CO. It can be failure of the left ventricle, right ventricle, or both. The most common cause of cardiogenic shock is myocardial infarction and its acute complications (see Chapter 17), ventricular dysrhythmias, myocarditis, cardiac contusion, and proximal aortic dissection. Physiologic presentation of cardiogenic shock includes hypotension, a low CO despite adequate volume status, elevated PAP and PA occlusion pressure (PAOP), and clinical signs of hypoperfusion.

3. **Distributive shock** is characterized by decreased vascular tone resulting in arterial vasodilatation, venous pooling, and redistribution of blood flow. It may be caused by live bacteria and their byproducts during **septic shock,** by mediators of the systemic inflammatory response syndrome (**SIRS**), by vasoactive

155

Table 8-1. Hemodynamic parameters in shock

Type of Shock	Systemic BP	CVP/PAOP	CO/SV
Hypovolemic	⇓	⇓	⇓
Cardiogenic	⇓	⇑	⇓
Distributive			
Septic	⇓	⇔	⇓
Anaphylactic	⇓	⇓	⇔
Neurogenic	⇓	⇓	⇔
Obstructive	⇓	⇑	⇓

We assumed for simplicity that the right and left sides of the heart are similarly affected by these conditions, thus moving the CVP and PAOP in the same direction. BP, blood pressure; CVP, central venous pressure; PAOP, pulmonary occlusion pressure; CO, cardiac output; SV, stroke volume.

compounds during **anaphylactic shock,** or by loss of vascular tone during **neurogenic shock** or adrenal apoplexy. Distributive shock is characterized by a low BP and high CO.

4. **Obstructive shock** is associated with a mechanical impediment to venous return and/or arterial outflow of the heart. Causes include tension pneumothorax, pulmonary embolism, pericardial tamponade, abdominal compartment syndrome and, occasionally, positive-pressure ventilation, positive end-expiratory pressure (PEEP), and auto-PEEP (see Chapter 3). Obstructive shock is characterized by decreased BP and CO with an elevated CVP. The hemodynamic presentation of the various types of shock is summarized in Table 8-1.

B. **The physiologic basis of shock** is the development of **tissue hypoperfusion** secondary to prolonged hypotension and/or decreased oxygen delivery. Tissue hypoperfusion leads to tissue hypoxia, anaerobic metabolism, and disruption of cellular integrity. Compensatory mechanisms initially help to maintain perfusion to vital organs, and they include the following:

1. **Neurohumoral responses:** increased sympathetic discharge, which enhances myocardial contractility and peripheral vasoconstriction, and release of stress hormones such as epinephrine, glucagon, aldosterone, cortisol, and antidiuretic hormone.

2. **Metabolic responses:** release of anti-insulin hormones (see prior discussion), which promotes insulin resistance, hyperglycemia, and lipolysis.

3. Release of **inflammatory mediators** causes muscle proteolysis, providing amino acids necessary to sustain protein synthesis essential for host defense (e.g., acute-phase reactants). This generalized catabolic state may cause muscle wasting, weakness, poor wound healing, loss of gastrointestinal mucosal integrity,

hypoalbuminemia, and anergy. Cellular injury can also be caused by tissue reperfusion when oxygen, local metabolites, and oxidative enzymes generate oxygen free radicals and other cytotoxic products.

C. **Signs and symptoms of individual organ dysfunction** secondary to inadequate end-organ flow include the following:

1. **Central nervous system:** altered mental status.
2. **Cardiac:** chest pain, ischemia on electrocardiogram (ECG), wall motion abnormalities on echocardiography, hemodynamic instability.
3. **Renal:** decreased urine output, increased blood urea nitrogen and serum creatinine concentration.
4. **Gastrointestinal:** abdominal pain and distension, decreased bowel sounds, and hematochezia.
5. **Periphery:** cool limbs, poor capillary refill, weak pulses.

D. **Monitoring**

1. **Standard monitors** include continuous ECG, pulse oximetry, noninvasive measurement of systemic blood pressure, urinary output, and core body temperature.
2. **Monitoring tissue perfusion.** Blood pressure measurement has been the foundation of assessing the adequacy of tissue perfusion (see Chapter 1). Patients with unstable hemodynamics should have an indwelling **arterial cannula** for pressure monitoring because it is the most reliable method for measuring BP (see Chapter 1). These patients will also frequently require **central venous access** for CVP monitoring and for delivery of vasoactive drugs. A **pulmonary artery (PA) catheter** allows for measurement of CO and assessment of volume status in the systemic and pulmonary circulation. However, traditional blood pressure monitoring is complex, is affected by variables other than the volume status of the circulation, and is a relatively insensitive method for assessing tissue perfusion (see Chapter 1). Additional monitoring methods are described in Chapter 2, and several metabolic indicators of the adequacy of tissue perfusion have been proposed as alternatives or as a complement to blood pressure monitoring (see Table 8-2):

   a. **Metabolic acidemia** may be a sign of anaerobic metabolism and definitely is an important sign of inadequate tissue perfusion. However, it is nonspecific and relatively late in its onset.
   b. **Serum lactate** is a measurable byproduct of anaerobic metabolism, hence a logical indicator of tissue hypoperfusion. Although a number of studies have suggested a direct correlation between the level of lactate in blood and the severity of shock, others have not, and its diagnostic/predictive value in individual patients is inconsistent.

Table 8-2. Clinical markers of tissue hypoperfusion and cellular dysfunction

Low arterial blood pressure and cardiac output, low urine output, decreased skin turgor, changes in mental status
Metabolic acidemia, base deficit, low serum bicarbonate
Increased serum lactate
Low intra gastric pH
Low mixed venous Po_2

c. **Mixed venous Po_2 (Pvo_2) or saturation (Svo_2)** is affected by the degree of tissue O_2 extraction. Hence, it could indicate an increased energy utilization or even a harmful **"oxygen debt."** However, changes in **Pvo_2** occur for other physiologic reasons, which are summarized in Table 8-3. To understand the clinical significance of a decreased Pvo_2, one has to measure **Pao_2** and **CO,** which requires invasive monitoring. Clinical studies are divided on the usefulness of Pvo_2 or Svo_2 as a tissue perfusion marker. However, a recent study of septic patients admitted to a large emergency department suggested that targeting the Svo_2 measured continuously via a central venous catheter (not strictly *mixed* because it is measured before full mixing of venous blood) may be of value in guiding initial resuscitation.

d. Gastric mucosal pH estimates the **intracellular pH (pH_i)** in the stomach by measuring the pCO_2 in a saline-filled balloon part of a special nasogastric (NG) tube. This pCO_2 should be in equilibrium with the pCO_2 gastric mucosa where the balloon sits. A pH value is then calculated through the Henderson-Hasselbach equation (see Chapters 3 and 7) using the arterial concentration of bicarbonate. The main shortcoming of this method is its high operator dependence, its predisposition to be affected by variables other than splanchnic perfusion, such as the use of acid secretion blockers, and its theoretical flaws, such as the use of the arterial as a surrogate of the gastric mucosal bicarbonate concentration.

Table 8-3. Determinants of mixed venous Po_2

Cardiac output
Pao_2
O_2 dissociation curve shift
Tissue O_2 consumption ($\dot{V}o_2$)

E. **Management of shock**
  1. **General measures** immediately undertaken include supportive therapies and diagnostic studies.
    a. Adequate **intravenous (IV) access** should be secured, including large-bore peripheral IV lines along with central access, with the goal to ensure rapid volume administration.
    b. **Evaluation of the airway** should be undertaken because endotracheal intubation and mechanical ventilation may be necessary due to hypoxemia, hypercarbia, airway edema, or altered mental status.
  2. **Volume replacement** is the cornerstone of treatment of hypotension and shock, particularly hypovolemic and distributive shock (see section **II.A**). Patients diagnosed with other types of shock also need evaluation and optimization of their fluid status. Appropriate volume replacement requires understanding of hemodynamics and the choice of the appropriate monitoring system (see Chapters 1 and 2). Unfortunately, no single parameter can be used to reliably guide volume resuscitation, as discussed in section **II.D.** Inadequate resuscitation may result in tissue hypoperfusion, whereas excessive volume replacement may lead to tissue edema, congestive heart failure, metabolic derangements, and coagulopathy.
    a. **Crystalloids.** The most commonly used crystalloid solutions are **lactated Ringer's** and **normal saline**. These solutions are nearly isotonic (see also Chapter 7), rapidly leave the intravascular space, and a volume equal to three to four times the intravascular deficit is required to restore circulating volume. The advantages of crystalloid solutions include low cost, easy storage, and availability. Dextrose-containing solutions should not be used for volume resuscitation because of the dangers of hyperglycemia (Chapter 27) and the difficulty of monitoring blood glucose levels closely during volume resuscitation. A small volume of **hypertonic saline** (3% NaCl) can replete the intravascular volume without significantly increasing the extravascular volume and may be useful in the resuscitation of patients with and patients without a head injury (see also Chapter 13).
    b. **Colloids** increase plasma oncotic pressure and maintain circulating volume longer than crystalloids. They include natural and synthetic solutions.
      (1) **Human albumin** is derived from pooled human plasma and is available as 5% and 25% solutions in normal saline. Heat treatment eliminates the risk of transmission of viral infections.
      (2) Allogenic blood products like packed **red blood cells** and **fresh-frozen plasma** are not recommended for pure volume expansion because of

their potential for transmission of viral disease (albeit low), immunosuppression, and their limited availability and high cost (see Chapter 10).

   (3) **Dextran** is a solution of synthetic glucose polymers of either 40 kd (D-40) or 70 kd (D-70). The main disadvantage of dextran is a high incidence of anaphylactic reactions (1%–5%). They have been almost entirely substituted by starch-based compounds (see later discussion).

   (4) **Hydroxyethyl starch (HES)** is a high-polymeric glucose compound available in various preparations and concentrations. Anaphylactoid reactions with HES are much less frequent than with the dextran-based solutions. HES has a dose-dependent effect on factor VIII levels, thus impairing platelet function. A maximum dose of 1,500 ml per 24 hours has been suggested to minimize negative side effects.

   c. There is no evidence to support that one type of fluid is better than another in the resuscitation of shock. Although several experimental studies have suggested the superiority of one solution over another in regard to specific outcomes, such as cell function, bowel edema, and gas exchange, the only large, prospective, and randomized trial of colloid (human albumin) versus crystalloid for volume resuscitation in a heterogeneous ICU population showed no advantage in using the colloid. Given the significant difference in cost, we recommend crystalloids as the main solution to use for general volume resuscitation.

3. **The "oxygen delivery/oxygen consumption" controversy**

   a. A series of studies conducted in the 1980s suggested that reaching a "supranormal" hemodynamic status (i.e., high filling pressures, high CO, and high oxygen delivery [$\mathbf{Do_2}$]) by aggressive volume resuscitation and use of inotropes improves the outcome of patients in shock. Furthermore, a subgroup of patients may have a "pathologic dependence" of oxygen consumption ($\dot{V}o_2$) on $\dot{D}o_2$, that is, the $\dot{V}o_2$ increases almost indefinitely as the $\dot{D}o_2$ is pharmacologically increased, indicating a "hidden oxygen debt" associated with a particularly high mortality.

   b. Subsequent investigations described major flaws of this theory and of the design of these clinical trials, and the enthusiasm for the "supranormal" resuscitation declined. However, recent studies conducted with more rigorous methodology suggest that aggressive, **early** resuscitation with volume and vasopressors of patients with septic shock and in candidates of major surgery may indeed improve outcome. Although controversy persists on whether it is necessary to reach "supranormal" values, these

studies underscore the importance of resuscitating patients in shock early and fully.
4. **Specific treatments**
   a. **Hypovolemic shock** mandates early and adequate volume resuscitation. Dilutional coagulopathy and hypothermia can accompany administration of larges volume of fluid or blood products.
   b. **Cardiogenic shock** is the result of acute, severe myocardial systolic dysfunction, most commonly due to an acute myocardial infarction. The mortality of this condition reaches 30% to 60%. Treatment of acute myocardial infarction and cardiogenic shock, including the use of intraaortic balloon counterpulsation **(IABP),** is described in Chapters 17 and 38.
   c. **Septic shock** is the result of an infection complicated by a severe systemic response to live bacteria, bacterial endotoxins, and products of inflammation, characterized by **hypotension** and signs of **organ system failure.** Hemodynamically, it is a classic example of distributive shock (see section **II.A.3**), with low vascular tone and high cardiac output. The mainstay of therapy is appropriate antibiotic administration, surgical drainage of accessible infections, and supportive measures to increase vascular tone and optimize tissue perfusion (see later discussion). Pathogenesis and treatment of septic shock, including specific therapies such as **corticosteroids** and **activated protein C,** are discussed in Chapter 11.
   d. **Anaphylactic shock** is an acute, immunoglobulin E (IgE)-mediated reaction that causes release of mediators from mast cells and basophils and occurs on reexposure to an antigen in previously sensitized individuals. Common causes of anaphylaxis include antibiotics and other drugs, radiographic contrast agents, and latex. Clinically, this syndrome includes vasodilatation and hypotension accompanied by flushing, urticaria, increased capillary permeability, airway edema, and bronchoconstriction. Treatment requires immediate identification and discontinuation of the suspected antigen, support of the circulation with volume and vasoactive drugs, and pharmacologic therapy directed at the immune mediators including **epinephrine,** the **histamine H_1-** and **histamine H_2-receptor blockers diphenhydramine** and **ranitidine,** and **corticosteroids.**
   e. **Obstructive shock** requires specific interventions depending on the cause. Tension pneumothorax is treated with needle decompression followed by tube thoracostomy (see Chapter 33). Abdominal compartment syndrome is treated with surgical decompression of the abdomen (see Chapter 33). Pulmonary embolism is treated with supportive care

and may involve the use of thrombolysis or surgical embolectomy; cardiac tamponade is treated with pericardiocentesis.

III. **Pharmacologic therapies of hypotension and shock.** When appropriate fluid replacement fails to restore adequate blood pressure and organ perfusion, vasopressor therapy must be initiated. Vasopressor therapy may also be required to maintain organ perfusion in the face of life-threatening hypotension even when a fluid challenge is in progress and hypovolemia has not yet been fully corrected. The appropriate drug is chosen based on the etiology and pathophysiology of the type of shock suspected in a given patient (Table 8-4).

A. **Inotropic agents** enhance cardiac contractility.

1. **Dopamine** is an immediate precursor of norepinephrine and epinephrine. At low doses, it affects vascular δ_1-dopamine receptors (renal and mesenteric) leading to vasodilation. At higher doses, it recruits β_1-adrenergic receptors associated with positive inotropic and chronotropic effects. At further high doses, it recruits α_1-adrenergic receptors associated with vasoconstrictive effects. Dopamine is frequently chosen as a first-line agent for shock because of its potentially beneficial effects on the renal circulation

Table 8-4. Commonly used inotropic and vasopressor agents

Drug	Target Receptor	Effects
Catecholamines		
Dopamine	$\delta, \beta_1, \alpha_1$	⇑CO, ⇑BP, ⇑HR, ⇑renal perfusion
Epinephrine	$\beta_1, \beta_2, \alpha_1$	⇑CO, ⇑BP, ⇑HR, bronchodilation
Norepinephrine	β_1, α_1	⇑BP, ⇑CO
Synthetic catecholamines		
Dobutamine	$\beta_1, \beta_2,$	⇑CO, ⇑HR, ⇔/⇓ BP
Dopexamine	δ, β_1, β_2	⇑CO, ⇑HR, ⇑renal perfusion
Ephedrine	$\beta_1, \beta_2, \alpha_1$	Like epinephrine, but less potent
Phenylephrine	α_1	⇑BP, ⇓HR ⇑/⇓/⇔CO
Phosphodiesterase-III inhibitors		
Milrinone	Cyclic GMP mediated	⇑CO, ⇑HR, BP ⇔/⇓
Hormones		
Vasopressin	G protein mediated	⇑BP

BP, blood pressure; CO, cardiac output; HR, heart rate.

and CO, but its predictable chronotropic and pro-dysrhythmic effects limit its use in patients with on-going or underlying myocardial ischemia.

2. **Dobutamine** also stimulates β-adrenergic receptors, but has no δ- and α-mediated effects. Hence, it enhances cardiac contractility and decreases vascular tone. The combination of these two effects makes dobutamine an excellent agent for the treatment of cardiogenic shock. Limitations to the use of dobutamine are its intrinsic vasodilator effect, which may cause systemic hypotension, and a moderate chronotropic effect.

3. **Dopexamine** is a synthetic derivative of dopamine with δ and β_2 greater than β_1 activity and no α activity, thus reducing the chronotropic and pro-dysrhythmic effects typical of dopamine. Dopexamine is not approved for clinical use in the United States, and its use in Europe is somewhat hindered by its high cost.

4. **Epinephrine** is a potent catecholamine that stimulates α-, β_1-, and β_2-adrenergic receptors. It is still a mainstay of cardiopulmonary resuscitation (see Chapter 14). Its effect on BP is due to a positive inotropic and chronotropic effect and to vasoconstriction in vascular beds, especially the skin, mucosae, and kidney. Its strong β_2 effect promotes bronchodilation and blocks mast-cell degranulation, making it the drug of choice for **anaphylaxis.** In adults, IV administration of 0.1 to 0.5 mg (0.1–0.5 ml of a 1:1,000 solution) of epinephrine is a common initial dose for the appropriate, severely hypotensive patient, followed by a continuous infusion of 1 to 4 μg/min.

5. **Norepinephrine** is also a catecholamine, with both α- and β-adrenergic activity. Its potent vasoconstrictive and inotropic effects make it the drug of choice in our ICU to treat hemodynamic instability in patients who require the support of both vascular tone and myocardial contractility. Typical examples are patients in septic shock who have some degree of preexistent or acute myocardial dysfunction. Compared to epinephrine, norepinephrine lacks β_2 activity.

6. **Phosphodiesterase-III (PDE-III) inhibitors. Amrinone** and **milrinone** exert their hemodynamic effects through the inhibition of PDE-III, which increases the availability of cyclic guanosine monophosphate (GMP) to the endothelium, thus increasing myocardial contractility and diastolic relaxation and decreasing vascular tone. These effects are useful in treating **systolic heart failure.** Intravenous infusions are started by a loading dose and followed by an infusion. Amrinone has been largely replaced by milrinone due to its shorter duration of action and easier titratability. Milrinone is administered as a load of 50 μg/kg followed by a continuous infusion of 0.25 to 1.0 μg/kg/min. Its elimination half-life is 30 to

60 minutes, compared to the 2 to 3 hours of amrinone. Hypotension and tachycardia are the main side effects that limit its use.

B. **Vasopressors**
   1. **Phenylephrine** is a selective α_1 agonist that causes pure arterial vasoconstriction. It rapidly increases BP, associated with a reflex bradycardia. It is a useful drug for treatment of pure and moderate vasodilatation, such as following the administration of potent hypnotic drugs or epidural local anesthetic or in the presence of a mild to moderate infection. Due to its rapid onset and ease of titration (it is not as potent as norepinephrine), phenylephrine is often used through peripheral IV access as a first line-treatment of hypotension to rapidly reestablish an adequate BP. However, the appropriateness of its use needs to be revised after stability has been achieved. Because of its pure vasoconstrictive effect, phenylephrine may be detrimental in patients with compromised left ventricular function.
   2. **Vasopressin (VP)** is a hormone synthesized in the hypothalamus and stored in the posterior pituitary. It is also known as **antidiuretic hormone (ADH)** and it is primarily involved in the osmotic and volume homeostasis as well as the regulation of other hormones (see Chapter 27). It is also a **direct vasoconstrictor** without inotropic or chronotropic effects. Recent studies have shown that hypovolemic and septic shock are associated with a biphasic VP response. Early, VP levels are appropriately high as the body releases all of its stored VP in an attempt to vasoconstrict and to hold on to sodium and water to defend blood pressure. As shock progresses, VP levels may fall for reasons that are unknown. Administration of low doses of VP ("replacement" therapy) in this subpopulation of patients with septic shock increases BP, decreases the need for other vasopressors such as norepinephrine, and may be associated with improved outcomes. Vasopressin also increases cortisol production, which could be relevant in patients with septic shock. Low-dose vasopressin therapy for septic shock consists of 0.04 units/min. This dose has not been associated with myocardial or other end-organ ischemia and decrease in cardiac output.
   3. **Ephedrine** is an indirect α- and β-agonist that causes an increase in heart rate and cardiac output with modest vasoconstriction.

IV. **Hypertension.** High BP may require aggressive treatment in the ICU in two main circumstances: to avoid damage from an acute vascular derangement such as aortic dissection or rupture and in the presence of a hypertensive crisis.

A. **Major hypertensive vascular emergencies**
   1. **Acute aortic dissection** occurs when the intima of the vessel is torn and separates from the media, causing the development of a false vessel lumen. Presenting symptoms include abrupt onset of chest or back

pain, a pulse deficit in a particular limb, myocardial infarction (MI), and syncope. Clinical signs include acute aortic insufficiency (diastolic murmur), congestive heart failure, Horner's syndrome, cardiac tamponade, hemothorax, ECG changes, and mediastinal widening on chest x-ray. The differential diagnosis includes acute conditions such as MI, pericarditis, pulmonary embolism, and expanding aortic aneurysm. The diagnosis is based on imaging studies: the intimal flap and false lumen need to be visualized by aortic angiogram, computed tomography, or magnetic resonance imaging angiogram. Transesophageal echo can also be helpful. Dissections involving the ascending aorta are **surgical** emergencies. Dissections in the descending aorta are treated by a combination of medical and (at times) surgical interventions.

2. **Contained ruptures of aortic aneurysms** (see Chapter 36) and traumatic aortic ruptures (see Chapter 33) are surgical emergencies. If the patient is hemodynamically stable, a period of stabilization in the ICU may be indicated. During that time, similar considerations apply as discussed in the previous section.

3. **Management** of these major vascular emergencies involves invasive BP monitoring, **pain control, reduction of the systolic blood pressure** to 100–120 mm Hg or the lowest tolerated, and **reduction of the heart rate** to approximately 60 beats per minute. This is frequently accomplished by **narcotics** for pain control, **IV** β-**blockers,** and further **vasodilators** if necessary. See the next subsection for a more detailed discussion of the antihypertensive agents.

B. **Hypertensive crisis** is a severe, acute increase in systolic and diastolic blood pressure associated with end-organ damage. Presenting signs and symptoms include headache, nausea/vomiting, seizures, hemorrhagic stroke, visual disturbances, oliguria, unstable angina/acute MI, and pulmonary edema. The objective of the initial therapy is to **limit ongoing organ damage.** It is important to remember that most of these patients are hypertensive at baseline, and rapid normalization of arterial pressure may compromise organ perfusion. A 20% immediate reduction of BP is a reasonable initial target, with a more gradual lowering over the ensuing 24 to 48 hours. Antihypertensive therapy is started with an IV agent that is short acting and easy to titrate (e.g., labetalol, nitroglycerine, or nitroprusside).

1. **General therapeutic considerations.** Appropriate IV access and intraarterial hemodynamic monitoring must be rapidly established. History and physical examination focus on the patient's premorbid status, etiology of hypertension, and signs of end-organ injury.

2. **Pharmacologic therapy**
   a. **Nitrates**
      (1) **Nitroglycerine (NTG)** is both a venous and arterial vasodilator. It decreases primarily

venous tone, but also ventricular end-diastolic pressure and arterial tone. Overall, these effects may improve systolic function. NTG also dilates large coronary vessels, relieving coronary spasm and redistributing myocardial blood flow from the epicardium to the subendocardium. **IV administration** of NTG is easy to titrate to effect, and is the preferred route for critically ill patients. Common IV rates range from 25 to 1,000 μg/min. Because NTG is absorbed by polyvinyl chloride IV tubing, its dose may decrease after 30 to 60 min, once the IV tubing is fully saturated. **Hypotension, reflex tachycardia,** and **headache** are common. **Tachyphylaxis** is the rule. In critically ill patients, a common strategy is simply to increase the rate of administration, generally over a period of a few days, until a ceiling effect is noted (usually at doses of about 1,000–1,200 μg/min). Nitroglycerine administration may **worsen hypoxemia** during acute respiratory failure by increasing pulmonary blood flow to poorly ventilated areas of the lung, which can worsen ventilation-perfusion mismatch and shunt.

   (2) **Sodium nitroprusside (SNP)** is a more potent arterial than venous vasodilator; it increases venous capacitance, but a reflex tachycardia often compensates for decreased venous return. **Central venous administration** is preferred. The normal dose range is 20 to 200 μg/min. The rapid onset and short duration of action make it ideal for continuous infusion. Because it is photodegradable, protection with foil wrapping is necessary. **Adverse effects** include cyanide toxicity from nitrosyl moieties that liberate free **cyanide** ions (CN^-), which bind to cytochrome oxidase and uncouple oxidative metabolism, causing tissue hypoxia. At low infusion rates, cyanide can be converted to thiocyanate (by thiosulfate and rhodanase), which is less toxic than CN^-. The risk of cyanide and thiocyanate toxicity is dose dependent and increases with renal impairment. Signs of cyanide toxicity include tachyphylaxis, increased mixed venous Po_2, and metabolic acidosis. It is treated by discontinuing the infusion of SNP and administering thiosulfate. **Rebound hypertension** may occur when SNP is abruptly discontinued. Like all nitrates, SNP blunts hypoxic pulmonary vasoconstriction and may cause **hypoxemia**.

   b. **Adrenergic-blocking agents**
   (1) **Labetalol** is a mixed α- and β-antagonist when administered IV. Initial IV doses of 5 to 10 mg

can be increased to 15 to 20 mg in 5-minute intervals and followed by a continuous infusion of 1 to 5 mg/min.

(2) **Esmolol** is a short-acting β-blocker that allows for easy titration as an IV infusion to maintain a low HR and BP in the setting of an aortic dissection.

(3) **Metoprolol and propranolol** are longer-acting agents generally used to continue β-blockade orally once the target heart rate has been reached.

(4) **Fenoldopam** is a dopamine agonist that is short acting and easily titratable. Its onset is within 5 minutes and its duration of action is 30 to 60 minutes. It activates δ receptors and results in renal and systemic vasodilation and natriuresis. At very low doses (up to 0.04 μg/min) it is devoid of systemic hemodynamic effects, whereas it should maintain its renal vasodilator effect. At higher doses, fenoldopam has significant systemic effects and can be effective in the treatment of hypertensive crisis.

c. **Hydralazine** is an arterial vasodilator that is generally administered in boluses rather than continuous infusion because of its slightly longer duration of effect than other available drugs. It is often used on a as-needed basis (10–20 mg IV) as an additional means of controlling BP high points.

SELECTED REFERENCES

Boyd O, Grounds M, Bennett D. Preoperative increase of oxygen delivery reduces mortality in high-risk surgical patients. *JAMA* 1993;270:2699.

Cochrane Injuries Group Albumin Reviewers. Human albumin administration in critically ill patients: systematic review of randomized controlled trials. *Br Med J* 1998;317:235–240.

Gattinoni L, Brazzi L, Pelosi P, et al. A trial of goal-oriented hemodynamic therapy in critically ill patients. *N Engl J Med* 1995;333: 1025–1032.

Hochman J. Cardiogenic shock complicating acute myocardial infarction: expanding the paradigm. *Circulation* 2003;107:2998–3002.

Holmes C, Patel B, Russell J, et al. Physiology of vasopressin relevant to management of septic shock. *Chest* 2001;120:989–1002.

Levy B, Bollaert P, Charpentier C, et al. Comparison of norepinephrine and dobutamine to epinephrine for hemodynamics, lactate metabolism and gastric tonometric variables in septic shock: a prospective, randomized study. *Intensive Care Med* 1997;23:282–287.

Levy M, Mitchell F, Marshall J, et al. 2001 SCCM/ESICM/ACCP/ATS/ SIS International Sepsis Definitions Conference. *Crit Care Med* 2003;311:250–256.

Martin C, Viviand X, Leone M, et al. Effect of norepinephrine on the outcome of septic shock. *Crit Care Med* 2000;28:2758–2765.

Patel B, Chittock D, Russell J, et al. Beneficial effects of short-term vasopressin infusion during severe septic shock. *Anesthesiology* 2002;96:576–582.

Rivers E, Nguyen B, Havstad S, et al. Early goal-directed therapy in the treatment of severe sepsis and septic shock. *N Eng J Med* 2001;345:1368–1377.

Rizoli S. Crystalloids and colloids in trauma resuscitation: a brief overview of the current debate. *J Trauma* 2003;54:S82–S88.

Russell JA, Pheng PT. The oxygen delivery/consumption controversy. Approaches to management of the critically ill. *Am J Respir Crit Care Med* 1994;149:533–537.

Sandham JD, Hull RD, Brant RF, et al. A randomized, controlled trial of the use of pulmonary-artery catheters in high-risk surgical patients. *N Engl J Med* 2003;348:5–14.

The SAFE Study investigators. A comparison of albumin and saline for fluid resuscitation in the intensive care unit. *N Engl J Med* 2004;350:2247–2256.

Varon J, Marik P. The diagnosis and management of hypertensive crises. *Chest* 2000;118:214–227.

Nutrition

Stephen V. Panaro and Thomas W. Felbinger

I. Introduction

A. Malnutrition is defined as "a nutritional deficit associated with an increased risk of adverse clinical events and with a decreased risk of such events when corrected." It is the result of underprescribing, low delivery, low tolerance of nutrition, or hypercatabolism. In critically ill patients, malnutrition is recognized as a clinically relevant problem with prevalence up to 40% in modern intensive care units (ICUs). Malnutrition is associated with impaired immune function, prolonged ventilatory dependence, increased length of stay, and increased mortality.

B. Benefits of nutrition include improved wound healing, improved gastrointestinal (GI) function (immune and structural), and decreased catabolic response to injury, resulting in decreased hospital stay and decreased mortality. However, inadequately high administration of enteral or parenteral substrates can also be associated with detrimental consequences.

C. Practice of nutritional support varies widely, as does the literature on nutritional support. Evidence-based clinical practice guidelines have been created that should provide an efficient structure and consistency to the field. The implementation of evidence-based nutritional support has been associated with improved clinical outcomes.

II. Metabolic changes during catabolic conditions

A. Starvation and stress metabolism both are catabolic states. However, the hormonal and metabolic consequences of starvation are reversible after reinstitution of nutritional support; in contrast, stress metabolism after injury and critical illness is a more complex state that is not simply resolved by administering adequate nutrition.

B. Hormonal and metabolic responses to injury and critical illness are classically divided into three phases (ebb phase, flow phase, and recovery), but each is ill defined and variable depending on the type, degree, and duration of the injury.

1. The **ebb phase** is a short, hypometabolic and hypothermic response (12–24 hours) with absolute insulin deficiency and increased incretion of the counterregulatory hormones, such as catecholamines and glucagon. This phase probably evolved as a mechanism to provide energy and substrate metabolism.

2. The **flow phase** is a longer; hypermetabolic phase characterized by normal or even enhanced insulin secretion. Counterregulatory hormones still are significantly increased and determine a catabolic state. Aldosterone and antidiuretic hormone (ADH) are increased, resulting in sodium and water retention. Over prolonged periods, this phase leads to severe depletion of body energy stores. Besides hormonal mediators, changes in circulating proinflammatory mediators (e.g., tumor necrosis factor [TNF]-α and interleukin-1 and -6) and neurotransmitters, changes in regional blood flow, and the lack of physical activity are all part of the metabolic response observed in this phase. Effects of this catabolic phase include an increased protein breakdown and decreased muscle protein synthesis in addition to lipolysis, glycogenolysis, and gluconeogenesis. The increase in hepatic glucose production and the decrease in insulin-mediated glucose utilization (especially in skeletal muscle and adipose tissue) often lead to **hyperglycemia.** Endogenous lipids represent the main energy store in critical illness. In adipose cells, **triglycerides are hydrolyzed to free fatty acids,** which are oxidized in the periphery to generate energy. In muscle, **protein breakdown** serves as a source of free amino acids and glutamine, serving as fuel in the viscera and immune system. The excess of amino acids is oxidized in the liver and in muscle and the resulting nitrogen is excreted.

3. The **recovery** is marked by normalization of glucose levels, reabsorption of interstitial fluid into intravascular compartment with diuresis, attendant to the resolution of other signs of acute illness such as leukocytosis and fever. Counterregulatory hormones return to normal levels. The late **anabolic phase,** often lasting for months, is characterized by return of muscle and adipose stores.

III. **Evaluation of the nutritional status**
A. **Forms of malnutrition**
1. **Adult marasmus** (calorie deficiency) is defined as loss of greater than 10% of body weight (BW) over 6 months or the development of a BW less than 85% of the ideal BW.
2. **Adult kwashiorkor** (protein deficiency) is defined as hypoalbuminemia (albumin <2.1 g/dl) and total lymphocyte count of less than 800/mm^3 in the absence of infection, radiation, or chemotherapy.
3. **Protein-calorie malnutrition** is a combined form of malnutrition often present in patients after major injury or surgery.
B. **Assessment of the nutritional status** is of importance to identifying malnutrition. It helps in determining the need for instituting and monitoring the success of nutrition. However, most tools that assess nutritional status (triceps skinfold thickness, mid-arm

circumference, grip strength, body bioimpedance analysis, etc.) have limitations.

C. **A subjective global assessment** of the nutritional status combines a history of change in weight, dietary intake, functional capacity, and physical examination and is easily obtained.

D. The **body mass index** (BMI) is a useful screening tool for both underweight and obesity:

$$BMI = weight\ (kg)/height^2\ (m^2)$$
$$BMI = weight\ (lb)/height^2\ (in^2) \times 703$$

A BMI of less than 18.5 kg/m^2 is considered underweight, a BMI between 25 and 30 kg/m^2 is considered overweight, and a BMI of greater than 30 kg/m^2 defines obesity. In critically ill patients, BMI should be used with caution due to rapidly changing fluid balances.

E. **Laboratory analysis** can be helpful in the diagnosis of malnutrition.

1. Low levels of serum proteins may reflect decreased synthesis, increased catabolism, dilution, or simply sequestration into the extravascular space.

2. Serum albumin is highly correlated with mortality. However, its long half-life (20 days) makes it irrelevant in nutritional assessment. Serum albumin levels can be depressed during catabolic states despite adequate nutritional status.

3. **Prealbumin** and **transferrin** (half-lives of 2 and 8 days, respectively) are more useful parameters for monitoring nutritional support.

IV. **Indications for nutritional support.** Precise indications for the timing of initiation of nutritional support are surprisingly lacking. Common sense and sparse data suggest the following general principles.

A. **Patients without malnutrition** who will be expected to be fasting for 5 to 7 days or more should be considered for nutritional support.

B. **Malnutrition** of any degree should be treated with early-initiated nutrition. In patients with severe cachexia, preoperative nutrition may improve outcome.

C. **Hypermetabolism** (e.g., trauma, burn, sepsis) should likewise lead to prompt initiation of nutritional support.

V. **Route of nutrition.** Enteral nutrition is generally recommended over total parenteral nutrition (TPN).

A. **Advantages of** enteral nutrition include fewer infectious complications, fewer metabolic derangements (especially hyperglycemia), higher safety, and lower cost. There are actually few contraindications to enteral nutrition. Small-bowel feeds delivered with a soft feeding tube placed distal to the pylorus may be preferable to gastric feeds, especially in patients at high risk for aspiration of gastric contents into the lungs. Gastroparesis, colonic ileus, diarrhea, the absence of bowel sounds, flatus, and stool are not absolute contraindications to initiating postpyloric feeds.

B. **Early enteral nutrition** (defined as initiation within 24–48 hours) when compared to delayed nutrition is beneficial in a heterogeneous patient population and demonstrates a trend toward decreased mortality. This effect has in particular been shown when combined with interventions aimed at optimizing delivery, such as delivery of small-bowel feeds, use of motility agents, and so on.

C. The term **trophic feeds** refers to the infusion of a small amount of elemental tube feeds (10–20 ml/h) in a patient otherwise intolerant of enteral feeding. Although not sufficient to provide full nutrition, this practice may prevent loss of mucosal villi function, disruption of tight junctions, bacterial translocation, and a loss of gut immune function. For this reason, trophic feeds are often administered in association with TPN.

D. **Parenteral supplementation** to enteral nutrition does not result in better outcome compared to enteral nutrition alone when the gastrointestinal tract is intact. There is no evidence of the benefit of starting TPN in these patients at the same time as enteral nutrition. Strategies should aim first at optimizing delivery of enteral nutrition (by using prokinetics, proper positioning, postpyloric placement of the feeding tubes, etc.) before considering supplemental parenteral nutrition. In patients with severe malnutrition or during severe catabolic response to the stress of surgery, trauma, or infection, the decision for supplemental parenteral nutrition should be made as a case-by-case basis. Data supporting the addition of supplemental parenteral nutrition are based in part on outdated practices that did not include tight blood glucose control and used first-generation fat emulsions.

E. **Contraindications for** enteral nutrition, where TPN should be started, are summarized in Table 9-1.

VI. **Determination of energy requirements**

A. Determination of energy requirements is necessary because both underfeeding and overfeeding can have

Table 9-1.   Contraindications for enteral nutrition

Absolute contraindications
  Intestinal perforation
  Mechanical bowel obstruction
  Mesenteric ischemia
  Paralytic small bowel ileus
Relative contraindications
  Gastrointestinal bleeding
  Severe short-bowel syndrome
  High-output enteral fistula
  Severe necrotizing pancreatitis
  Severe prolonged diarrhea

negative effects on the outcome in critically ill patients. During critical illness, endogenous gluconeogenesis and protein breakdown are not completely blocked by nutritional support. Hence, determination of the **resting energy expenditure (REE)** should serve as an upper limit of substrate supply rather than as a mandatory goal of energy intake. In severely catabolic patients, substrate supply sometimes has to be decreased to avoid metabolic derangements.

B. **Measuring REE by indirect calorimetry** (see also Chapter 3). Indirect calorimetry measures oxygen consumption ($\dot{V}O_2$) and carbon dioxide production ($\dot{V}CO_2$). This allows calculating the respiratory quotient (RQ), **RQ = $\dot{V}O_2/\dot{V}CO_2$,** providing knowledge of net substrate oxidation. Including the nitrogen excretion in the urine (UUN), one can calculate REE using the Weir equation:

$$REE = (3.94 \times \dot{V}O_2 + 1.1 \times \dot{V}CO_2) \times 1.44 - 2.17 \times UUN$$

Indirect calorimetry should be used for patients with concomitant severe starvation and stress metabolism (e.g., cachectic tumor, patient with sepsis), patients difficult to wean from the ventilator, or patients not responding adequately to nutritional intervention. This technique becomes less reliable in patients ventilated with a fraction of inspired oxygen (FiO_2) greater than 0.6. Endotracheal suctioning, positioning, and dressing changes may significantly influence the results when the measurements are done within 2 hours after these interventions. A limitation of indirect calorimetry is that the 10- to 30-minute measurement period might not be representative of the mean REE during the next 24 hours or the time until the next measurement. Given the complexity of indirect calorimetry in critically ill patients, it is often substituted by the measurement of $\dot{V}CO_2$; although less precise than calorimetry, measurement of $\dot{V}CO_2$ is simple and highly reproducible (see Chapter 3).

C. **Calculation of REE by the Harris-Benedict formula.** The Harris-Benedict formula is the most commonly used of a number of formulas devised to calculate energy expenditure. Despite its multiple assumptions, there is no evidence that more precise metabolic measurements (i.e., indirect calorimetry) result in improved outcomes. The Harris-Benedict equations for basal energy expenditure (BEE) are:

Men: $BEE = 66 + (13.7 \times W) + (5 \times H) - (6.8 \times A)$ (kcal/d)

Women: $BEE = 665 + (9.6 \times W) + (1.7 \times H)$
$- (4.7 \times A)$ (kcal/d)

$$REE = BEE \times Stress\ factor \times Activity\ factor$$

where W = weight, H = height, and A = age. The stress factor is 1.0 to 1.3 for most ICU patients and 1.0 to 1.7 for sepsis or severe burn. The activity factor is 1 to 1.3 for out of bed and walking; fever adds 5% to 10% per degree centigrade). Some data suggest that Harris-Benedict formula often overestimates actual caloric requirements.

D. Estimation of REE. For daily routine for many ICU patients, REE can most easily be estimated with clinically acceptable accuracy by

$$REE = 25 \text{ kcal/kg per day}$$

(obese patients: −20%; malnourished patients: +20%.). For the majority of ICU patients, 2,000 kcal/d should be an appropriate energy supply.

VII. Substrates

A. Protein. Average protein provides 4 kcal/g of calories when used as a fuel (RQ = 0.8). The recommended daily allowance (RDA) is 1 g/kg (6.25 g of protein = 1 g of nitrogen). Multiplied by a stress factor, the usual maximum daily administration is **1.5 g/kg** but can be higher with large weeping wounds or with severe burns (2 g/kg). There is insufficient evidence to support specific amino acid solutions for TPN. Most likely, **adequate protein administration is more important than meeting goals for energy supply.**

B. Carbohydrates. Anhydrous glucose yields 4 kcal/g, whereas hydrous glucose (dextrose) yields 3.4 kcal/g (RQ of 1.0). From 40% to 60% of nonprotein calories should be administered as carbohydrates. During acute catabolic states, 3 to 4 g/kg per day is an acceptable upper limit for glucose supply. Greater amounts only lead to hyperglycemia and promote the development of fatty liver. **Hyperglycemia increases mortality in critically ill patients** who have been in the ICU for more than 5 days (see Chapter 27).

C. Lipids. Triglycerides yield 9 kcal/g (RQ of 0.7). Up to 30% of a patient's nonprotein calories should be supplied as lipids. Most severely injured patients cannot metabolize more than 1 to 1.5 g/kg of lipids per day. Propofol can be an unaccounted source of fat in ICU and contains 1.1 kcal/ml. There is insufficient evidence to support specific types of lipids in TPN or low-fat, high-carbohydrate enteral feeds or the converse. Because of the possibility of increased infectious complications, lipid-free TPN may be considered in patients not malnourished and in whom length of TPN may be limited (<10 days).

VIII. Electrolytes and micronutrients. Malnutrition, catabolic response, and nutrition all are associated with major changes in electrolyte or micronutrient balance.

A. Sodium, potassium, magnesium chloride, acetate, and phosphorus should all be closely followed and replenished based on measured serum levels. In addition, calcium, magnesium, and phosphorus should be administered based on measured serum levels. Basic electrolyte requirements areas follow:

1. **Sodium:** 100 to 120 mEq/d (increased in gastrointestinal [GI] losses, decreased in cardiopulmonary diseases).
2. **Potassium:** 30 to 120 mEq/d (requirement depends on the rate of glucose and amino acid application).
3. **Chloride:** Replenish based on serum level. To maintain electrical neutrality for patients with metabolic alkalosis, chloride should be aggressively replenished in the form of sodium or potassium chloride.
4. **Acetate:** For patients with metabolic acidosis due to, for example, bicarbonate loss in a GI fistula or diarrhea, acetate should be used in favor of chloride for electroneutrality. Acetate is converted to bicarbonate in the liver; caution must be used when administering acetate ion in patients with impaired liver function.

B. **Electrolytes, vitamins,** and **trace elements** are contained in sufficient amounts in enteral solutions, but need to be added to TPN formulas (Tables 9-2 to 9-4). If enteral nutrition cannot be administered at goal, a multivitamin/mineral supplement should be added.

C. The effect of adding high dose antioxidant elements such as selenium is currently under investigation.

IX. **Application of nutritional support**

A. **TPN**

1. Due to the high osmolarity of TPN (>900 mOsm/L, dextrose $>10\%$), central vein access is necessary. A dedicated port should be reserved for TPN to decrease the risk of bacterial contamination.
2. Substrate composition of a routine TPN formula is as follows: carbohydrates, 50% to 60%; proteins, 15% to 25%; lipids, 20% to 30%. From day one of TPN, proteins should be given as a standard solution (15%) or as a glutamine-containing solution where indicated (see section **XIII.A**) and available. The amount of carbohydrates sometimes needs to be slowly adjusted over a few days to avoid severe hyperglycemia. For short-term application (<10 days), TPN should be

Table 9-2. **Electrolyte supplementation to parenteral nutrition**

Electrolyte	RDA	Usual Dose Range
Potassium (mEq/L)	30	0–120
Sodium (mEq/L)	30	0–150
Phosphate (mmol/L)	15	0–20
Magnesium (mEq/L)	5	0–16
Calcium (mEq/L) (as gluconate)	4.7	0–9.4
Chloride (mEq/L)	50	0–150
Acetate (mEq/L)	40	0–100

RDA, recommended daily allowance.

Table 9-3. Vitamin supplementation to parenteral nutrition

Vitamin	RDA	MGH PN
Ascorbic acid (vitamin C) (mg)	60	600
Vitamin A (retinol) (IU)	3,300	3,300
Vitamin D (ergocalciferol) (IU)	400	200
Thiamine (B_1) (mg)	1.5	3
Pyridoxine (B_6) (mg)	2	4
Riboflavin (B_2) (mg)	1.7	3.6
Niacin (as niacinamide) (mg)	20	40
Pantothenic acid (mg)	10	15
Vitamin E (DL-α-tocopherol acetate) (IU)	30	10
Biotin (μg)	100	60
Folic acid (μg)	400	400
Vitamin B_{12} (cyanocobalamin) (μg)	2	5
Vitamin K, phytonadione (vitamin K_1)[a]		

MGH, Massachusetts General Hospital; PN, parenteral nutrition; RDA, recommended daily allowance.
[a] 10 mg every Monday (contraindicated in patients receiving warfarin).

applied as hypocaloric TPN, withholding lipids. For long-term TPN (>10 days), high-energy and intravenous (IV) lipids should be included.

3. **Insulin** sliding scale should be ordered to maintain blood sugar concentration within very close limits, for example, 80 to 120 mg/dl. Insulin can also be added directly to the TPN solution (minimum: 10 IU/ bag). Half of the insulin dose administered on the previous day as part of the sliding scale can be added to the solution.

4. Because TPN is less complete than enteral nutrition in its composition, special attention has to be given to adequate substitution of electrolytes and micronutrients (see Tables 9-2 to 9-4).

Table 9-4. Trace elements supplementation to parenteral nutrition

Trace Element Solution	RDA (Oral)	RDA (Intravenous)	MGH PN
Zinc (mg)	15	2.5–5	5
Copper (mg)	2	0.5–1.5	1
Manganese (mg)	2.5–5	0.15–0.8	0.5
Chromium (μg)	0.02	0.01–0.015	10
Selenium (μg)	0.07		60

Reduce all trace elements 50% in chronic renal failure. Add zinc for prolonged diarrhea and impaired wound healing; withhold manganese and copper in liver failure.
MGH, Massachusetts General Hospital; PN, parenteral nutrition; RDA, recommended daily allowance.

5. Reassessment of the possibility of administering calories via the enteral route should be performed frequently. If no enteral nutrition is tolerated, glutamine (0.3–0.4 g/kg/d IV) should be added to the TPN solution.

B. Enteral nutrition via gastric or jejunal tube should be started within 24 to 48 hours if possible. It should be administered as a full-strength polymeric formula at 25 ml/h and advanced to goal by 20 ml/h every 8 hours if tolerated. Target feed rate should be reached within 48 to 72 hours.

1. Gastric enteral nutrition requires monitoring of gastric residuals every 4 hours. If residuals are greater than 250 ml, feeding should be held for 1 hour and residual rechecked. If rechecked residuals continue to be greater than 250 ml, the rate of feeds should be decreased (e.g., by 25 ml/h) after optimizing the use of prokinetics (**metoclopramide,** 10–20 mg IV every 6 hours, or **erythromycin,** 125–250 mg every 6 hours). Even if further decrease of the rate of administration is necessary, one should always try to administer a minimum of 10 to 20 ml/h (**trophic feeds**). Because a high percentage of critical care patients suffer from gastroparesis, the head of the bed should always be elevated greater than 30 degrees if not contraindicated by spinal injuries, pelvic instability, and so on. Small bowel feeds should be considered if high gastric residuals continue. Commonly used enteral formulas and their differences are shown in Table 9-5.

2. Jejunal enteral nutrition can be achieved by endoscopic, fluoroscopic, or surgical placement of nasojejunal tubes (e.g., at the time of laparotomy). In patients at high risk for pulmonary aspiration (prone or strictly supine position), jejunal feeding should be considered from the beginning. Jejunal enteral nutrition is not followed clinically based on the amount of gastric residuals. When jejunal nutrition is poorly tolerated, it is generally shown by the development of abdominal distension. Changing the enteral formula to an elemental diet may help to increase tolerance. The need to have an experienced person to do endoscopy is the most important factor that hampers the use of jejunal tubes. Nasogastric tube should be kept in place for gastric decompression while feeding into the jejunum. For planned long-term enteral nutrition (>4 weeks) surgical feeding jejunostomy or gastrojejunostomy should be initiated early.

X. Monitoring nutritional support

A. Plasma glucose concentration should be monitored often in particular during initiation of enteral nutrition and/or TPN because tight glucose control is associated with decreased mortality in critically ill patients (see Chapter 27).

Table 9-5. Composition of enteral formulas

	Osmolite HN	Osmolite	Jevity Plus	Ensure Plus HN	Suplena	TwoCal HN	Vivonex Plus	Promote w Fiber
Nature of formula	High protein	Low protein	Fiber 12 g/L	High protein	Low protein	High protein	Elemental	High fiber
cal/ml	1.6	1.06	1.2	1.5	2.0	2.0	1.0	1.0
Osmolarity mOsm/kg	300	300	450	650	600	690	650	380

B. Standard **chemistry** values (CHEM-7), phosphate, magnesium, and calcium concentration, liver function tests, triglycerides, cholesterol, **prealbumin,** and transferrin should be monitored weekly in particular during TPN.

C. One of the difficulties in providing nutrition to the critically ill is defining and assessing the goals of therapy. Catabolism cannot be completely reversed in critically ill patients, but further protein breakdown for gluconeogenesis has to be prevented. Meeting absolute caloric goals may be of secondary importance. During acute catabolic response a positive nitrogen balance often cannot be achieved and should not be targeted. A positive nitrogen balance often reflects more an improvement in the patient's status than a response to nutrition.

1. **Nitrogen-balance** analysis can estimate the degree of protein breakdown and assess the adequacy of protein replacement. The nitrogen balance can be calculated as

$$\text{N loss (g/d)} = 1.2 \times [\text{UUN (mg/dl)} \times \text{urine output (ml/d)} \\ \times 1 \text{ g}/1{,}000 \text{ mg} \times 1 \text{ dl}/100 \text{ ml}] + 2 \text{ g/d}$$

2. The extra 2 g/d corrects for skin and stool losses. Weekly measurements are reasonable.

D. Only 50% of the healthy population has a resting energy expenditure within 10% of that predicted by the Harris-Benedict equation. Meeting 100% of a critical care patient's energy needs is not a necessary primary goal. Only in head trauma patients has aggressive enteral nutrition with caloric intake at goal been shown to be beneficial.

E. During enteral nutrition, clinical monitoring of the gastrointestinal system (abdominal distension, pain, tenderness, gastric residuals) becomes more important than laboratory analysis. Abdomen should be examined at least every 8 hours during initiation of enteral nutrition in critically ill patients.

XI. Complications of TPN

A. TPN is associated with higher rate of infectious complications than enteral nutrition. The reasons are related to line access, loss of barrier, and immune gut function as well as increased likelihood of hyperglycemia or high content of ω-6-lipid emulsions. Patients on TPN have higher rates of sepsis and a trend toward higher mortality than patients on enteral nutrition.

B. Most complications of TPN are **metabolic derangements.** Excess carbohydrate administration can lead to increased CO_2 production and possible difficulty in weaning from ventilatory support and hepatic steatosis. Excess fat administration can lead to hyperlipidemia, reduced reticuloendothelial function, and decreased immune function. Excess fluid administration can also be a consequence of TPN. Hyperglycemia as a particular consequence of TPN is associated with increased mortality in critically ill patients.

XII. Complications of enteral nutrition

   A. Early enteral nutrition can be associated with high gastric residuals and bacterial colonization with the increased risk of aspiration of gastric contents and the development of ventilator-associated pneumonia (see Chapters 12 and 28).

   B. Surgically placed jejunostomy tubes have a measurable rate of mechanical problems including dislodgement, torsion of the small bowel, intussception, and internal hernia.

   C. Localized site abscess is very common, as are leaks, clogs, and so on. Jejunostomy feeds can also in rare instances cause intestinal ischemia. Causes for this severe complication may be multifactorial, but are probably related to intestinal hypoperfusion and to hyperosmolality of the enteral formula.

   D. Diarrhea (see also Chapter 26).

      1. Definition: more than three to five bowel movements per day, or greater than 300 to 500 ml of liquid stool per day, indicating an impaired function of the GI tract.

      2. Common reasons for diarrhea in the critically ill patient include change in intestinal bacterial overgrowth, antibiotics, high magnesium or sorbitol content in enteral nutrition, too rapid progression in rate or volume of enteral nutrition, malabsorption, and *Clostridium* (*C.*) *difficile* toxin.

      3. Treatment of diarrhea (before discontinuing enteral nutrition):

         a. Discontinue hyperosmolar medications and change oral to IV route when possible.

         b. Rectal check, manually de-impact if necessary.

         c. Send stool for *C. difficile* toxin analysis.

         d. Treat underlying disease (pancreatitis, short-bowel syndrome, inflammatory bowel disease).

         e. Consider fiber-containing diet if applicable (may lead to abdominal distension during early enteral nutrition).

         f. Discontinue enteral nutrition when abdominal distension and pain develop.

   E. Constipation (see also Chapter 26).

      1. Major causes for severe constipation:

         a. Lack of fiber.

         b. Low fluid intake.

         c. Antimotility effects of drugs such as opioids and anticholinergics agents.

      2. Treatment:

         a. Reduce opioids to minimum, and consider the use of regional anesthesia if applicable.

         b. Generously hydrate if medically possible.

         c. Mobilize the patient.

       d. Ogilvie's syndrome: after conservative treatment for 48 to 72 hours without success, or if the cecal diameter is greater than 12 cm, consider interventional decompression or explorative laparotomy.

XIII. Immunonutrition

Specific nutrients such as glutamine, arginine, and ω-3-fatty acids have been shown in experimental models to improve immune function. These nutrients are incorporated into enteral formulas, but are difficult to assess clinically. In a compilation of heterogeneous surgical patient populations using different formulations, recent meta-analyses suggest a benefit from these preparations.

    A. Glutamine is an amino acid used preferentially as an energy source for intestinal mucosa, in lymphocytes, and as a precursor for gluconeogenesis in the liver. Via the enteral route, it should be considered in burn and in trauma patients. As a parenteral supplement (0.3–0.4 g/kg per day) it has been shown to improve outcome in patients on TPN who are not able to tolerate enteral nutrition.

    B. Arginine as a supplement for enteral diets **did not** demonstrate benefit in critically ill patients, although it might be beneficial in perioperative surgical patients. Data do not support the use of arginine-containing diets in critically ill patients.

    C. ω-3-fatty acids, together with borage oils and **antioxidants** (vitamin E, vitamin C, β-carotene, taurine, L-carnitine) improved outcome in one study in patients with acute respiratory distress syndrome (ARDS).

XIV. Nutrition for organ failure

    A. Renal failure

        1. Patients in both acute and chronic renal failure are sensitive to volume overload. The amount of free water in TPN should be minimized. Serum levels of potassium, phosphorus, and magnesium need to be monitored closely. The amount of acetate in the formula may need to be increased. With worsening uremia during chronic renal failure without dialysis, protein needs to be decreased to 0.5 to 0.8 g/kg per day.

        2. Acute renal failure requiring renal replacement therapy (hemodialysis or continuous hemofiltration) often results in hypermetabolism due to the release of proinflammatory mediators such as TNF, interleukin-1, complement fractions, and bradykinins. Additional losses of carbohydrates and amino acids (peritoneal dialysis, 40–60 g/d; hemodialysis or hemofiltration, 3–5 g/h) are possible and must be accounted for, and should be maintained or even increased.

    B. Hepatic failure

        1. Chronic liver failure may result in hypoalbuminemia and elevated levels of ADH and aldosterone. Consequently, salt and water retention as well as losses of potassium, magnesium, and zinc may occur. Fluid and salt restriction helps to manage edema and ascites.

2. Decreased endotoxin clearance in acute liver failure may lead to hypermetabolism, whereas chronic liver failure may be associated with decreased energy expenditure.

3. Standard amounts of carbohydrate may prevent hypoglycemia, which often is a negative prognostic sign in the course of severe liver dysfunction. However, hypoglycemia may occur in these patients when glucose supply is abruptly stopped (e.g., transport out of the ICU for a diagnostic test).

4. Protein administration should be restricted to around 1 g/kg or even less in the face of worsening hepatic encephalopathy. The administration of **lactulose** and **neomycin** has long been used in the treatment of encephalopathy to decrease the production and absorption of ammonia. Hepatic encephalopathy has also been associated with elevated aromatic amino acids and diminished **branched-chain amino acids.** Formulas that contain elevated amounts of branched-chain amino acids and reduced amounts of the aromatic and sulfur-containing amino acids may be beneficial for patients with encephalopathy.

5. Lipids can be safely used during liver failure when monitored closely.

C. **Respiratory failure**

1. Acute respiratory failure or ARDS is associated with hypermetabolism, fluid intolerance, and difficulties in oxygenation and CO_2 elimination.

2. Protein insufficiency can lead to loss of diaphragmatic and accessory muscle strength, whereas excessive protein administration can lead to increases in the respiratory drive in patients with chronic weaning failure.

3. Excessive carbohydrate calories can lead to enhanced O_2 consumption and CO_2 production. Because the oxidation of lipid produces less carbon dioxide than the oxidation of carbon dioxide, some advocate that as much as 50% to 70% of calories should be from fat in these patients. However, CO_2 production may depend more on the total amount of energy supplied than on the carbohydrate–lipid ratio.

4. In ARDS, the enteral administration of eicosapentaenoic acid, gamma-linolenic acid, and antioxidants improved outcome in one clinical trial.

D. **Pancreatitis**

1. Enteral nutrition may be administered safely in these patients under careful clinical and laboratory monitoring and may be superior to TPN. Postpyloric tubes can be placed reliably with fluoroscopic techniques and endoscopically and may enhance

tolerance of enteral nutrition and applicability during severe pancreatitis.
2. However, in patients with necrotizing pancreatitis accompanied by circulatory shock and dependence on vasopressors, parenteral nutrition should be implemented.
3. Antioxidants might be of benefit during acute and chronic pancreatitis.

SELECTED REFERENCES

Beale RJ, Bryg DJ, Bihari D. Immunonutrition in the critically ill: A systematic review of clinical outcome. *Crit Care Med* 1999;27:2799–2805.

Biolo G, Grimble G, Preiser JC, et al. Position paper of the ESICM Working Group on Nutrition and Metabolism: metabolic basis of nutrition in intensive care unit patients: ten critical questions. *Intensive Care Med* 2002;28:1512–1520.

Cerra FB, Benitez MR, Blackburn GL, et al. Applied nutrition in ICU patients: a consensus statement of the American College of Chest Physicians. *Chest* 1997;111:769–778.

Giner M, Laviano A, Meguid NM, et al. In 1995 a correlation between malnutrition and poor outcomes in critically ill patients still exists. *Nutrition* 1996;12:23–29.

Heyland DK. Nutritional support in the critically ill patient: a critical review of the evidence. *Crit Care Clin* 1998;14:423–440.

Heyland DK, Dhaliwal R, Drover JW, et al. Canadian clinical practice guidelines for nutrition support in mechanically ventilated, critically ill adult patients. *JPEN J Parenter Enteral Nutr* 2003;27:355–373.

Heyland DK, MacDonald S, Keefe L, et al. Total parenteral nutrition in the critically ill patient: a meta-analysis. *JAMA* 1998;280:2013–3019.

Heyland DK, Novak F, Drover J, et al. Should immunonutrition become routine in critically ill patients? A systematic review of the evidence. *JAMA* 2001;286:944–953.

Kalfarentzos F, Kehagias J, Mead N, et al. Enteral nutrition is superior to parenteral nutrition in severe acute pancreatitis: results of a randomized prospective trial. *Br J Surg* 1997;87:695–707.

Klien S, Kinney J, Jeejeebhoy K, et al. Nutritional support in clinical practice: review of published data and recommendations for future research directions: National Institutes of Health, American Society of Parenteral and Enteral Nutrition, and American Society of Clinical Nutrition. *JPEN J Parenter Enteral Nutr* 1997;21:133–156.

Lobo DN, Memon MA, Allison SP, et al. Evolution of nutritional support in acute pancreatitis. *Br J Surg* 2000;87:695–707.

Van Den Berghe G, Wouters P, Weekers F, et al. Intensive insulin therapy in critically ill patients. *N Engl J Med* 345;19:1359–1367.

Transfusion Therapy and Anticoagulation

Rae M. Allain and Richard M. Pino

I. **Indications for transfusion therapy.** Blood component transfusion is usually performed because of decreased production, increased utilization/destruction or loss, or dysfunction of a specific blood component (red cells, platelets, or coagulation factors).

A. **Anemia**

1. **Red cell mass.** The primary reason for transfusion is to maintain oxygen-carrying capacity to the tissues by the normal mass of red blood cells. Healthy individuals or individuals with a chronic anemia can usually tolerate a hematocrit (Hct) of 20% to 25%, assuming normal intravascular volume. The Hct assumes red blood cell normocytosis and appropriate hemoglobin (Hgb) content. A patient with hypochromic normocytic anemia may have a Hct within normal range but a decreased oxygen-carrying capacity. For this reason, many institutions use Hgb (g/dl) in lieu of Hct (%) as an indicator of red blood cell mass. Modern techniques assay total red cell Hgb and the red blood cell count to calculate the Hct instead of measuring the packed cell volume by centrifugation.

2. If a patient is anemic, the etiology should be clarified. It may be **secondary to decreased production** (marrow suppression), **increased loss** (hemorrhage), or **destruction** (hemolysis).

3. Anemia in critically ill adults is common, but the Hgb level that should prompt red blood cell transfusion is controversial. Results from a large, controlled study of critically ill patients suggested that a "restrictive" transfusion policy (i.e., maintaining a Hgb level of 7.0–9.0 g/dl) improved hospital survival when compared to a more traditional transfusion regimen (i.e., maintaining Hgb at 10–12 g/dl). A cautious approach is recommended for patients with acute coronary syndromes, where clinical practice has been to transfuse to maintain Hgb of approximately 10 g/dl.

4. Estimating the volume of blood to transfuse can be calculated as follows:

$$\text{Volume to transfuse} = (\text{Hct}_{\text{desired}} - \text{Hct}_{\text{present}}) \times \text{BV}/\text{Hct}_{\text{transfused blood}}$$

where BV is blood volume, which may be estimated at 70 ml/kg ideal weight in male adults and 65 ml/kg in female adults.

B. Thrombocytopenia. Spontaneous bleeding is unusual with platelet counts above 5,000 to 10,000/μl, but in the immediate postoperative period, counts above 50,000 are preferable. Thrombocytopenia is due to either decreased bone marrow production (e.g., chemotherapy, tumor infiltration, and alcoholism) or increased utilization or destruction (e.g., hypersplenism, idiopathic thrombocytopenia purpura, and drug effects such as with heparin, histamine-2 blockers, and ticarcillin). It is also seen with massive blood transfusion.

C. Coagulopathy. Bleeding associated with documented factor deficiencies or prolonged clotting studies (prothrombin time, partial thromboplastin time) mandates replacement therapy to maintain normal coagulation function.

1. Coagulation studies. The most important clue to a clinically significant bleeding disorder in an otherwise healthy patient remains the **history.** Prior surgical bleeding, gingival bleeding, easy bruising, epistaxis, or menorrhagia should raise concern. There are many tests available to assess the coagulation, but no single test measures the integrity of the entire coagulation system.

a. Partial thromboplastin time (PTT) is performed by adding particulate matter to a blood sample to activate the intrinsic coagulation system. Normal values for the PTT are between 25 and 37 seconds and depend on normal levels of clotting factors in the intrinsic coagulation system. The test is sensitive to decreased amounts of coagulation factors and is elevated in patients on heparin therapy. The PTT will also be abnormal if there is a circulating anticoagulant present (e.g., lupus anticoagulant, antibodies to factor VIII). The clinician should remember that an abnormal PTT does not necessarily correlate with clinical bleeding. Aggressive correction of an abnormal PTT in surgical patients is not always indicated unless the patient is actively bleeding.

b. Prothrombin time (PT) is a measure of the extrinsic coagulation system and is measured by adding a thromboplastin reagent to a blood sample. Whereas both PT and PTT are affected by levels of factor V, factor X, prothrombin, and fibrinogen, the PT is specifically sensitive to deficiencies of factor VII. The PT is normal in deficiencies of factors VIII, IX, XI, and XII, prekallikrein, and high-molecular-weight kininogen. The **INR** (International Normalized Ratio) standardizes PT values to permit comparisons of PT value among laboratories or within one laboratory but at different times for patients anticoagulated with warfarin. The INR is the ratio of patient PT to control PT that would be obtained if international reference reagents had been used to perform the test. Warfarin therapy may be guided by a target INR value that is independent of laboratory variability. **Use of the INR is limited to warfarin anticoagulation therapy** and is not valid in the assessment of a prolonged PT unrelated to inhibition of vitamin K–dependent factors.

c. **Activated clotting time (ACT)** is a modified whole-blood clotting time in which diatomaceous earth or kaolin is added to a blood sample to activate the intrinsic clotting system. The ACT is the time until clot formation. A normal ACT is between 110 and 130 seconds. The ACT, a relatively easy and expedient test to perform, is useful in monitoring heparin therapy when immediate results are required.

d. **The bleeding time** is thought to be a crude assay of platelet function. Results are poorly reproducible and do not correlate with clinical observations of hemostasis in the perioperative period. This test is no longer recommended for assessment of coagulation status.

e. **Fibrinogen** may be depleted by excessive consumption as in massive hemorrhage or disseminated intravascular coagulation (DIC). A normal fibrinogen level is 170 to 410 mg/dl. It is an acute-phase reactant and is often elevated in postoperative patients or following trauma or inflammation. For extensive surgical procedures associated with bleeding or in cases of massive transfusion, it is prudent to maintain the fibrinogen level above 100 mg/dl.

f. **Fibrin(ogen) degradation products (FDPs)** are peptides produced from the action of plasmin on fibrinogen or fibrin monomer. They are measurable by serum assays and may aid in the diagnosis of primary fibrinolysis or DIC. FDPs modulate further clotting/lysis by interfering with fibrin monomer polymerization and by impairing platelet function. FDPs are often elevated in severe hepatic disease due to failed clearance from the circulation.

g. **D-dimer** is a specific fragment produced when plasmin digests cross-linked fibrin (clot). It is measurable by serum assay and is elevated in pulmonary embolism, in DIC, and in patients receiving surgery within the preceding 48 hours.

h. **Factor assays** are specialized tests that quantitate the activity of individual coagulation factors. Most of these are performed in the setting of an unexplained coagulopathy that has not improved after attempted repletion of coagulation factors, and are usually obtained in concert with a clinical pathology or hematology consultation. Classically, factor assays are used to confirm the diagnosis of hemophilia A or B.

II. Blood typing and cross-matching

A. Donor blood and recipient blood are typed in the red-cell surface **ABO** and **Rh systems** and screened for antibodies to other cell antigens. **Cross-matching** involves directly mixing the patient's plasma with the donor's red cells to establish that hemolysis does not occur from any undetected antibodies. An individual's red cells have either A, B, AB, or no surface antigens. If a person's red cells are lacking either surface antigen A or B, then antibodies will be produced against it. A person who is type B will have anti-A antibodies in the serum, and a type O individual, that is, a person having neither A nor B surface antigens, will have circulating anti-A and anti-B antibodies. Consequently, a person who is type AB will not have antibodies to either A or B and can receive red blood cells from a person of any blood type. Type O blood has neither A nor B surface antigens, and a person with this blood type is a universal red cell donor and can donate blood cells to persons of any other blood type.

B. Rh surface antigens are either present (Rh-positive) or absent (Rh-negative). Individuals who are Rh-negative will develop antibodies to the Rh factor when exposed to Rh-positive blood. This is not a problem with the initial exposure, but hemolysis will occur due to the circulating antibodies with subsequent exposures. This can be a particular problem during pregnancy. The anti-Rh antibodies are immunoglobulin (IgG) and freely cross the placenta. In Rh-negative mothers who have developed Rh antibodies, these antibodies are transmitted to the fetus. If the fetus is Rh-positive, massive hemolysis will occur, termed hemolytic disease of the newborn. **Rh-immune globulin,** an Rh-blocking antibody, prevents the Rh-negative patient from developing anti-Rh antibodies. Rh-immune globulin is routinely administered to Rh-negative women pregnant with Rh-positive fetuses and should be given to Rh-negative individuals who receive Rh-positive blood, especially women of childbearing age. The recommendation is one dose (approximately 300 μg/vial) for every 15 ml of Rh-positive blood transfused.

III. Blood component therapy

A. Whole blood

1. Whole blood has been largely replaced by component therapy because of storage impediments and no demonstrable superiority of the former. The one exception may be for children younger than 2 years of age undergoing complicated cardiovascular surgery, where whole blood may have an outcome benefit in

Table 10-1. Transfusion compatibility

| | Donor | | | | | |
Recipient	A	B	O	AB	Rh+	Rh−
1. Red blood cells						
A	X		X			
B		X	X			
O			X			
AB	X	X	X	X		
Rh+					X	X
Rh−						X
2. Fresh-frozen plasm						
A	X		X			
B		X	X			
O	X	X	X	X		
AB				X		
Rh+					X	X
Rh−					X	X

Compatible transfusions are marked by X.

reduced transfusions. Overall, component therapy is far more efficient and practical for transfusion.

  2. Whole blood must be ABO and Rh identical.

B. **Red blood cells (RBCs)**

  1. One unit of packed RBCs (hematocrit about 70%, volume about 250 ml) will usually raise the hematocrit of a euvolemic adult by 2% to 3% once equilibration has taken place.

  2. RBCs must be ABO compatible (Table 10-1). If an emergency blood transfusion is needed, type-specific (ABO) red cells can usually be obtained within minutes if the patient's blood type is known. If type-specific blood is unavailable, type O Rh-negative red cells should be transfused. Type-specific blood should be substituted as soon as possible to minimize the amount of type O plasma (containing anti-A and anti-B antibodies) transfused.

C. **Platelets**

  1. One unit of random donor platelets increases the platelet count by 5,000 to 10,000/μl. If thrombocytopenia is due to increased destruction (e.g., due to development of antiplatelet antibodies), platelet transfusions will be less efficacious. A posttransfusion platelet count drawn 10 minutes after completion of platelet transfusion confirms platelet refractoriness if the count fails to increase by 5,000/μl per random donor unit transfused.

  2. **ABO-compatible platelets** are not required for transfusion, although they may provide a better

response as measured by the posttransfusion platelet count. **Single-donor platelets** are obtained from one individual by platelet pheresis; one unit is equivalent to approximately six random donor units. Single-donor platelets may be used to reduce exposure to multiple donors or in cases of poor response to random donor platelets where destruction is suspected. In cases where alloimmunization causes platelet refractoriness, **HLA-matched platelets** may be required for effective platelet transfusion. **Rh-negative women** of childbearing age should receive Rh-negative platelets if possible because some RBCs are transfused with platelets. If this is impossible, Rh-immune globulin may be administered.

D. **Fresh-frozen plasma (FFP)** in a dose of 10 to 15 ml/kg will generally increase plasma coagulation factors to 30% of normal.

1. Factors V and VIII are most labile and quickly become depleted in thawed FFP. Fibrinogen levels increase by 1 mg/ml of plasma transfused. Acute reversal of warfarin requires only 5 to 8 ml/kg of fresh-frozen plasma.

2. ABO-compatible FFP transfusion (Table 10-1) is required, but Rh-negative patients may receive Rh-positive FFP.

3. Six units of platelets contain the equivalent of one unit of fresh-frozen plasma.

4. Volume expansion in itself should not be an indication for FFP transfusion.

E. **Cryoprecipitate** is the material formed from thawing FFP at 1°C to 6°C.

1. Each unit of cryoprecipitate contains a minimum of 80 international units of factor VIII and approximately 200 to 300 mg of fibrinogen. It also contains factor XIII, von Willebrand's factor, and fibronectin.

2. **Indications for cryoprecipitate** include hypofibrinogenemia, von Willebrand's disease, hemophilia A (when factor VIII is unavailable), and preparation of fibrin glue. The dose of cryoprecipitate is one unit per 7 to 10 kg, which raises the plasma fibrinogen by about 50 mg/dl in a patient without massive bleeding.

3. ABO compatibility is not required for transfusion of cryoprecipitate, but it is preferred because of the presence of 10 to 20 ml of plasma per unit.

F. **Factor concentrates.** Individual coagulation factors are available for patients with discrete factor deficiencies. These may be derived from pooled human plasma or synthesized by recombinant gene technology.

1. For an intractable coagulopathy with seemingly adequate factor replacement, some clinicians have used **factor IX complex** (Konyne 80), which contains factors II, VII, IX, and X in a small volume. This product should be used extremely cautiously in patients with

liver disease due to the risk of widespread thrombosis occurring because of impaired hepatic clearance of activated clotting factors from the circulation.

  2. **Activated recombinant factor VII (rFVIIa)** was originally developed to control bleeding in patients with hemophilia A or B who had developed circulating inhibitors to factors VIII and IX. Subsequently, this drug has been successfully used to treat hemorrhage related to trauma, severe postpartum disseminated intravascular coagulation, and perioperative bleeding associated with prostatectomy, spinal fusion, or cardiac surgery. This factor may work by complexing with a tissue factor after endothelial injury and subsequent stimulation of the coagulation cascade. The half-life is approximately 2 hours, thromboembolic complications are rare, and only 20 to 40 μg/kg is needed to reverse a coagulopathy. However, because the cost of this drug is prohibitive, it should only be used in life-threatening circumstances.

G. Technical considerations

  1. **Compatible infusions.** Blood products should not be infused with 5% dextrose solutions, which will cause hemolysis, or with lactated Ringer's, which contains calcium and may induce clot formation. Sodium chloride 0.9%, albumin 5%, and fresh-frozen plasma are all compatible with RBC.

  2. **Blood filters** (80 μm) should be used for all blood components except platelets to remove debris and microaggregates. **Leukocyte filters** may be used to remove white blood cells to prevent transmission of cytomegalovirus in the immunocompromised, to prevent alloimmunization to foreign leukocyte antigens, and to diminish the incidence of febrile reactions. **Platelets** should be transfused through a 170-μm blood filter.

IV. Plasma substitutes. Various colloid products are available commercially. Their main limitations are their cost and the dilution of red cells and coagulation factors that occurs with their administration. Volume resuscitation with colloid versus crystalloid solutions is a topic of ongoing controversy and study within critical care practice.

  A. Albumin is available as either an isotonic 5% or a hypertonic 20% or 25% solution. Under normal circumstances, administered albumin has an intravascular half-life of 10 to 15 days. The wisdom of routine infusion of albumin for volume repletion in critically ill patients has been called into question by a Cochrane Group meta-analysis and the recent Saline versus Albumin Fluid Evaluation (SAFE) (see Selected References) trial demonstrating no difference in outcome when albumin was compared to crystalloid resuscitation.

  B. Hydroxyethyl starch (HES) is manufactured from amylopectin. After infusion, HES is stored in the reticuloendothelial cells of the liver for a prolonged time.

Amylase excretion by the kidneys is diminished by attachment to HES, which may result in an elevated serum amylase for several days after HES infusion, which should not be confused with pancreatitis. Although a decrease in factor VIII levels and a prolonged PTT can be seen, HES doses of less than 1.5 L have not been associated with clinical bleeding in most studies. Anaphylactoid reactions are rare. HES is available in the United States as a high-molecular-weight 6% preparation in either 0.9% sodium chloride solution (Hespan) or balanced electrolyte solution containing lactate (Hextend).

V. Pharmacologic therapy

A. **Erythropoietin** increases red cell mass by stimulating proliferation and development of the erythroid precursor cells. It has been used to correct anemia in patients with chronic renal failure and increase preoperative hematocrits and red cell mass prior to preoperative autologous donation. In addition, a recent controlled trial of weekly erythropoietin in critically ill patients demonstrated a diminished transfusion rate for those who received erythropoietin (dosing regimen was 40,000 units subcutaneously [SQ] weekly for 3 weeks initiated on ICU day 3, and patients also received supplemental iron, 150 mg elemental per day, in a liquid enteral formulation). A less clear-cut use for erythropoietin may be in the severely anemic patient who refuses blood transfusion (see section **XI.B**). In addition to iron, folate supplementation is also recommended for patients taking erythropoietin. Initial recommended doses in renal patients range from 50 to 100 IU/kg IV or SQ three times a week.

B. **Granulocyte colony-stimulating factor (GCSF) and granulocyte-macrophage colony-stimulating factor (GMCSF)** are myeloid growth factors useful for shortening the duration of neutropenia induced by chemotherapy. GCSF is specific for neutrophils, whereas GMCSF increases production of neutrophils, macrophages, and eosinophils. Administration of these drugs enhances not only neutrophil counts, but also killing by neutrophils. As such, they are frequently used for the treatment of febrile neutropenia. Treatment results in an initial brief decrement in the neutrophil count (due to endothelial adherence), then a rapid (usually after 24 hours) sustained leukocytosis that is dose dependent. Recommended doses are GCSF 5 μg/kg/d SQ or GMCSF 250 μg/m^2/d SQ until absolute neutrophil count is greater than 10,000/μl.

C. **Desmopressin,** or 1-desamino-8-D-arginine vasopressin (**DDAVP**), is a vasopressin analogue with a more potent and longer duration of action. **DDAVP** increases endothelial cell release of von Willebrand's factor, factor VIII, and plasminogen activator and thus has utility in certain bleeding disorders, including hemophilia A (factor VIII deficiency), classic von Willebrand's disease, and **uremic bleeding.** The dose is 0.3 μg/kg IV *slowly*, because rapid administration may cause hypotension. Repeat dosing at intervals of 12 to 24 hours may be necessary, but tachyphylaxis usually occurs after three or four doses.

D. **Conjugated estrogens** may be used for diminishing bleeding in patients who are uremic. The mechanism is unknown. Unlike desmopressin, the duration of hemostatic effect is long lasting, on the order of 10 to 15 days. The onset of effect is delayed compared to the immediacy of desmopressin. Estrogen may be administered intravenously, 0.6 mg/kg/d, or orally, 50 mg/d, for a course of 4 to 7 days. Hormonal side effects from this short course of therapy are unusual.

E. **The lysine analogues aminocaproic acid** (Amicar) and **tranexamic acid** inhibit fibrinolysis, the endogenous process by which fibrin clot is broken down. They act by displacing plasminogen from fibrin, diminishing plasminogen conversion to plasmin, and preventing plasmin from binding to fibrinogen or fibrin monomers.

1. **Aminocaproic acid** is used to provide prophylaxis for dental surgery in hemophiliacs, prevent bleeding in prostatic surgery, and reduce hemorrhage in cases of excessive fibrinolysis (e.g., during orthotopic liver transplantation). Because cardiopulmonary bypass can initiate fibrinolysis, aminocaproic acid has been used during cardiac surgery to diminish postoperative bleeding, but its effects on transfusion requirements have been variable. The dose is 10 g IV load over 1 hour followed by 1 to 2 g/h IV.

2. **Thrombotic risks** of aminocaproic acid have been suggested via case reports, but have not been substantiated by clinical trial. Nevertheless, because normal function of the coagulation cascade involves a balance between pro- and anticoagulant effects, using aminocaproic acid in circumstances where uninhibited clotting may be disastrous (e.g., DIC) is ill advised and should be undertaken only with expert guidance.

F. **Aprotinin** is a serine protease inhibitor used to decrease blood loss from complicated cardiac procedures and perhaps major surgeries associated with massive hemorrhage, including orthotopic liver transplantation.

1. Aprotinin inhibits trypsin, plasmin, and kallikrein. In clinical practice, aprotinin helps to prevent the platelet dysfunction seen with cardiopulmonary bypass, but the mechanisms for this effect are poorly understood. One of these mechanisms involves protecting the glycoprotein Ib receptor on platelets, thereby preserving platelet adhesive capability.

2. **Complications** of aprotinin treatment include potential **anaphylactic reaction.** The incidence is approximately 0.1% and is greatest in the first 6 months of repeat exposure. **Toxicity** is primarily renal due

to extensive binding and metabolism in renal tubular cells; these effects appear to be reversible and dose related. Just as with aminocaproic acid, **thrombotic complications** related to aprotinin use are feared. These fears have generally not been borne out by clinical evidence, but the risks make use of the drug for treatment of DIC very controversial.

3. **Because of the risk of allergy**, an initial intravenous test dose of 10,000 kallikrein-inactivating units (KIU) is recommended. For cardiac surgery, a "high-dose" regimen of aprotinin (2 million KIU IV load, 2 million KIU cardiopulmonary bypass pump prime, and 500,000 KIU/h IV infusion) and a "low-dose" regimen (one half of the preceding) have been described. Advantages to low-dose therapy appear to be preserved blood conservation with potentially less renal toxicity. For orthotopic liver transplantation, similar regimens are employed without the pump prime.

4. Aprotinin appears to be more efficacious when it is used prophylactically as opposed to "hemostatic salvage" in the face of massive hemorrhage and coagulopathy. Continuous intravenous infusion at up to 500,000 KIU/h may be continued postoperatively until bleeding has stopped.

5. **Celite ACTs** are artificially prolonged following heparin administration to patients receiving aprotinin. Kaolin-activated ACTs remain accurate.

VI. **Blood conservation and salvage techniques.** Blood transfusion of critically ill patients is common, with approximately 30% to 37% of patients being transfused during an ICU stay. Those patients who are older and stay longer in the ICU are more likely to receive a transfusion. Recent research focusing on possible deleterious effects of homologous blood transfusion in critically ill patients has sparked an interest in techniques to diminish or eliminate the need for blood transfusion.

A. **Phlebotomy losses** from critically ill patients can be significant, ranging from 40 to almost 400 ml/24 h, with higher losses in surgical units versus medical units. Patients with more severe illnesses and a greater number of dysfunctional organs suffer higher phlebotomy losses due to a greater number of blood draws. Techniques demonstrated to reduce phlebotomy losses include (a) a "closed" system of blood sampling where the initial aspirated blood is reinjected into the patient instead of discarded, (b) use of small-volume phlebotomy tubes, and (c) "point-of-care" testing at the bedside, which frequently requires less blood than the clinical laboratory. Finally, the presence of both arterial and central venous catheters in critically ill patients is correlated with higher phlebotomy losses, suggesting another reason to repeatedly evaluate the need for such catheters with respect to hemodynamic monitoring or medication/nutritional support administration.

B. **Surgical drain salvage devices** allow the reinfusion of shed blood. Most commonly used in patients with blood collected from chest tubes, these are useful for reducing homologous transfusions in the immediate postoperative period. Use of these devices requires skilled nursing for proper administration and sterile technique. They are contraindicated in conditions where the drained cavity is infected. A potential danger is hyperkalemia from reinfusion of hemolyzed cells, which is occasionally life threatening.

VII. **Complications of blood transfusion therapy**
    A. **Transfusion reactions**
        1. **Acute hemolytic transfusion reactions** are estimated to occur in 1 in 250,000 transfusions, and are usually due to clerical errors. Symptoms include anxiety, agitation, chest pain, flank pain, headache, dyspnea, and chills. Nonspecific signs include fever, hypotension, unexplained bleeding, and hemoglobinuria. Table 10-2 describes the steps to be taken if a transfusion reaction is suspected.
        2. **Nonhemolytic transfusion reactions** are usually due to antibodies against donor white cells or plasma proteins. These patients may complain of anxiety, pruritus, or mild dyspnea. Signs include fever, flushing, hives, tachycardia, and mild hypotension. The transfusion should be stopped and a hemolytic transfusion reaction ruled out (see prior discussion).
            a. If the reaction is only urticaria or hives, the transfusion should be slowed, and antihistamines (**diphenhydramine,** 25–50 mg IV) and glucocorticoids (**hydrocortisone,** 50–100 mg IV) may be administered.
            b. In patients with known febrile or allergic transfusion reactions, leukocyte-poor red cells (leukocytes removed by filtration or centrifugation) may be given and the patient pretreated with antipyretics (**acetaminophen,** 650 mg) and an antihistamine.

Table 10-2. Treatment of suspected acute hemolytic transfusion reaction

1. Stop transfusion
2. Send remaining donor blood and fresh patient sample to blood bank for re–cross-match
3. Send patient sample to laboratory for free hemoglobin, haptoglobin, Coombs' test, DIC screen
4. Treat hypotension with fluids and/or vasopressors as necessary
5. Consider use of corticosteroids
6. Consider measures to preserve renal function and maintain brisk urine output (intravenous fluid, furosemide, mannitol)
7. Monitor patient for DIC

DIC, disseminated intravascular coagulation.

c. **Anaphylactic reactions** occur rarely and may be more common in patients with an IgA deficiency. These reactions are usually due to plasma protein reactions. Patients with a history of transfusion anaphylaxis should only be transfused with washed red cells (plasma free).

B. **Metabolic complications of blood transfusions**

1. **Potassium (K^+)** concentration changes are common with rapid blood transfusion, but seldom of clinical importance. With storage, red cells leak K^+ into the extracellular storage fluid. This is rapidly corrected with transfusion and replenishment of erythrocyte energy stores.

2. **Calcium** is bound by citrate, which is used as an anticoagulant in stored blood products. Rapid transfusion (one unit of packed red blood cells in 5 minutes) may decrease the ionized calcium level. An equal volume of an FFP transfusion is more likely to cause citrate toxicity compared with packed RBCs because citrate tends to concentrate in plasma during blood processing. Usually, the decreased ionized calcium level is transient because the citrate is rapidly metabolized by the liver. Severe hypocalcemia, manifested as hypotension, QT segment prolongation on the electrocardiogram, and narrowed pulse pressure, may occur in patients who are hypothermic, who have impaired liver function, or who have decreased hepatic blood flow. Ionized calcium levels should be monitored during rapid transfusions, and calcium replaced intravenously with calcium gluconate (30 mg/kg) or calcium chloride (10 mg/kg) if signs or symptoms of hypocalcemia are present.

3. **Acid-base status.** Although banked blood is acidic due to citrate anticoagulant and accumulated red cell metabolite, the actual acid load to the patient is minimal. Acidosis in the face of severe blood loss is more likely due to hypoperfusion and will improve with volume resuscitation. Alkalosis (from metabolism of citrate to bicarbonate) is common following massive blood transfusion.

C. **Infectious complications** of blood transfusions have been markedly reduced due to improved testing of donated blood. Recent changes to U.S. blood bank screening for viral pathogens include addition of specific nucleic acid testing of small pooled donated samples to enhance detection of hepatitis C virus (HCV) and human immunodeficiency virus (HIV) before serologic antibody conversion has occurred. Pooled products (e.g., cryoprecipitate) have an increased risk of infection proportional to the number of donors.

1. **Hepatitis B.** The current risk of HBV transmission is estimated to be 1 in 220,000 units transfused. Although the majority of infections are asymptomatic, with approximately 35% of infected individuals demonstrating acute disease, about 1%

to 10% become chronically infected with potentially significant long-term morbidity.

2. **Hepatitis C.** Institution of routine testing for antibody to HCV in 1990 and more recently nucleic acid testing has reduced the risk of transfusion-related HCV to approximately 1 in 800,000 units. Risks of HCV infection are more serious than those with HBV, however, because 85% of patients suffer chronic infection, 20% develop cirrhosis, and 1% to 5% of infections cause hepatocellular carcinoma.

3. **HIV.** Because of improved screening and testing, the risk of transfusion-associated HIV has been estimated to be about 1 in 1.4 million units transfused in the United States.

4. **Cytomegalovirus (CMV).** The prevalence of antibodies to CMV in the general population is approximately 70% by adulthood. The incidence of transfusion-associated CMV infection in previously noninfected patients is quite high. CMV infection in healthy individuals is usually asymptomatic, but immunosuppressed patients, such as those who have received bone marrow or stem cell transplantation, are at high risk for serious complications, including death. Prevention of CMV infection in high-risk individuals who are exposed to cellular blood elements through transfusion is extremely important. Thus, the American Association of Blood Banks recommends that either CMV-seronegative or leukoreduced blood be administered to transplant recipients who are CMV-negative and to patients undergoing chemotherapy with severe neutropenia an expected consequence.

5. **Bacterial infections.** Exclusion of donors with evidence of infectious disease and the storage of blood at 4°C reduce the risk of transmitted bacterial infection. However, the necessity of room-temperature storage of platelets to maintain functional integrity creates an ideal medium for bacterial growth. Infection rates for platelets are estimated at 1 in 1,000 to 2,000 units, with an estimated 15% to 25% of infected transfusions causing severe sepsis. Organisms likely to infect platelet concentrates include *Staphylococcus aureus,* coagulase-negative *Staphylococcus,* and diphtheroids. Red blood cells are much less likely to become contaminated with bacteria, but the most commonly cultured organism is *Yersinia enterocolitica,* and the mortality rate from transfusion-acquired sepsis is a striking 60%.

D. **Transfusion-related acute lung injury (TRALI)** is a syndrome of severe hypoxemia, dyspnea, and pulmonary edema, often accompanied by fever and hypotension, which is associated with blood transfusion. The pathophysiology is incompletely understood, but clearly involves an increased pulmonary capillary permeability resulting in lung edema. Leading theories for the mechanism of injury include (a) donor blood containing WBC antibodies to recipient WBC antigens resulting in granulocyte or lymphocyte activation and subsequent pulmonary endothelial injury and (b) donor blood containing biologically active lipids, which similarly activate granulocytes. Symptom onset is usually within 4 hours of receiving a blood transfusion, and the clinical findings fulfill criteria for acute lung injury/acute respiratory distress syndrome (see Chapter 20). Incidence of TRALI is estimated at 1 to 2 in 5,000 transfusions. Any transfused product that contains plasma may cause TRALI, but the most commonly reported causative products are RBCs, FFP, and whole blood. Mortality from TRALI is approximately 5%. Treatment is the same as for other forms of acute lung injury and frequently requires mechanical ventilation. Resolution is often rapid given the initial severe oxygenation impairment. Most patients show dramatic clinical improvement within 48 hours and radiographic clearing of edema within 4 days.

VIII. Coagulopathies

A. Massive transfusion is arbitrarily defined as the administration of at least 8 to 10 units of blood transfused within a 12-hour period.

1. Following the administration of 1 to 1.5 blood volumes (assuming a blood volume equals 75 ml/kg), **dilutional thrombocytopenia** can result in diffuse oozing and failure to form clot. Platelets should be readily available and transfused if there is clinical evidence of bleeding. In adults, the usual starting dose is six units.

2. The normal human body has tremendous reserves of clotting factors, and adequate hemostasis generally occurs with a plasma clotting factor concentration as low as 30% of normal. Small amounts of the stable clotting factors also are present in the plasma of each unit of red cells transfused. Bleeding from factor deficiency during a massive transfusion is usually due to diminished levels of fibrinogen and labile factors (V, VIII, and IX). Bleeding from hypofibrinogenemia is unusual unless the fibrinogen level is below 75 mg/dl. Labile clotting factors are administered in the form of fresh-frozen plasma.

3. **Additional complications of massive transfusion** include hypothermia from the rapid infusion of blood, citrate toxicity (see section **VII.B.2**), and dysrhythmias (secondary to hypocalcemia or hypomagnesemia). If ongoing bleeding is present, hypotension secondary to hypovolemia and metabolic acidemia secondary to organ hypoperfusion are to be expected. Hypotension may also be a result of ischemic- or septic-mediated myocardial depression.

4. In addition to transfusion of appropriate blood products, the strategy for massive transfusion includes maintaining intravascular volume, administering

calcium as needed to offset the effects of citrate, and the use of vasopressors with inotropic properties as a *temporizing* measure to maintain systemic arterial pressure until euvolemia has been established. A pulmonary artery catheter may be useful to assess cardiac output and stroke volume. Ongoing surgical bleeding is an indication for operative correction. Antifibrinolytic agents may be considered and employed if fibrinolysis is contributing to bleeding. Frequent laboratory measures of coagulation status are indicated because these parameters change rapidly in the setting of massive hemorrhage and transfusion. Finally, direct communication with the blood bank is important to expedite component preparation.

B. Disseminated intravascular coagulation refers to the abnormal, diffuse systemic activation of the clotting system (Table 10-3). Its presentation can range from mild and asymptomatic to severe and marked by massive hemorrhage, thrombosis, and multiorgan failure.

    1. Etiologies of DIC include infection, shock, trauma, complications of pregnancy (e.g., amniotic fluid embolism, placental abruption, septic abortion), burns,

---

Table 10-3. Causes of disseminated intravascular coagulation

Acute
  Sepsis
  Shock
  Trauma
    Head injury
    Crush injuries
  Pregnancy complications
    Placental abruption
    Amniotic fluid embolism
    Septic abortion
  Hemolytic transfusion reaction
  Extensive burns
  Fat embolism
  Cholesterol emboli
  Acute respiratory distress syndrome
  Liver disease
    Obstructive jaundice
    Acute hepatic failure
  Extracorporeal circulation

Chronic
  Malignancy
  Liver disease
  Aortic dissection/aneurysm
  Retained dead fetus
  Peritoneovenous shunt
  Intraaortic balloon pump

---

fat embolism, and cholesterol embolism. Endothelial cell damage with exposure of collagen may be the cause of DIC seen in shock and infections. DIC is common in extensive **head injury** because of the high content of thromboplastin in brain tissue. **Chronic causes of DIC** include cirrhotic liver disease, aortic aneurysm (particularly with intramural thrombus), aortic dissection, and malignancies.

2. **The pathophysiology of DIC** involves excessive formation of thrombin resulting in fibrin formation throughout the vasculature, platelet activation, fibrinolysis, and consumption of coagulation factors.

3. **Clinical features** include petechiae, ecchymoses, bleeding from venipuncture sites, and hemorrhage from operative incisions. The bleeding manifestations of DIC are most obvious, but the diffuse microvascular and macrovascular thromboses are common, difficult to treat, and frequently life threatening because of ischemia to vital organs. Bradykinin release during DIC may also cause hypotension.

4. **Laboratory features of DIC** include an **elevated D-dimer,** indicating fibrin degradation by plasmin, in all cases. The PT and PTT are prolonged in the majority of cases. FDPs are elevated, but this is not specific to DIC because FDPs may be present from the formation of fibrin by fibrinogen or from the degradation of fibrinogen by plasmin. **Serial measurements** demonstrating a **falling fibrinogen level and platelet count** are characteristic of DIC. Serial measurements are more useful than a single measurement because each may be abnormal at baseline in the critically ill patient. Examination of the peripheral blood smear in the patient with DIC reveals schistocytes in approximately 50% of cases; these are formed from the shearing of RBCs by intravascular fibrin strands.

5. **Treatment**
   a. The primary treatment of DIC involves treating the precipitating cause.
   b. **Transfusion** of appropriate blood components is indicated to correct bleeding. Fibrinogen levels should be maintained above 50 to 100 mg/dl by infusion of FFP (if also indicated for replacement of consumed coagulation factors) or cryoprecipitate.
   c. **Pharmacologic treatment** of DIC is controversial. In cases associated with inappropriate thrombosis rather than bleeding, **heparin therapy** to decrease fibrin formation can be considered, but cautious administration is warranted because this treatment risks life-threatening bleeding. Low-dose heparin treatment has been effective for chronic DIC with thrombosis. Clinical circumstances where heparin treatment of DIC may be beneficial include malignancy with

thrombosis, ischemic digits or skin, amniotic fluid embolus with ongoing passage of amniotic fluid into the vasculature, and stable aortic aneurysm scheduled for elective repair. In cases of large vessel thrombosis, full-dose heparin therapy is indicated. The efficacy of heparin is defined by an increase in fibrinogen levels without exogenous replacement.

   d. Inhibitors of fibrinolysis administered during DIC have some theoretical value but are risky given the possibility of diffuse intravascular thrombosis. In this respect, aminocaproic acid and aprotinin are generally contraindicated for DIC, although aprotinin would likely be more appropriately considered because of its kallikrein-inhibiting and platelet-sparing effects.

   e. Experimental unproved treatments for DIC include anti-thrombin-III (AT III) concentrate, protein C and S concentrates, and direct thrombin inhibitors, such as hirudin and argatroban.

C. Chronic liver disease. With the exception of factor VIII and von Willebrand's factor, which are manufactured by the endothelium, coagulation factors are synthesized by the liver. Patients with hepatic dysfunction may have decreased production of coagulation factors and decreased clearance of activated factors. Patients may have an ongoing consumptive coagulopathy, similar to DIC, if circulating activated clotting factors are increased. Because the liver is also instrumental in removing the byproducts of fibrinolysis, circulating FDPs may be increased. Patients with liver disease frequently have a prolonged PT due to decreased synthesis of clotting factors. Many, however, will respond to vitamin K (see **section VIII.D**) and thus should receive a trial of vitamin K therapy. Failed response to vitamin K and the immediate need to correct coagulopathy require FFP transfusions until the PT has normalized or bleeding has stopped. Thrombocytopenia also occurs frequently in liver disease due to splenic sequestration of platelets. This may be treated with platelet transfusion.

D. Vitamin K deficiency. Vitamin K is required by the liver for production of factors II, VII, IX, and X and proteins C and S. Because vitamin K cannot be synthesized by humans, interference with vitamin K absorption will cause a coagulopathy and a prolonged PT. This can be treated with vitamin K, 2.5 to 25 mg SQ once or 10 mg SQ once daily for 3 days. Intravenous administration of vitamin K can correct the PT slightly faster, but is accompanied by a rare risk of anaphylaxis. If used, intravenous vitamin K should be administered very slowly. If faster correction of PT than with vitamin K is required, fresh-frozen plasma (5–8 ml/kg) can be used.

IX. Anticoagulation. Indications include the prevention or treatment of deep venous thrombosis (DVT), pulmonary embolus (PE), intracardiac thrombus in atrial fibrillation or severe ventricular dysfunction, and vascular graft thrombosis. Anticoagulation also may be required for renal replacement therapy (dialysis or hemofiltration), extracorporeal circulation (ECMO), or cardiac support (intraaortic balloon pump).

A. **Heparin** is a naturally occurring anticoagulant produced from bovine lung or porcine intestine that acts by accelerating the effect of AT III. Structurally, heparin is a heterogeneous mixture of glycosaminoglycans with molecular weights ranging from 3,000 to 30,000 daltons. A repetitive pentasaccharide glucosamine sequence that is present in only one-third of the heparin molecules is necessary for AT III binding. The heparin–AT III complex inactivates several factors in the coagulation cascade, but most importantly thrombin (factor II) and factor X. Longer heparin chains are required for thrombin inhibition than for X inhibition.

1. **For full anticoagulation,** as in the treatment of DVT or PE, heparin may be administered by a continuous intravenous infusion, sometimes after an initial bolus. Efficacy is measured by the PTT, which is prolonged to 60 to 85 seconds. The PTT is determined every 6 hours until the level of anticoagulation is stable. Heparin has a short life (approximately 90 minutes). Stopping a heparin infusion for approximately 2 to 4 hours will usually reverse the effect. If faster reversal is required, **protamine,** a natural antagonist, may be used. Protamine (1 mg for every 100 units of heparin remaining in the patient) should be given slowly because adverse reactions (e.g., hypotension, pulmonary hypertension, hypersensitivity reactions) are common. Institution-wide heparin protocols facilitate adequate anticoagulation.

2. **"Heparin resistance"** occurs frequently in critically ill patients because circulating acute-phase reactants nonspecifically bind heparin and limit its anticoagulant effect. The resulting tachyphylaxis to heparin can usually be overcome with increasing doses of the drug. Occasionally, AT III levels may be depleted in critically ill patients, also contributing to heparin failure. If AT III levels are low, AT III concentrate or, alternatively, FFP may be administered to replete AT III and restore heparin efficacy. Of note, **heparin-induced thrombocytopenia (HIT;** see section **X.B.3**) should always be considered in the differential diagnosis of heparin tachyphylaxis.

1. **Heparin may be administered subcutaneously** in low dose for DVT prophylaxis. The usual dose is 5,000 units SQ every 12 hours. This dose usually does not prolong the PTT.

B. **Low-molecular-weight heparins (LMWH)** are commercially prepared by fractionating heparin into molecules of 2,000 to 10,000 daltons. Most of these lower-molecular-weight molecules are incapable of cross-linking to both antithrombin and thrombin and thus exert their anticoagulant effect primarily by inhibiting factor X. Treatment with LMWH generally does not prolong the PTT and usually does not require laboratory monitoring of anticoagulation. The anticoagulant effect may be assessed by measuring anti-Xa levels, if desired.

1. **Advantages.** LMWH has been shown to be superior to standard heparin in DVT prophylaxis of certain high-risk patients, including patients undergoing elective hip or knee replacement or hip replacement due to fracture. Studies also support a therapeutic advantage in trauma and spinal cord–injured patients. LMWH has a more predictable dose–response relationship for anticoagulation than unfractionated heparin. This occurs because LMWH has much less nonspecific binding to acute-phase reactants than unfractionated heparin. The more predictable effect of LMWH decreases or eliminates the need for laboratory monitoring of drug effect. LMWH anticoagulation may be associated with fewer bleeding complications than standard heparin. Finally, the incidence of HIT is less with LMWH than with unfractionated heparin.

2. **Disadvantages** of LMWH include its long half-life (4 hours), incomplete reversal with protamine, renal clearance, and expense.

3. **Several commercially available preparations of LMWH** are available with slightly different mean molecular weights and anti-Xa activity. LMWH may be administered intravenously, but excellent bioavailability and long half-life permit convenient subcutaneous dosing. Dosing for DVT prophylaxis is 30 mg SQ every 12 hours for **enoxaparin** and 2,500 to 5,000 anti-Xa units SQ once daily for **dalteparin.** Dosing for DVT treatment is 1 mg/kg SQ every 12 hours for enoxaparin and 100 units/kg SQ every 12 hours for dalteparin.

C. **Fondparinux** is a pentasaccharide molecule that selectively inhibits factor Xa by binding to antithrombin and inducing a conformational change that increases antithrombin's binding affinity for Xa. The drug is administered subcutaneously, has a long half-life (14 to 16 hours), and has a predictable anticoagulant effect. Prophylactic doses (2.5 mg daily) normally do not prolong the PT or PTT, and laboratory monitoring of anticoagulant effect is usually unnecessary. In critically ill patients, the drug may be used for either prophylaxis or treatment of DVT. Fondaparinux does not induce HIT, but fears of possible (but unproven) cross-reactivity with HIT antibodies prevent recommending its routine use in patients with demonstrated HIT. Disadvantages to use of fondaparinux in the critically ill include its irreversibility and diminished clearance in the elderly and patients with renal dysfunction.

D. **Warfarin (Coumadin)** inhibits vitamin K epoxide reductase. This produces a deficiency of vitamin K, preventing the hepatic carboxylation of factors II, VII, IX,
   and X and proteins C and S to the active form. The
   half-life of warfarin is approximately 35 hours, requiring days for reversal. If quick reversal of warfarin is
   required, active factors can be given in the form of FFP
   (5–15 ml/kg). **Vitamin K** (2.5–25 mg IV or SQ) can also
   be given for warfarin reversal, but its effect requires 6 or
   more hours. Warfarin may be administered enterally or
   parenterally once daily. Anticoagulation does not occur
   for approximately 3 to 4 days and may require a week
   or more to achieve a stable level. Therapy is guided by
   measurement of the PT or, more usefully, the INR (see
   section **I.C.1.b**). Cautious dosing should be undertaken
   in patients who are vitamin K depleted to avoid over-
   anticoagulation and possible bleeding complications.
E. **Hirudin and argatroban** are specific, direct thrombin inhibitors that may be used for the treatment of
   or as alternative anticoagulants in HIT. Hirudin was
   originally isolated from the salivary gland of leeches,
   but is now produced by recombinant genetic technology
   and marketed as lepirudin. Argatroban is a small, synthetic molecule derived from L-arginine. Both agents act
   independently of cofactors (e.g., AT III) to inhibit not
   only circulating thrombin, but also clot-bound thrombin, thereby inhibiting clot enlargement. Dosage of the
   direct thrombin inhibitors is guided by prolongation of
   the ACT or PTT to therapeutic range. The short half-
   lives (80 minutes for lepirudin, 40 minutes for argatroban) of these agents allow relatively rapid reversal of
   anticoagulation by stopping the drug. Both hirudin and
   argatroban are approved by the Food and Drug Administration for treatment of HIT complicated by thrombosis; argatroban is approved for prophylaxis against
   thrombosis in patients with HIT. Table 10-4 reflects
   current dose guidelines for this indication. Lepirudin
   undergoes renal excretion, and thus its use should be
   avoided or the dose carefully adjusted in patients with
   renal failure due to the risk for bleeding. Argatroban
   undergoes hepatobiliary excretion and requires dose adjustment in patients with hepatic dysfunction. Argatroban prolongs the INR, complicating assessment of
   warfarin anticoagulant effect when patients are transitioned from parenteral to enteral anticoagulation.
   Argatroban has a greater pharmacodynamic predictability than lepirudin and may have a greater safety
   profile in critically ill patients due to its reliable excretion even in moderate renal failure. In addition, argatroban crosses the blood–brain barrier and may serve a
   role in the treatment of ischemic or thrombotic stroke.
   Neither lepirudin nor argatroban, however, has a reversal agent. Another new drug in the category of direct
   thrombin inhibitors is **bivalirudin,** a hirudin analogue
   with a short (25 minute) half-life that is administered

Table 10-4. Dosing guidelines for treatment of heparin-induced thrombocytopenia (HIT)

Drug	Initial dose	Adjustment	Comment
Argatroban	1–2 μg/kg/min	Titrate to target PTT 1.5–3.0 times baseline	Diminish initial dose to 0.5 μg/kg/min if hepatic dysfunction
Lepirudin	Bolus 0.4 mg/kg, then infuse 0.15 mg/kg/h	Titrate to target PTT 1.5–2.5 times baseline	Consider omission of the bolus to reduce risk of bleeding; consider argatroban if renal dysfunction

PTT, partial thromboplastin time.

via intravenous infusion for percutaneous coronary interventions. Anecdotal reports suggest its efficacy in the treatment of patients with HIT, but there is insufficient data about the drug to recommend its routine use in HIT.

F. **Thrombolytic agents** act by dissolving thrombi via conversion of plasminogen to plasmin, which lyses fibrin clots. They are intended to reverse thrombosis and recanalize blood vessels. These agents are used to treat acute occlusion of coronary, cerebral, pulmonary, and peripheral arteries, typically in combination with heparin to prevent reocclusion. Three thrombolytic agents, **tissue plasminogen activator (tPA), streptokinase,** and **urokinase,** are used commonly in clinical practice, each with slightly different pharmacodynamic and side effect profiles. Each of these drugs results in a hypofibrinogenemic state and carries a substantial risk of bleeding. They are generally contraindicated perioperatively. If emergent surgery is required following thrombolytic therapy, the effect may be reversed by administration of aminocaproic or tranexamic acid. Additionally, the fibrinogen level may be restored by transfusion of cryoprecipitate or FFP (see sections **III.D** and **III.E**).

G. **Platelet inhibitors** may be useful for reducing thromboembolic events in patients with arterial vascular disorders (e.g., carotid stenosis), prosthetic heart valves, or recent invasive arterial procedures (e.g., percutaneous coronary angioplasty or stenting). **Aspirin** and **nonsteroidal antiinflammatory drugs** (NSAIDs) inhibit platelet aggregation by interfering with the cyclooxygenase pathway. Aspirin permanently inhibits the pathway for the lifespan of the platelet. Because the half-life of platelets in circulation is approximately 4 days, at least 10 days is required before platelet function returns to normal after aspirin. The other NSAIDs reversibly inhibit the cyclooxygenase pathway; their effects dissipate within 3 days of discontinuing the drug. **Ticlopidine** and **clopidogrel** are newer oral antiplatelet agents that inhibit ADP-mediated platelet aggregation and are frequently used following percutaneous coronary interventions. The intravenous glycoprotein IIb/IIIa receptor inhibitors **abciximab** and **eptifibatide** are drugs that bind to the key platelet receptor that mediates aggregation. Fibrinogen, von Willebrand's factor, and other adhesive molecules are thereby blocked from binding to the platelet, inhibiting platelet aggregation and resulting in anticoagulation. Both drugs may be used for treatment of acute coronary syndromes or during percutaneous coronary interventions. Abciximab remains in the circulation bound to platelets 15 days following dosing, although platelet function is usually recovered within 48 hours after a dose. Eptifibatide has a reversible antiplatelet effect that normalizes approximately 4 hours after discontinuation of the infusion. **The use of glycoprotein IIb/IIIa receptor inhibitors is contraindicated within 6 weeks of major surgery** or trauma due to bleeding risk. Immediate reversal of platelet inhibitors may require platelet transfusion, although even this treatment may result in only partial reversal of the effect (see section **III.C**).

X. **Abnormalities of hemostasis**

A. **Bleeding disorders**

1. **Classic hemophilia or hemophilia A** is due to an abnormality of factor VIII. The incidence in the United States. is 1 in 10,000. It is a sex-linked recessive trait, affecting male individuals almost exclusively.

   a. **Clinical features.** The diagnosis should be suspected in a patient with the appropriate history and an elevated PTT but normal PT. Bleeding episodes are related to the level of factor VIII activity (normal is 100%):

   (1) Less than 1% activity: spontaneous bleeding.

   (2) From 1% to 5% activity: bleeding after minor trauma.

   (3) Greater than 5% activity: infrequent bleeding.

   b. Because these patients have normal platelet function, they are able to form an initial clot, and they will have normal bleeding times. Because they are unable to stabilize the blood clot, however, bleeding will recur.

   c. **Treatment** consists of lyophilized factor VIII, rFVIIa, cryoprecipitate, or desmopressin. A dose of 1 unit/kg of factor VIII will increase the activity of factor VIII by approximately 2%. Activity levels of 20% to 40% are recommended prior to surgery. The half-life of factor VIII is 8 to 12 hours. Because up to 20% of patients will eventually develop resistance due to antibodies against factor VIII, factor VIII activity levels should be measured before and after transfusion. Patients with resistance must then be treated with high-dose factor VIII, activated factor IX, or plasmapheresis. Because many hemophiliacs have received multiple transfusions over their lifetimes, many are seropositive for HIV and hepatitis.

2. **Hemophilia B, or Christmas disease,** is due to a factor IX abnormality. It also is sex linked, occurring almost exclusively in male individuals, and has an incidence of 1 in 100,000. These patients present similarly to patients with classic hemophilia, and have an abnormal PTT and a normal PT. Therapy consists of factor IX concentrates, rFVIIa, or fresh-frozen plasma. For surgical hemostasis, activity levels of 50% to 80% are necessary (0.5–0.8 units/ml). A dose of 1 unit/kg of factor IX will increase the activity of factor IX by about 1%. The half-life of factor IX is approximately 24 hours.

3. **von Willebrand's disease** is associated with abnormalities of von Willebrand's factor, a glycoprotein manufactured by megakaryocytes and endothelial cells that has multiple functions. It serves as an anchor for platelet adhesion to collagen, it interlinks platelets (aggregation) in clot formation, and it protects and stabilizes VIII. von Willebrand's disease is most commonly inherited in an autosomal dominant pattern with variable penetrance.

   a. **Clinical features.** The bleeding tendency of these patients is quite variable. Most commonly, these patients have episodes of mucocutaneous bleeding such as epistaxis.

   b. The most common laboratory finding is a prolonged bleeding time, although the PTT may also be prolonged.

   c. **Treatment** for these individuals includes desmopressin (see **section V.C**) and/or cryoprecipitate. Plasma products may also be required for an actively bleeding patient. Cryoprecipitate is preferred; but fresh-frozen plasma may be used if cryoprecipitate is unavailable. In patients with acquired von Willebrand's disease, high-dose IV gamma globulin (1 g/kg for 2 days) has been used successfully.

4. **Other rare factor deficiencies** that predispose patients to bleeding have been described, including deficiencies of fibrinogen, factor II (prothrombin), factor V, factor VII, factor X, factor XI, and factor XIII. Treatment usually consists of factor concentrate or

blood component replacement, and is best guided by expert hematology consultation.

B. **Clotting disorders**
   1. **Congenital hypercoagulability abnormalities,** which predispose to clotting, may cause thrombosis and concurrent critical illness. Many specialized tests are available for diagnosing these abnormalities and guide therapy, which usually consists of lifelong anticoagulation. Test results may affect not only the patient, but also family members because many of these disorders are genetically transmitted. For patients presenting with **venous thromboembolism,** consideration should be given to testing for factor V Leiden (activated protein C resistance), AT III defects, protein C and S deficiency, antiphospholipid antibodies, and hyperhomocysteinemia. The exact tests to be performed may be best determined by patient and family history. Many of these tests are unreliable during an acute illness because of the presence of acute-phase reactants. For these reasons, a clinical pathology or hematology consultation is advisable when a congenital hypercoagulable state is suspected.
   2. **Acquired disorders**
      a. **Surgery, pregnancy, and trauma** all predispose to thrombosis. The cause is multifactorial. In surgical patients, venous stasis during perioperative immobility contributes. In addition, surgery and trauma produce a systemic response marked by an increase in acute-phase reactants, including increases in fibrinogen, factor VIII, and alpha-1-antitrypsin. Fibrinolytic proteins and coagulation inhibitors are decreased. Platelet activation and aggregation is enhanced. All of the preceding events promote a hypercoagulable state in surgical and trauma patients and mandate aggressive prophylaxis for thromboembolism (see Chapter 12). Prophylaxis may include pneumatic compression boots, early ambulation, and treatment with heparin, LMWH, heparinoids, or warfarin (see Section **IX**).
   3. **HIT** occurs in two forms:
      a. **HIT type I,** a common, non–immune-mediated phenomenon, is a benign drop in platelet count within 5 days of institution of heparin therapy. Platelet counts rarely fall to less than 100,000 and recover to normal after approximately 5 days. **HIT type I does not require discontinuation of heparin and does not carry a risk of thrombosis.**
      b. **HIT type II,** hereafter referred to as **HIT,** is an immune-mediated thrombocytopenia triggered by IgG antibodies, which may form against heparin–platelet factor 4 (PF 4) complexes. The

heparin–PF 4 complexes are seen as "antigens" and are bound to the Fc receptor on the platelet, activating the platelet and causing platelet aggregation and further PF 4 release. The result is thrombocytopenia, platelet aggregation, and the potential for arterial and venous thromboses.

(1) The spectrum of HIT is best described by the "iceberg model," which suggests that a significant number of patients who are exposed to heparin develop the heparin–PF 4 complex antibody; a subset of these develop platelet aggregation and thrombocytopenia, and a small fraction of this subset develop vascular thrombosis. Data suggest that up to 50% of cardiac surgery patients and 15% of orthopedic surgery patients who are exposed to unfractionated heparin develop the HIT antibody as assessed by the enzyme-linked immunosorbent assay (ELISA). Of these, approximately 1% and 3%, respectively, go on to develop clinical HIT with thrombosis. The risk for HIT is greater with use of bovine versus porcine unfractionated heparin and may be dramatically reduced by use of low-molecular-weight heparins. Use of fondaparinux or the direct thrombin inhibitors for parenteral anticoagulation is not associated with development of HIT.

(2) The diagnosis of HIT should be suspected in a patient noted to have a greater than 50% drop in platelet count from baseline, with the onset of the drop usually occurring 5 to 14 days after heparin exposure, but potentially sooner if the patient has a circulating antibody and is reexposed to heparin. The heparin exposure may occur in any form, including subcutaneous prophylactic dosing, heparin flushes for indwelling catheters, or heparin coatings on indwelling central lines (e.g. pulmonary artery catheters). **Unexplained tachyphylaxis or resistance to heparin anticoagulation may be suggestive of HIT, as may recovery of the platelet count after discontinuing heparin.** The diagnosis is usually easy to make with ELISA testing in the proper clinical setting. Confirmation with a functional test of platelet aggregation such as the platelet serotonin release assay may be desirable because of the imperfect specificity of ELISA, but is in general impractical because of the limited availability of this test outside research settings.

(3) The clinical course of HIT is notable for a median nadir of the platelet count of 50,000.

Despite the thrombocytopenia, the hallmark of the syndrome is platelet activation, aggregation, and a cascade of procoagulant effects resulting in thrombosis.

(4) Treatment of suspected or diagnosed HIT consists of (a) discontinuing all heparin exposure, including stopping heparin flushes and removing heparin-coated vascular catheters, and (b) initiating alternate anticoagulation, usually with a direct thrombin inhibitor. Prophylactic platelet transfusions are contraindicated and usually unnecessary because thrombosis is a far greater clinical problem than bleeding. The importance of alternate anticoagulation in these patients must be emphasized because approximately 40% of patients with HIT will develop thrombotic complications with resultant amputation in 10% to 20% and death in 30% to 50%.

(5) Thromboses due to HIT most commonly present as DVT or PE, but mesenteric venous and cerebral sinus thromboses have been reported. In addition, clotting of arterial vasculature may occur, particularly at sites of severe atherosclerosis or recent arterial trauma (e.g., vascular access catheters). Arterial thromboses may present as mesenteric or limb ischemia, stroke, or myocardial infarction.

(6) No consensus exists as to the required **duration** of anticoagulant therapy for HIT, but most consultants recommend at least 6 weeks of treatment with an endpoint possibly marked by disappearance of the HIT antibody on ELISA. Oral anticoagulation should not be used to treat acute HIT and should not be initiated until the platelet count is greater than 100,000. When initiating oral anticoagulation, it is critical to overlap therapy with a direct thrombin inhibitor because warfarin treatment is associated with an initial brief period of hypercoagulability due to decreased levels of protein C preceding adequate suppression of prothrombin levels. Thus, initiation of warfarin without overlapping anticoagulation can trigger venous limb gangrene. Reference to an algorithm for the transition to oral anticoagulation in HIT or consultation with a hematologist is recommended.

XI. **Special considerations**

A. **Sickle cell (SC) disease** has a prevalence of approximately 1% in the African-American population of the United States. Sickle cell disease is caused by the substitution of valine for glutamic acid at the sixth position on the beta chain of hemoglobin. Homozygotes for this substitution (as well as double heterozygotes for SC or beta-thalassemia) have clinical sickle cell disease.

1. **Clinical features.** The abnormal hemoglobin polymerizes and causes a sickling deformity of the red cell under certain conditions (e.g., hypoxia, hypothermia, acidosis, and dehydration). Sickled cells cause microvascular occlusion with tissue ischemia and infarction. A sickle cell crisis typically presents with excruciating chest or abdominal pain, fever, tachycardia, leukocytosis, and hematuria. The red cells have a shortened survival time of 12 days (normal being 120 days), leading to anemia and extramedullary hematopoiesis. Neonates are usually protected from sickle crisis for the first few months of life due to persistent fetal hemoglobin (hemoglobin F). Patients with sickle cell trait are usually asymptomatic.

2. **The perioperative management** of these patients remains controversial. It had been common practice to give patients preoperative RBC transfusions to increase the Hct and decrease the relative proportion of Hgb S. Past guidelines suggested transfusing to an endpoint of having 70% Hgb A and less than 30% Hgb S cells as measured by hemoglobin electrophoresis prior to major surgery. Recently, this practice has been questioned, and routine preoperative transfusion of asymptomatic patients is not recommended. Perioperative care should be directed at reducing the risk of sickling. Because hypoxia is a known precipitant of sickling, these patients should be well oxygenated at all times. Acidosis should be avoided. Patients should be well hydrated to maintain intravascular volume and ensure adequate tissue perfusion (preventing systemic acidosis). Hypothermia should also be avoided because it can precipitate sickle cell crises, probably due to increased blood viscosity and stasis.

B. **Jehovah's Witness patients** generally may refuse to receive blood or blood products (e.g., fresh-frozen plasma, platelets, cryoprecipitate, or albumin) based on their religious beliefs even if such refusal results in death. Some patients may accept autotransfused or chest tube salvaged autologous blood, especially if it remains in contiguous circulation with their vasculature.

1. Special considerations regarding homologous transfusion may apply if the patient is a minor, is incompetent, or has responsibilities for dependents and in certain emergency circumstances. An ethical dilemma may present when unexpected hemorrhage is encountered in the operating room or critical care unit following a preoperative agreement not to transfuse. Careful documentation of preoperative discussions and informed consent is mandatory.

Legal precedent generally supports patient autonomy regarding the acceptance of transfusion.

2. **In the critically ill Jehovah's Witness who refuses blood transfusion,** blood conservation measures are extremely important. Efforts to minimize iatrogenic blood loss, including minimizing phlebotomies, should be employed. Erythropoietin (which contains a small amount of human albumin) is sometimes used in combination with iron to increase red cell mass perioperatively. In extreme circumstances of anemia, measures to diminish oxygen consumption via sedation, pharmacologic paralysis, and hypothermia may be attempted. Hypothermia, however, may contribute to coagulopathy and cause further bleeding. Finally, hyperbaric oxygen therapy has been used in these patients to increase tissue oxygenation, but improved outcome has not been demonstrated.

SELECTED REFERENCES

American Society of Anesthesiologists Task Force on Blood Component Therapy. Practice guidelines for blood component therapy. *Anesthesiology* 1996;84:732–747.

Boehlen F, Morales MA, Fontana P, et al. Prolonged treatment of massive postpartum haemorrhage with recombinant factor VIIa; case report and review of the literature. *BJOG* 2004;111:284–287.

Cochrane Injuries Group Albumin Reviewers. Human albumin administration in critically ill patients: systematic review of randomized controlled trials. *BMJ* 1998;317:235–340.

Corwin HL, Gettinger A, Pearl RG, et al. Efficacy of recombinant human erythropoietin in critically ill patients. *JAMA* 2002;288:2827–2835.

Dutton RP, Hess JR, Scalea TM. Recombinant factor VIIa for control of hemorrhage: early experience in critically ill trauma patients. *J Clin Anesth* 2003;15:184–188.

Fowler RA, Berenson M. Blood conservation in the intensive care unit. *Crit Care Med* 2003;31(Suppl.):S715–S720.

Goodnough LT. Risks of blood transfusion. *Crit Care Med* 2003;31 (Suppl.):S678–S686.

Hebert PC, Wells G, Blajchman MA, et al. A multicenter, randomized, controlled clinical trial of transfusion requirements in critical care. *N Engl J Med* 1999;340:409–417.

Lake CL, Moore RA, eds. *Blood: hemostasis, transfusion, and alternatives in the perioperative period.* New York: Raven Press, 1995.

O'Connell NM, Perry DJ, Hodgson AJ, et al. Recombinant FVIIa in the management of uncontrolled hemorrhage. *Transfusion* 2003;43:1711–1716.

The SAFE Study Investigators. A comparison of albumin and saline for fluid resuscitation in the intensive care unit. *N Engl J Med* 2004;350:2247–2256.

Warkentin TE. Heparin-induced thrombocytopenia: pathogenesis and management. *Br J Haematol* 2003;121:535–555.

General Considerations in Infectious Disease

Catherine Valentine and Judith Hellman

I. Introduction

  A. Diagnosis of infection in intensive care unit (ICU) patients can be difficult because they often develop clinical signs of infection (e.g., fever, hemodynamic instability, etc.) from noninfectious causes and often have multiple potential sites of infection (Table 11-1). A systematic, thorough evaluation is essential to localize site(s) of infection and to exclude noninfectious etiologies so that appropriate intervention(s) can be initiated.

  B. There are many risk factors for development of serious infections in the ICU (Table 11-2). **Nosocomial infections** are hospital-acquired infections occurring after 48 hours of hospitalization. Nosocomial infections tend to be caused by organisms with increased antimicrobial resistance.

  C. Infections are caused by a variety of microorganisms, including bacteria, fungi, viruses, and parasites. Common organisms are shown in Table 11-3.

II. Antibacterial agents

  A. *β*-**Lactam** antimicrobial agents, including **penicillins, cephalosporins, monobactams,** and **carbapenems,** interfere with bacterial cell wall synthesis. The spectrum of various *β*-lactams varies widely. *β*-lactam agents have bactericidal activity against susceptible organisms. However, they have only bacteriostatic activity against *Enterococcus* species (spp). A synergistic combination of a *β*-lactam (or vancomycin) plus an aminoglycoside is necessary for bactericidal activity against *Enterococcus* spp. **Resistance** to *β*-lactams results from production of *β*-lactamase, altered binding to penicillin-binding proteins, and/or decreased antibiotic penetration into the bacteria. Treatment of *Enterobacter* spp, *Citrobacter* spp, and *Acinetobacter* spp with *β*-lactams, especially cephalosporins, may be complicated by rapid development of resistance because they harbor an inducible chromosomal *β*-lactamase.

  1. Penicillins (penicillin, nafcillin, ampicillin, ticarcillin, piperacillin)

  a. Spectrum

  (1) Penicillin and **nafcillin** are active against aerobic and anaerobic gram-positive bacteria. **Penicillin** is active against gram-positive cocci such as *Streptococcus* spp, gram-positive rods such as *Listeria monocytogenes,* and many anaerobes. *Staphylococcus (S.) aureus* and *S.*

Table 11-1. Potential sites of infection in intensive care unit patients

Site	Infection
Surgical	Superficial and deep wound infection, anastamotic breakdown, abscess
Chest	Pneumonia, tracheobronchitis, mediastinitis, lung abscess, empyema, endocarditis
Abdomen	Peritonitis, abscess, cholecystitis, cholangitis, urinary tract infection, *Clostridium* (*C.*) *difficile* colitis
Head and neck	Sinusitis, parotitis, central nervous system infection, periotonsillar abscess
Indwelling catheters	Urinary, intravascular

epidermidis are often resistant. **Nafcillin** is effective against *S. aureus,* excluding methicillin-resistant *S. aureus* (MRSA). Nafcillin is less active than penicillin against *Streptococcus* spp.

(2) **Ampicillin** is active against many gram-positive cocci and enteric gram-negative bacilli, including *Escherichia coli, Proteus* spp, and *Serratia* spp. The addition of the β-lactamase inhibitor sulbactam to ampicillin **(Unasyn)** increases the activity against *S. aureus* (not MRSA), β-lactamase producing gram-negatives, and anaerobes.

(3) **Ticarcillin** and **piperacillin** are active against gram-positive, gram-negative, and anaerobic bacteria. Their resistance to β-lactamase confers broader gram-negative coverage than ampicillin and can include *Pseudomonas* spp and *Enterobacter* spp. **Piperacillin** is also active against some species of *Klebsiella.* Although these antipseudomonal penicillins are active against many gram-positives,

Table 11-2. Risk factors for infections in the intensive care unit

1. Age >70 years
2. Shock
3. Major trauma
4. Coma
5. Prior antibiotics
6. Mechanical ventilation
7. Drugs affect the immune system (steroids, chemotherapy)
8. Indwelling catheters
9. Prolonged intensive care unit stay (>3 days)
10. Acute renal failure

Table 11-3.   Classification of microorganisms causing infections in the intensive care unit

General Groups	Specific Microorganisms
Bacteria: gram-positive aerobes	*Staphylococcus aureus (S. aureus), S. epidermidis* (coagulase-negative staphylococcus), *Streptococcus* spp, *Enterococcus* spp
Bacteria: enteric gram-negative aerobes and facultative anaerobes	*Escherichia coli (E. coli), Klebsiella pneumoniae, Proteus mirabilis, Enterobacter cloacae (E. cloacae)* and other *Enterobacter* spp, *Acinetobacter* spp, *Citrobacter* spp, *Serratia marcescens, Salmonella* spp
Bacteria: nonenteric gram-negative aerobes and facultative anaerobes	*Pseudomonas aeruginosa, Burkholderia* (previously known as *Pseudomonas) cepacia, Neisseria* spp, *Haemophilus (H.) influenzae H. parainfluenzae*
Bacteria: anaerobes (gram-positive and gram-negative)	*Bacteroides fragilis* and other *Bacteroides* spp, *Clostridium (C.) difficile* and other *Clostridium* spp, *Peptostreptococcus* spp
Fungi	*Candida* spp, *Aspergillus* spp, *Histoplasma capsulatum, Pneumocystis carinii*
Viruses	Varicella zoster virus (VZV), herpes simplex virus (HSV) I and II, cytomegalovirus (CMV), Epstein-Barr virus (EBV)

S. aureus is often resistant. The addition of the β-lactamase inhibitor clavulanate to ticarcillin **(Timentin)** and the addition of tazobactam to piperacillin **(Zosyn)** broaden the spectrum to include *S. aureus* (except MRSA), *Bacteroides fragilis,* and some aerobic β-lactamase–producing gram-negatives.

   b. **Adverse reactions** to penicillins include hypersensitivity reactions ranging from rash to anaphylaxis, bleeding due to impaired platelet function (ticarcillin), volume overload or hypernatremia due to a large salt load (ticarcillin, piperacillin), interstitial nephritis (especially nafcillin), neutropenia (nafcillin at high doses), fever, and central nervous system (CNS) toxicity. A history of **"allergy"** to penicillin is often elicited in patients without clear documentation that an actual allergic reaction has occurred. **Skin testing** may be useful in diagnosing true allergy to β-lactams. **Desensitization** may be an option if a β-lactam is essential for optimal treatment of a life-threatening bacterial infection in a patient with a history of a severe β-lactam allergy. Rapid desensitization may be achieved by intravenous administration of escalating doses of the desired antibiotic in a carefully monitored setting. Because of the potential for serious complications, a physician who is trained in this procedure should perform the desensitization.

2. **Cephalosporins**
   a. **Spectrum**
      (1) **First-generation cephalosporins** such as **cefazolin** are active against many gram-positive and some gram-negative bacteria. Enteric gram-negative rods such as *E. coli,* some *Klebsiella* spp, and gram-positive oral anaerobes are often susceptible. *Enterococcus* spp, methicillin-resistant *S. epidermidis* (MRSE), and gram-negative anaerobes such as *Bacteroides* spp are resistant to cefazolin.

      (2) **Second-generation cephalosporins** are more active against gram-negatives and less active against gram-positives than are first-generation agents. There are two major subgroups of second-generation cephalosporins. One group, which includes **cefuroxime,** is active against *Haemophilus* (*H.*) *influenzae.* The other group, which includes **cefoxitin** and **cefotetan,** is active against anaerobes such as *Bacteroides* spp.

      (3) **Third-generation cephalosporins** have greater activity against gram-negative bacilli than do second-generation agents. They are active against most enteric and some nonenteric (*H. influenzae* and *Neisseria* spp) gram-negative bacilli. *Enterobacter* spp, *Citrobacter* spp, and *Acinetobacter* spp often become resistant to third-generation cephalosporins because of inducible production of β-lactamase. **Ceftazidime** has strong activity against *Pseudomonas* spp, but is poorly active against gram-positives. **Ceftriaxone** and **cefotaxime** have activity against some gram-positives (not *Enterococcus* spp, *Listeria monocytogenes,* MRSA, or MRSE), but are often ineffective against *Pseudomonas* spp. Third-generation cephalosporins have good CNS penetration and are often used for treatment of bacterial meningitis.

      (4) **Fourth-generation cephalosporins** such as **cefepime** have a similar spectrum to ceftriaxone against gram-positive cocci, but broader gram-negative coverage that includes bacteria with inducible β-lactamase, such as *Enterobacter* spp, and *Citrobacter* spp. They may also be active against some ceftazidime-resistant *Pseudomonas aeruginosa.*

   b. Adverse reactions to cephalosporins include hypersensitivity reactions (5%–10% incidence of cross-reactivity with penicillin allergy) and bleeding due to inhibition of vitamin K–dependent coagulation factor synthesis (cefotetan).

3. **Carbapenems** have broad antibacterial activity. They offer the advantage of extensive coverage of gram-positives, gram-negatives, and anaerobes. It is prudent to reserve carbapenem agents for treating documented nosocomial infections due to antibiotic-resistant bacteria.

   a. The spectra of **imipenem/cilastatin** and **meropenem** are similar. They are active against most gram-negatives, many gram-positives, and anaerobes. Although they have the broadest spectrum of the β-lactams, some pathogenic strains remain resistant. Resistant gram-negatives have included *Stenotrophomonas maltophilia, Burkholderia* (previously known as *Pseudomonas*) *cepacia,* and occasionally *Pseudomonas aeruginosa, Enterobacter cloacae,* and *Serratia marcescens.* Resistant gram-positives have included some *Enterococci* spp, MRSA, *Corynebacterium* spp, and *Bacteroides* spp. **Ertapenem** is a newer carbapenem with a similar spectrum to imipenem/cilastatin and meropenem, except that it has limited activity against *Pseudomonas* and *Acinetobacter* species. Therefore ertapenem is not recommended for use as empiric therapy in nosocomial infections, but rather for directed treatment of a sensitive pathogen. Ertapenem offers the advantages that it does not require dose adjustment for renal insufficiency and it can be administered once a day.

   b. Adverse reactions include seizures and hypersensitivity reactions. Safety data from clinical trials using meropenem suggest that it may be less frequently associated with seizures than imipenem/cilastatin. Ertapenem also has a reported decreased incidence of seizure activity relative to imipenem/cilastatin.

4. **Monobactams**

   a. Spectrum. Aztreonam is active against many gram-negative bacteria. It is not active against gram-positive bacteria or anaerobes. Some nonenteric gram-negatives can be resistant, including *S. maltophilia* and *Acinetobacter* spp, and *P. aeruginosa.*

   b. Adverse reactions include hypersensitivity reactions. Despite the β-lactam structure, aztreonam seems to have very little cross-reactivity with other β-lactams and is often used in patients who have had minor allergic responses to β-lactams. There is a theoretical concern that patients with anaphylaxis to ceftazidime may also react to aztreonam because both drugs have a side chain in common; however, clinical data supporting this are sparse.

B. Glycopeptides, including **vancomycin** and **teicoplanin,** interfere with bacterial cell wall synthesis.

1. Spectrum. Glycopeptides are bactericidal for most gram-positive bacteria. They are active against the highly resistant staphylococcal strains, MRSA and MRSE, as well as *Enterococcus* spp and *Streptococcus* spp. As with the β-lactams, vancomycin is not bactericidal for *Enterococcus* spp, and should be combined with an aminoglycoside for synergistic coverage if bactericidal activity is required.

2. Adverse reactions to vancomycin include "red man syndrome," rash, ototoxicity, nephrotoxicity, and neutropenia. "Red man syndrome" is a histamine-release syndrome characterized by flushing of the face, neck, and trunk and variable degrees of hypotension. This reaction is not truly allergic (not immunoglobulin E [IgE] mediated) in nature, occurs frequently, is generally mild and transient (20 minutes), and can be minimized by delivering the drug in a large volume, reducing the dose, slowing the rate of infusion, and/or premedicating with an antihistamine. The other adverse effects listed are rare. Ototoxicity often is not reversible and may be associated with a gait disturbance.

3. Vancomycin-resistant gram-positive bacteria. Vancomycin-resistant isolates of *Enterococcus* (VRE) have become very common. Of great concern is the emergence over the last several years of vancomycin-intermediate and rare vancomycin-resistant strains of *S. aureus*. Thus, vancomycin should be used cautiously and for clear indications.

C. Linezolid, an oxazolidinone, is bacteriostatic and acts by inhibiting bacterial protein synthesis. It is approved for treatment of VRE, hospital- and community-acquired pneumonia, and infections of the skin and skin structures. Enteral absorption of linezolid is excellent, with equivalent bioavailability to intravenous administration.

1. Spectrum: active against highly resistant gram-positive bacteria, including MRSA, penicillin-resistant *Streptococcus pneumoniae,* and VRE, including vancomycin-resistant *Enterococcus faecalis.*

2. Adverse reactions: headache, diarrhea, tongue discoloration. With prolonged therapy, mild reversible anemia, thrombocytopenia, and leucopenia.

3. Drug interactions. Because linezolid reversibly inhibits monoamine oxidase, it has the potential for interaction with adrenergic and serotonergic agents.

D. Quinupristin/dalfopristin (Synercid) is a mixture of streptogramin A and B antibiotics that act by inhibiting bacterial protein synthesis. It is approved for treatment in adults of vancomycin-resistant *Enterococcus faecium* bacteremia or complicated infections of the skin and skin structures.

1. **Spectrum:** active against MRSA, methicillin-resistant coagulase-negative staphylococci, *Streptococcus pneumoniae,* and most strains of *Enterococcus faecium. Enterococcus faecalis* may be resistant.

2. **Adverse reactions:** discomfort/swelling at the infusion site, nausea, vomiting, diarrhea, rash, myalgias, arthralgias, increased bilirubin, increased gamma-glutamyl transferase. Rarely Synercid causes increased serum creatinine, thrombocytopenia, and anemia.

3. **Multiple drug interactions:** cyclosporine, carbamazepine, calcium-channel blockers, diazepam, midazolam, dysopyramide, lidocaine, methylprednisolone, astemizole, cisapride, statins.

E. **Daptomycin** is a relatively new bactericidal cyclic lipopeptide that has been approved by the Food and Drug Administration for treatment of complicated skin and skin structure infections due to gram-positive bacteria.

1. **Spectrum.** Daptomycin is active *in vitro* against methicillin-resistant *S. aureus* and *S. epidermidis* as well as VRE species.

2. **Adverse reactions:** gastrointestinal (GI) effects such as nausea, diarrhea, and constipation and elevated creatine phosphokinases.

F. **Aminoglycosides** are bactericidal agents that interfere with bacterial protein synthesis. **Gentamicin, tobramycin,** and **amikacin** are the most commonly used aminoglycosides in the ICU.

1. **Spectrum.** Aminoglycosides are active primarily against gram-negatives, although they are synergistic with the cell wall–active agents (β-lactams, vancomycin) against *Enterococcus* spp, *Staphylococcus* spp, and *Streptococcus viridans.* Most enteric gram-negatives are sensitive. *Pseudomonas aeruginosa* is often sensitive, but *B. cepacia* and *Stenotrophomonas maltophilia* are often resistant.

2. **Adverse reactions** include nephrotoxicity, ototoxicity, weakness, and potentiation of neuromuscular blockade. Nephrotoxicity is generally mild, nonoliguric, and reversible. Risk factors for nephrotoxicity include advanced age, overall debilitation, baseline renal dysfunction, hypotension, hypovolemia, and concomitant administration of other nephrotoxins. These risk factors are not absolute contraindications to aminoglycoside administration. Aminoglycosides can be extremely useful in some life-threatening infections (e.g., endocarditis caused by *Enterococcus* spp or *Pseudomonas* spp), and in some situations may be indicated despite the potential for renal toxicity.

3. **Low pH and low oxygen tension** significantly diminish aminoglycoside antibacterial activity. Thus,

they are not considered to be effective in acidic fluids (such as ascites) or under anaerobic conditions (such as within abscesses and poorly perfused tissues).

4. **Tissue concentrations** of aminoglycosides are variable. Low concentrations are achieved in tracheo-bronchopulmonary secretions, and CNS penetration is poor.

5. **Monitoring aminoglycoside levels.** Peak serum concentrations are often measured to verify that bactericidal levels are achieved, and trough levels are measured to assure adequate clearance of the drug in the hopes of preventing renal toxicity.

6. **Once-a-day administration** may have some advantages, including less renal toxicity, maximization of concentration-dependent bactericidal activity, and a "postantibiotic effect" whereby bacterial growth is suppressed even after the serum level drops below the minimal inhibitory concentration. Although studies have not conclusively shown improved eradication of serious infections in adults, multiple laboratory and clinical studies have demonstrated a trend toward decreased nephrotoxicity with a single daily dose. Studies are incomplete in patients with abnormal or changing renal function.

G. **Fluoroquinolones** are bactericidal agents that act by inhibiting DNA synthesis. Enteral absorption of **ofloxacin** and **levofloxacin** is excellent (approaching 95%), but is decreased by concomitant administration of iron, zinc, antacids (particularly those containing aluminum and magnesium), and sucralfate. Fluoroquinolones are concentrated in the urine, prostate, kidney, bowel, and lung. They are potentially useful for many conditions, including bone and joint infections, complicated urinary tract infections, bacterial gastroenteritis, and intraabdominal infection.

1. **Spectrum. Ciprofloxacin, ofloxacin,** and **levofloxacin** are primarily active against aerobic gram-negative bacilli, including *Pseudomonas aeruginosa.* Levofloxacin is active against some gram-positives, including penicillin-resistant *Stretococcus pneumoniae,* but are not consistently active against anaerobes. **Levofloxacin** is often used in combination with agents that cover gram-positives and anaerobes, such as clindamycin. Fluoroquinolones are also active against atypical bacteria such as *Legionella* spp, *Chlamydia* spp, and some *Mycobacterial* spp.

2. **Adverse reactions** include GI upset, neurologic dysfunction (headache, dizziness, confusion, hallucinations, seizures), and hypersensitivity reactions. Administration of ciprofloxacin to patients taking theophylline can result in theophylline toxicity. Metabolism via the hepatic P-450 enzyme system predicts extensive drug interactions that merit consideration.

H. **Metronidazole** is bactericidal and acts by cleaving bacterial DNA. It is well absorbed from the GI tract and is metabolized in the liver.
   1. **Spectrum.** Metronidazole is only active against anaerobes. It is often used alone for the treatment of pseudomembranous (*C. difficile*) colitis and in combination with other agents for treatment of peritoneal infections arising from the GI tract.
   2. **Adverse reactions** are uncommon and include GI symptoms (metallic taste, anorexia, nausea) and neurologic dysfunction (peripheral neuropathy, seizures, ataxia, vertigo).

I. **Clindamycin** is bacteriostatic and inhibits bacterial protein synthesis. It is well absorbed from the GI tract and is metabolized in the liver.
   1. **Spectrum.** Clindamycin is active against most anaerobes and gram-positive aerobes. Resistant organisms include gram-negative aerobes and facultative anaerobes, *Enterococcus* spp, and some isolates of *Bacteroides fragilis*. Clindamycin may be used alone or with other agents for the treatment of aspiration pneumonia or for thoracic or abdominal infections originating from the upper GI tract.
   2. **Adverse reactions** include GI upset, rash, and elevated liver enzymes. Clindamycin is the antibiotic most commonly associated with development of *C. difficile* colitis.

J. **Macrolides** are bacteriostatic and work by inhibiting bacterial protein synthesis. **Erythromycin** is well absorbed from the GI tract and undergoes hepatic metabolism and biliary excretion. The main indication for erythromycin in critically ill patients is atypical pneumonia. Newer agents of this class (e.g., **azithromycin, clarithromycin**) have a similar spectrum of activity with increased activity against *H. influenzae* and are much better tolerated with fewer GI side effects.
   1. **Spectrum.** Erythromycin is active against many gram-positives (especially *Streptococcus* spp), *Legionella* spp, *Listeria monocytogenes, Chlamydia pneumoniae* (TWAR), and *Mycoplasma pneumoniae.*
   2. **Adverse reactions.** GI upset with enteral administration, thrombophlebitis with intravenous administration, tinnitus, and transient deafness (rare).

K. **Chloramphenicol** inhibits protein synthesis.
   1. **Spectrum.** Chloramphenicol is active against a wide range of gram-positive and gram-negative aerobic and anaerobic organisms.
   2. **Adverse reactions.** Because of the rare but serious side effect of aplastic anemia, chloramphenicol is rarely used. Current indications include serious infections that cannot be treated with alternative regimens, such as meningitis or endocarditis due to VRE. Chloramphenicol can cause adverse hematologic effects, ranging from dose-dependent but reversible bone marrow depression to fatal aplastic anemia

(approximately 1 per 25,000–50,000). Other adverse effects include GI upset, hypersensitivity reactions, and optic neuritis.

III. **Antifungal agents**
   A. **Amphotericin B** exerts its antifungal effect by creating pores in the cell membrane. It is administered via intravenous or intrathecal routes and by local instillation into the bladder. Amphotericin B is still considered the treatment of choice for empiric therapy of suspected life-threatening fungal infections.

   1. **Spectrum.** Amphotericin B is broadly active against most *Candida* spp, including non-*albicans Candida* (*glabrata* and *krusei*), and many isolates of *Aspergillus.*

   2. **Adverse reactions**
      a. **Fever and rigors** are common with administration of amphotericin B. Hypotension and/or hypoxemia also occur. **Pretreatment** with acetaminophen, antihistamines, low-dose corticosteroids, and/or meperidine decreases the incidence and severity of these side effects. In some cases, reduction of the daily dose is necessary to allow continued treatment.

      b. Some degree of **renal dysfunction** occurs in most patients treated with amphotericin B. Adverse renal effects include azotemia, renal tubular acidosis, impaired ability to concentrate urine, electrolyte imbalances (hypokalemia, hypomagnesemia), and decreased production of erythropoietin. Severe renal failure occurs primarily in patients receiving other nephrotoxic drugs, patients with preexisting renal disease or renal transplantation, and severely ill patients who are hypotensive and/or hypovolemic. Alternate-day dosing and administration of saline (1 L/d in excess of baseline fluid requirements) may be of benefit in preventing or blunting renal toxicity.

      c. **Other** adverse effects include anemia and GI upset.

      d. **Test dose.** Some physicians favor administration of a 1-mg intravenous (IV) test dose given over 15 minutes followed by close observation for 1 hour. An unfavorable reaction to the test dose should not prompt a dose reduction in a critically ill patient, but rather prolongation of infusion time, increases in the volume of fluid used to administer the drug, and treatment of symptoms.

   3. **Lipid formulations** of amphotericin B include **amphotericin B lipid complex (Abelcet), amphotericin B colloidal suspension (Amphotec),** and **liposomal amphotericin B (Ambisome).** In clinical trials, lipid formulations have been demonstrated to be as effective as standard amphotericin. The cost difference is significant: The liposomal formulation is approximately 50-fold more expensive that standard formulation. Indications for use are generally limited to

patients with preexisting renal insufficiency (baseline serum creatinine of >2.5 mg/dl or creatinine clearance of ≤40 ml/min) and not maintained on chronic hemo- or peritioneal dialysis, or patients with known intolerance of standard amphotericin B therapy. Patients who develop a 1.5-mg/dl rise in serum creatinine or intolerable side effects while on standard therapy may also be switched to the liposomal formulation.

B. **Triazoles,** including **fluconazole** and **voriconazole,** act by inhibiting fungal membrane sterol synthesis. Potential uses of fluconazole include prophylaxis against invasive fungal infections in immunocompromised hosts (e.g., leukemia, HIV infection, organ transplant recipients), treatment of candidemia, and treatment of invasive fungal infections in stable patients due to *Candida* spp, excluding *krusei* and most *glabrata*. Preliminary noncontrolled studies in patients with candiduria suggest that fluconazole may be more effective in preventing dissemination and sepsis than amphotericin B bladder irrigation. Enteral absorption of fluconazole is excellent (≥90%) in patients that are tolerating enteral feedings, and CNS penetration is reasonably good. Voriconazole is a new triazole antifungal agent that has excellent enteral bioavailability and a broad spectrum of activity.

1. **Spectrum.** Triazoles are active against many *Candida* spp (*albicans, parapsilosis,* and *tropicalis*) and *Cryptococcus neoformans. krusei* and *glabrata* are frequently resistant. The newer agent, voriconazole, has a broader spectrum, which includes molds such as *Aspergillus.*

2. **Adverse reactions.** GI upset, rash, headaches, increased hepatocellular enzyme levels, exfoliative dermatitis (rare), and severe hepatotoxicity (rare).

3. **Drug interactions**
   a. **Coumadin.** Further prolongation of the prothrombin time.
   b. **Phenytoin** and **cyclosporine** levels are increased by fluconazole.
   c. **Rifampin** increases fluconazole levels.
   d. **Cisapride** administration with fluconazole can cause QT prolongation on the electrocardiogram and, rarely, polymorphic ventricular tachycardia.

C. **5-Fluorocytosine** is an antimetabolite that inhibits fungal protein and DNA synthesis. It is sometimes used with amphotericin B for synergistic treatment of severe systemic candidiasis or cryptococcal meningitis. Toxicity (primarily hematologic) correlates with high serum levels.

D. **Caspofungin** is an echinocandin that inhibits the synthesis of β-(1,3)-D-glucan, a component of fungal cell walls.

1. **Spectrum.** Caspofungin is active against *Candida* spp, including those that are resistant to fluconazole, and *Aspergillus.*

2. **Uses.** Treatment of candidal and *Aspergillus* infections in patients who are intolerant to or are refractory to traditional agents (fluconazole or amphotericin B, depending on the fungal infection).

3. **Adverse effects.** Caspofungin is relatively nontoxic. Reported adverse effects include increase in transaminases and pruritis at the infusion site.

IV. **Antiviral agents**

A. **Acyclovir** is available in enteral and parenteral formulations. Parenteral administration is recommended for treatment of serious infection such as varicella pneumonia or herpes encephalitis.

   1. **Spectrum.** Acyclovir is active against herpes simplex virus (HSV) I and II and varicella-zoster virus (VZV).

   2. **Uses.** Intravenous acyclovir is the treatment of choice for serious infections with HSV and VZV. Oral acyclovir can be used for treatment of mucocutaneous HSV.

   3. **Adverse reactions** include renal dysfunction, particularly in hypovolemic patients or those with preexisting renal disease. Neurotoxicity also occurs (confusion, tremulousness, seizures).

B. **Famciclovir and valacyclovir** are newer antiviral agents with a similar spectrum as acyclovir. Only enteral formulations are available.

C. **Ganciclovir**

   1. **Spectrum.** Ganciclovir is active against HSV, VZV, and cytomegalovirus (CMV).

   2. **Uses.** CMV infections, including retinitis, colitis, and pneumonitis in immunocompromised patients. Ganciclovir is also used as prophylaxis against CMV infections in transplant recipients.

   3. **Adverse reactions.** Myelosuppression and nephrotoxicity are the major adverse effects of ganciclovir.

   4. **Alternatives. Foscarnet** and **cidofovir** are also active against CMV, but nephrotoxicity is common.

V. **Sepsis and septic shock.** Sepsis is an important cause of morbidity and mortality in the ICU. Sepsis is caused by a variety of microorganisms, including bacteria, fungi, and rarely viruses, that originate from virtually any site of infection. The mortality of septic shock is extremely high ($\geq$30%) despite the multitude of available antibiotics and improved supportive care in the ICU.

A. **Definitions**

   1. **The systemic inflammatory response syndrome (SIRS)** has infectious and noninfectious etiologies (e.g., pancreatitis, major trauma, transfusion reaction, etc.). Criteria for SIRS include (a) fever ($>38°C$) or hypothermia ($<36°C$), (b) tachypnea (respiratory rate >20 breaths/min), hypocarbia ($Paco_2 <32$ mm Hg) or mechanical ventilation, (c) tachycardia (heart rate >90 beats/min), and (d) leukocytosis ($>12,000/\mu l$), leukopenia ($<4,000/\mu l$), or greater than 10% immature (band) forms.

2. **Sepsis** is the systemic inflammatory response to infection.
3. **Severe sepsis** is sepsis with hypotension or hypoperfusion and acute dysfunction of at least a single organ (acute respiratory failure, acute renal failure, metabolic acidosis, mental status changes).
4. **Septic shock** refers to severe sepsis with hypotension that does not promptly respond to fluid administration. Septic shock can progress to **refractory septic shock** when hypotension persists for more than 1 hour despite appropriate fluid resuscitation.
5. **Multiple organ dysfunction syndrome (MODS)** refers to the failure of more than organ, requiring external support to maintain stability (i.e., dialysis for renal failure, mechanical ventilation for acute respiratory failure).

B. **Pathophysiology**
   1. **Microbial toxins** such as endotoxin and secreted exotoxins trigger a complex inflammatory cascade in the host.
   2. **Host responses** against infection are crucial, but can have deleterious effects. A variety of mediators are involved, including cytokines, vasodilator substances such as nitric oxide, arachidonic acid metabolites, reactive oxygen intermediates, and so on.

C. **Manifestations and complications of sepsis.** Early signs include hyperventilation, tachycardia, fever, and disorientation. Fever is not always present. Later signs include shock with hypotension, obtundation, respiratory failure, acute renal failure, and disseminated intravascular coagulation (DIC). **Vascular endothelial injury** leads to extravasation of intravascular fluid into the extravascular space, microthrombosis, and activation of the coagulation/fibrinolytic system.
   1. **Shock** results from vasodilation, myocardial dysfunction, and intravascular hypovolemia.
   2. **Respiratory failure.** Arterial oxygenation can decline due to extravasation of fluid across leaky alveolar capillaries. The **acute respiratory distress syndrome** (ARDS) is common in severe sepsis and septic shock.
   3. **Renal dysfunction** ranging from mild oliguria to acute renal failure requiring dialysis can result from hypotension leading to impaired renal perfusion or from direct damage to the kidneys (ATN).
   4. **Metabolic acidosis** is common in sepsis, although initially patients may be alkalemic from hyperventilation.
   5. **DIC** can lead to microcirculatory problems resulting in ischemic necrosis of the digits.
   6. **MODS.** The mortality of MODS is high.

D. **Basic management** includes antibiotics, source control, and supportive care. A thorough evaluation for and prompt infection source control is crucial.

1. **Antibiotics.** Empiric broad-spectrum coverage is often used initially until culture data become available. Specific choices will depend on the suspected origin and potential pathogens. Antibiotics should then be adjusted based on culture and sensitivity data.
2. **Source control.** Choice of surgery, catheter drainage, or other invasive procedures will depend on the source. Abscesses are often drained with percutaneous catheters, whereas open peritoneal contamination requires surgical intervention.
3. **Supportive care**
   a. **Hemodynamic management** should focus on restoration of intravascular volume and tissue perfusion. Usually this requires administration of a combination of intravenous fluids and vasopressors (pressors).
      (1) **Fluids.** Patients initially may require massive volumes of intravenous fluid to offset "third-space" losses.
      (2) **Pressors** are added when fluid administration fails to restore adequate perfusion pressure. Vasopressors, including norepinephrine, dopamine, vasopressin, phenylephrine, and/or dobutamine, can be used depending upon the hemodynamic profile of each individual patient (see Chapter 8). Generally, **norepinephrine** or **dopamine** is used. Recently, low-dose **vasopressin** (0.01–0.04 U/min) has been suggested to have specific utility in patients with septic shock. Although the doses of vasopressin used in septic shock should be well below the doses that cause compromise of coronary or splanchnic blood flow, there are still concerns that low-dose vasopressin may have some effect on splanchnic blood flow.
      (3) **Early goal-directed therapy (EGDT) for sepsis.** Early optimization of hemodynamic and fluid management to balance oxygen delivery with oxygen demand is important in the management of septic patients. A recent clinical trial showed improved outcome with very early initiation of goal-directed therapy in the emergency department. Because very early initiation of aggressive therapy seems to dramatically improve outcome, many institutions have or are developing standardized protocols for EGDT. These protocols target therapy to physiologic and laboratory parameters including central venous pressure, mean arterial pressure, central venous oxygen saturation, and lactate levels, and include some combination of aggressive fluid administration and pressors or vasodilators and dobutamine if goals are not met with fluids and pressors/vasodilators.

    b. Mechanical ventilation (see Chapter 5) is frequently necessary and may be required well beyond resolution of the episode of sepsis and ARDS.

    c. Hemodialysis or **hemofiltration** may be required if severe acidemia, hyperkalemia, uremia, or hypervolemia complicates acute renal failure (see Chapter 24).

    d. Severe DIC is treated with transfusions of fresh-frozen plasma and platelets as indicated by coagulation profile and platelet count, whether or not the patient is bleeding, and the need for procedures.

E. Recombinant activated protein C (rAPC) (Drotrecogin alfa, Xigris) has recently been approved by the Food and Drug Administration for the treatment of patients with severe sepsis (sepsis with organ dysfunction) who have a high risk of death (e.g., high APACHE [acute physiologic and chronic health evaluation] score). APC is an endogenous protein that is an important modulator of the coagulation and inflammation associated with severe sepsis. Administration of rAPC in clinical trials resulted in a 6% absolute reduction in mortality.

    1. Many institutions have developed guidelines for use of rAPC. The **Massachusetts General Hospital guidelines** include severe sepsis with (a) three or more SIRS criteria and (b) vasopressor-dependent shock **or** sepsis-induced dysfunction of two or more organs.

    2. Contraindications include hypersensitivity, active internal bleeding, recent hemorrhagic stroke (within 3 months), recent severe head trauma or intracranial or intraspinal surgery (within 2 months), intracranial neoplasm or mass lesion, evidence of cerebral herniation, presence of an epidural catheter, or trauma with an increased risk of life-threatening bleeding.

    3. Dosing. rAPC is administered as a continuous IV infusion at 24 μg/kg/h for 96 hours.

    4. Monitoring/adverse effects/clearance. Patients should be monitored closely for signs of **bleeding,** which is the major adverse effect of rAPC. Plasma levels are nondetectable within 2 hours of stopping the infusion.

F. Steroids in sepsis. Although the role of exogenous steroids in the treatment of sepsis remains somewhat controversial, recent studies suggest that more-physiologic doses of steroids may be of benefit in some patients with septic shock, as evidenced by lower and shorter duration of pressor requirements and improved survival. The best responders appear to be a subset of patients with **"relative adrenal insufficiency,"** which is characterized by an inadequate adrenal response to the stress of sepsis. Relative adrenal insufficiency is diagnosed using an adrenocorticotropic hormone stimulation test. Serum cortisol levels are measured just prior to and 60 minutes after administration of cosyntropin (250 μg IV). Relative adrenal insufficiency is indicated by a baseline cortisol level less than or equal to 9 μg/dl and/or failure of the level to rise by more than 9 μg/dl. Recommended replacement therapy is hydrocortisone 50 mg IV every 6 hours and fludrocortisone 50 μg enterally every day. Studies are underway to verify the utility of, and to optimize the steroid replacement regimen in, sepsis.

G. **Glycemic control.** A large trial demonstrated improved survival in critically ill patients treated with insulin drips to maintain tight glycemic control. Many institutions have set up protocols that use insulin to maintain blood glucose levels at less than about 150 mg/dl in critically ill septic patients.

H. **Experimental therapies** developed for adjunctive treatment of sepsis target microbial toxins (i.e., antilipopolysaccharide antibodies, bactericidal/permeability-increasing protein, etc.) or intervene in the inflammatory cascade triggered by the infection (i.e., antibodies against tumor necrosis factor [TNF]-alpha, soluble TNF receptors, etc.). Many of these therapies were protective in experimental models, but they have not been convincingly effective in clinical trials.

VI. **Infections in immunocompromised hosts.** Immunocompromised hosts are at increased risk of community-acquired, nosocomial, and opportunistic infections. Prompt intervention is required to successfully treat these infections, but their diagnosis often is difficult because of the lack of clear localizing signs. A thorough search for the source of infection must be undertaken. This, at minimum, includes cultures of blood, urine, and sputum and a chest radiograph. There are many causes of immunocompromise, including immunosuppressive therapy, burns, malignancy, HIV infection, chemotherapy, corticosteroids, and severe malnutrition. Because different aspects of the immune response may be altered in these conditions, the infectious disease complications are variable. The most common site of infection in the immunocompromised patient is the lung.

A. **Infections in neutropenic patients**

1. **Neutropenia** (neutrophil count <500 cells/mm^3 or <1,000 cells/mm^3 with anticipated decrease of >500 cells/mm^3 within 48 hours) most often results from leukemia, chemotherapy, or bone marrow transplantation, and less frequently is due to drug reactions or aplastic anemia. Bacteria, particularly enteric and nonenteric gram-negatives and gram-positives, and fungi (*Candida* spp, *Aspergillus* spp, *Torulopsis glabrata*) characteristically cause infection in neutropenic patients, although severe viral infections (HSV, CMV, Epstein-Barr virus) may also occur.

2. **Fever** in patients with severe neutropenia (absolute neutrophil count [ANC] <100/μl) should be assumed to be due to infection.

3. **Treatment of neutropenic fever**

   a. **Initial treatment. Broad-spectrum antibacterial agents** directed against gram-positive and gram-negative bacteria, including *Pseudomonas* spp, should be administered initially. Antibiotics should be continued for a minimum of 10 days or until the ANC rises above 500/μl (whichever is later).

  (1) Monotherapy using a broad-spectrum agent such as a third- or fourth-generation cephalosporin (ceftazidime, cefepime), a carbapenem (imipenem, meropenem), or an antipseudomonal penicillin/β-lactamase combination (piperacillin/tazobactam) may be appropriate in patients who are not critically ill.

  (2) Combination therapy should be administered to critically ill patients, using agents that are likely to treat nosocomial antibiotic-resistant organisms and organisms such as *Enterobacter* spp and *Citrobacter* spp that rapidly become resistant to β-lactams. Potential combinations include a third- or fourth-generation cephalosporin (ceftazidime, cefepime), a carbapenem (imipenem, meropenem), or an antipseudomonal penicillin/β-lactamase combination, plus either an aminoglycoside or a fluoroquinolone. Aminoglycosides may be problematic, particularly in patients who have renal dysfunction or are receiving cyclosporine. Vancomycin should be added if there is suspicion of infection due to resistant gram-positive bacteria.

  b. Subsequent treatment. Ongoing fever for 4 to 7 days despite broad antibacterial therapy warrants consideration of antifungal treatment with amphotericin B.

B. Infections in transplant recipients. Transplant recipients are most susceptible to life-threatening infections during the first 6 months after organ transplantation. During this time they are maximally immunosuppressed, are exposed to many nosocomial organisms, and may be experiencing allograft rejection or graft-versus-host disease (GVHD). Infections are caused by bacteria, fungi, viruses, protozoa, parasites, and mycobacteria. Bacterial infections are caused by aerobic gram-positive and gram-negative bacteria. Fungal infections are most commonly caused by *Candida* and *Aspergillus* spp. Some infections, such as CMV infection, are transmitted from the organ to the recipient or via transfused blood products. Fever in the absence of localized findings is often the first manifestation of infection. Short courses of parenteral antibiotics are generally given before and after solid-organ transplantation. Patient and environmental factors dictate antibiotic choice. Some antibiotics have significant interactions with immunosuppressive agents. Metabolism of cyclosporine (CSA) by the cytochrome P-450 system can be increased or decreased by administration of fluoroquinolones, macrolides, fluconazole, rifampin, and isoniazid. Aminoglycosides, amphotericin B, vancomycin, pentamidine, and high-dose trimethoprim/sulfamethoxazole enhance the nephrotoxicity of CSA. CSA levels should be monitored in patients receiving these agents.

1. **Solid-organ transplantation**

   a. **In the first month** posttransplantation, infections are usually caused by the same bacteria and fungi that cause infections in immunocompetent postsurgical patients. **Early posttransplant infections** are usually nosocomial, occurring at the surgical site or as a result of indwelling catheters or prolonged endotracheal intubation.

   b. **Between 1 and 6 months,** viral and opportunistic infections, such as *Pneumocystis carinii* pneumonia and aspergillosis, predominate.

   c. **After 6 months,** infections depend on the degree of immunosuppression and environmental exposures. Patients on minimal immunosuppressive therapy develop similar infections as normal hosts. High doses of immunosuppressive agents predispose patients to infections with opportunistic pathogens such as *P. carinii, L. monocytogenes, Aspergillus fumigatus,* and *Cryptococcus neoformans*. Preexisting viral infections may progress and cause damage to infected organs. CMV infection can cause isolated fever, hepatitis, pneumonitis, hypotension, enterocolitis and glomerulonephritis. Manifestations of CNS infections (generally caused by *L. monocytogenes* or opportunistic pathogens) can be atypical. Computed tomography (CT) of the head and lumbar puncture are necessary for transplant patients with unexplained fever or headache. Chest CT may be useful in evaluating transplant patients with pulmonary symptoms because the typical radiographic signs of inflammation are often attenuated.

2. **Bone marrow transplantation.** Allogeneic and autologous bone marrow transplants are performed for the treatment of acute and chronic leukemias, lymphoma, solid tumors, multiple myeloma, and severe aplastic anemia. There are three phases of infectious disease complications after bone marrow transplantation:

   a. **The first month** is characterized by ongoing neutropenia from prior chemotherapy. Bacterial, fungal, and viral infections occur. Bacterial infections are caused by gram-positive aerobes, including coagulase-negative *Staphylococcus, Streptococcus viridans, Staphylococcus aureus,* and *Corynebacterium* spp, and enteric and nonenteric gram-negative aerobes and facultative anaerobes. Reactivation of HSV can also occur. **Empiric antibiotic therapy** for febrile neutropenic bone marrow transplant patients should include agents that cover gram-negative and gram-positive bacteria. Antipseudomonal coverage should be included. Empiric coverage is often undertaken using a combination of β-lactams (one antipseudomonal cephalosporin and one antipseudomonal penicillin such as piperacillin or mezlocillin) or an antipseudomonal β-lactam plus vancomycin, or a carbapenem (imipenem or meropenem) plus vancomycin. **Antifungal coverage** should be considered if fevers persist despite broad antibacterial coverage.

   b. **From 1 to 3 months,** patients are prone to viral infections (CMV), opportunistic infections, and grampositive and gram-negative bacterial infections.

   c. **Late infections occur after 3 months.** Late infections often involve the respiratory tract and are caused by respiratory viruses and encapsulated organisms such as *Streptococcus pneumoniae* and *H. influenzae.* Mucocutaneous damage due to GVHD also predisposes these patients to infections with skin flora.

C. **Human immunodeficiency virus (HIV).** Progress in antiretroviral therapy and prophylaxis against opportunistic infections has resulted in longer survival of patients infected with HIV and in improved survival of HIV-infected patients in the ICU. Similarly, survival in HIV-infected patients admitted to the ICU has improved considerably. The **T4-helper (CD4)** count is an accurate predictor of sites and organisms involved in infection in HIV patients, as indicated in Table 11-4. Infection with HIV predisposes patients to opportunistic infections and increases susceptibility to infection with encapsulated bacteria, including *Streptococcus pneumoniae* and *H. influenzae.*

   1. **Pulmonary infections** in the HIV patient are caused by a variety of microorganisms. In patients with normal CD4 counts, pneumonia may be due to community-acquired organisms. As the CD4 count drops, the likelihood that pulmonary infection is due to opportunistic

Table 11-4. Relationship of CD4 count to infection in HIV patients

CD4 Count (per μl)	Microbiologic Predisposition
>800	Community-acquired organisms
<800	*Mycobacterium tuberculosis* (pulmonary)
<500	*Candida* species, *Cryptococcus neoformans, Histoplasma capsulatum, Coccidioides* species
<300	*Pneumocystis carinii*
<100	*Mycobacterium avium intracellulare, Mycobacterium tuberculosis* (disseminated), *Cryptosporidium,* cytomegalovirus

infections, particularly *Pneumocystis carinii* and CMV, increases. Evaluation for the etiology of pneumonitis should be prompt, and should include induced sputum examination, deep aspiration, or bronchoscopy with bronchoalveolar lavage. Empiric antibiotic therapy should cover most likely pathogens based on the CD4 count and geographic location. Above a CD4 count of roughly 200 to $300/\mu l$, antibiotics should cover community-acquired organisms. Below a CD4 count of 200, treatment also should cover *Pneumocystis carinii*.

2. **CNS infections,** such as brain abscess, meningitis, and encephalitis, can be caused by a variety of organisms, including bacteria, fungi, viruses, and parasites, in patients with HIV. Evaluation for CNS infections, including CT scans or magnetic resonance imaging of the brain and lumbar puncture, should be performed if CNS infection is suspected, and empiric antibiotics should be administered while awaiting the results.

SELECTED REFERENCES

Ambrose PG, Owens RC, Quintiliani R, et al. Antibiotic use in the critical care unit. *Crit Care Clin* 1998;14:283–308.

Annane D, Sebille V, Charpentier C, et al. Effect of treatment with low doses of hydrocortisone and fludrocortisone on mortality in patients with septic shock. *JAMA* 2002;288:862–871.

Cohen J, Powderly WG. *Infectious diseases,* 2nd ed. New York: Elsevier, 2004.

David N, Gilbert RC, Moellering GM, et al. *The Sanford guide to antimicrobial therapy,* 34th ed. Vienna, VA: Antimicrobial Therapy, 2004.

Dellinger RP, Carlet JM, Masur H, et al. Surviving Sepsis Campaign guidelines for management of severe sepsis and septic shock. *Crit Care Med* 2004;32:858–873.

Fishman JA, Rubin RH. Infection in organ-transplant recipients. *N Engl J Med* 1998;338:1741–1751.

Hotchkiss RS, Karl IE. The pathophysiology and treatment of sepsis. *N Engl J Med* 2003;348:138–150.

Mora-Duarte J, Betts R, Rotstein C, et al. Comparison of caspofungin and amphotericin B for invasive candidiasis. *N Engl J Med* 2002;347:2020–2029.

Rivers E, Nguyen B, Havstad S, et al. Early goal-directed therapy in the treatment of severe sepsis and septic shock. *N Engl J Med* 2001;345:1368–1377.

van den Berghe G, Wouters P, Weekers F, et al. Intensive insulin therapy in the critically ill patients. *N Engl J Med* 2001;345:1359–1367.

Wunderink RG, Rello J, Cammarata SK, et al. Linezolid vs vancomycin: analysis of two double-blind studies of patients with methicillin-resistant *Staphylococcus aureus* nosocomial pneumonia. *Chest* 2003;124:1789–1797.

Prophylaxis

Kathryn Brush and Ulrich Schmidt

Critically ill patients have a high morbidity and mortality. Prophylactic measures decrease morbidity and mortality in the intensive care unit (ICU). Three core issues have been identified as important to reducing the risk of the sequelae of critical illness and the risk associated with the treatment of critical illness: **infection control, prophylaxis of deep venous thrombosis,** and prophylaxis of **gastrointestinal (GI) bleeding.** Guidelines in these areas have been developed; there is evidence that hospitals that have implemented such guidelines have been able to decrease ICU morbidity and mortality.

I. **Infection Control in the ICU**
   Patients in the ICU have an increased risk for nosocomial infection. Pneumonia, urinary tract infection, and bloodstream infection are the most common. Both host factors and environmental factors are important in the development of nosocomial infections (Table 12-1). Elderly patients and immunosuppressed patients are at increased risk of acquiring infections. Chronic diseases increase the risk of site-specific infections. Patients with underlying lung disease are more likely to develop pneumonias, and patients with chronic renal disease and diabetes are prone to develop urinary tract infections. Environmental factors impair host defenses. Antibiotics shift the endogenous colonizing flora. Instrumentation of the airway for the delivery of mechanical ventilation constitutes a port of entry for nosocomial pathogens and compromises clearing of bronchial secretions. Invasive monitors break the skin and mucosal barriers. These impaired host defenses facilitate transmission of microorganisms to patients by personnel, equipment, or ventilation systems.
   A. **General infection control.** Microorganisms are transmitted in hospitals by contact, droplet, airborne, and contaminated items.
      1. **Contact.** Spread of microorganisms can occur by direct and indirect contact. Transmission by hand to body surface is much more common than indirect contact to a contaminated surface. For example, almost all cases of methicillin-resistant *Staphylococcus aureus* are transmitted by hand contamination of health care providers.
      2. **Droplets** are particles greater 5 μm in diameter. Droplets can only be transmitted over a short distance—less than 3 feet. They are transmitted through coughing and sneezing. Droplets transmit microorganisms including *Neisseria meningitidis, Haemophilus influenzae, Mycoplasma pneumoniae,* adenovirus, and rubella virus.

**Table 12-1.   Risk factors for
infections in the intensive care unit**

Patient Factors	Environmental Factors
Age >70 years	Prior antibiotics
Malnutrition	Mechanical ventilation
Immunocompromised states	Drugs that suppress the immune system
Chronic disease	Indwelling catheters
	Length of intensive care unit stay (>3 days)

3. **Airborne particles** are smaller (<5 μm) than droplets and can remain in the air for a long period of time. **Tuberculosis (TB), measles, varicella,** and **disseminated varicella-zoster virus** are spread by airborne particles.
4. **Contaminated items.** Infection by contaminated items is rare. However, improper sterilization of bronchoscopes and endoscopes has led to infection with microorganisms such as *Pseudomonas aeruginosa* and *Serratia marescens.*

B. **Specific infection control measures** decrease the risk of nosocomial infection and prevent transmission of pathogens from ICU staff to patients and vice versa. The Centers for Disease Control and Prevention (CDC) has implemented a system based on standard precautions and transmission-based precautions (Table 12-2).
1. **Standard precautions** are intended for all patients. They decrease the risk of infections for patients and health care workers. They include the following:
   a. **Hand washing.** Lack of hand hygiene constitutes a major factor for transmission of infectious disease in the hospital setting. Recent surveys show that only 20% of health care providers wash their hand before and after patient contact. Hand hygiene should take place prior to patient contact and prior to contact with surfaces in patients' rooms. In addition, hand cleansing is warranted immediately after removal of gloves and/or contact with the patient or surfaces within the patient's environment. Hand washing with soap and water should take place if hands are visibly soiled. Hand disinfections with alcohol-based hand rubs are indicated for all situations and after hand washing.
   b. **Gloves** are recommended in working with all ICU patients. **Gowns and protective eye wear** should be worn in situations where exposure to blood and body secretions is likely.
   c. **Safe disposal of sharps** in specially designed, safe containers is warranted. According to the Occupational Safety and Health Administration (OSHA), 600,000 to 800,000 needle stick injuries occur annually in hospitals throughout the United

Table 12-2.   Precaution for transmission of infectious diseases

Standard precautions	All hospitalized patients	Hand washing Gloves, gowns, eye protection Safe disposal of sharps Safe disposal of contaminated material
Airborne precautions	Tuberculosis, measles, varicella, varicella-zoster virus	Isolation room Special mask
Droplet precautions	*Neisseria meningitidis, Haemophilus influenzae, Rubella Mycoplasma,* adenovirus, severe acute respiratory syndrome	Private room Face mask for contact
Contact precautions	Multidrug-resistant bacteria	Nonsterile gloves and gowns Hand washing

States. The most important pathogens transmitted include human immunodeficiency virus (**HIV**), hepatitis B virus (**HBV**), and hepatitis C virus (**HCV**). OSHA requires all health care facilities to implement plans **to decrease the transmission of blood-borne pathogens.** These include the following measures:

   (1) Annual education for health care workers regarding the minimization of transmission of blood-borne pathogens.
   (2) Standard precautions for working with all patients.
   (3) Hepatitis B immunization as preexposure prophylaxis.
   (4) Engineering tools to reduce the risk of injury with sharps (needle systems, special containers, etc.).

   d. Following exposure to blood, tissue, or other body fluids, the health care worker should undergo an immediate evaluation. This evaluation includes documentation of the incidence. In addition, blood both from the health care worker and from the source should be tested for HBV, HBC, and HIV. For details of postexposure prophylaxis refer to regularly updated CDC guidelines (**www.cdc.gov/ncidod/hip/**).

   e. Soiled material should be placed in special bags. Feces and urine should be discarded in sanitary toilets.

2. **Airborne precautions** are used in patients with suspected or confirmed infection with *Mycobacterium tuberculosis,* varicella, and disseminated varicella-zoster

virus. A single, **negative-pressure isolation room** is required for patients with airborne precautions.

a. **Special considerations for TB**

(1) **Negative-pressure rooms** should have 12 or more exchanges of air per hour, should be exhausted to the exterior, and should have anterooms to effectively separate them from the rest of the ward.

(2) **Respiratory protection mask** are designed to filter inhaled air. They filter small particles (<1 μm) with at least 95% efficiency **(N95).** These masks should be fitted to each person's face in advance to assure optimal fit and limit leakage. Persons in contact with the patient should wear respiratory protection masks. In contrast, the patient should wear a surgical mask when leaving the isolation room. Surgical masks are designed to prevent secretions from entering the environment.

(3) **Discontinuation of TB isolation.** The patient can be transferred to a regular room when TB is ruled out or when the patient is felt to have been treated effectively. Treated patients must show clinical signs of improvement and have three consecutive sputum samples that are negative for acid-fast bacilli.

b. **Severe acute respiratory syndrome (SARS).** The following precautions should be taken in patients with a suspected diagnosis of SARS:

(1) The patient must be placed in a negative-pressure room. Contact by health care providers and visitors should be limited to an absolute minimum.

(2) All persons entering the isolation room must wear a respiratory protection mask (N95) that has been fitted to the individual and tested.

(3) All persons entering the isolation room must wear gloves, gowns, and eye protection. They must wash hands before leaving the room.

(4) Transport of patient with SARS should be kept to an absolute minimum. If patients need to leave the room, they should disinfect hands and wear a surgical mask, gown, and gloves. For intubated patients, a bacterial expiratory filter should be placed at the end of the endotracheal tube.

(5) Patients must stay in negative pressure isolation rooms until SARS is not longer suspected. SARS isolation precautions should be discontinued only after consultation with the local public health authorities.

3. **Droplet precautions** are used to limit the spread of infectious agents that are transmitted over a short distance by coughing and sneezing. Patients should be placed in a single room. Personnel and visitors that

come in close proximity to patients on droplet precautions must wear a surgical mask.

4. **Contact precautions** minimize spread of microorganisms from direct contact or indirect contact with environmental surfaces.
   a. They are used for patients colonized or infected with antibiotic-resistant bacteria.
   b. Patients should be placed in private rooms.
   c. Health care providers must wear gloves and gowns to minimize direct contact with patients and surfaces.

C. **Prevention of intravascular catheter-related infections.** More than 200,000 incidents of catheter-related nosocomial bloodstream infections are reported annually. These line infections have 12% to 25% mortality and bear a significant financial burden (the appendix to this chapter shows the protocol for central line placement used in our surgical ICU). The following measures have been shown to significantly reduce the rate of line infections.

1. **Limitation of number and duration of central access:** To decrease complications, central access should only be obtained when medically necessary. Early discontinuation of central access decreases the number of line infections.

2. Strict **aseptic technique** is recommended for the insertion of central venous catheters. The importance of infection control practices should be included in the training of health care providers. Operators should disinfect their hands. It is recommend that sterile gloves, gowns, caps, and surgical masks be worn for insertion of central lines. Larger sterile barrier drapes should be used. The observance of sterile technique should be supervised.

3. **Skin preparation** with 2% aqueous **chlorhexidine** has been shown to decrease the number of central line infections. It is recommended to switch to chlorhexidine-containing solutions.

4. **Catheter site selection.** Central lines are placed mainly in internal jugular, subclavian, and femoral veins. Subclavian-vein catheters have the lowest risk of infection.

5. **Selection of catheters.** The material and coating of catheters influence the incidence of line infection.
   a. **Material.** Bacterial adherence is decreased in catheters made from polyurethane, Teflon, and silicone elastomers. It is therefore recommended to use catheters made form one of these materials.
   b. **Coating. Heparin sodium** bonding decreases the incidence of catheter-related thrombus as a possible source of infection. Heparin-bonded catheters reduced the incidence of catheter infection.
   c. **Chlorhexidine/silver sulfazidine**–impregnated catheters lead to a significant reduction in catheter colonization and catheter-related bacteremia.

  d. Minocyclin/rifampin-impregnated catheters decrease the rate of line infections. The impregna-
  tion does not cause changes in antibiotic resistance.
  Both types of catheters are cost effective.
  e. Number of catheter lumens. Multilumen
  catheters have a higher number of infections. When
  possible, it is recommended to insert catheters
  with a lower number of lumens.
6. Change of central lines: Routine change of central
  lines either by new stick or guide wire change does not
  seem to decrease the incidence of line infection. Instead of scheduled line changes, it is recommended to
  evaluate the patient for line infection on a continuous
  basis.
**7. Percutaneously inserted central catheters
  (PICC)** are inserted centrally via peripheral arm
  veins, generally at the antecubital fossa. Insertion
  carries a low risk, and the catheters have a low risk
  of infection. Therefore these lines are preferred for
  infusion of drugs or parenteral nutrition when central
  monitoring is not necessary.
**D. Prevention of catheter-associated urinary tract in-
  fections.** Urinary tract infections affect about 600,000
  patients per year in acute care hospitals. About 1% of
  these patients develop severe gram-negative sepsis.
1. Catheter placement and removal: Indwelling urinary catheters should be placed only in patients
  for whom frequent measurement of urinary output
  would prove beneficial. The benefit of the catheter
  should be discussed daily. Alternatives to indwelling
  devices such as condom catheters or intermittent
  catheterization should be considered. Indwelling urinary catheters must be placed under strict aseptic
  technique by trained personnel. For most adult patients 14 to 18 French catheters are an appropriate
  size. Smaller catheters are preferable in terms of infection prevention.
2. Catheter maintenance: Clinicians should wash
  their hands and wear gloves prior to handling the indwelling catheter or drainage tubing. Closed drainage
  systems should be utilized. The incidence of urinary
  tract infection increases with breaks in the drainage
  system. Catheters should be secured to the patient's
  leg to prevent movement or traction of the catheter.
  Catheters should not be changed unless there is frequent occlusion of the catheter that requires frequent
  irrigation. Routine irrigation should be avoided. The
  most often cited strategies for avoiding catheter-
  associated urinary tract infections are the following:
  a. Removal of the urinary catheter as soon as possible.
  b. Discussing on daily rounds whether the patient
  needs an indwelling device.
  c. Use of closed drainage systems.
**E. Prevention of ventilator-associated pneumonia
  (VAP).** VAP is one of the most common nosocomial

infections within the ICU, resulting in increased mortality, length of stay, and overall cost of care. Pathogenesis, diagnosis, and treatment of VAP are outlined in Chapter 28. Prevention strategies are aimed at minimizing aspiration and prevention of colonization of the airway and the gastrointestinal (GI) tract with pathogens. Commonly used pharmacologic and nonpharmacologic approaches and their efficacy are summarized in Table 12-3.

1. **Positioning**
    a. **Semirecumbent position** decreases the incidence of aspiration and VAP. It is therefore recommended to keep the head of the bed elevated at greater than 30 degrees whenever possible.
    b. **Kinetic therapy.** Altering a patient's position has been shown to enhance mobilization of secretions and decrease atelectasis. There is evidence that systematic mechanical rotation of patients decreases the incidence of ventilator-associated pneumonia. Based on this, rotating beds have been introduced in clinical praxis. Due to high costs we recommend restricting the use of these beds to patients who are difficult to mobilize.
2. **Airway management**
    a. **Duration of intubation.** Intubation of the airway is a prerequisite for developing VAP. Noninvasive ventilation (see Chapter 5) has emerged as a successful alternative to intubation especially in patients with congestive heart failure and chronic obstructive pulmonary disease (COPD). Development of VAP increases with the duration of mechanical

Table 12-3. Prevention of ventilator-associated pneumonia (VAP)

Approach		Recommendation
Nonpharmacologic		
Positioning	Semirecumbent position	++
	Kinetic beds	+
Airway manipulation	Short intubation	++
	Oral intubation	++
	Subglottic suctioning	+
	Infrequent change of humidifier	+
Pharmacologic	No stress ulcer prophylaxis in low-risk patients	+
	Gastrointestinal decontamination	+
	Restriction of antibiotics	+

Note: ++, strong evidence, +, some evidence supporting the recommendation.

ventilation. Strategies to shorten time on the ventilator have the potential to decrease VAP.

b. **Route of intubation.** Nasal intubation is associated with a higher incidence of VAP. In addition, the presence of nasogastric tubes promotes sinusitis and VAP. Therefore the oral route for intubation is recommended.

c. **Subglottic suctioning.** Most intubated patients have secretions in the upper airways that tend to pool above the balloon of the endotracheal tube. Constant microaspiration occurs. Strategies for decreasing these secretions may aid in preventing VAP. Special endotracheal tubes with a separate dorsal hole allowing continuous suction have been developed. Use of these tubes has decreased the incidence of VAP in some studies. Because the ultimate benefit of these tubes remains to be seen, thoroughly intermittent suction of the back of the throat is recommended.

3. **Stress ulcer prophylaxis.** Decreasing intragastric acidity by histamine-2 blockers or proton-pump inhibitors may increase the incidence of VAP. However, intubated patients are at increased risk of developing GI bleeding. It is therefore recommended that prophylaxis for GI bleeding be continued in these patients.

4. **Prevention of colonization of GI tract.** Colonization of the oropharynx is major pathophysiologic factor in the development of VAP.

a. **Oral decontamination** is effective for decreasing the incidence of VAP. Treatment with chlorhexidine in patients intubated for more than 24 hours showed reduction in the development of VAP. Topical oral antibiotics have also been shown to decrease the incidence of VAP. The use of topical antibiotics has been associated with emergence of antibiotic resistance. Their universal use can therefore not be recommended.

b. **Selective decontamination** of the digestive tract **(SDD)** uses a combination of topical and nonabsorbable antibiotics to eradicate pathogenic organisms from the GI tract. It has been shown to decrease nosocomial pneumonia and ICU mortality. However, there is concern that SDD may promote the emergence of antibiotic resistance. Due to these concerns SDD is not widely used in the United States.

5. **Antibiotics.** The use of antibiotics in general is associated with the emergence of antibiotic-resistant bacteria. This is associated with an increase of antibiotic-resistant VAP. The following strategies have been shown to decrease the incidence of pneumonia by antibiotic-resistant bacteria.

a. **Prophylactic antibiotics.** Prolonged use of prophylactic antibiotics is associated with an increased incidence of VAP; therefore, it is recommended to limit the duration of prophylactic antibiotics to 24 hours or less.

  b. **Antibiotic change.** Antibiotic cycling has been shown to decrease the incidence of VAP. This strategy should be part of a wider strategy to limit the emergence of antibiotic-resistant infections.

  c. **Shortening the course of empiric antibiotic** therapy has been shown to decrease the emergence of resistant bacteria. This approach may help to reduce the incidence of subsequent infections including VAP.

II. Prophylaxis of GI bleeding

The majority of patients admitted to the ICU develop mucosal damage of the gastrointestinal tract. Clinically significant gastrointestinal bleeding develops in about 2% to 15% of critically ill patients and carries a high mortality. Mechanical ventilation of greater than 48 hours and coagulopathy have been identified as major risk factors for GI bleeding. The following strategies are used to decrease the incidence of gastrointestinal bleeding.

  A. **Antacids** decrease gastric acidity by direct neutralization of stomach acid. The efficacy of these drugs in critically ill patients is questionable. In addition, these drugs have to be given in large volume (30–60 ml) every 1 to 2 hours. In general antacids are not recommended in the ICU population.

  B. **Cytoprotection.** Sucralfate is a polysaccharide that provides protection of gastric mucosa by coating the surface. In mechanically ventilated patients sucralfate was less effective than ranitidine in preventing clinically important GI bleeding. However, sucralfate is less expensive and has not been associated with an increase in VAP. Prostaglandin analogues have also been shown to be cytoprotective. There are not enough data to support their widespread use in critically ill patients.

  C. **Histamine-2 (H-2)–receptor antagonists** decrease the stimulatory effects of histamine on acid production. H-2 blockers decrease the incidence of gastrointestinal bleeding in the ICU. They can be given in enteral and intravenous (IV) form. Continuous infusion has the best control over gastric pH. The use of H-2 blockers is limited by the development of tolerance. It is unclear whether H-2 blockers increase the risk of VAP.

  D. **Proton-pump inhibitors (PPIs)** inactivate the hydrogen–potassium ATPase pump and thereby decrease gastric pH. PPIs are effective in decreasing GI bleeding. In contrast to H-2 blockers, there is no tolerance development against proton-pump inhibitors. To date, no trials prove the superiority of PPIs over ranitidine in the prevention of gastrointestinal bleeding. In addition, PPIs, especially in IV form, are expensive.

  E. **Enteral feeding** may decrease the incidence of bleeding in critically ill patients. The mechanism is unknown. In patients with risk for GI bleeding it is recommended to combine enteral feeding with pharmacotherapy.

III. For the prophylaxis of **deep venous thrombosis and pulmonary embolism,** see Chapter 22.

APPENDIX

Protocol for Infection Prevention in the Placement of Central Venous and Pulmonary Artery Catheters in the ICU

These Guidelines apply to patients over 2 years of age.

I. Line Selection
  A. Line selection is based on access/therapeutic needs.
  B. Use a central venous catheter (CVC) with the minimum number of ports or lumens necessary for management of the patient.

II. Placement
  A. Each new catheter will be inserted at a new site when possible.
  B. Catheter exchange over a guidewire is allowed when there is no evidence of infection at the site, and a new insertion is felt to carry an increased risk of complications, because of, e.g., coagulopathy or difficult anatomy.
  C. For *non-emergent* line placements, the medical and nursing staff will mutually arrange the time of insertion.
  D. Competent MD staff and fellows will supervise trainees.
  E. An RN or second clinician will be present for the entire procedure.
  F. An RN or second clinician will monitor for breaks in sterile technique.

III. Site Selection
  A. Weigh the risk and benefits of placing a device at a recommended site to reduce infectious complications against the risk for mechanical complications.
  B. Selection of the insertion site is determined by the patient's physical characteristics, availability of sites, anticoagulation status, and experience of the physician. The internal jugular and subclavian veins are commonly used. The femoral vein is an option.
  C. A subclavian site rather than a jugular or femoral site in adult patients is preferred to minimize infection risk, although other factors (e.g., the potential for complications) should also be considered.

IV. Pre-Procedure Preparation
  A. The patient will be medicated and sedated as necessary.
  B. The insertion site will be clean and free of blood or other bioburden.
  C. The area selected for insertion will be set-up to establish a clean, clear workspace (e.g., head of the bed removed, ventilator tubing moved, absorbable material ("chux") placed underneath the patient to protect the mattress from fluids).
  D. Insertion tray will be set up on an appropriate flat surface.
  E. Such surface will be cleaned with hospital-approved disinfectant and dried prior to set up of sterile field.
  F. Steps will be taken to minimize traffic in the area, e.g., close door or pull curtains.
  G. An ultrasound imaging monitor should be available for all line placements. Its routine use is encouraged.

V. Insertion Protocol

A. Maximal barrier precautions and appropriate aseptic technique will be utilized during catheter insertion and guidewire exchanges.

B. Mask, head cover, and eye protection will be donned.

C. Hands will be decontaminated with an alcohol-based hand disinfectant (*Cal Stat* or equivalent) prior to donning sterile gloves.

D. Sterile gloves will be donned.

E. The insertion site (skin must be clean) will be prepped with 2% chlorhexidine gluconate in 70% isopropyl alcohol, (e.g., Chloraprep).

F. Alternatively, a wide prep with alcohol, followed by a narrow prep with 2% tincture of iodine is acceptable.

G. Sterile gloves will be discarded after skin prep is complete.

H. Sterile gowns and a new set of sterile gloves will be donned by the operator, supervisor and any other clinician involved in the insertion.

I. Double gloving will be employed if a PA catheter is to be placed.

J. Use a sterile sleeve to protect pulmonary artery catheter during insertion.

K. The bed should be fully draped, utilizing sterile half sheets.

L. The insertion site is then draped with a large sterile impervious barrier with a minimum area exposed.

VI. After Insertion

A. Blood is withdrawn from the thin-walled needle for culture if needed.

B. If a PA catheter is to be placed, the outer pair of sterile gloves is removed and the insertion site is further covered with sterile drapes to only expose the tip of the introducer.

C. The nurse or MD in some settings will apply the final occlusive dressing.

SELECTED REFERENCES

Abraham E. Acid suppression in a critical care environment: state of the art and beyond. *Crit Care Med* 2002;30(6 Suppl):S349–S350.

Arroliga AC, Budev MM, Gordon SM. Do as we say, not as we do: healthcare workers and hand hygiene. *Crit Care Med* 2004;32:592–593.

Cook DJ, Reeve BK, Guyatt GH, et al. Stress ulcer prophylaxis in critically ill patients. Resolving discordant meta-analyses. *JAMA* 1996;275:308–314.

Dellinger RP, Carlet JM, Masur H, et al. Surviving Sepsis Campaign guidelines for management of severe sepsis and septic shock. *Intensive Care Med* 2004;30:536–555.

Kollef MH. Prevention of hospital-associated pneumonia and ventilator-associated pneumonia. *Crit Care Med* 2004;32:1396–1405.

Kunin CM. Nosocomial urinary tract infections and the indwelling catheter: what is new and what is true? *Chest* 2001;120:10–12.

OSHA revises bloodborne pathogen standard—mandates sharps safety devices. *Infect Control Hosp Epidemiol* 2001;22:182–183.

Neurocritical Care

Neeraj Badjatia and Lee H. Schwamm

I. **Neuroprotection** is the goal of neurocritical care.
  A. **Common presenting symptoms** that require neurocritical care intervention include weakness, cognitive dysfunction, reduced alertness with or without impaired airway reflexes, uncontrolled seizures, and respiratory muscle failure.
  B. **Diagnoses** likely to produce these symptoms include subarachnoid, subdural, or intracerebral hemorrhage, ischemic stroke, brain tumor, infectious or inflammatory meningoencephalitis, traumatic brain or spinal cord injury, status epilepticus, toxic-metabolic encephalopathy, amyotrophic lateral sclerosis, myasthenia gravis and acute myopathies, and polyneuropathies.
  C. Because cerebral ischemia and hypoxemia are the most common mechanisms of secondary brain injury, a thorough understanding of the regulation of cerebral blood flow is necessary. In addition, familiarity with the neurologic examination of the critically ill patient is required for early recognition of secondary brain injury and subsequent evaluation of the efficacy of therapeutic interventions.
  D. Three aspects distinguish hemodynamic management in neurocritical care from that of other critically ill patients:
    1. Assessment of end-organ perfusion is at times more difficult to determine.
    2. Because of the lack of local energy reserves, the interval to end-organ failure under adverse conditions is more rapid.
    3. Unlike most other organs, injury to even small regions of brain can have devastating consequences.

II. **Intracranial hemodynamics**
  A. **Intracranial compliance.** The skull is a rigid box filled with incompressible brain parenchyma. When the volume inside the skull increases, there is evacuation of cerebrospinal fluid (CSF) into the extracranial subarachnoid space followed by a rapid rise in intracranial pressure (ICP; see Fig. 13-1). **Intracranial pressure** is normally less than 10 mm Hg; transient elevations up to 30 mm Hg are well tolerated. When ICP rises above 20 mm Hg (or **cerebral perfusion pressure [CPP]** falls below 60 mm Hg) cerebral blood flow may be inadequate.
  B. **Cerebral blood flow (CBF)** equals the (CPP) divided by the cerebrovascular resistance (CVR), according to Ohm's law. The CPP is the difference between the mean

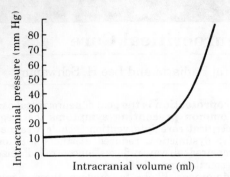

Fig. 13-1. Intracranial compliance curve. In the normal intracranial pressure (ICP) range; increases in intracranial volume produce minimal changes in ICP initially. Further small increases in intracranial volume at the "elbow" of the curve, however, can produce an abrupt increase in ICP.

intracerebral artery pressure (hard to measure) and mean ICP (easy to measure). The CVR (hard to measure) is the ability of the precapillary arterioles to dilate and constrict in response to changes in pressure or metabolic factors. Because CBF is cumbersome to measure directly and CBF is held relatively constant over a mean arterial pressure (MAP) between 50 and 150 mm Hg in healthy, young individuals, a CPP of 60 to 90 mm Hg likely provides appropriate CBF (see Fig. 13-2).

C. **Autoregulation of cerebral blood flow is often impaired** in patients with acute cerebral injury. In this setting, reductions in CPP below 60 mm Hg may decrease CBF and cause cerebral ischemia. Increases in CPP above 80 mm Hg may increase CBF and cause vasogenic edema and increased ICP. An optimal CPP goal should therefore include both a minimum and a maximum range.

D. **Tissue oxygen delivery.** Because brain energy metabolism is dependent on continuous tissue oxygen influx, the primary focus should be optimal tissue oxygen delivery. Over a wide range of temperature and pH, oxygen delivery is proportional to the oxygen saturation, hemoglobin content, and cardiac output. Cardiac output may be compromised due to hypovolemia, sepsis, and impaired myocardial contractility or cardiac dysrhythmia as a complicating factor of brain or spinal cord injury.

E. **Oxygen extraction.** The immense energy requirements of the brain demand a system for oxygen delivery that can tolerate sudden increases in demand (e.g., seizures) or decreases in supply (e.g., hypotension and hypoxemia). Unlike other organs, a system of "oxygen reserve" exists in which the brain can vary its oxygen

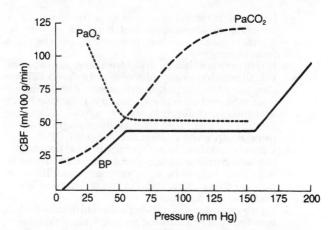

Fig. 13-2. Autoregulation maintains a constant level of cerebral blood flow (CBF) over a wide range of carotid artery mean blood pressures (BPs). Independent of this effect, CBF is elevated by hypercarbia (Paco₂) and hypoxemia (Pao₂); hypocarbia diminishes CBF.

extraction from a baseline of approximately 30% to an extreme of 70% under conditions of oligemia (CBF 20–30 ml/100g/min) or hypoxemia. It is only when CBF decreases below 20 ml/100g/min that electrical and chemical cellular functions are interrupted and ischemic symptoms develop. Increased oxygen extraction can be demonstrated with radiolabeled oxygen species using positron emission tomography (PET) or single photon emission computed tomography (SPECT) imaging (not practical in the management of most critically ill patients), or as a decrease in **cerebral mixed venous oxygen saturation** via cerebral venous jugular bulb sampling (Sjvo₂). The latter has been used at the bedside as a measure of inadequate CBF in patients with traumatic brain injury or those undergoing cardiopulmonary bypass. Recently developed fiberoptic sensors of brain partial pressure of oxygen may be useful in defining targets for resuscitation.

F. **Medications that influence ICP**
   1. **Vasodilators** such as **hydralazine, sodium nitroprusside (SNP), nitroglycerin,** and, to a lesser degree, **nicardipine** can induce cerebral vasodilation. In patients with poor intracranial compliance, this can increase ICP.
   2. **β-adrenergic blockers** such as **labetalol** or **propranolol** have minimal direct effect on CBF or ICP and are easily titrated. Because labetalol also blocks α-adrenergic tone, it may reduce sympathetically mediated large vessel vasoconstriction. This

better simulates the endogenous mechanisms of lowering blood pressure and helps to prevent regional ischemia as blood pressure is lowered pharmacologically.

3. **Barbiturates** such as **thiopental** and **pentobarbital,** although typically administered to lower ICP, are also potent antihypertensive agents, decreasing venous tone and cardiac contractility. This usually undesirable side effect may require the use of α- and/or β-adrenergic agonists such as **phenylephrine** and **norepinephrine** to maintain adequate CPP.

4. **Catecholamines** have an unpredictable potential to increase cerebral metabolic rate and CBF. These effects are likely to be more pronounced as BP is increased above normal and in the presence of blood–brain barrier disruption.

5. **Hypo-osmolar and iso-osmolar solutions** such as lactated Ringer's solution and half- normal saline in 5% dextrose (D5 1/2 NS) may exacerbate brain edema in the setting of osmotic diuretic therapy. **Glucose-containing solutions** may produce hyperglycemia and may lead to neurologic worsening after brain ischemia.

G. **Other factors that influence ICP**

1. Intracranial pressure is increased by many of the complications of **central venous access** including pneumothorax, carotid puncture, painful stimulation, and body position (e.g., Trendelenburg, lateral head rotation, jugular compression). Patients should be kept in optimal position for ICP management until the last possible moment prior to puncture.

2. **Noxious stimuli** can increase ICP, CBF, and cerebral metabolic rate and should be prevented and treated aggressively.

III. **Extracranial hemodynamics.** The primary goal of systemic blood pressure management is defined by the type of central nervous system (CNS) or systemic injury present. An optimal CPP must be maintained at all times. Because the MAP decreases to the same extent (<20%) between the aortic root and the distal middle cerebral arteries or the radial arteries, conventionally measured systemic MAP is a reasonable surrogate for mean intracerebral artery pressure.

A. **Reduced CPP.** In the case of reduced CPP, the primary objective should be the lowering of ICP, but systemic MAP may need to be pharmacologically augmented while the ICP reduction strategies are initiated. The first choice in patients with adequate myocardial contractility should be a pure α-**adrenergic agonist** such as **phenylephrine** because it is well tolerated and causes minimal cerebrovascular vasoconstriction. If this does not produce sufficient blood pressure elevations or there is inadequate contractility to support the increased systemic vascular resistance, then additional inotropic support is required.

B. Excessive CPP. When there is evidence of excessive CBF because of severe hypertension or impaired autoregulation or blood–brain barrier permeability (e.g., eclampsia, brain neoplasm), MAP should be reduced in a reliable and highly titratable manner. Hypertension alone in the absence of excessive CBF or myocardial dysfunction should not be treated because it often reflects a homeostatic response to acute cerebral ischemia. Reductions in blood pressure can provoke cerebral ischemia in this setting.

1. **Sympathetic antagonists** such as **labetalol** reduce the systemic effects of the high-catecholamine-output states frequently associated with CNS injury, including arterial hypertension, tachycardia, cardiac irritability, neurogenic pulmonary vascular injury, and large-vessel vasoconstriction.
2. Often, additional agents are necessary, and **nicardipine** and **SNP** provide a reliable and titratable response. Both agents may lead to significant cerebral vasodilation and therefore raise ICP.
3. **Avoid sublingual administration** of short-acting calcium-channel blockers, which lower pressure unpredictably without reducing sympathetic output.

C. Cardiac dysrhythmias

1. In large strokes and subarachnoid hemorrhage, **ST segment changes** may be seen on the electrocardiogram (ECG), but these do not predict future cardiovascular morbidity. Electrocardiographic changes may be diffuse or confined to a cardiovascular territory. Myocardial ischemia should always be excluded.
2. **Sympathetic outflow** associated with brain injury may provoke ventricular dysrhythmias in patients with coronary artery disease, and **Guillain-Barré syndrome** may produce an autonomic cardioneuropathy.
3. **Cervical spine injury** may cause sympathetic cardiac denervation and unopposed vagal tone, leading to bradydysrhythmias.

IV. Airway and ventilation

A. Indications for endotracheal intubation. Impairment of airway reflexes occurs frequently in the brain-injured patient and predisposes to aspiration and poor clearance of secretions. **Neuromuscular respiratory failure** may be seen in amyotrophic lateral sclerosis, myasthenia gravis, acute inflammatory demyelinating polyneuropathy, and critical care myopathy or polyneuropathy. **Transient apnea** in the setting of a self-limited generalized convulsion is not an indication for intubation or assisted ventilation.

B. Complications of endotracheal intubation include hypotension, reduced CBF, and paradoxically increased ICP due to increased transthoracic pressures. An experienced anesthesiologist should be present at the intubation of a patient with intracranial hypertension or hemorrhage.

C. Permissive hypercapnia is often used in the ventilatory management of acute respiratory failure to limit mechanical lung injury (see Chapter 20). However, hypercapnia may result in unacceptable elevations of the ICP, and it is not recommended in patients with intracranial hypertension or blood–brain barrier injuries.

D. Spontaneous or induced hyperventilation causes acute cerebral vasoconstriction in a brain in which CO_2 reactivity is preserved. This decreases cerebral blood volume (CBV) and thereby ICP. If pressure autoregulation is preserved, the increased CPP may restore adequate CBF.

1. **The brain quickly equilibrates** to changes in P_{CO_2}. A new steady state is established within 3 to 4 hours in most patients. This is accomplished by both carbonic anhydrase and nonbicarbonate buffer systems.

2. **With excessive hypocapnia,** excessive vasoconstriction may produce regional or generalized cerebral ischemia.

3. **A rapid return to baseline** P_{CO_2} may produce cerebral vasodilation, causing increased CBV and a further deleterious rise in ICP. Therefore, hyperventilation should be used as a temporizing measure until more effective and durable measures can be initiated.

4. **Lack of response to hyperventilation** is a poor prognostic sign.

V. Sodium and water homeostasis

A. The goal of fluid resuscitation in the brain-injured patient is to maintain **hyperosmolar euvolemia.** This is accomplished with the use of osmotic diuretics (e.g., **mannitol, 23.4% NaCl**) and hyperosmolar intravenous fluid replacement (e.g., normal saline, **3% NaCl**). It is important to note that the distinction between 23.4% NaCl as an osmotic diuretic rather than a hyperosmolar intravenous fluid replacement is due to the predominant diuretic action of 23.4% NaCl when given as a bolus. Brain injury may disturb sodium balance in several different ways, sometimes simultaneously. Rapid shifts in subacute plasma sodium may produce demyelination or aggravate cerebral edema.

1. **Hyponatremia**

a. Cerebral injury may cause release of **natriuretic factors,** leading to profound **salt wasting,** that may require up to 200 ml/h of normal saline replacement or use of 3% solution in continuous infusion in addition to fludrocortisone (0.1–0.3 mg by mouth once or twice a day) This is seen most often in vasospasm after subarachnoid hemorrhage.

b. **Syndrome of inappropriate antidiuretic hormone (SIADH)** release should be treated aggressively with normal or **hypertonic saline** (3% solution) and loop diuretics when intravascular volume repletion is essential and fluid restriction is contraindicated.

    c. High-dose osmotic diuretic administration (mannitol $\geq$50 g intravenously [IV] every 4 hours) rarely may demand renal solute excretion to such a degree that it causes paradoxical free water retention. This is easily treated with small doses of loop diuretic to degrade the renal-concentrating ability.

    d. Intravascular volume depletion remains the most common cause of hyponatremia in the neurocritical care unit. Bladder catheterization and monitoring of central venous pressure (CVP) and plasma sodium are essential.

  2. Hypernatremia due to diabetes insipidus (DI) may be seen after pituitary tumor resection, traumatic brain injury, central herniation syndromes, and, occasionally, vasospasm following subarachnoid hemorrhage. **Hypotonic fluids and vasopressin** therapy may be indicated, and hourly monitoring of urine output and specific gravity is required.

B. Osmotic balance

  1. Plasma osmolality = $(2 \times [Na^+]) + [BUN]/2.8 + [Glucose]/18$, where BUN is blood urea nitrogen, and is normally 280 to 290 mOsm/kg.

  2. When plasma osmolality is increased above normal for more than 48 hours, intracellular osmotic particles are generated (idiogenic osmoles) and a new steady state is achieved to restore cell volume. Any rapid correction of plasma osmolality after this will result in a shift of free water into the intracranial compartment. Therefore, once osmotic agents have been initiated with sustained osmolality, they must be withdrawn gradually to permit excretion of these idiogenic osmoles. This is true regardless of the osmotic agent.

  3. Mannitol (0.5–1.0 g/kg IV bolus every 4–6 hours) should be given to attain the minimum osmolality sufficient to produce the desired effects, which often results in a stepwise increase in osmolar gap (osmolar gap = measured mOsm – calculated mOsm; normal $\leq$10). The goal of therapy is to continue until the osmolality gap is equal to or greater than 15. Osmolality in excess of 320 mOsm/kg with mannitol does not produce incremental benefits and is often associated with an increased osmolar gap and acute renal failure.

  4. Hypertonic saline may also be used to reach a desired osmolality by directly affecting plasma sodium levels. When administering hypertonic saline solutions, frequent serum Na assessments are required to avoid a rapid change in plasma Na concentration. Hypertonic saline solutions may exacerbate or contribute to the development of congestive heart failure and should be used with caution in patients at risk.

3% NaCl can be given as either a bolus of 150 ml every 4 to 6 hours or as a continuous infusion of 0.5 to 1.0 ml/kg/h. One administers **23.4% NaCl** as a 30- to 60-ml IV bolus every 6 hours.

VI. Glucose control

A. Elevated blood glucose levels after acute brain and spinal cord injury increases tissue acidosis and edema in and around injured tissue and impairs endogenous antiinflammatory mechanisms of repair. **Hyperglycemia** ($\geq$200 mg/dl) has been shown to be a predictor of poor outcome in the intensive care unit (ICU) population and in many forms of acute brain injury. Hypoglycemia (<60 mg/dl) can also lead to focal neurologic deficits, and glucose levels should be acutely restored with a bolus of **50% dextrose solution (D50)** along with 100 mg IV of **thiamine** to avoid the complication of Wernicke's encephalopathy. Overall, the goal for care is to achieve normoglycemia (80–140 mg/dl) with the administration of insulin.

VII. Temperature regulation

A. The occurrence of **hyperthermia** after brain injury is very common and has been shown to increase the release of excitatory neurotransmitters, further the breakdown of the blood–brain barrier, and worsen the clinical outcome. Once the source of fever has been properly investigated and appropriate therapy initiated, antipyretic measures, such as the administration of acetaminophen 650 mg every 4 to 6 hours, surface cooling (cooling blankets, ice packs), and/or intravascular cooling catheters should be instituted. **Normothermia** (temperature 37°C) should be the goal for all patients in the neuro-ICU.

B. **Induced hypothermia** has been shown to be neuroprotective in global ischemic brain injury after cardiac arrest but not in focal brain injury such as traumatic brain injury, ischemic stroke, and intracerebral hemorrhage. Due to the potentially significant adverse effects, including electrolyte disturbances, cardiac arrhythmias, and coagulopathy, induced hypothermia has limited application.

VIII. Hypothesis-driven neurologic examination

A. The **neurologic exam** of the critically ill patient should document cortical, brainstem, and spinal cord function in a simple and easily reproducible manner that can be recognized by a colleague at a later point in time.

1. **Avoid confusing acronyms** and empty summaries (e.g., "MS nonfocal").

2. **Report the neurologic exam** in the following order: cognitive functions (alertness, orientation, attention, language), cranial nerves, strength, sensation, deep-tendon reflexes, and other.

3. **Use a minimal stimulus** first, then escalate as needed (e.g., speak before yelling, yell before pinching).

4. **Coma** is produced by bilateral cortical or bilateral brainstem dysfunction.
B. **Cortical function. Language and attention** are lateralized in the human brain, and essentially all right-handed individuals and 85% of left-handed individuals process language in the left hemisphere and attention in the right hemisphere. The **motor cortex** (pre-central gyrus) controls the contralateral limbs and directs voluntary gaze (saccades) to the contralateral field. **Sensation** is processed in the post-central gyrus of the contralateral hemispheres. **Inattention** is common in critically ill patients (a hallmark of delirium) and often is due to medication or metabolic insults. However, the presence of a lateralizing hemiparesis, sensory loss, or gaze deviation should trigger urgent investigation. Cortical injury often produces face and arm weakness due to their large area of representation on the brain's surface.
C. **Brainstem function.** The brainstem controls involuntary eye movements, pupillary function, facial sensation, and vital functions. Knowledge of its functions is critical in the evaluation of the comatose patient and the posterior circulation acute stroke syndromes (see Table 13-1).
D. **Spinal cord function.** In contrast to brainstem and cortical injury, spinal cord injury of any type (vascular, traumatic, demyelinating) often produces bilateral, symmetric impairment of the limbs but never facial

Table 13-1. **Common findings in brainstem lesions**

Lesion Level	Common Findings	Anatomic Pathway
Midbrain	Mid-position fixed pupils	Light reflex pathways
		Oculomotor nuclei
	Ophthalmoplegia	Cerebral peduncles
	Hemiparesis, Babinski sign	
High pons	Pinpoint, reactive pupils	Sympathetic fibers
	Internuclear ophthalmoplegia	Medial longitudinal fasiculus
	Facial weakness	Facial nerve
	Reduced corneal sensation	Trigeminal nerve
Low pons	Horizontal reflex gaze paralysis	Abducens nerve, horizontal gaze center
	Hemiparesis, Babinski sign	Corticospinal, corticobulbar tracts
Medulla	Disordered breathing	Respiratory center
	Hypotension, hypertension, dysrhythmias	Vasomotor center

weakness. Always distinguish anterior column function (strength, sensation of pin/temperature) from posterior column function (sensation of vibration, proprioception) and document sacral functions (anal sphincter tone, bulbocavernosus reflex). The **anterior spinal artery** receives contributions from the vertebral arteries in the cervical region and the artery of Adamkiewicz (a branch of the abdominal aorta) in the thoracolumbar region. This anatomy creates a "watershed" vascular territory, which is prone to hypoperfusion, in the high thoracic cord.

1. **Brown-Sèquard syndrome** of hemicord dysfunction is characterized by ipsilateral loss of motor and proprioceptive functions and contralateral loss of pain and temperature.
2. **Central cord syndrome** is characterized by weakness in arms more than legs and variable sensory, bladder, and bowel dysfunction. This predilection for arm involvement is due to the medial lamination of arm fibers in the descending corticospinal tracts.
3. **Anterior spinal artery syndrome** is characterized by bilateral symmetric motor weakness and disassociated sensory loss, with impairments in pain and temperature sensation and preservation of proprioception and vibration.
4. **Cauda equina syndrome** is characterized by variable degrees of bilateral lower motor neuron weakness in the legs (sparing the arms), sensory loss of the lower extremities and sacrum, and dysfunction of bowel and bladder.
5. **Mixed tract syndromes** occur commonly in traumatic injury of the spinal cord. The aim of localization is to identify the highest level of injury (see Chapter 34).

IX. **Neuroimaging.** Recent advances in **computed tomography (CT)** and **magnetic resonance (MR)** make it possible to noninvasively image neurovascular structures and identify sites of venous sinus thrombosis, arterial occlusion, nonocclusive dissection, focal tissue ischemia, and diffuse axonal injury (Fig. 13-3). Areas of mismatch between tissue hypoperfusion (oligemia) and tissue ischemia can be identified to measure tissue at risk. Spinal cord compression or ischemia can also be rapidly evaluated. With appropriate planning, MR imaging can be performed in the presence of a halo vest or invasive monitoring. Extra lengths of rigid tubing can pass from the patient, through a small hole placed in the shielding wall, and to monitoring equipment and infusion pumps located in the MR control room. **Nuclear medicine blood flow imaging** is useful for assessing cerebral perfusion in cases of suspected brain death, especially when factors that confound the clinical evaluation are present. **Transcranial Doppler ultrasound imaging** can identify regions of increased blood flow velocity consistent with focal arterial narrowing (e.g., atherosclerosis, vasospasm), retrograde flow (which provides information

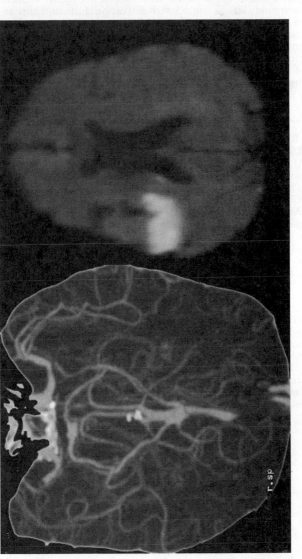

Fig. 13-3.   Computed tomography angiographic image (*left*) demonstrates an acute occlusion of the right middle cerebral artery. Diffusion-weighted magnetic resonance image (*right*) identifies an area of hyperintensity reflecting hyperacute ischemia. These techniques have revolutionized acute stroke management by providing rapid identification of vascular occlusion and early tissue injury.

about collateral circulation), or absent blood flow (which may indicate complete occlusion).

X. Coagulation disturbances. Due to the release of large quantities of brain tissue thromboplastin, massive brain injury may be associated with activation of the clotting cascade, disseminated intravascular coagulation, and subsequent clinical hemorrhage or clotting. Fresh-frozen plasma and recombinant coagulation factors (factor VII and IX) may be administered to treat coagulopathies in the setting of intracerebral hemorrhage (see Chapter 29). Brain tumors, coma, and paraplegia place patients at high risk for deep vein thrombosis (see Chapters 12 and 22).

SELECTED REFERENCES

Adams RD, Victor M. *Principles of neurology*. New York: McGraw-Hill, 1993.

Arieff AI, Kerian A, Massry SG, et al. Intracellular pH of brain: alterations in acute respiratory acidosis and alkalosis. *Am J Physiol* 1976;230:804–812.

Fisher CM. The neurological examination of the comatose patient. *Acta Neurol Scand* 1969;45(Suppl 36):1–56.

Guarantors of Brain. *Aids to the examination of the peripheral nervous system*. London: Bailliere Tindall, 1986.

Paulson OB, Standgaard S, Edvinsson L. Cerebral autoregulation. *Cerebrovasc Brain Metab Rev* 1990;2:161–192.

Plum F, Posner JB. *Diagnosis of stupor and coma,* 3rd ed. Philadelphia: FA Davis, 1982.

Ropper AH. *Neurological and neurosurgical intensive care,* 4th ed. New York: Raven Press, 2003.

Schwamm LH, Koroshetz WJ, Sorensen AG, et al. Time course of lesion development in patients with acute stroke: serial diffusion- and hemodynamic-weighted magnetic resonance imaging. *Stroke* 1998;29:2268–2276.

Suarez JI, ed. *Critical care neurology and neurosurgery*. New York: Humana Press, 2004.

Wijdicks EF. *The clinical practice of critical care neurology*. New York: Lippincott-Raven, 1997.

Adult and Pediatric Resuscitation

Shyam Parekh and Richard M. Pino

I. **Overview.** The intensivist is frequently called on to assist with **advanced cardiopulmonary resuscitation (CPR)** throughout the hospital. This chapter provides basic information for adult and pediatric resuscitation. Formal training in these areas is encouraged and is often mandated by institutional policy. The protocols described here follow the evidence-based Guidelines 2000 for Cardiopulmonary Resuscitation and Emergency Cardiovascular Care, with modifications for the clinician in a hospital setting. Table 14-1 lists the classifications for the quality of evidence used to support most of the protocol interventions presented in this chapter. The algorithms presented serve as a useful starting point when confronted with a cardiac arrest. It is important to remember that the responsibilities of the intensivist during a cardiac emergency include managing people and resources effectively in addition to knowledge of **advanced cardiac life support (ACLS).** To achieve this goal, the intensivist must maintain global awareness in an event, delegate tasks to appropriate personnel, and instill a sense of calmness and order.

II. **Cardiac arrest**
   A. **The diagnosis of cardiac arrest** is made swiftly in the intensive care unit (ICU) because of the high nurse-to-patient ratio, continuous monitoring of the electrocardiogram (ECG), routine arterial-pressure monitoring, and the use of central monitoring stations. The ECG might reveal ventricular tachycardia **(VT),** ventricular fibrillation **(VF),** or asystole. In pulseless electrical activity **(PEA),** an organized ECG is present without a blood pressure. The absence of a palpable pulse in a major artery (e.g., carotid, femoral) in an unconscious, unmonitored patient is diagnostic of a cardiac arrest.
   B. **Etiologies.** Cardiac arrest may be due to underlying primary cardiac or pulmonary disease or result from metabolic and physical abnormalities such as the following:
      1. Hypoxemia.
      2. Acid-base disturbances.
      3. Derangements of potassium, calcium, and magnesium serum concentrations.
      4. Hypovolemia.
      5. Adverse drug events.
      6. Pericardial tamponade.
      7. Tension pneumothorax.

Table 14-1. Evidence classification for interventions

Class	Evidence	Clinical Use
I	Excellent	Definitely recommended
IIa	Good/very good	Acceptable, safe, useful
IIb	Fair/good	Acceptable, safe, useful
Indeterminate	Preliminary research stage	May be used
III	Positive evidence absent	None

       8. Pulmonary embolus.
       9. Hypothermia.
      10. Myocardial infarction.
   C. Pathophysiology. With the onset of cardiac arrest, effective blood flow ceases and tissue hypoxia, anaerobic metabolism, and accumulation of cellular wastes result. Organ function is compromised and permanent damage ensues unless the condition is reversed within minutes. Acidosis from anaerobic metabolism may cause systemic vasodilation, pulmonary vasoconstriction, and a decreased responsiveness to the actions of endogenous and exogenous catecholamines. Following resuscitation, organ dysfunction may be exacerbated by reperfusion injury.

III. Adult resuscitation
   A. Basic life support (BLS) is the foundation of using resuscitation to maintain vital organ perfusion. The **ABCDs** (airway, breathing, circulation, defibrillation) of resuscitation should be evaluated for all patients in arrest. **ACLS** is the definitive treatment of a cardiac arrest with airway management, electrical cardioversion and defibrillation, and pharmacologic intervention.
     1. Airway and breathing. If the trachea is not already intubated, the airway should be evaluated for patency using the head tilt/chin lift or an oropharyngeal/nasopharyngeal airway as needed. Hemoglobin saturation can be readily monitored with pulse oximetry. If adequate spontaneous ventilation is still absent, bag-valve mask ventilation with 100% oxygen should be initiated until spontaneous ventilation returns. For example, a patient who has transient ventilatory depression shortly after the administration of a narcotic or a patient with hypotension related to a supraventricular tachycardia that resolves quickly with pharmacologic therapy or cardioversion might only require transient mask ventilation. When a secure airway is needed, intubation is performed by the most experienced

person with a minimal disruption of resuscitative measures. Correct placement of the endotracheal tube should be confirmed by auscultation and the presence of **end-tidal CO_2**. The latter can be monitored by capnography or via a colorimetric change in an indicator paper. End-tidal CO_2 may not be detectable when pulmonary blood flow is absent or when cardiac compressions are inadequate. The use of a self-inflating bulb (the esophageal detector) attached to the endotracheal tube and direct visualization by fiberoptic bronchoscopy have been suggested as alternative means of assessing proper placement of the endotracheal tube. **Epinephrine, lidocaine, naloxone,** and **atropine** may be administered by the endotracheal route if intravenous access has not been established. In adults, dilution of these drugs in 5 to 10 ml of sterile saline ensures their more complete delivery. Higher doses (two to three times) may be warranted with endotracheal administration to achieve adequate peak concentrations.

2. **Circulation.** The circulation is assessed by palpation of the carotid artery pulse for 5 to 10 seconds. In the absence of a palpable pulse, artificial circulation should be instituted with external **chest compressions.** (The presence of a pulse does not necessarily mean that an "adequate" mean arterial pressure is present.) Although the ACLS protocols consider a systolic blood pressure of less than 90 mm Hg as unstable in a variety of scenarios, the precise value for an individual patient must be considered with respect to coronary and cerebral perfusion pressures. Noninvasive blood pressure monitoring should be quickly employed in the absence of an arterial line. If the patient is pulseless or has an inadequate blood pressure, artificial circulation should be provided by external chest compressions. The patient must be on a firm surface (e.g., backboard or CPR position for a bed with an inflatable mattress) with the head at the same level as the thorax. The person doing chest compressions places the heel of one hand on the patient's sternum, two fingerbreadths above the xiphoid process. The other hand may either sit on top of the first, interlocking the fingers, or it may grasp the wrist of the first hand. The shoulders should be directly over the patient, with the elbows locked for effective compressions. The sternum is depressed 1.5 to 2.0 inches in a normal-sized adult with **the compressions accounting for 50% of each compression–relaxation cycle, delivered at 100 per minute, and at a 5:1 ratio with ventilation.** The return of spontaneous cardiopulmonary activity should be checked after the first four cycles and every several minutes thereafter.

3. **Defibrillation** within 3 minutes in the hospital (evidence Class I) and 5 minutes after calling the emergency medical system (EMS) is the major determinant of a successful resuscitation of a cardiac arrest secondary to VF because it becomes more difficult to treat with time. Until recently, defibrillation was taught only to ACLS providers. Public-access defibrillation programs (PADs) have now enabled "level I" responders (e.g., fire personnel, police, security guards, airline attendants) to employ readily **accessible automated external defibrillators (AEDs).** AEDs are small, lightweight defibrillators that use adhesive electrode pads for sensing and delivering shocks. The AED, after analysis of the ECG signal, *advises* either "shock indicated" or "no shock indicated." The AED is manually triggered and does not automatically defibrillate the patient. AEDs are now standard on most hospital defibrillators to allow immediate treatment of lethal dysrhythmias by all health care providers.

   a. **Biphasic waveform defibrillators** possess the most recent technology for delivering energy that flows in a positive direction for a specified number of milliseconds followed by reversal of flow in the negative direction. Although the optimum biphasic energy to terminate VF has not been determined, repeated shocks at company-specific energy levels appear to be at least as effective as monophasic sequential 200, 300, and 360 J. The newest biphasic defibrillators, in addition to manual modes for cardioversion and defibrillation, often have AED and transcutaneous pacing features. It is the responsibility of the person operating the defibrillator to ensure that members of the resuscitation team are not in contact with the patient during defibrillation.

   b. **Monophasic waveform defibrillators** deliver a unidirectional current. Although biphasic defibrillators in many hospitals have replaced this mode, knowledge of monophasic defibrillators is needed because they are still widely in use. The energy level for the initial series of unsynchronized monophasic damped sinusoidal (MDS) shocks is 200 J followed by 300 J, and 360 J, if needed. Subsequent shocks at 360 J are repeated after every pharmacologic intervention. For recurrent VF following a successful defibrillation, the lowest energy level that was previously useful should be tried first.

4. **Diagnosis and cardioversion of dysrhythmias.** Symptomatic hypotension may be the result of bradycardia, multiple forms of supraventricular tachycardia (including atrial fibrillation [AF] and flutter), and VT. Although adenosine (section **III.7.a**) can be used

to diagnose (Fig. 14-1) and possibly convert to normal sinus rhythm a supraventricular tachycardia, it is often difficult to differentiate a wide-complex supraventricular tachycardia from VT. An atrial electrogram is useful for this purpose. An atrial electrogram can be obtained via connection of intraoperatively placed transthoracic pacing wires to lead I of the ECG (assuming that the patient is not dependent on atrial pacing). A second method takes advantage of the proximity of the esophagus to the atrium. A transesophageal pacer can be used as a sensing electrode for this purpose (Fig. 14-2). If not readily available, a transvenous pacing wire can be placed into the esophagus via a No. 4.0 endotracheal tube used as a conduit. Synchronized biphasic and monophasic shocks beginning at 50 J are used for supraventricular dysrhythmias such as paroxysmal supraventricular tachycardia (PSVT) (Fig. 14-3), AF, and atrial flutter. Many clinicians feel that AF and flutter are more resident to cardioversion and necessitate 100- to 150-J synchronous biphasic shocks. Hemodynamically stable VT and atrial fibrillation can be cardioverted using 100 J as the starting point. Once the rhythm is cardioverted, it is necessary to

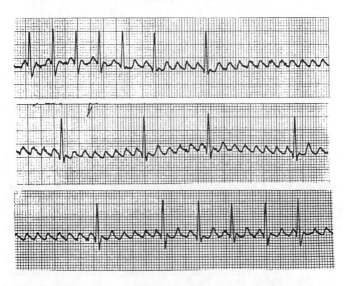

Fig. 14-1.   Diagnosis of a rhythm with adenosine. The initial ventricular response of 180 beats/min disappears after atrioventricular conduction is inhibited by adenosine, revealing an underlying rhythm of atrial flutter (300 beats/min, *top*), followed by a 6 to 8:1 block (*middle*), then a 2 to 3:1 block of atrial flutter with a ventricular rate of 120 beats/min.

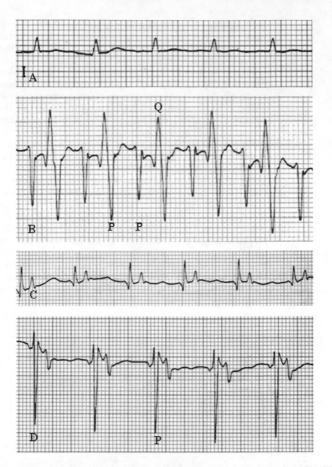

Fig. 14-2.   Suspected atrial flutter with a 2:1 block. A. Standard lead I of the ECG: The flutter waves are not distinct. B. Atrial electrogram obtained through an esophageal lead, showing an atrial rate of 300 beats/min with P waves (P) and Q waves (Q) easily seen. The polarity of the P wave is inverted because of the positioning of the esophageal probe. C. After treatment with amiodarone and cardioversion, normal sinus rhythm is seen on the standard ECG and the atrial electrogram (D).

attempt correction for possible underlying causes of the dysrhythmia, for example, electrolyte abnormalities.

5. **Pacing.** High-grade heart block with profound bradycardia is one etiology of cardiac arrest. Temporary pacing should be used when the heart rate does not increase with pharmacologic therapy. Transcutaneous pacing is the easiest method of increasing the ventricular rate, though sedation of the patient

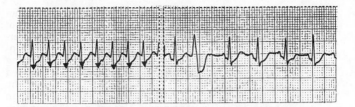

Fig. 14-3. Synchronous cardioversion of a supraventricular tachycardia. Arrowheads (*left*) indicate synchrony of the defibrillator with the patient's rate (300 beats/min) prior to cardioversion (*right*) to a rate of 140 beats/min that was followed with pharmacologic therapy.

may be necessary. Esophageal pacing is efficacious for sinus bradycardia with maintained atrioventricular (AV) conduction and is useful intraoperatively for bradycardia-related hypotension in otherwise stable patients. Transvenous pacing via a temporary wire into the right heart is a third option to increase heart rate, though technically more difficult. It has the added advantage of being more secure and reliable for longer periods of time than the first two options. Special pacing pulmonary artery catheters are capable of AV pacing.

6. **Intravenous access** is imperative for a successful resuscitation. The most desirable route is within the central circulation. Many patients in the ICU will have some form of central access in place. Internal or external jugular, subclavian, femoral, or long peripheral lines may be used. The **internal jugular** and **femoral veins** are desirable because of the relative ease of insertion, fewer complications, and minimal interruption of resuscitative efforts during insertion. The antecubital veins are the next most desirable and are fairly effective if the extremity is elevated and a large volume of intravenous fluid is used to flush the medication toward the central circulation. One should not overlook the utility of existing subcutaneous central venous ports or dialysis catheters. Peripherally inserted central catheters (PICC lines) are usually not suitable for extended resuscitation because of the high resistance to flow. Fluid replacement with crystalloids or blood products is indicated for patients with known or suspected intravascular volume depletion. In the usual cardiac arrest scenario, fluids are used only to keep intravenous lines open and to flush drugs toward the central circulation.

7. **Drugs.** The drugs to be described are used in ACLS protocols for the treatment of hemodynamic instability, myocardial ischemia and infarction, and dysrhythmias. It is crucial to know which drugs are infusing into a patient at the time of an arrest. For

example, stopping a dopamine infusion in a hemodynamically stable patient with a sudden onset of supraventricular tachycardia might be the best therapeutic option. Similarly, trying to revive a hypotensive patient with VT would be difficult if a continuing infusion of nitroglycerin is not recognized. Discussed are drugs that are commonly used to support the circulation; they are listed in alphabetical order to assist in quick referencing. Also refer to the **supplemental drug information** in Appendix 1. The doses of drugs used for **pediatric advanced life support (PALS)** are in brackets.

a. **Adenosine,** an endogenous purine nucleotide with a half-life of 5 seconds, slows AV nodal conduction and interrupts AV node reentry pathways to convert narrow-complex tachycardias and wide-complex tachycardias with *confirmed* supraventricular origin to a sinus rhythm. It also assists with the diagnosis of supraventricular tachycardias (e.g., atrial flutter with a rapid ventricular response versus PSVT; see Fig. 14-1). Adenosine is not effective for common ventricular dysrhythmias or for atrial fibrillation/flutter. Although adenosine has short-lived vasodilatory effects, hypotension has been reported in patients inappropriately given adenosine for VT. Other potential adverse effects include angina, bronchospasm, and dysrhythmia. The initial dose is a 6-mg *rapid* IV bolus. A brief asystole ensues, followed by P waves, flutter waves, or AF that are initially without ventricular responses. PSVT is sometimes converted to a sinus rhythm with an initial dose of 6 mg. A second injection of 12 mg may terminate PSVT if the first administration is unsuccessful. Recurrent PSVT will require drugs of longer half-life for definitive treatment. These doses are based on the peripheral administration of adenosine and compensate for its rapid degradation. When given via a central route the first dose should be 3 mg followed by 6 mg if needed. The dose of adenosine should be increased in the presence of methylxanthines (competitive inhibition) and decreased if dipyridamole (potentiation via blockage of nucleoside transport) has been administered. [**PALS:** 0.1 mg/kg; repeat dose 0.2 mg/kg; maximum dose 12 mg.]

b. **Amiodarone** is the most versatile drug in the ACLS algorithms. It has the properties of all four classes of antiarrhythmics (lengthening of the action potential, sodium-channel blockade at high frequencies of stimulation, noncompetitive antisynaptic actions, negative chronotropism) and is preferable for patients with severely impaired cardiac function because of its efficacy and comparative lower incidence of proarrhythmic effects. Amiodarone is indicated for persistent unstable VT and for VF after defibrillation and epinephrine treatment (Evidence Class IIb); rate control of stable monomorphic VT, polymorphic VT (Evidence Class IIb), and AF (Evidence Class IIa) to sinus rhythm; ventricular rate control of rapid atrial arrhythmias when digitalis is ineffective (Evidence Class IIb) and secondary to accessory pathways (Evidence Class IIb); and as an adjunct to electrical cardioversion of refractory PSVTs (Evidence Class IIa) and atrial tachycardia (Evidence Class IIb). The dose for the treatment of unstable VT and VF is 300 mg diluted in 20 to 30 ml of saline or 5% dextrose in water (D5W) administered rapidly. For the treatment of more stable disorders, the dose is 150 mg administered over 10 minutes, followed by an infusion of 1 mg/min for 6 hours, then 0.5 mg/min. The maximum daily dose is 2 g. Immediate side effects include bradycardia and hypotension, which can be managed by slowing the rate of infusion or administering fluids or pressors. With chronic use, hypothyroidism, elevation of hepatic enzymes, alveolar pneumonitis, and pulmonary fibrosis may occur. [**PALS:** loading dose, 5 mg/kg; maximum dose, 15 mg/kg/d.]

c. **Atropine** is useful in the treatment of hemodynamically significant bradycardia (Evidence Class I) or AV block occurring at the nodal level (Evidence Class IIa). It increases the rate of sinus node discharge and enhances AV node conduction by its vagolytic activity. The dose of atropine for bradycardia or AV block is 0.5 mg repeated every 3 to 5 minutes to a total dose of 0.04 mg/kg. For asystole, atropine is given as a 1-mg bolus repeated in 3 to 5 minutes if needed. Atropine should not be used when Mobitz type II block is suspected. Full vagal blockade is obtained at a cumulative dose of 3 mg. [**PALS:** 0.02 mg/kg; minimum dose, 0.1 mg; maximum single dose, 0.5 mg in child, 1.0 mg in adolescent.]

d. **Beta-adrenergic blocking drugs (atenolol, metoprolol, propranolol)** have established utility (Evidence Class I) for patients with unstable angina and myocardial infarction. These drugs reduce the rate of recurrent ischemia, nonfatal reinfarction, and postinfarction VF. In the absence of contraindications, β-blockers should be given to all patients with suspected acute myocardial infarction or high-risk unstable angina. In contrast to calcium-channel blockers, β-blockers are not direct negative inotropes. Esmolol, a very short acting agent, in addition to other β-blockers, is useful for the acute treatment of PSVT, AF, and atrial flutter (Evidence Class I) and ectopic atrial tachycardia (Evidence Class IIb). Initial and subsequent IV doses, if tolerated, are: **atenolol,** 5 mg over 5 minutes, repeated once at 10 min; **metoprolol,** 5 mg every 5 minutes times 3 doses; **propranolol,** 0.1 mg/kg divided into three doses given every 2 to 3 minutes; **esmolol,** 0.5 mg/kg over 1 minute followed by an infusion starting at 50 μg/min and titrated as needed to 200 μg/min. Contraindications include second- or third-degree heart block, hypotension, and severe congestive heart failure. Caution should be used in patients with preexisting sinus bradycardia or sick-sinus syndrome. Atenolol and metoprolol, because of their relatively specific β_1-adrenergic blockade, are preferable to propranolol in patients with a history of reactive airway disease. There is a small number patients who will exhibit bronchospasm with the administration of any β-blocker. Most patients with chronic obstructive pulmonary disease, however, are able to tolerate β-blockers.

e. **Calcium** is indicated during cardiac arrest only when hyperkalemia, hypermagnesemia, hypocalcemia, or toxicity from calcium-channel blockers is suspected. Calcium chloride, 2 to 4 mg/kg IV, can be repeated as necessary. [**PALS:** 20 mg/kg.]

f. **Dopamine** has dopaminergic (generally at doses <2 μg/kg/min), β (2–5 μg/kg/min), and α (5–10 μg/kg/min) activities. Although these are "traditional" doses, in practice, α and β effects can be present at the lowest dose levels. Therefore, the drug should be started at a low dose (e.g., 150 μg/min) and titrated until the desired effect (e.g., increased urine output, increased heart rate/inotropy, increased blood pressure) is seen or undesired side effects (e.g., a tachyarrhythmia) occur. Dopamine is indicated for bradycardia in which atropine is ineffective, replacing isoproterenol due to a better side-effect profile.

g. **Epinephrine** has been the mainstay of pharmacologic therapy for cardiac arrest. Its **α-adrenergic vasoconstriction of noncerebral and noncoronary** vascular beds produces compensatory shunting of blood toward the brain and the heart. The β-adrenergic effects of increased work and possible ischemia are potentially harmful during resuscitation, especially when used in high doses. It is now Evidence Class Intermediate when used during cardiac arrest. Studies have failed to show a significant improvement in the rate of survival to hospital discharge after an arrest when high-dose epinephrine was used. The recommended dose is 1.0 mg IV (10 ml of a

1:10,000 solution), repeated every 3 to 5 minutes, or administered by an infusion of 1 to 4 μg/min. Intratracheal epinephrine given at 2 to 2.5 times the IV dose appears to have good bioavailability and is therefore a reasonable option when intravenous access has not been established. Epinephrine used for symptomatic bradycardia is Evidence Class IIb. [**PALS:** bradycardia, 0.01 mg/kg; pulseless arrest, 0.01 mg/kg with subsequent doses up to 0.1 mg/kg.]

h. **Ibutilide** is used for the acute conversion of AF or flutter, either alone or with electrical cardioversion. It prolongs the duration of the action potential and increases the refractory period. The dose of 1 mg given over 10 minutes can be repeated in 10 minutes. The dose for patients weighing less than 60 kg is 0.01 mg/kg. Continuous monitoring of the patient is required during its administration and for at least 6 hours thereafter because the major side effect of ibutilide is polymorphic VT (including torsades de pointes), especially in patients with impaired left ventricular function.

i. **Isoproterenol** is a β_1 and β_2 agonist. It is a rarely used second-line drug used to treat hemodynamically significant bradycardia that is unresponsive to atropine and dopamine in the event that a temporarily pacemaker is not available (Evidence Class IIb). Its β_2 activity can cause hypotension. Isoproterenol is administered by IV infusion at 2 to 10 μg/min, titrated to achieve the desired heart rate.

j. **Lidocaine,** the mainstay of ventricular arrhythmia treatment in previous years, has been relegated to an Evidence Class Indeterminate status and is considered a **second choice** compared with amiodarone, procainamide, and sotalol. It may be useful for the control (not prophylaxis) of ventricular ectopy during an acute myocardial infarction. The initial dose during a cardiac arrest is 1.0 to 1.5 mg/kg IV and may be repeated as a 0.5- to 0.75-mg/kg bolus every 3 to 5 minutes to a total dose of 3 mg/kg. A continuous infusion of lidocaine at a rate of 2 to 4 mg/min is instituted after successful resuscitation. The lidocaine dose should be decreased for patients with reduced cardiac output, hepatic dysfunction, prolonged lidocaine infusion, or advanced age. [**PALS:** 1 mg/kg; infusion, 20 to 50 μg/kg/min.]

k. **Magnesium** is a cofactor in a variety of enzyme reactions including Na^+K^+-ATPase. Hypomagnesemia can precipitate refractory VF as well as exacerbate hypokalemia. Magnesium replacement is effective for the treatment of drug-induced torsades de pointes even in the absence of magnesium deficiency. The dose for emergent administration is 1 to 2 g in 10 ml of D5W over 1 to 2 minutes. Hypotension and bradycardia are side effects of rapid administration. [**PALS:** 25 to 50 mg/kg; maximum dose, 2 g.]

l. **Oxygen.** Because of profound tissue hypoxia, 100% O_2 should be provided by positive-pressure ventilation to all cardiac arrest victims. For hemodynamically stable patients with dysrhythmias, oxygen can be administered via a face mask. The benefit of providing oxygen to a patient with chronic obstructive pulmonary disease clearly outweighs the theoretical suppression of ventilation.

m. **Procainamide** can convert AF and atrial flutter to sinus rhythm (Evidence Class IIa), control the ventricular response to SVT secondary to accessory pathways (Evidence Class IIb), and convert wide-complex tachycardias of unknown origin (Class IIb). The loading dose is a continuous infusion of 20 to 30 mg/min that is terminated when the arrhythmia is suppressed, hypotension occurs, the QRS complex is widened by 50% of its original size, or a total dose of 17 mg/kg is reached. When the arrhythmia is suppressed, a maintenance infusion of 1 to 4 mg/min should be initiated, with reduced dose considered in the presence of renal failure. An ECG should be examined for QRS widening and prolonged QT at least daily. The therapeutic blood level is the sum of procainamide and its active metabolite, N-acetylprocainamide (NAPA). [**PALS:** 15 mg/kg.]

n. **Sodium bicarbonate** administration is detrimental in most cardiac arrests because it creates a paradoxical intracellular acidosis (Evidence Class III) among other potentially harmful effects. The few justifications for use are when the standard ACLS protocol has failed in the presence of severe preexisting metabolic acidosis and for the treatment of hyperkalemia, tricyclic antidepressant, or phenobarbital overdose. The initial dose of bicarbonate is 1 mEq/kg IV, with subsequent doses of 0.5 mEq/kg given every 10 minutes (as guided by arterial blood pH and $Paco_2$). [**PALS:** 1 mEq/kg.]

o. **Sotalol** is a class III antiarrhythmic agent with nonselective β-blocking properties that is used for both ventricular and supraventricular dysrhythmias. Like amiodarone, it prolongs the duration of the action potential. IV sotalol is administered at a rate of 10 mg/min to total dose of 1 to 1.5 mg/kg, and must be administered slowly or bradycardia and hypotension may occur. As a result, sotalol may be impractical for use in emergent situations.

Intravenous sotalol is not available in the United States.

p. **Vasopressin,** a neurohypophyseal antidiuretic hormone (see Chapter 27) and is an Evidence Class IIb intervention that is an alternative to epinephrine for the **treatment of VF.** Endogenous levels of vasopressin are increased in patients undergoing CPR who eventually survive in comparison to those who do not. Vasopressin constricts vascular smooth muscle when used in high doses. It is more effective than epinephrine in maintaining the coronary perfusion pressure and has a longer half-life of 10 to 20 minutes. It is administered as a single dose of **40 units IV** as an alternative to epinephrine. Although no definitive data exist to support the use of vasopressin in asystole or pulseless electrical activity (PEA), it may be effective for use in these arrest states.

q. **Verapamil** and **diltiazem,** calcium-channel blockers that depress AV nodal conduction, are used to treat hemodynamically stable narrow-complex PSVTs that are unresponsive to vagal maneuvers and adenosine. These drugs are also useful in rate control of AF. The initial verapamil dose is 2.5 to 5.0 mg IV, with subsequent doses of 5 to 10 mg IV administered every 15 to 30 minutes. Diltiazem is given as an initial bolus of 20 mg. An additional dose of 25 mg and an infusion of 5 to 15 mg/h can be administered if needed. Their vasodilator and negative inotrope properties can cause hypotension, exacerbation of congestive heart failure, bradycardia, and enhancement of accessory conduction in patients with Wolff-Parkinson-White syndrome. The hypotension can often be reversed with calcium chloride, 0.5 to 1.0 gm IV, while the heart rate control is maintained.

8. **Specific ACLS protocols**
   a. Ventricular fibrillation (Fig. 14-4).
   b. Asystole (Fig. 14-5).
   c. Pulseless electrical activity (PEA) (Fig. 14-6).
   d. Unstable tachycardia (Fig. 14-7).
   e. Stable tachycardia (Fig. 14-8).
   f. Bradycardia (Fig. 14-9).

9. **Open-chest direct cardiac compression** is an intervention used at institutions with appropriate resources to manage penetrating chest trauma, abdominal trauma with cardiac arrest, pericardial tamponade, hypothermia, and pulmonary embolism. Direct cardiac compressions also are indicated for individuals with anatomic deformities of the chest that prevent adequate closed-chest compression. The ICU may be the optimal setting outside of the operating room for considering open-chest cardiac compression during an arrest.

Ventricular Fibrillation

Cardiac arrest
↓
BLS algorithm
↓
Assess rhythm
↓
VF/pulseless VT
↓
Defibrillate, 150 J biphasic (200, 300, 360 J monophasic)
[PALS: 2 to 4 J/kg]
↓
CPR if VF, pulseless VT
Secure airway
Differential diagnoses
↓
Establish IV access
↓
Epinephrine 1:10,000, 1 mg IV, q 3-5 min[a]
[PALS: 0.01 mg/kg]
or
Vasopressin 40 units IV X 1
↓
Defibrillate[b]
↓
Amiodarone 300 mg IV push[c]
[PALS: 5 mg/kg]
↓
Magnesium sulfate, 1-2 g IV
[PALS: 25-50 mg/kg; max. 2 g]
(hypomagnesemia; polymorphic VT [torsades de pointes])
↓
Defibrillate
↓
Procainamide, 20-30 mg/min IV[d]
(refractory VF)

[a] Defibrillate after each epinephrine administration.
[b] Use the lowest energy that was successful with initial defibrillation.
[c] Amiodarone is diluted in 20-30 ml saline or D5W. If successful, an infusion of 1 mg/min for 6 hours followed by 0.5 mg/h is given. An additional dose of 150 mg IV push can be administered if VF or pulseless VT recurs. The maximum dose is 2.2 g over 24 hours.
[d] The maximum dose is 17 mg/kg or termination with arrhythmia suppression, hypotension, or QRS width of 50%. If successful, infuse 2 mg/kg/h.

Fig. 14-4. Protocol for ventricular fibrillation. BLS, basic life support; VF, ventricular fibrillation; VT, ventricular tachycardia; PALS, pediatric advanced life support; CPR, cardiopulmonary resuscitation; IV, intravenous; q, every; D5W, 5% dextrose in water.

Asystole

Cardiac arrest
↓
BLS algorithm
↓
Assess rhythm
↓
If rhythm is unclear and possible ventricular
fibrillation, defibrillate as for VF
↓
Asystole
↓
Secure airway
↓
Establish IV access
↓
Transcutaneous pacing
↓
Epinephrine 1:10,000, 1 mg IV q 3-5 min
↓
Intubate when possible
↓
Atropine, 1 mg IV q 3-5 min
(total: 0.04 mg/kg)

Fig. 14-5. Protocol for asystole. BLS, basic life support; VF, ventricular fibrillation; IV, intravenous; q, every.

10. **Termination of CPR.** There are no absolute guidelines to determine when to stop an unsuccessful resuscitation, but there is an exceedingly low probability of survival after 15 minutes. It is at the discretion of the intensivist or other physician in charge to determine when the failure of the cardiovascular system to respond to adequately applied BLS and ACLS indicates that the patient has died. There should be a meticulous documentation of the resuscitation including the reasons for terminating the effort.

11. The advanced directive **"do not resuscitate" (DNR)** places the intensivist in a key position with respect to perioperative and postoperative care. It is often incorrectly *assumed* that a DNR order is suspended in the perioperative period. Each institution's written guidelines should be reviewed. In advance of a procedure, physicians and the patient with

Pulseless Electrical Activity

Organized ECG activity without pulse
↓
CPR, IV access, intubation
↓
Consider underlying cause:

Hypovolemia (give volume)
Tension pneumothorax (relieve pressure)
Hypoxemia (oxygen)
Cardiac tamponade (pericardiocentesis)
Hypokalemia (give potassium)
Bicarbonate-responsive metabolic acidosis (bicarbonate)
Drug overdose (treatment appropriate to substance)
Myocardial infarction (heparin, thrombolysis, IABP)
↓
Epinephrine 1:10,000, 1 mg IV q 3-5 min
[PALS: 0.01 mg/kg]
↓
Atropine 1 mg IV (if slow PEA rate)
(total: 0.04 mg/kg)

Fig. 14-6. Protocol for pulseless electrical activity. ECG, electrocardiogram; CPR, cardiopulmonary resuscitation; IV, intravenous; IABP, intraaortic balloon pump; q, every; PALS, pediatric advanced life support; PEA, pulseless electrical activity.

the DNR status or the patient's health care proxy should clarify any resuscitative measures that would be compatible with the patient's wishes. For example, the use of a pressor to control hypotension following a hip replacement with a spinal anesthetic might be permitted, in contrast to defibrillation and CPR for spontaneous VF that might be prohibited. When asked to perform an emergent intubation outside of the operating room, the intensivist should ask about the patient's code status and is ethically and legally bound to follow a known decision to limit treatment.

IV. **Pediatric resuscitation**
   A. **Basic life support.** The need for CPR in the pediatric age group is rare after the neonatal period. The majority of cardiac arrests occur in infants less than 1 year of age. Pediatric cardiac arrests usually result from **hypoxemia linked to respiratory failure or airway obstruction.** Initial efforts should be directed toward the establishment of a secure airway and adequate ventilation. For children 8 years of age or older, basic considerations for resuscitation are the same as for the

Unstable Tachycardia

Tachycardia
↓
Ventricular tachycardia
Wide complex of unknown type
Paroxysmal supraventricular tachycardia
Atrial fibrillation
Atrial flutter
↓
Consider unstable if:
Chest pain
Dyspnea
Hypotension
Decreased level of consciousness
Pulmonary edema
Congestive heart failure
Acute myocardial infarction
Hypoxemia
Ventricular rate >150 bpm
↓
Appropriate sedation and resuscitation equipment present
↓
Synchronous cardioversion
50, 100, 150 J biphasic (50–360 J monophasic)

Fig. 14-7. Protocol for unstable tachycardia in adults.

adult. The "phone-first" rule applies to children younger than 8 years of age and any child with suspected drowning, traumatic arrest, or drug overdose or at high risk for dysrhythmias. Modifications of the rate and magnitude of compressions and ventilations as well as of the hand position for compressions are necessary because of anatomic and physiologic differences (Table 14-2). The differences between pediatric and adult resuscitation techniques are as follows.

1. **Airway and breathing.** Maneuvers to establish an airway are the same as in the adult, with a few caveats. For children less than 1 year old, abdominal thrusts are not used because the gastrointestinal tract can be damaged easily. Hyperextension of an infant's neck for the head tilt/chin lift may lead to airway obstruction because of the small diameter and ease of compression of the immature airway. Submental compression while performing the chin lift can also lead to airway obstruction by pushing the tongue into the pharynx. Ventilations should be

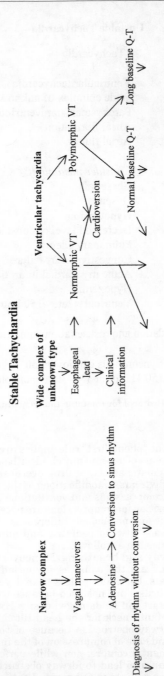

Atrial fibrillation Atrial flutter	Rhythm	Supraventricular tachycardia EF ≥ 40%	EF < 40%	EF ≥ 40%	EF < 40%	EF ≥ 40%	Consider torsades
Rate control Diltiazem β-blocker Digoxin	Junctional	Amiodarone β-blocker Diltiazem/verapamil	Amiodarone	Preferred: Procainamide Sotalol	Amiodarone (150 mg) or lidocaine (0.5-0.75 mg/kg)	Treat ischemia	
	Paroxysmal	Diltiazem/verapamil β-blocker Digoxin DC cardioversion Consider: procainamide, amiodarone, sotalol	Amiodarone Digoxin Diltiazem			Correct electrolytes	Correct electrolytes
Rate control/ conversion Amiodarone Procainamide				Acceptable: Amiodarone Lidocaine	Synchronized cardioversion	One of the following: β-blocker Lidocaine Amiodarone Procainamide Sotalol	One of the following: Magnesium Overdrive pacing Isoproterenol Phenytoin Lidocaine
Conversion DC cardioversion Ibutilide	Ectopic or multifocal atrial	Diltiazem/verapamil β-blocker Amiodarone	Amiodarone Diltiazem				

Fig. 14-8. Protocol for stable tachycardia in adults. VT, ventricular tachycardia. EF, ejection fraction; DC, direct current.

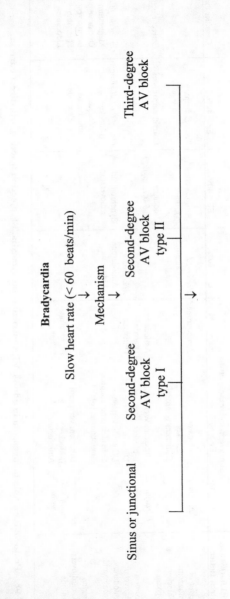

Bradycardia

Slow heart rate (<60 beats/min)

Mechanism

Sinus or junctional

Second-degree
AV block
type I

Second-degree
AV block
type II

Third-degree
AV block

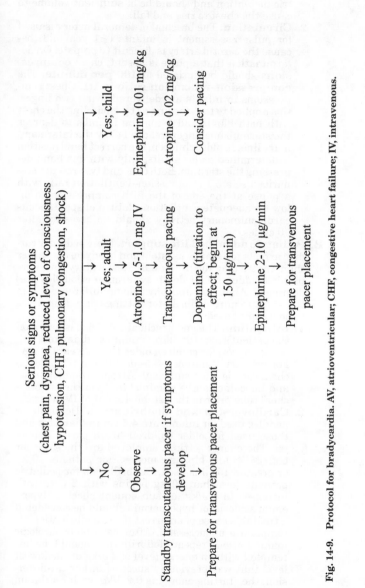

Serious signs or symptoms
(chest pain, dyspnea, reduced level of consciousness
hypotension, CHF, pulmonary congestion, shock)

No → Observe → Standby transcutaneous pacer if symptoms develop → Prepare for transvenous pacer placement

Yes; adult → Atropine 0.5-1.0 mg IV → Transcutaneous pacing → Dopamine (titration to effect; begin at 150 µg/min) → Epinephrine 2-10 µg/min → Prepare for transvenous pacer placement

Yes; child → Epinephrine 0.01 mg/kg → Atropine 0.02 mg/kg → Consider pacing

Fig. 14-9. Protocol for bradycardia. AV, atrioventricular; CHF, congestive heart failure; IV, intravenous.

given slowly with low airway pressures to avoid gastric distention and should be of sufficient volume to cause the chest to rise and fall.

2. **Circulation.** The brachial or femoral artery is used for pulse assessment in infants (<1 year old) because the carotid artery is difficult to palpate. On determination that a pulse is absent, chest **compressions** should be initiated at **100 per minute.** The **compression–relaxation ratio is 1:1.** Chest compressions in infants are delivered using two fingertips applied to the sternum or by encircling the chest with both hands and using the thumbs to depress the sternum one fingerbreadth below the intermammary line. In older children, the correct hand position is determined as for adults, only with one hand depressing the sternum. Both one- and two-rescuer scenarios use a 5:1 compression–ventilation ratio with a pause at the end of the fifth compression to allow for adequate ventilation. Return of spontaneous cardiopulmonary activity should be assessed after 10 cycles.

B. **Pediatric advanced life support.** Most pediatric cardiac arrests present as asystole and bradycardia rather than ventricular dysrhythmias. Respiratory and idiopathic (sudden infant death syndrome) etiologies predominate. Anatomic and physiologic differences from the adult require defibrillator settings and drug doses to be weight based.

1. **Intubation.** The endotracheal tube size is based on the patient's age: tube size (mm inner diameter [ID]) = 4 + (age/4) for children older than 2 years of age. For younger children, a 3.5- or 4.0-mm-ID endotracheal tube is often sufficient. Atropine, epinephrine, and lidocaine can be administered via the endotracheal tube prior to the establishment of IV access.

2. **Cardioversion and defibrillation.** Defibrillator paddles used for infants are 4.5 cm in diameter and those used for older children are 8 cm in diameter. The energy settings employed are the same for both MDS and biphasic modes. For patients 40 kg or greater, 150 J is used. Defibrillation for pediatric patients less than 40 kg begins with 2 J/kg with increases to 4 J/kg for subsequent shocks. Hypoxemia, acidosis, or hypothermia should be considered a treatable cause of an arrest if the defibrillation attempts are unsuccessful. After each pharmacologic manipulation, repeat defibrillation should be attempted with an energy level of 4 J/kg or the lowest level that was previously successful. For cardioversion, the starting energy is 0.2 J/kg, with escalation to 1.0 J/kg if needed.

3. **Intravenous access.** Central venous access is preferred, but existing peripheral IVs should be used without delay. The femoral vein can be used with a catheter of suitable length. The intraosseous route

Table 14-2. **Adult and pediatric cardiopulmonary resuscitation: basic life support**

Age	Ventilations/Min	Compressions/Min	Ventilation-to-Compression Ratio	Depth of Compressions (in)
Neonate	30–60	120	3:1	1/3–1/2 chest depth
Infant (<1 yr)	20	>100	5:1	0.5–1
Child (1–8 yr)	20	100	5:1	1–1.5
Adult and child >8 yr	12	100	5:1	1.5–2

Tachycardia in Children

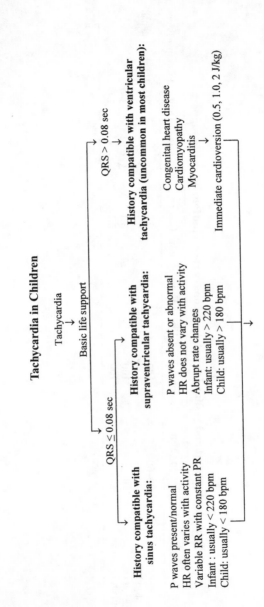

Tachycardia
↓
Basic life support

QRS ≤ 0.08 sec

History compatible with sinus tachycardia:

P waves present/normal
HR often varies with activity
Variable RR with constant PR
Infant : usually < 220 bpm
Child: usually < 180 bpm

History compatible with supraventricular tachycardia:

P waves absent or abnormal
HR does not vary with activity
Abrupt rate changes
Infant: usually > 220 bpm
Child: usually > 180 bpm

QRS > 0.08 sec

History compatible with ventricular tachycardia (uncommon in most children):

Congenital heart disease
Cardiomyopathy
Myocarditis
↓
Immediate cardioversion (0.5, 1.0, 2 J/kg)

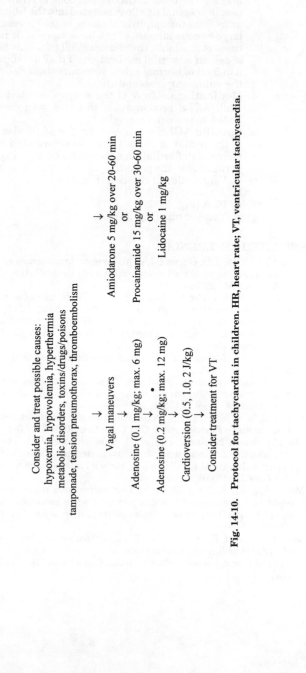

Consider and treat possible causes:
hypoxemia, hypovolemia, hyperthermia
metabolic disorders, toxins/drugs/poisons
tamponade, tension pneumothorax, thromboembolism

Vagal maneuvers →

Adenosine (0.1 mg/kg; max. 6 mg) →

Adenosine (0.2 mg/kg; max. 12 mg) →

Cardioversion (0.5, 1.0, 2 J/kg) →

Consider treatment for VT

→ Amiodarone 5 mg/kg over 20-60 min

or

Procainamide 15 mg/kg over 30-60 min

or

Lidocaine 1 mg/kg

Fig. 14-10. Protocol for tachycardia in children. HR, heart rate; VT, ventricular tachycardia.

may also be used in children. A bone marrow biopsy needle or spinal needle is inserted into the tibial shaft away from the epiphyseal plates to gain access to the large venous sinuses of the bone marrow. If none of these is available, the endotracheal tube may be used to deliver essential medications if they are diluted in 2 to 5 ml of normal saline to ensure their delivery to the pulmonary vasculature.

4. **Medications.** Many of the drugs described in the adult ACLS section apply to PALS with doses adjusted to the child's weight.

5. **Specific ACLS protocols** for the adult also apply to the pediatric patient with weight-related adjustments of defibrillation energies and drugs. Protocols pertaining to the pediatric patient are as follows:
   a. Ventricular fibrillation (Fig. 14-4).
   b. Asystole (Fig. 14-5).
   c. PEA (Fig. 14-6).
   d. Tachycardia (Fig. 14-10).

SELECTED REFERENCES

Bunch TJ, White RD, Gersh BJ, et al. Long-term outcomes of out-of-hospital cardiac arrest after successful early defibrillation. *N Engl J Med* 2003;348:2626–2634.

Caffrey SL, Willoughby PJ, Pepe PE, et al. Public use of automated external defibrillators. *N Engl J Med* 2002;347:1242–1247.

Dorian P, Cass D, Schwartz B, et al. Amiodarone as compared with lidocaine for shock-resistant ventricular fibrillation. *N Engl J Med* 2002;346:884–890.

Eisenberg MS, Mengert TJ. Cardiac resuscitation. *N Engl J Med* 2001;344:1304–1313.

International Consensus on Science. Guidelines 2000 for cardiopulmonary resuscitation and emergency cardiovascular care. *Circulation* 2000;102(Suppl I):1–376.

Luce JM, Weil MH, Tang W, eds. Wolf Creek V Conference on Cardiopulmonary Resuscitation. *Crit Care Med* 2000;28:N181–N235.

Mayr A, Ritsch N, Knotzer H, et al. Effectiveness of direct-current cardioversion for treatment of supraventricular tachyarrhythmias, in particular atrial fibrillation, in surgical intensive care patients. *Crit Care Med* 2003;31:401–405.

Mittal S, Ayati S, Stein KM, et al. Comparison of a novel rectilinear biphasic waveform with a damped sine wave monophasic waveform for transthoracic ventricular defibrillation. *J Am Coll Cardiol* 1999;34:1595–1601.

Mittal S, Ayati S, Stein KM, et al. Transthoracic cardioversion of atrial fibrillation. Comparison of rectilinear biphasic versus damped sine wave monophasic shocks. *Circulation* 2000;101:1282–1287.

15

Ethical and End-of-Life Issues

Rae Allain, Sharon Brackett, and
William E. Hurford

I. **Introduction.** Care of the critically ill patient necessarily involves acknowledgment that some patients will die despite best medical therapy. Mortality rates in intensive care units (ICUs) vary widely depending on practice type and patient population, but a minimum 10% mortality rate is typical. Observational studies reveal that **most deaths in ICUs today are preceded by decisions to withhold or withdraw some form of therapy.** Thus, imminent death is usually a predictable event that has been discussed among the critical care team, patient's family, and patient, if possible. In this setting, ethical and end-of-life issues come to the forefront and sometimes provoke conflict. This chapter explores the ethical and end-of-life issues that frequently arise in the intensive care unit and offers suggestions for avoiding and resolving conflicts. Customs, laws, ethical beliefs, and religious practices differ considerably in different cultures and societies. This chapter describes the prevailing practice at the Massachusetts General Hospital (MGH) and is meant to be thoughtful rather than definitive.

II. **Treatment decisions**
  A. U.S. society highly values patient **autonomy** (i.e., respect for an individual's preferences) as a guiding ethical principle in medicine. Competent adults can and may choose to accept or refuse medical therapies offered. If a patient's competence is questionable, a psychiatrist should evaluate the patient to determine whether he or she has decision-making capacity. This requires an ability to receive and understand medical information, to discern the various options presented, and to choose a course based on the information offered and one's values.
  B. Autonomy is best preserved by obtaining the patient's **informed consent** for procedures (e.g., endotracheal intubation) and therapies (e.g., intravenous vasopressors) whenever possible. Frequently, however, critically ill patients are incompetent to make medical decisions because of the gravity of their illness or because of sedative/analgesic medications employed to diminish suffering.
    1. An **advance directive,** a legal document specifying the patient's health care wishes should he or she become unable to speak for himself or herself, is very useful in this circumstance. Advance directives include the **health care proxy,** the **durable power of attorney for health care,** and the **living will.**

The form of advance directives honored in each of the U.S. states varies.

  a. A patient may designate a **surrogate** who is charged with executing the patient's wishes should he or she become incompetent. The surrogate must offer **substituted judgment** for the patient, providing decisions that the patient would make if competent. If the patient has not designated a surrogate prior to becoming incompetent, the next of kin may become the de facto surrogate. In some circumstances where no family is living or available, a trusted friend may act as the patient's surrogate.

  2. A court-appointed legal **guardian** may be necessary in rare instances where no family member or friend is able to make decisions in the best interest of the patient.

C. **Communication with the family**

  1. **Discussions** with family members regarding treatment of an incompetent patient are best conducted in a quiet, private **environment** in an unhurried fashion. Physicians should refrain from such discussions in the ICU or in hospital corridors because real or apparent distractions and breaches of confidentiality will threaten to destroy the family's confidence in the critical care team. A comfortable conference room near the ICU is the ideal setting.

  2. **Attendants** to the family meeting should include the following:

    a. The patient's close family, including the **health care proxy** or person who will serve as surrogate.

    b. The patient's **primary care physician** or alternate physician with whom the patient has had a long-term, trusting relationship.

    c. The **ICU attending physician and ICU nurse.** Occasionally, it may be helpful to have adjuvant team members (e.g., respiratory therapist, physical therapist, or occupational therapist) present.

    d. **Consulting specialists,** if needed to present information regarding the patient's condition, therapeutic options, or prognosis.

    e. Ancillary support staff, including **social worker** and **chaplain,** when appropriate.

  3. **The goals of ICU therapy** should be confirmed with the family. For many patients, the obvious goals will include preventing imminent death, "curing" the acute disease, preventing/relieving pain and suffering, discharging the patient from the ICU, and eventually returning the patient to his or her premorbid level of function. Some patients may only hope to delay the disease process sufficiently to gain a few more months or years of meaningful living. Occasionally, ICU care is requested to prolong a patient's life long

enough for close relatives to arrive to pay last respects or consent to organ donation.

a. **The prognosis** of the patient is very important to setting realistic therapeutic goals. For example, a family may consent to a brief trial of dialysis for a patient who had previously been opposed to chronic dialysis if the prognosis for recovery of renal function is good. Alternatively, a grim prognosis may allow family members to abandon insistent demands for continued aggressive care. It is important for the health care team to discuss the patient's prognosis and arrive at a consensus before meeting with the family. Variant opinions about a patient's prognosis only serve to confuse the family, often resulting in delayed decisions, additional anguish, and sometimes hostility toward the care team. If opinions of consulting specialists differ, the intensivist or trusted primary physician should assume responsibility for summarizing the patient's overall condition for the family. Presenting a poor prognosis can be devastating to the family; care should be taken to express compassion and empathy. Time should be allowed for the family to contemplate what has been said and to ask questions. Often the first response is denial of the loved one's condition. The intensivist should gently reaffirm what has been presented and allow family members to express their grief. Acceptance of a poor prognosis may require several discussions over days or even a few weeks.

b. Once the prognosis has been discussed, the family may request or the physician may suggest a **limitation of life-sustaining treatment** status for the patient, also defined as **"do not resuscitate" (DNR).** The DNR status seeks to clarify what therapies will be offered to the patient in case of acute, life-threatening instability that requires immediate treatment to prevent death. Clear instructions should be given and documented in the chart regarding preferences for specific interventions such as cardiopulmonary resuscitation, endotracheal intubation, electrical therapy, and medical therapy in case of sudden cardiac or respiratory failure. The simple phrase "DNR" in the physician's orders is insufficient because the meaning will vary to different caregivers. When discussing limitations to treatment with the family, physicians should use their best clinical judgment to describe each therapy, including the potential risks and benefits and the expected outcome or prognosis for recovery. This step is important: one study of the elderly showed that individuals revise their decisions regarding CPR once the procedure is described to them with outcome data. Many of those who would have requested to receive CPR will forgo this treatment when presented with information about odds for full recovery. Notably, any agreed limitation of treatment status does not signify that a patient's condition is hopeless or that therapies other than those specifically discussed will be withheld. In this sense, the term "DNR" has been associated by patients and caregivers with a general withdrawal of care and often carries an ominous implication. Families may need to be reassured that current therapies intended to improve the patient's health will be continued unless a further decision to withdraw or withhold therapy has been made (see later discussion).

c. Eventually, a decision to **withdraw** or **withhold** therapies may be made. Most critically ill patients are incompetent to make this decision, and, thus, a **surrogate** is involved. As in deciding the possible limitations of care, the patient's surrogate should approach this decision using substituted judgment or determining what type of care **the patient would have wanted for himself or herself.** The surrogate should refer to written indications of the patient's preferences or to past conversations concerning end-of-life wishes. Surrogates should refrain from incorporating their own preferences or values into decision making. If the patient's wishes regarding end-of-life care are unknown, the principle of relative **benefit versus burden** may be used. In this process, the potential helpful versus harmful effects of each therapy are weighed, resulting in a choice to accept or reject each therapy. Thus, a surrogate may choose, for example, to accept antibiotics for the patient in the hopes of curing pneumonia, but to reject a lung biopsy because of the pain associated with the procedure. Neither an ethical nor a legal distinction exists between withdrawing and withholding therapies, including hydration and nutrition, but some families may see a psychological advantage to withholding rather than withdrawing life-sustaining measures.

1. If the ICU team determines that ongoing care is **futile** (i.e., only serves to prolong the dying process), the team may advise that therapies be withdrawn to reduce the suffering of the dying patient. Determining futility may be problematic because technology can prolong the survival of patients with multiorgan failure and because few physicians are able to judge with unequivocal certainty that a patient will die in the ICU. All members of the ICU team should agree that further treatment of the patient is futile before meeting with the family. Again, patience and

compassion are paramount to the family's acceptance of this determination.

2. Once a decision has been made to withdraw or withhold life-sustaining measures, **maintaining the patient's comfort** becomes the primary goal of therapy. This may include discontinuing endotracheal suctioning, daily chest radiographs, and routine laboratory tests while adjusting the doses of sedative or analgesic medications to a desirable level.

3. Therapeutic goals will need to be reevaluated as the patient's condition changes. Communication with the family should be established early and continue throughout a patient's ICU course. **Conflict** is best resolved via ongoing discussion with individuals involved. ICU physicians must recognize and respect cultural differences that influence end-of-life decisions. Unresolvable conflict among family members, among health care team members, or between the family and the medical care team is best addressed by the institutional ethics committee (see later discussion).

D. **The pediatric patient** deserves special consideration. Legally, end-of-life decisions are deferred to the parents. Ethically, however, the child may participate in these decisions depending on his or her developmental level and decision-making capacity. If the child is too immature to participate in decisions, parents are relied on to make decisions in the child's best interest by weighing the benefit versus burden of each therapy. Pediatric intensivists must be sensitive to individual family dynamics and parenting styles when approaching end-of-life discussions for the pediatric ICU patient.

E. The **institutional ethics committee** is generally made up of a group of health care professionals trained in medical ethics.

1. **The purpose** of the ethics committee is to educate and advise clinicians regarding ethical dilemmas and to enable resolution of ethical conflicts. The ethics committee offers an objective analysis of the patient's case and may draw on basic ethical principles to guide the patient, clinicians, and family to a consensus about the therapeutic course. Ideally, the ethics committee should be accessible to all members of the health care team and to the patient and family. This diminishes inequalities of power present in the hospital environment and promotes a climate of respect for all viewpoints. When the ethics committee is requested to consult on a case, the question to be answered or the nature of the conflict should be clearly stated. The patient's condition and prognosis should be documented. An ethics committee consultation is never a substitute for communication with the family regarding end-of-life issues. Instead, the ethics committee serves to elucidate pertinent ethical issues and thereby aid conflict resolution.

Members of the ethics committee may help to organize and/or attend a family meeting to facilitate decision making.

2. The ethics committee uses guiding ethical principles to make recommendations to the health care team, the patient, and/or the family. The role is one of expert consultant, not arbiter in a dispute. In rare situations where irreconcilable differences exist between the physician and the patient and/or family and where the usual mechanisms for decision making (e.g., informal discussions, team/family meetings, assistance of social workers, clergy, or ethics consultants) have proven ineffective, an institutional **"resolving-conflict policy,"** which describes a stepwise process toward achieving accord, can be useful. Rarely, ultimate resolution may require transfer of care of the patient to another accepting physician or care team.

III. **Guidelines for withdrawing life-sustaining therapies**
   A. **Goals** for withdrawal of life-sustaining therapies include the following:
      1. Promoting comfort and respecting the wishes of the patient.
      2. Promoting comfort of the family.
      3. Maintaining or achieving the patient's ability to communicate.
      4. Withdrawing burdensome therapies.
      5. Allowing death to occur.
   B. All physician orders should be reexamined with a goal toward **palliative** and **comfort care.** Therapies that increase patient comfort or relieve pain, anxiety, or agitation should be continued or added (Table 15-1). Therapies directed toward supporting physiologic homeostasis or treating the underlying disease process are no longer indicated and may be discontinued. These include many of the "routine" procedures and interventions associated with being an ICU patient (Table 15-2). The benefit-to-burden ratio of each intervention should

---

Table 15-1. Examples of comfort and palliative measures

Clearance of oral secretions
Continuation of general nursing care and cleanliness
Offering of food/water to alert patients
Antiseizure or antiepileptic regimens
Narcotics
Sedatives
Antipyretics
Nonsteroidal antiinflammatory drugs
Prophylaxis for gastrointestinal bleeding
Antiemetics

Table 15-2.   Examples of routine measures that may be withdrawn during the process of withdrawing life-sustaining therapy

Frequent phlebotomy for laboratory tests
Frequent vital sign determinations
Placement of intravenous and central lines
Radiographic examinations
Aggressive chest physiotherapy and endotracheal suctioning
Debridement of wounds

be used to determine which interventions should be eliminated. The precise order of discontinuation is often determined by patient or family preference or the patient's situation. Most commonly, a stepwise approach is followed, with mechanical ventilation discontinued only after the withdrawal of vasopressors, antibiotics, or enteral feedings. There can be no substitute for the continual presence of a concerned and caring medical staff, especially including the experienced physician, at the bedside. Clear plans for monitoring the patient's level of discomfort and intervening with additional medications should be made and shared with the family in attendance. The decision to withdraw life-sustaining treatment should be accompanied by an increase of vigilance and bedside attention, not withdrawal of the medical staff.

C. A large variability of **individual situations** should be anticipated. Each situation is unique. Paramount during the process are the wishes of the patient or the patient's surrogate. Patient autonomy must be respected. Immediately secondary to this is assurance of patient comfort and the comfort of the patient's family. Cultural practices and beliefs of the patient and the family should be identified and respected. In each situation, the process of withdrawal should be clearly explained. Practical wishes of the patient and family concerning the desirability of extubation can usually be easily accommodated. The anticipated rapidity of the dying process or realities of the patient's medical condition, however, may dictate specific choices concerning therapies to be withdrawn, the rate of withdrawal, and the ability to accommodate the requests of families. Such situations should be clearly explained to the family. When a rapid death is anticipated, it may not be possible to accommodate requests to extubate and communicate with the patient or hold prolonged vigils.

D. Specific life-sustaining therapies that may be withdrawn include the following:

1. **Vasopressor** and **inotropic** medications. Continuous chemical circulatory support can be discontinued without weaning. The gradual withdrawal of

circulatory support appears to offer no benefit for patient comfort.

2. **Extracorporeal support** therapies are usually considered quite invasive by the patient and family. They require maintenance of vascular cannulas and the presence of additional equipment and personnel at the bedside. Intermittent extracorporeal support (e.g., intermittent hemodialysis) may simply not be restarted. Continuous renal support (e.g., continuous venovenous hemofiltration, etc.) can be discontinued. Death is usually not immediate following the discontinuation of dialysis. Studies have reported mean survival to be 8 to 9 days following the discontinuation of dialysis. Continuous circulatory support (e.g., ventricular assist, extracorporeal membrane oxygenation, intraaortic balloon pump) can be discontinued and death anticipated soon after termination of support.

3. **Antibiotics** and other curative pharmacotherapy. Once the decision to terminate life-sustaining treatments is made, it is no longer consistent to consider therapies directed toward "curing" the patient. Such therapies include cancer chemotherapy, radiation therapy, steroids, and antibiotics. It is reasonable, however, to continue treatments such as topical antifungal agents used for oral hygiene or antibiotics aimed at treating painful lesions.

4. **Supplemental oxygen.** Because the avoidance of hypoxemia is no longer a therapeutic goal, supplemental oxygen may be discontinued and the patient returned to breathing room air. This is reasonable even if it is decided that mechanical ventilation will be continued. If the patient is removed from the ventilator but continues to have an artificial airway in place (e.g., endotracheal tube or tracheostomy), **humidified air** or oxygen can be administered to avoid the irritation of drying of the airway and tracheal secretions.

5. **Mechanical ventilation.** Several studies have suggested that mechanical ventilation is the most common therapy withdrawn when life-sustaining therapies are discontinued. Some physicians, however, prefer to withdraw therapies other than mechanical ventilation (such as vasopressors) with the expectation that the patient will die while still receiving mechanical ventilation. Similarly, during a prolonged illness, patients' families may have become comfortable with the surroundings of the ICU, the monitors, the artificial airway, and the mechanical ventilator. They may voice fears that the patient may suffer if mechanical ventilation or airway support is withdrawn. In such cases, it is reasonable to continue mechanical ventilation and airway support while discontinuing other life-sustaining therapies. Nevertheless, mechanical ventilation does not differ

morally from other life-sustaining treatments such as dialysis, and can be discontinued if the patient or his or her proxy believes that it represents unwanted therapy.

    a. Mechanical ventilation may be gradually withdrawn by decreasing the inspired oxygen to room air, decreasing positive end-expiratory pressure, and then slowly decreasing ventilatory rate. The rate of decrease is quite variable among practitioners. A relatively slow weaning process may prolong the dying process and may provide the family with a misleading hope for survival.

    b. Mechanical ventilation may be discontinued entirely and humidified air administered via T-piece, or the patient can simply be removed from the ventilator and the trachea extubated. Extubation may more quickly result in death compared with gradually decreasing the intensity of mechanical ventilation. It is important that extubation not appear to be objectively associated with greater discomfort or with the administration of greater doses of opioids. Each technique is applicable in certain situations. The ability of the patient to maintain a patent airway, the presence of secretions, the perceptions of the patient and family, and the confounding presence of anesthetic drugs and neuromuscular blocking agents all may dictate a particular method of discontinuing mechanical ventilation. Invasive monitoring and analysis of arterial blood gas tensions or oxygen saturation are unnecessary during withdrawal of mechanical ventilation.

    c. The **timing of death** after the withdrawal of mechanical ventilation is uncertain and depends on the etiology and severity of respiratory failure. Usually death occurs within a few hours to 1 day. In some studies, however, a small proportion of patients with chronic lung disease did well and were discharged alive from the hospital after deciding to forgo mechanical ventilation.

  6. Nutrition (enteral or parenteral), fluid resuscitation, blood replacement, and intravenous hydration are all therapies that have the goal of returning the patient to health and may be discontinued. Nasogastric and orogastric tubes may be discontinued. Case reports and controlled studies suggest that little, if any, discomfort accompanies the withdrawal of enteral nutrition and intravenous hydration.

E. Indications for pharmacologic intervention

  1. Presumption for **comfort measures.** Clinicians should not withhold comfort measures for fear of hastening death. Patients who are given large doses of opioids to treat discomfort during the withdrawal of life-sustaining treatments on average live as long as patients not given opioids, suggesting that it is the underlying disease process, not the use of palliative medications, that usually determines the time of death.

2. **Standard of care.** The administration of sedatives and analgesics during the withholding or withdrawal of life-sustaining treatments is consistent with the standard of care for critically ill patients. The majority of ICU patients do receive these medications during the withholding or withdrawal of support. Certainly, competent patients may refuse pharmacologic intervention to preserve lucidness. Drugs may not be indicated for patients who will gain no benefit (e.g., comatose patients).

F. **Specific indications**

1. **Pain.** The patient's report of pain or discomfort is certainly the best guide of treatment. Frequently, the patient is unable to communicate effectively. Other signs and symptoms of pain such as vocalizations, diaphoresis, agitation, tachypnea, and tachycardia may be valuable.

2. **Air hunger/dyspnea.** Especially with the withdrawal of supplemental oxygen and mechanical ventilatory support, discomfort should be expected and anticipatory doses of anxiolytics and opioids should be administered. Additional doses should be immediately available and opioids continued as a continuous infusion. Clinicians must be immediately and continuously available to assess the patient's level of comfort and provide additional medication as necessary.

3. **Death rattle.** Noisy, gargling breathing may occur in patients who are close to death, particularly in extubated patients. Although these sounds may be accompanied by dyspneic symptoms in the patient, they are usually more distressing to family members present. Treatment can include repositioning, gentle oropharyngeal suctioning, and anticholinergics to diminish oral and respiratory secretions.

4. **Anxiety.** Alert patients may display varying levels of anxiety at the prospect of termination of life support. Although nonpharmacologic means of allaying anxiety can be extremely effective, sometimes patients request to be deeply sedated or unconscious prior to the discontinuation of life-sustaining therapies such as mechanical ventilation. Although death may be hastened by deep sedation, such requests should be honored.

5. **Agitation or excessive motor activity.** Nonspecific motor activity may occur in some patients. Such activity is often interpreted as discomfort or distress by those attending the patient. It is reasonable that the level of sedation be increased in such situations. Neuromuscular blockade is never indicated because it does not treat the presumed underlying distress of the patient.

6. **Avoidance of drug withdrawal.** Often, patients are already receiving high doses of opioids or sedatives during the course of their illness. The patient's individual dose ranges can be used as a guide to provide increased amounts of opioids and sedatives during the discontinuation of support. Certainly, there appears to be little reason to decrease therapeutic doses of sedatives or opioids prior to the discontinuation of support for fear that the patient will not breathe adequately once the ventilator is discontinued.

IV. **Pharmacologic choices**
   A. **Opioids** are the first line of treatment for pain, dyspnea, or tachypnea during the discontinuation of life-sustaining measures. It is imperative that the route, dose, and schedule be individualized. Intravenous administration is by far the most common route of administration. Bolus administration is the fastest route for providing relief. An initial bolus dose may be followed by a continuous infusion with additional bolus doses available as needed. Commonly used opioids and their doses are summarized in Table 15-3. Additional details are available in Chapter 6. Opioid doses for **children** are not as well established as for adults. For babies and infants, continuous morphine infusions ($10–25\ \mu g/kg/h$) can be administered after an initial bolus ($0.1–0.2$ mg/kg IV as a starting point). Sometimes very large doses may be necessary to assure the absence of discomfort.
   B. **Benzodiazepines** (see also Chapter 6) are the drugs of choice for the treatment of anxiety. **Lorazepam** is a common choice because of its pharmacodynamic predictability in both intravenous and oral forms.
   C. **Haloperidol** (see also Chapter 6) may be indicated in the presence of delirium (acute confusional states) or agitation not controlled with benzodiazepines and opioids. In one survey of practitioners, haloperidol was used at least occasionally as an adjunct to the discontinuation of life-sustaining measures by 24% of physicians. Haloperidol does not affect the respiratory drive.

Table 15-3. **Examples of initial opioid doses**

Generic Name	Bolus Dose	Infusion
Dihydromorphone	0.02 mg/kg	—
Fentanyl	$0.5–1.5\ \mu g/kg$	$2–4\ \mu g/kg/h$
Methadone	0.1 mg/kg	—
Meperidine	0.5–1.0 mg/kg	0.5 mg/kg/h
Morphine	0.05–0.1 mg/kg	0.1–0.5 mg/kg/h

These represent typical initial doses for a patient without tolerance. Doses should be titrated to effect without regard to a maximal dose.

D. **Propofol** (see also Chapter 6) is a potent hypnotic agent that can be used for sedation or for rapid induction of unconsciousness. This may be helpful for procedures and to rapidly reach a desired level of sedation. Propofol has no analgesic properties. Dose-dependent decreases of arterial blood pressure and ventilatory drive should be expected.

E. **Barbiturates,** such as thiopental, are potent hypnotics that rapidly produce unconsciousness. Their pharmacodynamic effects are similar to those of propofol, but their pharmacokinetic profile is much less favorable. Hence, propofol has essentially substituted for the short-acting barbiturates in most ICUs.

F. **Anticholinergic medications,** such as **atropine, ipratropium bromide,** and **glycopyrrolate,** may be used to diminish copious oral and respiratory secretions that can produce death rattle. In general, atropine should be avoided because of its potential central nervous system side effects. Glycopyrrolate is a potent antisialogogue that may be administered intravenously or nebulized (5–10 μg/kg every 4 hours via either route).

G. **Neuromuscular blocking agents** (see also Chapter 6) are sometimes administered in the ICU to facilitate mechanical ventilation in patients with severe acute respiratory failure. **The indication for the use of neuromuscular blocking agents is lost** once the decision to forgo life-sustaining treatments is made. Neuromuscular blocking agents do not contribute to comfort of the patient and have no analgesic or sedative properties. Paralyzed patients are unable to express discomfort by attempting to communicate, move, or become tachypneic. The precise doses of opioids and anxiolytics necessary to avoid discomfort are then difficult to determine. Although it may be preferable to permit reversal of neuromuscular blockade prior to the withdrawal of mechanical ventilation, sometimes a prolonged drug effect that precludes adequate reversal or profound weakness is present. Many clinicians are uncomfortable with extubating a patient with no capability of maintaining spontaneous ventilation or a patent airway. In such cases, physicians may decide to forgo the withdrawal of mechanical ventilation or proceed only after administering high doses of sedatives and opioids to assure the absence of patient awareness.

H. **Euthanasia** is illegal in most states in the United States. Drugs should not be administered with the sole and express purpose of causing death. Such interventions include the administration of neuromuscular blocking agents to produce apnea or the administration of potassium chloride to produce asystole.

V. **Brain death**

A. **"Brain death"** is a term used to connote that death has been determined via evaluation of brain function and as such is distinct from cardiac death. Ethically and legally, brain death is equivalent to death, even when other organs, such as the heart, may still be functioning. Occasionally, this concept presents difficulties in patients and families from cultures and religions that do not consider the concept of brain death as outlined here. Because these patients are dead, we are obligated to end care, even though this may be stressful to the family. In our experience, families understand this concept, even though it may require the additional efforts of social workers and chaplains who are part of the same culture or religion and are trusted by the family. Practically, the diagnosis of brain death means that a patient can potentially become an organ donor if the conditions of consent (premortem by the patient or postmortem by the family) and medical acceptability are met.

    B. Locally accepted guidelines are used to establish the diagnosis of brain death. Our guidelines are outlined in Chapter 29.

VI. Organ donation. Traditionally, the majority of organ procurements derive from **heart-beating patients who have been declared brain dead.** Recently, however, a renewed interest in **donation after cardiac death (DCD)** has occurred due to the dramatic mismatch between the number of organs available for transplant and the number of patients on the waitlist. Often, critically ill patients are unable to become organ donors due to the nature of illness (e.g. sepsis) or due to failure of the vital organs, but because some are eligible and a significant number die in the ICU, the critical care unit is a natural environment to discuss the issue.

    A. Early contact with the organ procurement organization (OPO) is important. In an effort to increase the number of potential organ donors in the United States, the Centers for Medicare and Medicaid Services (formerly the Health Care Financing Administration) mandated in 1998 that hospitals must notify their local OPO about all deaths, including imminent deaths. Additionally, it was required that the local OPO be involved in collaboration with clinicians when families were approached regarding organ donation because it has been demonstrated that consent for donation is more likely to be obtained if presented by an experienced requester. OPO preferences regarding medications (such as vasopressors, diuretics), mechanical ventilator settings, and laboratory blood work after death should be known to the ICU team. The United Network for Organ Sharing publishes a convenient checklist for organ donors (both heart-beating and DCD) that is easily accessed at the website http://www.unos.org/resources/donorManagement.

    B. Approaching the family regarding organ donation must be done tactfully and in consultation with trained professionals from the OPO. In the case of DCD, ethical treatment of the patient mandates that discussion about organ donation occurs after the health care proxy or family has agreed on withdrawing life-sustaining therapies. Ideally, the discussion should be overseen by a physician with whom the family has developed a rapport. The topic may be introduced by asking the family whether the patient had ever expressed an opinion regarding use of his or her organs after death. Many families are consoled by the thought that their loved one's body parts may be life saving to another individual and may in some sense carry on the life that has been lost.

C. **Care of the patient** for organ donation is challenging. Physiologic problems frequently include hypotension, dysrhythmias, hypoxemia, and diabetes insipidus. If a successful donation is to occur, the vigilant attendance of the ICU team, in concert with direction from the organ procurement agency, is necessary. In the case of DCD, compassionate care aimed at assuring patient comfort, including the use of opioids and amnestic agents, supersedes the goals of organ preservation. DCD requires thoughtful consideration by the institution and is best guided by a written protocol which clearly stipulates the following:

1. The nonoverlapping roles of caregivers to the donor and the recipient, to avoid a conflict of interest.
2. The physician responsible for pronouncing cardiac death.
3. The time interval after asystole at which death is declared; currently, this is **5 minutes.**
4. The process for obtaining consent and administering medications/treatments necessary for organ procurement (e.g., heparin).
5. The process for enabling family presence at the time of death (either in the ICU or operating room).
6. The time interval after which organ procurement will not be attempted in the case of unexpected patient survival following withdrawal of life-sustaining therapies; currently this is **1 hour** at MGH.

D. If the institutional transplant team will participate in harvesting or transplanting organs, it is prudent to establish contact with the team and immediately apprise them of any change in the donor's condition that might warrant expedited harvest.

VII. **Supporting survivors**

A. **Support of the patient's survivors** during the dying process and following death begins with honest, frequent, and compassionate communication from physicians and nurses in the ICU. Families appreciate the guidance of experienced practitioners to prepare them for what to expect during the dying process, especially when life-sustaining therapies have been withdrawn. Reassurance should be given that measures will be taken to ensure the patient's comfort and that some sights (e.g., gasps) and sounds (e.g., gurgling) are normal during dying and may not be completely obliterated. The environment where death occurs should accommodate the wishes of the patient and family as much as possible.

1. **Privacy** is important for a dignified death. This may be achieved by closing ICU cubicles and shielding the dying patient and family from the routine commotion of a busy ICU. Alternatively, the patient or family may request to be moved to a private room on a hospital ward or to an in-hospital hospice unit to die. If the condition of the patient allows transfer before death will occur, these requests should be granted.

2. **Cultural background and individual values** will affect who is at the bedside of a dying patient. For some patients, one or two close family members may attend; for others, a vigil is maintained by a large extended family. The ICU staff should strive for flexibility when presented with each situation.

   a. The medical social worker may be an important source for understanding the family's religious and cultural background and for communicating the family's wishes to the medical care team.

   b. Many patients and families find solace in the presence of clergy at death. If so, arrangements can be made for the patient's religious representative or a hospital-based chaplain to attend.

B. **Support of the caring team** is also important. Members of the team (particularly trainees and junior staff) are often distressed by the process of allowing a patient to die. Very little is formally taught in medical schools about end-of-life situations, and doctors and nurses learn by experience. Debriefings with the whole team and the addition of senior staff and hospital ethicists are very helpful.

VIII. **Legal considerations.** Physicians who follow the preceding process regarding honest, open communication with patients and their families about ethics and end-of-life care should rarely find themselves resolving such issues in a court of law. Nevertheless, several recent judicial rulings have implications that may prove useful to the clinician when confronted with ethical and end-of-life issues.

A. **Patient autonomy** is primary in decision making. That patients may refuse life-sustaining or other therapies has been repeatedly affirmed. Wishes of the patient may be expressed via advance directives or, lacking this, via prior voiced opinion. The role of a surrogate in providing substituted judgment has been supported.

B. **Human life** has qualification beyond mere biologic existence. Thus, a surrogate's decision to withdraw care may be based on the potential for meaningful existence **(quality of life).**

C. **Care once rendered may be withdrawn.** The idea that a life-sustaining therapy that has been implemented can never be stopped is not valid.

D. **End-of-life decisions** are best addressed by the physician and the patient and/or family with help from institutional facilitators (e.g., ethics committee) as needed. Permission to withdraw therapies does not require a court order.

E. **Withdrawal of hydration or nutrition is not legally different** from withdrawal of other life support. In addition to legal decisions, this stance has been supported by numerous medical societies, including the American Medical Association and the American Academy of Neurology.

F. **Physicians are not bound to provide care that they deem futile.** Although still somewhat controversial, the latter was supported by a jury decision involving a patient at the Massachusetts General Hospital from whom ventilatory support was withdrawn despite the objection of one family member. It is advisable for a physician, however, to pursue every avenue of conflict resolution (see section **II.E.2**), including removing oneself from the care of a patient, before exercising this dictum against a family's wishes.

G. **For unusual or questionable cases,** it is appropriate to seek the advice of the institutional legal counsel before acting on decisions.

SELECTED REFERENCES

American College of Surgeons. Statement on advance directives by patients: "do not resuscitate" in the operating room. *Bull Am Coll Surg* 1994;79:29–31.

Asch DA, Hansen-Flachen J, Lanken PH. Decisions to limit or continue life-sustaining treatment by critical care physicians in the United States: conflicts between physicians' practices and patients' wishes. *Am J Respir Crit Care Med* 1995;151:288–292.

Brody H, Campbell ML, Faber-Langendoen KF, et al. Withdrawing intensive life-sustaining treatment—recommendations for compassionate clinical management. *N Engl J Med* 1997;336:652–656.

Burns JP, Mello MM, Studdert DM, et al. Results of a clinical trial of care improvement for the critically ill. *Crit Care Med* 2003;31:2107–2117.

Faber-Langendoen K. The clinical management of dying patients receiving mechanical ventilation: A survey of physician practice. *Chest* 1994;106:880–888.

Hurford W. Practical guidelines for the withdrawal of life-sustaining therapies. In: Braunwald E, Fauci AS, Isselbacher KJ, et al. *Harrison's online* 2.0. Available at: http://www.accessmedicine.com/.

Luce JM. Physicians do not have a responsibility to provide futile or unreasonable care if a patient or family insists. *Crit Care Med* 1995;23:760–766.

Luce JM. Withholding and withdrawal of life support: Ethical, legal, and clinical aspects. *New Horiz* 1997;5:30–37.

Meisel A. Legal myths about terminating life support. *Arch Intern Med* 1991;151:1497–1502.

Murphy DJ, Burrows D, Santilli S, et al. The influence of the probability of survival on patients' preferences regarding cardiopulmonary resuscitation. *N Engl J Med* 1994;330:545–549.

Prendergast TJ. Resolving conflicts surrounding end-of-life care. *New Horiz* 1997;5:62–71.

Schneiderman LJ, Jecker NS, Jonsen AR. Medical futility: its meaning and ethical implications. *Ann Intern Med* 1990;112:949–954.

Todres ID, Armstrong A, Lally P, et al. Negotiating end-of-life issues. *New Horiz* 1998;6:374–382.

Wilson WC, Smedira NG, Fink C, et al. Ordering and administration of sedatives and analgesics during the withholding and withdrawal of life support from critically ill patients. *JAMA* 1992;267: 949–953.

16

Evidence-Based Medicine in Critical Care

Henry Thomas Stelfox and Edward A. Bittner

I. **Evidence-based medicine** (EBM) is defined as the conscientious, explicit, and judicious use of current best evidence in making decisions about the care of individual patients. By encouraging physicians to explicitly explain their medical decision-making processes, including the evidence on which their decisions are based, we may improve decision making and patient care. Scientific evidence will never be available to guide all medical decisions, but a clear understanding of the benefits and boundaries of evidence-based medicine will help to optimize patient care. The practice of EBM can be organized into a four-step approach (Fig. 16-1).

  A. The practice of EBM begins by asking a **clinically relevant question.** The more precisely the question is framed, the more likely it is the physician will find an appropriate answer in the literature. Each question should specify:

   1. A patient or problem.
   2. An intervention or diagnostic test (if relevant).
   3. A comparison group (if relevant).
   4. An outcome.

  B. Once a question has been formulated, then the next step is to **search for the best evidence** that will provide an answer. The main databases for clinical medicine are Medline and the Cochrane Library.

   1. **Medline** indexes all the articles of the major medical journals since 1966 (www.Pubmed.gov).
   2. The **Cochrane Library** is a critical summary by specialty, updated periodically, of all relevant randomized, controlled trials and systemic reviews (www.Cochrane.org).

  C. **The evidence can be evaluated** by asking two simple questions:

   1. Is the evidence valid?
   2. What are the results?

  D. Once it has been established that the evidence is valid, we need to ask whether the results will help in caring for patients. Evaluating and **applying a specific piece of evidence** can be guided by asking additional questions depending on the exact nature of the evidence (Table 16-1).

   1. **Diagnostic studies.** Assigning a diagnosis is both crucial and subtle. Rarely does any symptom, sign, laboratory test, or any combination of them completely distinguish between those with and those

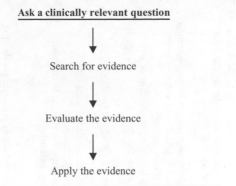

Fig. 16-1. An approach to evidence-based medicine.

without a disease. Instead, disease is generally defined using a gold standard, and formal approaches to studies evaluating diagnostic instruments are essential to solidifying the foundation for diagnostic decision making.

2. **Prognostic studies.** Prognosis is a prediction of the outcome of a disease process. It describes the duration, the timing, and the nature of the disease as it progresses along its clinical course.

3. **Treatment or prevention studies.** The course of disease may be greatly affected by the choice of treatment options. Not all therapies are equally effective, and in fact some may be deleterious.

4. **Systemic reviews, overviews, and meta-analyses.** The terms systemic review and overview are used for any summary of the medical literature, and meta-analysis is used for reviews that use quantitative methods to summarize results.

5. **Clinical decision analyses.** Decision making is the choosing of a course of action after weighing the benefits and harms of the alternatives. Clinical decision analysis is the application of quantitative methods to decision making under conditions of uncertainty.

6. **Economic analyses.** Clinicians are being increasingly asked to make decisions regarding patient care that not only weigh the benefits and harms, but also consider whether the benefits are worth the health care resources consumed. Economic analyses are quantitative methods used to compare alternative clinical strategies with respect to both outcomes and resource utilization.

7. **Clinical practice guidelines** are published recommendations that employ subject experts to synthesize the medical literature into practical recommendations for guiding clinical practice.

Table 16-1. A basic guide for systematically evaluating and applying evidence-based medicine

Study	Is the Evidence Valid?	What Are the Results?	Will the Results Help Me Care for My Patients?
Diagnostic	Was there an independent, blind comparison with a gold standard? Did the patient sample include an appropriate spectrum of patients? Was the gold standard applied to all patients?	Are likelihood ratios presented?	Will the test results be reproducible and applicable to patients in my clinical setting? Will the test results change my management?
Prognostic	Did the patient sample include a well-defined, appropriate spectrum of patients at a similar disease stage? Was there adequate follow-up? Were the outcome criteria objective? Were important prognostic factors measured and accounted for?	How large and precise (95% confidence interval) are the estimates of the likelihood of the outcome in a period of time?	Were the study patients similar to my own? Will the results change my management? Can I use the results to counsel my patients?
Treatment and prevention	Were patients assigned to treatments using randomization? Were all patients accounted for at the conclusion of the study? Were patients analyzed in the groups to which they were randomized (intention-to-treat analysis)?	How large and precise (95% confidence interval) are the estimates of the treatment effect?	Were the study patients similar to my own? Were all clinically important outcomes (positive and negative) considered? Are the benefits worth the harms and costs?

	Were patients, health workers, and study personnel blind to treatment? Were the study groups similar at the start of the study? Were the groups treated equally except for the assigned treatment?	How large and precise (95% confidence interval) are the results?	Were the study patients similar to my own? Were all clinically important outcomes considered? Are the benefits worth the harms and costs?
Systemic reviews	Was a focused clinical question asked? Were appropriate criteria used to select the individual articles? Is it likely that important studies were missed? Was the validity of the selected studies appraised? Were similar results found across the different studies?	How large and precise (95% confidence interval) are the results?	Were the study patients similar to my own? Were all clinically important outcomes considered? Are the benefits worth the harms and costs?
Clinical decision analyses	Were all important clinical strategies and outcomes examined? Was an explicit and reasonable process used to assign probabilities? Was an explicit and reasonable process used to assign utilities? Were sensitivity analyses performed to determine the potential impact of any uncertainty in the evidence?	Does one strategy result in a clinically important difference? How strong is the evidence used in the analysis? How much does allowance for uncertainty change the results?	Do the probability estimates approximate my patients' clinical features? Do the utilities reflect my patients' values?

(continued)

Table 16-1. *Continued*

Study	Is the Evidence Valid?	What Are the Results?	Will the Results Help Me Care for My Patients?
Economic analyses	Was a full economic comparison of different strategies provided? Were all costs and outcomes properly measured? Were allowances made for uncertainties? Are the costs and outcomes related to the baseline risk in the treatment population?	What were the incremental costs and outcomes of each strategy? Could the uncertainty in the evidence change the results?	Could my patients expect similar health outcomes and costs? Are the benefits worth the harms and costs?
Clinical practice guidelines	Were all important options and outcomes clearly specified? Was an explicit and reasonable approach used to identify, select, and combine evidence? Is the guideline reasonably up to date? Has the guideline been subject to peer review?	Are the recommendations practical and clinically relevant? What is the impact of uncertainty and of any value judgments?	Is the primary objective of the guidelines consistent with my goals? Are the recommendations applicable to my patients?

Adapted from Guyatt G, Rennie D. *User's guide to the medical literature: essentials of evidence-based clinical practice.* Chicago: American Medical Association, 2001.

II. Study design and measurement
A. Definitions

1. **Bias** is systematic error or deviation from the truth. We are generally concerned with two forms of bias in clinical studies, selection bias and information bias. Selection bias pertains to noncomparability in how subjects are selected. Information bias pertains to noncomparability in how information is obtained or reported.

2. **Confounding** is a mixing of effects between the study variable, the outcome, and a third factor that is associated with the study variable and independently affects the risk of developing the outcome. The extraneous factor is called a confounding variable.

3. **Effect modification** is a change in the magnitude of an effect according to the value of some third variable.

4. **Cointervention** is an intervention made in the intervention group, the control group, or both that is outside of the study protocol and that might contribute to a study's outcome.

5. **Efficacy** is the extent to which medical interventions achieve health improvements under ideal circumstances (e.g., clinical trials).

6. **Effectiveness** is the extent to which medical interventions achieve health improvements in real, practical settings.

7. **The _p_ value** is the probability _p_ of observing a particular result or one that is more extreme due solely to chance. It reflects the sample size and the magnitude of the association. By convention in most medical research, $p \leq 0.05$ is considered statistically significant.

8. The **confidence interval** is the estimated range of values within which the true magnitude of effect lies with a certain degree of probability or confidence. Confidence intervals provide information about statistical significance (a 95% confidence interval is the complement of $p = 0.05$) and data variability. By convention, 95% confidence intervals are generally employed in medical research.

9. **Type I error** is the probability that the null hypothesis is rejected when it is actually true (_p_ value or alpha).

10. **Type II error** is the probability of failing to reject the null hypothesis when it is in fact false (beta). A study's power is calculated by subtracting the probability of a Type II error from 1.

11. **Internal validity** is the extent to which an observed association between an exposure and outcome is valid.

12. **External validity** is the extent to which one can generalize the study conclusions to populations and settings outside the study.

B. **Epidemiologic studies** can be broadly divided in two groups, descriptive studies and analytic studies. Descriptive studies are designed to generate hypotheses, whereas analytic studies are designed to test hypotheses. There are three main types of descriptive studies: case reports or case series, correlational series, and cross-sectional studies. Analytic studies can be subdivided into observational studies (case–control studies and cohort studies) and experimental studies (intervention studies or clinical trials as they are generally called in medicine).

1. **Case reports and case series** document unusual medical occurrences and may represent the first clues in the identification of new diseases, adverse effects of exposures, or presence of an epidemic.
   a. Strength
      (1) Very useful for hypothesis generation.
   b. Limitations
      (1) Interpretation is limited by the lack of a comparison group.
      (2) Cannot be used to test for a valid statistical association.
      (3) Based on the experiences of a single individual or small group of individuals.
2. **Correlational studies** describe a variable of interest in relation to an outcome in an entire population.
   a. Strengths
      (1) Can often be performed quickly with minimal resources because the information is often already available.
      (2) May allow for geographic comparisons.
   b. Limitations
      (1) Inability to link exposure and outcome in individuals because the data are aggregated at a higher level (e.g., city, county, state).
      (2) Inability to control for confounding.
3. **Cross-sectional studies (prevalence studies)** assess both the exposure and outcome status of individuals at a specific point in time.
   a. Strength
      (1) Both exposure and outcome data are obtained from individuals.
   b. Limitations
      (1) Inability to establish temporal sequence between exposure and outcome.
      (2) Prevalent outcomes are assessed, so any association between the exposure and the outcome may reflect determinants of survival.
4. A **case–control study** is a type of observational study where study individuals are selected on the basis of whether they do (cases) or do not (controls) have a particular outcome. The groups are then examined for a history of an exposure or particular characteristic.

    a. Strengths
- **(1)** Good for studying rare outcomes.
- **(2)** Can evaluate multiple exposures.
- **(3)** Efficient from both a time and economic perspective.
- **(4)** Particularly well suited to studying diseases with long latent periods.

    b. Limitations
- **(1)** Does not allow a direct estimate of outcome rates.
- **(2)** Inefficient for evaluating rare exposures.
- **(3)** Susceptible to selection and information bias.
- **(4)** Temporal sequence of exposure and outcome may be difficult to establish.

5. Cohort studies are observational studies where disease-free individuals are selected and classified based on the presence or absence of exposure and then followed over time (retrospectively or prospectively) for the development of the outcome of interest.

    a. Strengths
- **(1)** Establish a temporal relationship between the exposure and outcome.
- **(2)** Allow a direct estimate of the incidence rate for the outcome.
- **(3)** Good for evaluating rare exposures.
- **(4)** Allow multiple outcomes to be evaluated.
- **(5)** Minimize bias in exposure assessment.

    b. Limitations
- **(1)** Prospective cohort studies have numerous feasibility considerations including the availability of participants, the ability to ensure complete follow-up, and the extensive time and cost required.
- **(2)** Retrospective cohort studies require access to sufficient numbers of adequate-quality records.
- **(3)** Not efficient for examining rare outcomes.

6. Clinical trials are generally considered the gold standard of clinical research because the investigator assigns exposure status. In most clinical trials participants are allocated to exposure groups at random.

    a. Strength
- **(1)** Provide the strongest causal evidence.

    b. Limitations
- **(1)** Ethical considerations make it difficult for many interventions to be evaluated in a clinical trial.
- **(2)** It may be difficult to find a sufficiently large population of individuals willing to forego an intervention that is believed to be beneficial even if there is no evidence to support this view.

Table 16-2. Data can be presented in two-by-two tables to facilitate the calculation of measures of association

Exposure	Outcome	
	Yes	No
Yes	A	B
No	C	D

  (3) Clinical trials generally have numerous feasibility considerations including being very resource intensive.

  (4) Findings may reflect the relationship between an exposure and an outcome in a clinical trial setting (efficacy), but not necessarily in the real-world setting (effectiveness).

C. Quantitative measures

 1. **Measures of association** are single summary parameters that estimate the association between an exposure and an outcome. They generally involve either calculating the ratio or the absolute difference of the measures of outcome frequency for two groups, which indicates on a relative or an absolute scale, respectively, how much more likely one group is to develop the outcome than the other (Table 16-2).

  a. **Relative risk** is the likelihood of developing the outcome in one group (e.g., treated patients) relative to another group (e.g., untreated patients):

$$[A/(A + B)]/[C/(C + D)]$$

  b. **Relative risk reduction** is the proportional reduction in event rates between two groups:

$$(1 - \text{Relative risk})$$

  c. **Absolute risk reduction** is the absolute difference in event rates:

$$[A/(A + B)] - [C/(C + D)]$$

  d. **Number needed to treat** is the number of patients who need to be treated to prevent one additional event:

$$1/(\text{Absolute risk reduction})$$

  e. **Odds ratio** is the ratio of the odds of exposure or outcome (depending on study design) between two study groups:

$$(A/B)/(C/D)$$

  f. When the outcome is undesirable, a relative risk or odds ratio of less than 1.0 represents a beneficial treatment.

Table 16-3. Two-by-two table for evaluating a diagnostic test

Test Result	Gold Standard	
	Disease Present	Disease Absent
Disease present	True positive (A)	False positive (B)
Disease absent	False negative (C)	True negative (D)

2. **The selection and interpretation of diagnostic tests** is a sequential process whose goal is to reduce uncertainty about a patient's diagnosis until either the threshold for treating or the threshold for not treating the patient is reached. A test result cannot be interpreted without considering the probability of disease before the diagnostic result was obtained. When the pretest probability of disease is high, a positive test result confirms the presence of disease, but a negative test result is insufficient to rule out disease. When the pretest probability of disease is low, a negative test result excludes the presence of disease, but a positive rest is insufficient to rule in disease (Table 16-3).

   a. **Sensitivity** is the proportion of patients with the disease who have a positive test result:

   $$A/(A + C)$$

   b. **Specificity** is the proportion of patients without the disease who have a negative test result:

   $$D/(B + D)$$

   c. **Positive predictive value** is the proportion of patients with a positive test result who have the disease:

   $$A/(A + B)$$

   d. **Negative predictive value** is the proportion of patients with a negative test result who do not have the disease:

   $$D/(C + D)$$

   e. **Likelihood ratio for a positive test result** is the relative odds of having the disease given a positive test result:

   $$[A/(A + C)]/[B/(B + D)]$$

   f. **Likelihood ratio for a negative test result** is the relative odds of having the disease given a negative test result:

   $$[C/(A + C)]/[D/(B + D)]$$

Table 16-4. Levels of evidence

Increasing strength of evidence ▲	Randomized, controlled trials
	All-or-none case series[a]
	Cohort studies
	Case–control studies
	Case series
	Expert opinion

Systemic reviews can be used to aggregate evidence when more than one study is available and can be particularly valuable if the studies included are of high quality and demonstrate consistent findings.

[a]All-or-none case series refer to clinical scenarios where rigorous scientific evaluation of new interventions was difficult because either all patients died before the treatment became available and some now survive or some patients died before the treatment became available but now none die (e.g., penicillin).

    g. Pretest odds are the odds that the patient has the disease before the test is carried out:

    (Probability of disease present):

        (1 − Probability of disease present)

    h. Posttest odds are the odds that the patient has the disease after the test is carried out:

    (Pretest odds) × (Likelihood ratio for the test result)

    i. Posttest probability is the proportion of patients with a particular test result who have the disease:

    (Posttest odds)/(Posttest odds + 1)

  3. Levels of evidence. Many different systems exist for grading the strength of a body of scientific evidence. Although there is no universal agreement on the best approach, there is general agreement that certain research methodologies are less likely to be subject to bias and are consequently apt to provide stronger levels of scientific evidence (Table 16-4). The Agency for Health Care Research and Quality has identified three important elements for any system used to grade the strength of scientific evidence:

    a. Quality is an aggregate measure of quality ratings for the individual studies based on the extent to which they minimize bias.

    b. Quantity is an aggregate measure of the magnitude of the overall effect based on the numbers of studies, the total sample size, or the overall power.

    c. Consistency is the extent to which similar findings are reported in different studies employing various methodologies.

III. Evidence-based medicine in the intensive care unit

  A. Severity-of-illness scoring systems use elements of the history, physical examination, and diagnostic tests to objectively gauge illness severity and determine prognosis. There are four main applications for these scoring systems: clinical research, performance assessment, resource allocation, and guidance in individual patient decisions. The most commonly used scoring systems for adult critical care medicine are the **Acute Physiology and Chronic Health Evaluation** system **(APACHE), the Simplified Acute Physiology Score (SAPS),** and the **Mortality Probability Model (MPM).** In addition, several organ dysfunction scores have been developed for use in the critically ill. Although these scores have been developed primarily to describe organ dysfunction, there is clearly a relationship between organ failure and patient outcomes.

1. **APACHE (I, II, and III)** is based on the premise that severity of illness on ICU admission is based on a patient's physiologic reserve (age and the presence of comorbidities) and the extent of any acute physiologic abnormalities (worst abnormalities within 24 hours of admission) (Table 16-5).

2. **SAPS (I and II)** was initially developed as a simplification of the APACHE I classification system. SAPS II uses 17 variables and performs similarly to APACHE II.

3. **MPM (I and II)** is a statistical modeling system that uses patient clinical variables to predict the probability of hospital mortality rather than to measure severity of illness.

4. **Trauma and Revised Injury Severity Score (TRISS)** is a severity-of-injury scoring system for trauma patients, but is not specific to ICU trauma admissions.

5. **Multiple Organ Dysfunction Score** is an organ dysfunction score that is calculated based on a patient's respiratory, renal, hepatic, cardiovascular, hematologic, and neurologic function.

6. **Sequential Organ Failure Assessment (SOFA)** is an organ dysfunction score that mainly differs from the MODS in that it includes therapeutic interventions in its assessment of a patient's cardiovascular function.

B. **Outcomes of special interest in the intensive care unit**

1. **In-hospital mortality** is the incidence of death in a particular population during the period of the hospitalization.

2. The **28-day mortality** is the incidence of death in a particular population during a specific period of time (28 days is commonly used).

3. **Hospital length of stay** is frequently assessed to examine the length of a patient's acute illness. It may be subdivided into length of stay in the intensive care unit, in the hospital, as well as any subsequent rehabilitation facilities.

Table 16-5.   The APACHE II severity-of-disease classification system

Physiologic Variable	High Abnormal Range				0	Low Abnormal Range			
	+4	+3	+2	+1		+1	+2	+3	+4
Temperature, rectal (°C)	≥41	39–40.9		38.5–38.9	36–38.4	34–35.9	32–33.9	30–31.9	≤29.9
Mean arterial pressure (mm Hg)	≥160	130–159	110–129		70–109		50–69		≤49
Heart rate (ventricular response)	≥180	140–179	110–139		70–109		55–69	40–54	≤39
Respiratory rate (nonventilated or ventilated)	≥50	35–49		25–34	12–24	10–11	6–9		≤5
Oxygenation: $P(A-a)O_2$ or PaO_2 (mm Hg) a. Fio_2 ≥0.5, record $P(A-a)O_2$ b. Fio_2 <0.5, record only $P(A-a)O_2$	≥500	350–499	200–349		<200 Po_2>70	Po_2 61–70		Po_2 55–60	Po_2<55
Arterial pH	≥7.7	7.6–7.69		7.5–7.59	7.33–7.49		7.25–7.32	7.15–7.24	<7.15
Serum sodium (mmol/L)	≥180	160–179	155–159	150–154	130–149		120–129	111–119	≤110

Serum potassium (mmol/L)	≥7	6–6.9		5.5–5.9	3.5–5.4	3–3.4	2.5–2.9		<2.5
Serum creatinine (mg/100 ml) (Double point score for acute renal failure)	≥3.5	2–3.4	1.5–1.9		0.6–1.4		<0.6		
Hematocrit (%)	≥60		50–59.9	46–49.9	30–45.9		20–29.9		<20
White blood count (thousands/mm³)	≥40		20–39.9	15–19.9	3–14.9		1–2.9		<1
Glasgow Coma Score (GCS): Score = 15 minus actual GCS									
[A] Total Acute Physiology Score (APS): Sum of the 12 individual variable points									
Serum HCO_3 (venous mmol/L) (Use if no ABGs)	≥52	41–51.9		32–40.9	22–31.9		18–21.9	15–17.9	<15

(continued)

Table 16-5. *Continued*

Physiologic Variable	High Abnormal Range				Low Abnormal Range				
	+4	+3	+2	+1	0	+1	+2	+3	+4

B Age points:
Assign points according to age as follows:

Age (yr)	Points
≤44	0
45–54	2
55–64	3
65–74	5
≥75	6

C Chronic health points
If the patient has a history of severe organ system insufficiency or is immunocompromised assign points as follows:
a. For nonoperative or emergency postoperative patients, 5 points.
b. For elective postoperative patients, 2 points.

APACHE II score
Sum of A + B + C

A APS points ____
B Age points ____
C Chronic health points ____
Total APACHE II ____

P(A-a)o$_2$, alveolar-arterial oxygen difference; ABG, arterial blood gas; APACHE, acute physiology and chronic health evaluation; Fio$_2$, inspired oxygen fraction; Pao$_2$, arterial oxygen partial pressure.

Organ insufficiency or immunocompromised state must have been evident prior to this hospital admission and conform to the following criteria:

Liver: biopsy-proven cirrhosis and documented portal hypertension; episodes of past gastrointestinal bleeding attributed to portal hypertension; or prior episodes of hepatic failure/encephalopathy/coma.

Cardiovascular: New York Heart Association class IV.

Respiratory: chronic restrictive, obstructive, or vascular disease resulting in severe exercise restriction, or documented chronic hypoxia, hypercapnia, secondary polycythemia, severe pulmonary hypertension (>40 mm Hg), or ventilator dependency.

Renal: receiving chronic dialysis.

Immunocompromised: the patient has received therapy that suppresses resistance to infection (e.g., chemotherapy, radiation, long-term or recent high-dose steroids) or has a disease that is sufficiently advanced to suppress resistance to infection (e.g., leukemia, lymphoma, acquired immune deficiency syndrome).

From Knaus WA, Draper EA, Wagner DP, et al. APACHE II: A severity of disease classification system. *Crit Care Med* 1985;13:818–829. With permission.

4. **Ventilator-free days** is a measure of the number of days that patients spend in the intensive care unit alive but not on a ventilator in a specified time period (e.g., 28 days). It is a commonly used measure because of the frequency of respiratory failure in most intensive care units.

SELECTED REFERENCES

Boyd CR, Tolson MA, Copes WS. Evaluating trauma care: the TRISS methodology. *J Trauma* 1987;27:370–378.

Guyatt G, Rennie D. *User's guide to the medical literature: essentials of evidence-based clinical practice*. Chicago: American Medical Association, 2001.

Knaus WA, Draper EA, Wagner DP, et al. APACHE II: a severity of disease classification system. *Crit Care Med* 1985;13:818–829.

Le Gall JR, Lemeshow S, Saulnier F. A new simplified acute physiology score (SAPS II) based on European/North American multicenter study. *JAMA* 1993;270:2957.

Lemeshow S, Teres D, Klar J, et al. Mortality probability models (MPM II) based on an international cohort of intensive care unit patients. *JAMA* 1993;270:2478.

Marshall JC, Cook DJ, Christou NV, et al. Multiple Organ Dysfunction Score: a reliable descriptor of a complex clinical outcome. *Crit Care Med* 1995;23:1638–1652.

Sackett DL, Strauss SE, Richardson WS, et al. *Evidence-based medicine: how to practice and teach EBM,* 2nd ed. Edinburgh: Churchill Livingstone, 2000.

Vincent JL, Moreno R, Takala J, et al. The SOFA (Sepsis-related Organ Failure Assessment) score to describe organ dysfunction/failure. *Intensive Care Med* 1996;22:707–710.

Specific Considerations

17

Coronary Artery Disease

Michael G. Fitzsimons

I. **Introduction.** Coronary artery disease (CAD) is the leading cause of morbidity and mortality among adults in the United States. More than 64 million Americans have some form of cardiovascular disease (CAD, congestive heart failure [CHF], hypertension, and stroke), and nearly 39% of all deaths in the United States are due to cardiovascular disease. Although approximately one-third of patients with acute myocardial infarction (MI) die, most deaths are due to fatal dysrhythmias in the early prehospital course. Identifying patients at risk and prevention of heart disease through risk modification and medical therapy should be the primary medical objectives. The major **risk factors** of CAD include hypertension, diabetes mellitus, smoking, dyslipidemia, obesity, elevated homocysteine levels, a sedentary lifestyle, and a family history of CAD.

A. **Definitions.** Although chest discomfort is the most common complaint of patients with ischemia, electrocardiographic changes without accompanying typical anginal symptoms ("silent" ischemia) are common, especially in diabetic, elderly, and postoperative patients. Typical angina pain may also be blunted by techniques such as epidural analgesia. The initial evaluation of patients presenting with chest pain or similar symptoms must determine whether a patient has an acute coronary syndrome, stable angina, or noncardiac chest pain because the management may be quite different.

1. **Angina pectoris** is chest discomfort (tightness, pressure, pain) that is generally located retrosternal, occurs at rest or is precipitated by physical or emotional stress, and lasts approximately 10 minutes or less. Pain can be referred to the back, jaw, arm, or shoulder. Angina generally occurs in patients with compromise of at least one epicardial artery. Associated symptoms include nausea, vomiting, diaphoresis, and shortness of breath. Angina is a manifestation of myocardial ischemia without myocardial necrosis. Angina can occur without CAD in patients with valvular heart disease, hypertrophic cardiomyopathy, or uncontrolled hypertension. The Canadian Cardiovascular Society Classification System grades angina from class I (ordinary physical exertion does not cause angina) to class IV (angina with minimal exertion or at rest).

2. **Stable angina** is a predictable form of angina pectoris that has not changed in frequency, duration, precipitating factors, or ease of relief within recent months. The etiology is commonly due to fixed coronary artery atherosclerosis.

3. **Unstable (crescendo) angina** refers to angina of recent onset (within 2 months) occurring with increasing frequency, intensity, progressively less effort, or at rest. Prognosis is poor because about 10% of these patients have left main CAD and up to 20% of patients will progress to acute MI within 3 months. Plaque rupture, platelet aggregation, coronary arterial thrombosis, and vasospasm are the underlying causes. The role of an ongoing inflammatory response and acute inflammatory reaction in chronic atherosclerosis and acute coronary syndrome is increasingly recognized.

4. **Prinzmetal's (variant) angina** is characterized by resting angina that is generally worse in the morning, lasts for several minutes, and is accompanied by transient ST-segment elevation and/or ventricular dysrhythmias. This form of angina can also be induced by exercise. It is caused by coronary vasospasm usually occurring within an atherosclerotic artery.

5. **Acute coronary syndrome** refers to a clinical scenario with potential myocardial ischemia, and may include unstable angina pectoris, ST-segment elevation MI (STEMI), or non–ST-segment elevation MI (NSTEMI).

B. **Pathophysiology**

1. **Myocardial oxygen supply–demand balance.** At rest, the myocardium extracts oxygen maximally such that during exertion or hemodynamic stress, oxygen delivery must be increased to meet the demand. Myocardial ischemia and infarction occur when oxygen demand exceeds delivery.

   a. **Myocardial oxygen supply** is determined by the following factors:

      (1) **Coronary blood flow,** which occurs mainly during diastole and is a function of the pressure gradient from aortic root to downstream coronary pressure. In normal coronary arteries, exercise or stress can increase coronary blood flow four- to fivefold. Stenoses in these arteries can reduce oxygen supply. Conditions such as hyperviscosity, polycythemia, and sickle cell disease may compromise coronary blood flow.

      (2) **Oxygen content** is determined by hemoglobin (Hgb) concentration, oxygen saturation (Sao_2), and dissolved oxygen concentration: **oxygen content (ml/dl)** $= [1.31$ ml $O_2 \times$ Hgb $\times Sao_2] + 0.003$ ml $\times Pao_2$. Oxygen content can be augmented mainly by increasing Hgb and Sao_2. The contribution from dissolved oxygen is small.

   b. **Myocardial oxygen demand** is determined by the following factors:

      (1) **Ventricular wall tension** is the product of transmural pressure and ventricular radius divided by two times ventricular wall thickness.

Increases in transmural pressure or ventricular radius will increase oxygen demand.

(2) **Heart rate** can promote increased oxygen consumption through associated increases in myocardial contractility. Tachycardia also decreases the duration of maximal coronary perfusion in the atherosclerotic vessels, thus limiting oxygen supply. Hyperthyroidism, sympathomimetic activity (cocaine use), or anxiety can increase demand.

(3) **Contractility** is directly proportional to oxygen demand.

2. **Etiologies of myocardial oxygen-demand imbalance.** The most common (90%) cause of myocardial ischemia and infarction is coronary atherosclerotic narrowing. Other etiologies include vasospasm, vasculitis, trauma, thromboembolism of the coronary artery, valvular heart disease (i.e., aortic stenosis), hypertrophic or dilated cardiomyopathies, and thyrotoxicosis.

II. **Myocardial ischemia.** The principal objectives of diagnosing myocardial ischemia are to identify the cause and assess the severity of CAD, guide therapeutic options, and minimize any future ischemic insult or MI.

A. **Diagnosis**

1. **History.** Risk factors of CAD should be noted. The character, location, duration, radiation, exacerbating factors (physical or emotional stress, eating, or cold weather), alleviating factors (rest or medications), accompanying symptoms, and change in pattern over the last few weeks should be sought. The type of angina should be identified based on the history. Historical factors associated with a high risk of death or nonfatal myocardial infarction as defined by the American Heart Association include prolonged rest pain (>20 minutes) that does not resolve with nitrates. Intermediate-risk factors include prolonged rest angina of greater than 20 minutes resolved with nitroglycerin, nocturnal angina, new-onset class III or class IV angina, or age greater than 65 years. Lower-risk factors include increased frequency, severity, or duration of angina or new-onset angina in the last 2 weeks to 2 months.

2. **Physical examination.** Although physical examination can be normal or nonspecific, physical distress, anxiety, tachycardia, hypertension, an S4 gallop, pulmonary rales, xanthomas, or evidence of peripheral atherosclerosis may be evident. Pulmonary edema, new or worsening murmur of mitral regurgitation, and angina with hypotension are associated with a high risk of death or nonfatal MI.

3. **Noninvasive studies**

a. **Resting electrocardiogram (ECG)** is normal in about one-half of patients with ischemia. ECG changes indicative of myocardial ischemia that may

Table 17-1. Location of ischemia or infarct by electrocardiographic criteria

Region	Leads	Vessel
Anterior	V_1–V_4	Left anterior descending
Anteroseptal	V_1–V_2	Left anterior descending
Anterolateral	I, aVL, V_1–V_6	Left anterior descending
Lateral	I, aVL, V_5–V_6	Circumflex
Inferior	II, III, aVF	Right coronary artery
Posterior	Large R wave in V_1, V_2, or V_3 with ST depression	Right coronary artery
Right ventricular	V_3R, V_4R	Right coronary artery

progress to MI include new ST-segment elevations at the J point in two or more contiguous leads that are 0.2 mV or greater in leads V_1 through V_3 and greater than 0.1 mV in all other leads. In patients without ST-segment elevation, ST depression or T-wave abnormalities may signal risk for MI. Isolated J-point elevation may occur as a normal variant in young, healthy adults. Ischemia secondary to coronary vasospasm may result in ST-segment elevation. Presence of significant Q waves is suggestive of prior MI. The presence of a bundle-branch block (BBB) or artificial pacer rhythm on the ECG increases the difficulty of detecting ST-segment or T-wave abnormalities. In general, reversibility of ECG changes after therapeutic interventions is highly suggestive of ischemia. Table 17-1 outlines the ECG changes associated with specific regions of ischemic myocardium.

b. **Exercise ECG.** Exercise stress testing involves monitoring blood pressure and ECG while an individual performs exercise on a treadmill or a bicycle. The indications for exercise stress testing include the diagnosis of obstructive CAD, risk assessment and prognosis in patients with symptoms or known CAD, asymptomatic patients with multiple risk factors, and certain post-revascularization situations. Most protocols involve a warm-up period followed by progressive increases in workload. Each level of exercise reflects increases on oxygen uptake or metabolic equivalents (METs). A single MET is 3.5 ml/kg/min. The test is continued until an individual's heart rate reaches 85% to 90% of his or her maximal predicted heart rate or maximum perceived exertion. A test may be considered positive or indicating a high likelihood of significant CAD in the presence of ST-segment elevation or depression, a fall in blood pressure with exercise, or the development of serious arrhythmias or of anginal chest pain with exercise. The test should be terminated when an individual requests its termination or there is a fall in blood pressure or the appearance of anginal symptoms, central nervous system symptoms, poor peripheral perfusion, or serious arrhythmias. The sensitivity of exercise ECG to detect obstructive CAD is dependent on the severity of stenosis and the extent of disease. The sensitivity is 86% and specificity is 53% for three-vessel or left main CAD. Patients with a positive stress test should be considered for cardiac catheterization to explore the potential of revascularization. Absolute contraindications of exercise stress testing include recent MI (within 2 days), severe aortic stenosis, symptomatic CHF, arrhythmias causing hemodynamic compromise, acute pulmonary embolus, pulmonary infarction, and aortic dissection. Relative contraindications include hypertension (systolic blood pressure >200 mm Hg or diastolic blood pressure >110 mm Hg), tachyarrhythmias or bradyarrhythmias, hypertrophic cardiomyopathy, high-grade atrioventricular block, and a physical or mental limitation to exercise. The sensitivity of exercise tolerance testing increases with increased coronary disease. ECG changes that occur at a lower workload are generally more significant than those occurring at higher workloads.

c. **Myocardial injury enzymes.** Patients with unstable angina or those suspicious of having evolving MI should have myocardial injury enzymes levels followed as part of their diagnostic evaluation. **Creatine phosphokinase (CPK)** and **troponin** are released during myocardial injury and necrosis. Changes in the serum concentration of the subfractions specific for cardiac muscle are CPK-MB isozyme and troponins I and T, and over time these are important for diagnosis of MI. Increases in these biomarkers indicate that myocardial injury has occurred, but do not indicate the mechanism.

(1) **CPK.** The time course of CPK-MB increase is between 4 and 6 hours, with a 2- to 10-fold peak in 18 to 24 hours and a return to normal within 2 to 3 days from the initial onset of symptoms if no further myocardial injury occurs. Other major causes of increased CPK-MB include muscle trauma, rhabdomyolysis, myopathies, and polymyositis. Generally, CPK with MB isozyme should be determined at 8- to 12-hour intervals for at least 24 hours or until the diagnosis is established. Generally, CPK enzymes are more reliable for the early diagnosis of myocardial infarction but may be less sensitive in the postoperative patient.

(2) **Troponin** is more sensitive and specific than CPK-MB for indicating myocardial cell

damage. Up to 30% to 40% of patients with unstable angina have elevated troponin levels, although CPK-MB levels are often normal. These patients generally have a less favorable prognosis. The time course of troponin I and troponin T increase is between 3 and 12 hours, peaks in 1 to 2 days, and returns to normal within 4 to 14 days. Troponin levels are of special value for ruling out MI in the immediate postoperative period (when CPK-MB may be elevated due to skeletal muscle injury), in patients with normal CPK-MB but high clinical suspicion of having an acute MI, and in patients with symptoms occurring days prior to presentation. Clinically, troponin level should be measured at baseline and repeated 12 to 24 hours later. Troponin may be more accurate in the diagnosis of a remote MI than CPK.

d. **Radionuclide perfusion imaging** provides a safe and effective method of assessing myocardial perfusion and function.

(1) **Exercise myocardial perfusion imaging.** Thallium-201 is a radioactive tracer that is injected intravenously during peak treadmill exercise and avidly extracted as a potassium analogue by viable myocardium in proportional to regional myocardial blood flow. Regions of perfusion defect correlate with severity of coronary artery stenosis supplying the regions. On delayed imaging, a fixed defect devoid of tracer represents an area of prior infarct, whereas a region with thallium redistribution is considered to be myocardium at risk of ischemia. The test has a sensitivity of 85% and a specificity of 90%.

(2) **Exercise radionuclide ventriculography.** Technetium-99m sestamibi is injected intravenously and accumulated in myocardium in proportion to blood flow. Using a first-pass technique, one obtains multiple ventricular images synchronized to the cardiac cycle at rest and during exercise. The occurrence of regional wall motion abnormalities and the inability to increase left ventricular (LV) ejection fraction (EF) during exercise are suggestive of myocardial ischemia.

(3) **Pharmacologic stress perfusion imaging.** Dipyrimadole and adenosine are coronary artery vasodilators commonly used in stress imaging. Adenosine is a direct-acting agent that causes coronary vasodilation and increases blood flow in areas without stenosis. This subsequently creates an area of apparent heterogeneous flow on imaging because stenotic areas will not dilate. Dipyridamole inhibits

cellular uptake and degradation of adenosine and thus indirectly increases coronary blood blow in nonstenotic vessels. Because the side effects of both agents include angina, headache, and bronchospasm, they should be used with caution in patients with severe obstructive pulmonary disease and asthma. Additionally, dobutamine is an inotropic agent that increases heart rate, systolic blood pressure, and contractility. Blood flow increases secondarily, and imaging may reveal heterogeneous blood flow due to stenotic areas, which cannot dilate.

e. **Echocardiography.** Transthoracic echocardiography (see Chapter 2) can detect valvular stenosis, valvular regurgitation, and hypertrophic cardiomyopathy. It may also be helpful in evaluating the consequences of myocardial infarction to include pericardial effusion, ventricular free wall rupture, or mitral regurgitation. Evidence of chronic myocardial ischemia seen on echocardiogram may include hypokinesis (reduced wall motion), akinesis (absence of wall motion), or dyskinesis (paradoxical wall motion). The locations of these abnormal wall motions can correlate with the distribution of CAD. Transesophageal echocardiography (TEE) provides better visualization of valvular function, the left atrial appendage, ascending aorta, mural or atrial thrombi, and aortic aneurysms than transthoracic echocardiography. Exercise echocardiography (dobutamine) has a sensitivity of approximately 85%.

4. **Invasive studies. Coronary angiography** remains the gold standard for identifying and quantifying the extent of CAD. Hemodynamic parameters, anatomy of the heart and coronary vessels, and wall motion abnormalities can be obtained. A coronary obstruction is clinically significant when more than 70% of the coronary artery luminal diameter is narrowed. Coronary angiography is not without risk, and the mortality rate is approximately 0.5%. Coronary angiography will determine the need for percutaneous coronary intervention (angioplasty, stenting, atherectomy), coronary artery bypass grafting, or medical management only.

B. **Differential diagnosis of chest pain** includes angina, MI, aortic dissection, pulmonary embolism, pneumothorax, costochondritis, pericarditis, anxiety disorder, peptic ulcer disease, gastroesophageal reflux disease, and acute cholecystitis.

C. **Management of myocardial ischemia**
1. **General approach.** The initial goals are to reduce myocardial oxygen consumption, improve oxygen supply, relieve pain, stabilize hemodynamics, and prevent coronary thrombosis. Supplemental oxygen should be provided. Routine vital signs should be monitored. Any

precipitating condition (e.g., tachycardia, dysrhythmias, hypertension, anemia, thyrotoxicosis) requires correction. Patients with unstable angina should be placed on bedrest with anxiolytic medication prescribed if needed. Intense antianginal pharmacologic therapy should be initiated. Serial ECGs and cardiac enzyme determinations are standard diagnostic tools. The patient should be referred for coronary catheterization.

2. **Medications.** See Appendix 1 to this book for additional pharmacologic information on most of these agents.

   a. **β-adrenergic antagonists** decrease exertional angina symptoms and mortality in patients with known CAD. In the setting of acute MI, they reduce ventricular ectopy, ventricular fibrillation, and infarct size. β-blockers also decrease death and nonfatal MI in patients who have received fibrinolytics, reduce myocardial oxygen demand, and relieve angina by lowering heart rate, blood pressure, and contractility. Generally, β-1–selective agents without intrinsic sympathomimetic activity (e.g., **metoprolol, atenolol, esmolol**) are better tolerated in patients with reactive airway diseases (asthma, chronic obstructive pulmonary disease). Low doses (e.g., atenolol 25–50 mg orally once daily, metoprolol 50–100 mg orally twice daily) initially are administered and titrated upward until a resting heart rate of 50 to 60 beats/min, or an exercise heart rate of less than 100 beats/min, is achieved or adverse effects are observed. The administration of β-blockers prior to surgical procedures has been shown to decrease mortality in patients felt to be at risk for perioperative cardiac events.

   b. **Nitrates** provide relief of angina primary by decreasing venous return and ventricular wall tension. Their other effects include coronary vasodilation, relief of coronary vasospasm, redistribution of coronary blood flow, and antiplatelet activity. The net effect is a reduction in myocardial oxygen demand and anginal symptoms. For acute anginal attacks, a rapidly acting sublingual preparation is preferred. The usual sublingual dose is 0.3 to 0.4 mg every 5 minutes, repeated up to three times if systolic blood pressure is greater than 90 mm Hg or heart rate is greater than 50 or less than 100 beats/min. The titratability of **intravenous (IV) nitroglycerin** is useful in the acute management of ischemia or unstable angina in combination with administration of β-blockers, heparin, and aspirin. The usual starting dose is 10 to 20 μg/min and is titrated upward by increments of 10 to 20 μg/min at 5- to 15-minute intervals, until symptoms resolve or adverse effects occur. Nitroglycerin may be continued for the initial 24 to 48 hours in patients with MI and congestive heart failure, large anterior wall MIs, persistent or recurrent ischemia, or hypertension. It may be continued beyond 48 hours for patients with recurrent angina or persistent pulmonary congestion.

c. **Calcium-channel antagonists** alleviate angina and improve the myocardial oxygen supply–demand ratio by inhibiting coronary vasospasm, dilating coronary arteries, reducing heart rate, and reducing peripheral vascular resistance. This class of agent is most effective in vasospastic angina, but is also useful in stable and the chronic treatment of unstable angina especially when β-blockers or nitrate therapy is not well tolerated. There is little evidence to support the routine use of calcium-channel blockers in the setting of acute myocardial infarction.

d. **Antiplatelet agents. Aspirin** prevents acute coronary syndromes and improves mortality and reinfarction rate primarily by its antiplatelet aggregation action (inhibition of thromboxane A_2). The usual dose is 160 to 325 mg daily. Aspirin prevents reocclusion and recurrent ischemic events after fibrinolytic therapy. Activation of the platelet-surface glycoprotein IIb/IIIa receptor is the final common pathway in the process leading to platelet aggregation. When the receptor is activated, it binds circulating fibrinogen and cross-links with adjacent platelets to create a platelet–fibrinogen matrix. **Glycoprotein IIb/IIIa inhibitors** block this physiologic pathway and may be used in patients who undergo percutaneous coronary interventions within 24 hours and in some patients who will be medically managed. Antiplatelet agents **ticlopidine** and **clopidogrel** inhibit adenosine diphosphate receptor–mediated platelet activation. Clopidogrel and aspirin administered together in patients with acute coronary syndromes are more effective than aspirin alone in preventing death from MI, stroke or cardiovascular causes, although there is an increased risk of bleeding.

e. **Opioids.** Pain not adequately responding to antianginal medications should be controlled by opioids such as **morphine sulfate** 2.5 to 5 mg IV every 5 to 10 minutes titrated to effect. Adverse effects of morphine in the patient with CAD include hypotension, which can be treated with supine positioning and fluid repletion, vagally mediated bradycardia, nausea and vomiting, which may be difficult to distinguish from the symptoms of evolving MI, and respiratory depression.

3. **Invasive approaches.** Revascularization procedures are indicated to manage patients who have incapacitating angina refractory to medical therapy, and they may improve survival in selected patient populations.

a. **Percutaneous coronary intervention (PCI).** Patients with normal ventricular function and one- or two-vessel disease refractory to medical therapy may benefit from PCI. Patients who are not candidates for PCI include those with minimal coronary stenosis (<60% narrowing), left main CAD, and severe diffuse multiple-vessel disease. Procedure-related complications include death (1%), MI (4%–5%), and emergency bypass surgery (4%–5%). Restenosis occurs in 25% to 30% of patients, usually within the first 6 months following the procedure. **Intracoronary stenting** in conjunction with **antiplatelet agents** (abciximab or ticlopidine) have substantially reduced the restenosis rate.

b. **Coronary artery bypass grafting (CABG)** improves survival compared to medical management in patients with greater than 50% left main CAD, three-vessel disease, depressed ventricular function (left ventricular EF <40%), residual angina following MI, and those with multivessel disease and proximal left anterior descending (LAD) artery involvement. Approximately 95% of patients will improve their anginal symptom after CABG and up to 75% of patients will remain symptom free for 5 years following CABG. The use of the internal mammary artery provides a 90% patency rate over 10 years. Perioperative mortality is about 1% to 3%, and perioperative MI is about 5% to 10%. Mortality risk decreases in centers with higher operative volume.

III. **Myocardial infarction.** Traditionally, a MI has been classified as Q-wave (transmural) infarction resulting from persistent occlusive thrombus or non–Q-wave (subendocardial) infarction resulting from incomplete or spontaneously recanalized thrombotic occlusions. Non–Q-wave infarcts were felt to have less extensive infarction but a higher risk of recurrent MI and arrhythmia. The current classification is based on the presence of ST-segment elevation in the presenting ECG. Patients presenting with ST elevation on their initial ECG benefit from immediate reperfusion therapy via thrombolysis or revascularization (section **II.C.3**). Fibrinolytic agents are not indicated in the absence of ST elevation.

A. **Diagnosis.** Two or more of the following features are required for the diagnosis of MI: (a) clinical history and physical examination suggestive of MI, (b) ECG evidence of myocardial injury, and (c) cardiac injury enzyme markers consistent with necrosis. The primary objective is to rapidly **identify patients who are candidates for thrombolysis** because survival benefit is lost after 12 hours from the initial onset of angina. The ideal time from arrival at the emergency room to time of thrombolysis should be less than 30 minutes. Patients with ST-segment elevations (≥ 1 mm) in at least two contiguous leads or new left BBB with symptoms for less than 12 hours and no contraindications for thrombolytic therapy should be referred for thrombolysis or PCI therapy immediately.

1. **History** of patients with acute MI is similar to those with ischemia. Most perioperative myocardial infarctions are silent.

2. **Physical examination** resembles that of patients with angina. In addition, signs of complications from the MI may include a new murmur (ventricular septal defect, mitral regurgitation), S_3 or S_4 gallop (noncompliant ventricle), pulmonary rales (left ventricular failure), jugular venous distention without pulmonary rales (right ventricular failure), pericardial rub (pericarditis), or dysrhythmias.

3. **Noninvasive studies**
   a. **Electrocardiogram.** The initial ECG should be obtained within 10 minutes of arrival in the emergency room. The presence of ST elevation will determine therapeutic options (see section **II.C.3**). Serial ECGs should be followed daily to assess response to therapy and detect any evidence of reinfarction or dysrhythmias. ST-segment elevations of 1 mm or greater imply injury to the epicardium. Symmetrically peaked T waves or inverted T waves are suggestive of ischemia or infarction. New BBB, dysrhythmias, or atrioventricular blocks are also suggestive of ischemia or infarction. The evolution to new Q waves is indicative of myocardial necrosis. In patients with inferior wall MI, a right-sided ECG may be necessary to rule out right ventricular MI. The occurrence of new ST-segment elevation has a sensitivity of 46% and a specificity of 91% for diagnosing MI. The presence of previous infarction decreases the sensitivity of ECG to detect MI, whereas electrolyte derangements and pericarditis decrease the specificity.

   b. **Myocardial injury enzymes** (see section **II.A.3.c**).

   c. **Chest radiography** may help to detect some complications resulting from MI. Pulmonary vascular redistribution, pulmonary edema, and pleural effusions are indicative of congestive heart failure. An enlarged cardiac silhouette implies a dilated heart or pericardial effusions.

   d. **Radionuclide perfusion imaging** (see section **II.A.3.d**) is useful when clinical history, ECG, and enzyme pattern are nondiagnostic for MI. In general, thallium-201 scintigrams lack specificity for an acute MI. Radionuclide imaging may reveal wall motion abnormalities but these may be due to an old MI, acute ischemia, stunned or hibernating myocardium, or a combination of these. Attenuation artifacts or inexperienced observers may lead to false-positive results. Exercise perfusion studies should not be employed to evaluate patients with an acute MI.

e. **Echocardiography** is helpful in patients with an equivocal diagnosis using the standard criteria. It identifies regional wall motion abnormalities as well as features due to complications of MI (e.g., mitral regurgitation, ventricular septal defect, ventricular free wall rupture, papillary muscle dysfunction). A limitation of echocardiography is its inability to differentiate between old and new infarctions.

B. **Management of acute myocardial infarction**

1. **General approach.** In addition to the goals described previously for myocardial ischemia, minimizing infarct size, preventing recurrent ischemia and MI, and early recognition and management of life-threatening complications are critical.

2. **Supportive measures.** Supplemental oxygen, IV access, routine vital signs and continuous ECG monitoring should be established. Unless CHF or hypoxemia (SpO_2 <90%) occurs, supplemental oxygen generally is required only in the initial 2 to 3 hours after an uncomplicated MI. Patients with severe CHF or cardiogenic shock may require endotracheal intubation and mechanical ventilation. Hemodynamically unstable patients may benefit from the use of a pulmonary artery catheter. Laboratory studies include electrolytes with magnesium, lipid profile, complete blood count to assess anemia, and pulse oximetry to evaluate oxygenation especially in patients with CHF or in cardiogenic shock.

3. **Medications.** See Appendix 1 for additional pharmacologic information on these agents.

a. **Aspirin** alone or in combination with certain thrombolytic therapies (e.g., streptokinase) improves survival. A dose of 160 to 325 mg should be given immediately and continued daily indefinitely. Chewable tablets provide quicker absorption, whereas the suppository form may be used in patients with nausea and vomiting. The effects of aspirin generally occur within 30 minutes and last the 3- to 7-day lifetime of the platelet. The beneficial action of aspirin is probably as much an effect of its antiinflammatory action as its antiplatelet mechanisms. Aspirin should be given to any patient with a suspected acute coronary syndrome unless specific contraindications exist. **Ticlopidine** or **clopidogrel** may be used in patients who are intolerant to aspirin. Reversible neutropenia is the most serious adverse effect of ticlopidine when used for more than 2 weeks. The addition of clopidogrel to aspirin in the initial management of acute coronary syndrome has proven beneficial but may worsen bleeding at the time of CABG.

b. β-adrenergic antagonists. β-blockers reduce infarct size, associated complications, and overall mortality during the initial and subsequent course. Patients without contraindications, especially in those with persistent/recurrent angina or tachydysrhythmias, should be placed on β-blockers within the first 12 hours of symptoms. Initially, **metoprolol** 5 mg IV every 5 min to a total of 15 mg may be given, if tolerated, and then metoprolol 50 mg orally every 6 to 12 hours can be administered for 2 days and then increased to 100 mg orally twice daily. Alternatively, **atenolol** may be administered on a similar graded dose schedule. Relative contraindications include heart rate (HR) less than 60 beats/min, systolic blood pressure less than 100 mm Hg, severe left ventricular failure, second-degree or third-degree atrioventricular (AV) block, and significant reactive airway diseases.

c. Nitrates. Clinical evidence does not support the routine long-term use of nitrate therapy in uncomplicated MI. Those patients with acute MI and CHF, large anterior infarction, persistent ischemia, or hypertension, however, may benefit from IV nitroglycerin for the first 24 to 48 hours. Those with continuing pulmonary edema, recurrent ischemia, or recurrent angina may benefit from more prolonged use of nitroglycerin. Nitroglycerin is generally not indicated in patients with hypotension or persistent bradycardia. The benefits of nitrates include a decrease in oxygen demand by decreasing preload and afterload and in addition an antiplatelet effect.

d. Heparin. Prior to the widespread use of thrombolytic therapy, heparin was shown to reduce mortality and reinfarction in patients with acute MI. Currently, the only additional survival benefit from heparin is when it is used in combination with **alteplase** (tissue plasminogen activator). Intravenous heparin should be titrated to keep the activated partial thromboplastin time at 1.5 to 2 times the normal range for 48 hours for patients receiving alteplase. Patients at high risk for developing thromboembolism (e.g., large or anterior MI, atrial fibrillation, previous embolus, or present of LV thrombus) will require IV heparin for prophylaxis of thrombotic complications. In patients with uncomplicated MI, subcutaneous heparin 7,500 U twice daily for 24 to 48 hours or until the patient ambulates is recommended. Heparin also is indicated in patients undergoing PCI or CABG. Low-molecular-weight heparin (**dalteparin** or **enoxaparin**) has been shown to reduce mortality in patients with non–Q-wave MI or unstable angina.

e. Administration of **angiotensin-converting-en-zyme inhibitors (ACEIs)** can improve mortality after acute MI, with the greatest benefit occurring among those with anterior infarction or history of MI, CHF, or tachycardia. The benefit of ACEIs may be from a limitation of left ventricular dysfunction and prevention of ventricular remodeling. Given no contraindications, ACEIs should be administered within the first 24 hours to patients with a suspected or documented MI and those with CHF without hypotension (systolic blood pressure >100 mm Hg). One graded-dose schedule recommended is to administer **captopril** 6.25 mg orally followed by 12.5 mg 2 hours later, then 25 mg 10 to 12 hours later, and then 50 mg twice daily. Alternative agents (e.g., lisinopril, enalapril, quinapril, ramipril) may be used. In patients with uncomplicated MI and preserved LV function, ACEIs can be discontinued after 4 to 6 weeks. ACEIs are contraindicated in angioedema, bilateral renal artery stenosis, hypersensitivity to ACEIs, and pregnancy.

f. **Calcium-channel antagonists** have not been shown to improve survival after MI or prevent secondary ischemia or infarction. When β-blockers are contraindicated or ineffective, verapamil or diltiazem may be used to treat atrial fibrillation with rapid ventricular response or persistent ischemia.

g. **Opioids** (section **II.C.2.c**) should be administered for analgesia and for further reduction of symptoms of pulmonary edema.

h. **Magnesium** might reduce mortality in high-risk patients if given early (<6 hours) after the initial symptoms, but the results of clinical studies are conflicting. Magnesium produces coronary vasodilation, antiplatelet activity, and suppression of automaticity, and may provide protection against reperfusion injury. Supplemental magnesium is currently recommended to correct hypomagnesemia and to treat torsades de pointes. Hypomagnesemia should be corrected with magnesium sulfate 2 g IV over 30 to 60 minutes, whereas torsades de pointes should be treated with 1 to 2 g IV over 5 minutes. Because magnesium is mostly intracellular, patients with hypomagnesemia may require multiple replacement doses to achieve normal levels. Prophylactic administration in acute MI is not indicated.

4. **Reperfusion therapy,** either pharmacologic or mechanical, reduces infarct size and mortality and improves function. Restoration of perfusion is possible even after a prolonged period. Temporary myocardial impairment ("stunned myocardium") may exist after the injury is reversed.

a. **Thrombolysis** is only indicated in the presence of ST-segment elevation. Thrombolysis produces greatest benefit when it is initiated within 6 hours of the onset of symptoms, although definite benefits still exist if administered within 12 hours. Response to therapy may be manifested as improvement in ST-segment elevation and resolution of chest discomfort. Persistent symptoms and ST-segment elevation at 60 to 90 minutes after thrombolysis should be considered indications for urgent coronary angiography and possible PCI. Thrombolytic treatment offers no clinical benefit to patients without ST-segment elevation or new BBB or those MIs complicated by heart failure or cardiogenic shock. Table 17-2 compares the commonly used thrombolytic agents. **Absolute contraindications** are suspected aortic dissection, active internal bleeding, known intracranial neoplasm, aneurysm, or malformation and any prior hemorrhagic stroke or cerebrovascular accident within 3 months. **Relative contraindications** include known bleeding diathesis or concurrent use of anticoagulants, recent trauma (within 2–4 weeks), prolonged cardiopulmonary resuscitation (>10 minutes), recent major surgery (<3 weeks), recent internal bleeding (within 2–4 weeks), severe hypertension (blood pressure >180/110 mm Hg), other

Table 17-2. Comparison of thrombolytic drugs

	tPA	Streptokinase	APSAC
Half-life (min)	6	20	100
Dose	100 mg[a]	1.5 million units	30 units
Administration (min)	90	30–60	5
Fibrin selective	Yes	No	Partial
Artery patency rate[b] (%)	79	40	63
ICH (%)	0.6	0.3	0.6
Lives saved/1,000 treated	35	25	25
Antigenic	No	Yes	Yes
Hypotension	No	Yes	Yes
Heparin required	Yes	No	No
Cost per dose (USD)	2,750	537	2,368

tPA, tissue plasminogen activator; APSAC, anisoylated plasminogen streptokinase activator complex; ICH, intracranial hemorrhage.

[a]15-mg bolus, then 0.75 mg/kg over 30 minutes (maximum 50 mg), then 0.5 mg/kg over 60 minutes (maximum 35 mg) to provide a total of 100 mg over 90 minutes.

[b]Artery patency rate at 90 minutes after treatment.

intracranial pathology, noncompressible vascular puncture sites, pregnancy, active peptic ulcer disease, or prior exposure (within 5 days to 2 years) to streptokinase or anisoylated plasminogen streptokinase activator complex (APSAC) treatment. **Patients requiring retreatment** who failed either streptokinase or APSAC should be managed with tissue plasminogen activator. Those who have contraindications to thrombolytic treatment should be considered for PTCA.

(1) **Tissue plasminogen activator (tPA)** increases plasmin binding to fibrin and provides relative clot-selective fibrinolysis without inducing a systemic lytic state. When coadministered with heparin, it has an early reperfusion rate that is slightly better than other agents. Compared with streptokinase, it is less likely to cause hemorrhage requiring transfusion, and has the greatest survival benefit (10 additional lives in 1,000 patients treated). It also has a modest increase in the incidence of hemorrhagic stroke (0.7% as compared to 0.5%). **Reteplase** and **tenecteplase** are genetically engineered tPA mutants with higher specificity for fibrin and may be easier to administer.

(2) **Streptokinase** is a bacterial protein, produced by alpha-hemolytic streptococci, that induces activation of free plasminogen and clot-associated plasminogen, eliciting a nonspecific systemic fibrinolytic state. It may decrease mortality rate by 18%.

(3) **Anisoylated plasminogen streptokinase activator complex** (Eminase or anistreplase) has clinical characteristics between those of tPA and streptokinase (see Table 17-2).

b. **PCI and stenting.** Atherectomy and stenting have improved patency rates above that of angioplasty alone. In addition to the absence of a thoracotomy and need for analgesia, there are fewer neurologic complications with PCI compared to a CABG. The primary constraint of PCI is the availability of personnel and supportive facilities, which are only available in about 20% of hospitals in the United States. Success rates are lower in operators who perform fewer than 60 to 75 procedures per year. Indications for PCI include acute ST-segment elevation or Q-wave MI and a contraindication to thrombolysis, rescue after failed thrombolysis, and cardiogenic shock complicating MI. PCI may also be indicated in patients with ventricular arrhythmias, CHF, and an ejection fraction less than 40% during their subsequent hospital stay after a MI. Several adjuncts to PCI that reduce coronary reocclusion include **IV heparin and antiplatelet agents** such as aspirin, ticlopidine, and abciximab. The benefit of low-molecular-weight heparin compared with unfractionated heparin is unclear. The addition of a glycoprotein **IIb/IIIa** inhibitor (abciximab) may improve the rate of death, recurrent MI, and need for urgent revascularization.

c. **Coronary artery bypass grafting** may be indicated on an emergency basis for patients with operable coronary anatomy who have failed medical management but are not candidates for PCI, failed PCI, and have persistent ischemia or hemodynamic instability, are in cardiogenic shock, or have surgically correctable mechanical complications (e.g., severe mitral regurgitation or ventricular septal defect [VSD]) from the MI. The mortality from emergent CABG is high.

5. **Intraaortic balloon counterpulsation** may be indicated for patients waiting for PTCA or CABG who are in cardiogenic shock or hemodynamically unstable despite medical therapy (see Chapter 38).

C. **Complications of myocardial infarction**

1. **Recurrent ischemia and infarction.** The most common causes of chest pain after MI are pericarditis, ischemia, and reinfarction. Up to 58% of patients after successful reperfusion will exhibit early recurrent angina. Reinfarction occurs in approximately 3% to 4% of patients during the first 10 days after treatment with thrombolysis and aspirin. Patients with reinfarction are at increased risk of developing cardiogenic shock, fatal dysrhythmias, or cardiac arrest. The initial approach should be optimize medical therapies while considering either repeat thrombolysis or PCI, if not already performed. Emergency CABG may be considered for those who are refractory to both medical treatment and PCI. Patients with active ischemia unresponsive to medical therapies may be placed on an IABP while waiting for coronary angiography to evaluate them for the appropriate therapeutic option.

2. **Mechanical complications**

a. **Mitral regurgitation** generally is secondary to papillary muscle rupture, which may occur between 3 and 5 days post-MI and is commonly associated with inferoposterior MI. Findings may include pulmonary edema, hypotension, cardiogenic shock, and a new apical systolic murmur. The pulmonary artery occlusion pressure waveform may exhibit large V waves. Ruptured papillary muscle and mitral regurgitation will be demonstrated with echocardiography. Treatment includes afterload reduction, inotropic agents, and, if ineffective, IABP while arranging for emergency surgical repair. Mortality with medical management is approximately 75% within the first 24 hours and is improved with prompt surgical correction.

b. **Ventricular septal rupture or defect** most commonly occurs between 3 and 5 days after anterior infarction. Clinical signs include new onset of a holosystolic murmur with systolic thrill and cardiogenic shock. An interventricular septal defect with left to right shunt will be seen on echocardiography. An increase or "step-up" of oxygen saturation between blood sampled from the right atrium and right ventricle can be confirmatory. Treatment includes afterload reduction, inotropic support, and intraaortic balloon counterpulsation. Hemodynamically stable patients may not require immediate surgical repair, but mortality in patients with cardiogenic shock is up to 90% without surgical intervention.

c. **Ventricular free wall rupture** accounts for about 10% of periinfarct death. Risk factors include sustained hypertension after MI, a large transmural MI, late use of thrombolysis, female gender, advanced age, and exposure to steroids or nonsteroidal antiinflammatory agents. It occurs most commonly in the first 2 weeks after the first MI, with a peak incidence between 3 and 6 days after infarction. Recurrent chest pain and acute onset of heart failure and cardiovascular collapse suggest free wall rupture. Death can occur rapidly, and the overall mortality rate is high. Diagnosis is by echocardiography. Volume expansion, pericardiocentesis to decompress tamponade, and IABP are temporizing measures while transferring the patient to the operating room for definitive emergency surgical repair.

d. **Ventricular aneurysm** is generally due to thinning of the infracted ventricular wall and is characterized by a protrusion of the ventricular scar that is associated with CHF, malignant dysrhythmias, and systemic embolism. Persistent ST-segment elevation may be evident on ECG; echocardiography confirms the diagnosis. Anticoagulation is required, especially in patients with documented mural thrombus. Surgical repair of ventricular geometry may be necessary.

e. **Pericarditis** is due to an extension of myocardial necrosis to the epicardium and occurs in about 25% of patients within several weeks after infarction. Pleuritic chest pain or positional discomfort, radiation to the left shoulder or scapula, a pericardial rub, ECG evidence of diffuse J-point elevation, concave ST-segment elevation, and reciprocal PR depression, and echocardiographic signs of pericardial effusion may be evident. The treatment of choice is **aspirin** 160 to 325 mg daily and increased to 650 mg every 4 to 6 hours if necessary. Indomethacin, ibuprofen, and corticosteroids should be avoided because of the potential for wall thinning within the zone of myocardial necrosis, which may predispose to ventricular wall rupture.

3. **Dysrhythmias** are common and have multiple etiologies including CHF, ischemia, reentrant rhythms, reperfusion, acidosis, electrolyte derangements (e.g., hypokalemia, hypomagnesemia, intracellular hypercalcemia), hypoxemia, hypotension, drug effects, and heightened reflex sympathoadrenal and vagal activity. Treatment of any correctable precipitating factors is prudent. Chapter 19 discusses emergency treatment of dysrhythmias.

   a. **Ventricular fibrillation (VF).** Primary VF is an important cause of mortality within the first 24 hours of an acute MI and occurs in about 3% to 5% of patients within 4 hours of infarction. Prophylactic treatment with lidocaine may reduce the incidence of VF, but increases the mortality rate and is not recommended. β-blockers are associated with a reduction in early VF and should be used if no contraindications exist. Maintaining normal levels of potassium (>4 mEq/L) and magnesium (>2 mEq/L) may reduce dysrhythmogenic causes of VF. Specific therapies are discussed in Chapter 14.

   b. **Ventricular tachycardia (VT). Premature ventricular contractions (PVCs)** are common after MI. Prophylactic therapy is not recommended. Treatment includes correction of abnormal electrolyte levels and continued β-blocker therapy (Chapter 14).

   c. **Accelerated idioventricular rhythm** occurs in about 10% to 20% of patients after MI. It may be due to an ectopic ventricular pacer, enhanced automaticity, or variable exit block. It is generally self-limiting within 48 hours, and treatment is not recommended unless the rhythm is associated with cardiovascular instability or precipitates VT/VF. In these cases, suppression with lidocaine, atropine, or overdrive atrial pacing is indicated.

   d. **Atrial fibrillation (AF).** Up to 10% to 16% of patients will develop transient AF within 24 hours of an acute infarction. Risk factors include anterior and inferior MI, advanced age, and large infarcts. Other precipitating factors include hypoxia, electrolyte derangements, chronic lung disease, sinus nodal ischemia, and increased sympathetic activity. In patients without hemodynamic instability, β-**adrenergic blockers** (metoprolol 2.5–5 mg IV every 5 minutes to a total of 15 mg) Alternatively, **verapamil** (2.5–5 mg IV over 2 minutes, may repeat with 5–10 mg in 30 minutes, maximum dose is 20 mg) or **diltiazem** (15–20 mg IV over 2 minutes, may repeat in 15 minutes with 20–25 mg IV followed by a maintenance infusion at 5–15 mg/h) may be used if beta-blockers are contraindicated or ineffective. Given their negative inotropic effects, these agents should not be considered as the first line of therapy for patients with compromised ventricular function. **Digoxin,** 10 to 15 μg/kg lean body weight followed by a maintenance dose based on body size and renal function, may be an acceptable alternative in patients with compromised ventricular function. In hemodynamically unstable patients, **synchronized cardioversion** may be needed and is discussed in Chapter 19.

e. **Bradycardia and AV blocks.** Sinus bradycardia is common after MI and frequently is associated with increased vagal tone, inferior wall infarct, and right coronary artery reperfusion. Myocardial infarction complicated by heart block increases in-hospital mortality. **Atropine** (0.5–1 mg up to 0.04 mg/kg) is considered a first-line agent in patients with symptomatic sinus bradycardia. Atropine may be beneficial in ventricular asystole or symptomatic AV block at the AV nodal level (second-degree type 1 or third-degree with a narrow complex escape rhythm). Patients with infranodal (type 2) or bilateral bundle-branch block are at risk of developing complete heart block or asystole in the setting of atropine. **Transcutaneous or transvenous pacing** should be considered when a patient is severely symptomatic in the setting of acute MI complicated by symptomatic sinus node dysfunction, type 2 second-decree heart block, third-degree heart block, new left, right, or alternating bundle-branch block, or bifasicular block.

4. **Heart failure and cardiogenic shock.** The incidence of cardiogenic shock after MI is approximately 7.5%. Mortality is extremely high. About 40% of the ventricular myocardium must be lost for cardiogenic shock to develop; other factors such as ventricular septal rupture, acute mitral regurgitation, tamponade, and right ventricular failure may be the cause. Management may involve hemodynamic support with pressors, intraaortic balloon counterpulsation, or immediate revascularization.

5. **Hypertension** increases myocardial oxygen demand and may worsen myocardial ischemia. Causes of hypertension include premorbid hypertension, CHF, and elevated catecholamines due to pain and anxiety. Treatment includes adequate antianginal therapy and analgesia, anxiolytic therapy if indicated, and IV nitroglycerin, β-blockers, and ACEIs. Calcium-channel blockers (verapamil or diltiazem) may be indicated in patents who have contraindications to other agents. Nitroprusside may be required if hypertension is severe.

SELECTED REFERENCES

Bypass Angioplasty Revascularization Investigation (BARI) Investigators. Comparison of coronary bypass surgery with angioplasty in patients with multivessels disease. *N Engl J Med* 1996;335:217–225.

Gottlieb SS, McCarter RJ, Vogel RA. Effect of beta-blockade on mortality among high-risk and low risk patients after myocardial infarction. *N Engl J Med* 1998;339:489–497.

Hennekens CH. Update on aspirin in the treatment and prevention of cardiovascular disease. *Am Heart J* 1999;137:S9–S13.

Lange RA, Hillis, LD. Antiplatelet therapy for ischemic heart disease. *N Engl J Med* 2004;350:277–280.

Libby P, Ridker PM. Inflammation and atherosclerosis. *Circulation* 2002;105:1135–1143.

Ryan TJ, Antman EM, Brooks NH, et al. 1999 Update: ACC/AHA guidelines for the management of patients with acute myocardial infarction: executive summary and recommendations. *Circulation* 1999;100:1016–1030.

Schoebel FC, Frazier OH, Jessurun GA, et al. Refractory angina pectoris in end-stage coronary artery disease: evolving therapeutic concepts. *Am Heart J* 1997;134:587–602.

Smith SC, Dove JT, Jacobs AK, et al. ACC/AHA guidelines for percutaneous coronary intervention (revision of the 1993 PTCA guidelines). Executive summary. *Circulation* 2001;103:3019.

The Clopidogel in Unstable Angina to Prevent Recurrent Events Trial Investigators. Effects of clopidogrel in addition to aspirin in patients with acute coronary syndromes without ST-segment elevation. *N Eng J Med* 2001;345:494–502. [Errata. *N Eng J Med* 2001;345:1506, 1716.]

The Joint European Society of Cardiology/American College of Cardiology Committee. Myocardial infarction redefined. A consensus document of the Joint European Society of Cardiology/American College of Cardiology Committee for the Redefinition of Myocardial Infarction. *J Am Coll Cardiol* 2000;36:959–969.

Valvular Heart Disease

John C. Klick and Theodore A. Alston

Each of the cardiac valves is subject to malfunction. Advances in portable echocardiography permit quantitative assessment of valvular function as an aid to management of critically ill patients.

I. **Aortic stenosis (AS)** is usually **valvular** but can be **supravalvular** or **subvalvular.** Rheumatic heart disease, congenital bicuspid valve, and senile degeneration are the primary causes of valvular AS.

   A. **Pathophysiology**

   1. As the valve orifice decreases, the heart maintains stroke volume through increased pressure generation. This results in **concentric hypertrophy** of the left ventricle (LV). Critical AS eventually results in LV dysfunction with pulmonary edema, myocardial ischemia, or sudden lethal dysrhythmias.

   2. There are a number of causes of morbidity in the patient with AS:

      a. Elevated intracavitary pressures can compress the subendocardium and impair perfusion. Ischemia may be difficult to treat. **Though afterload is increased, a high aortic pressure may be required to maintain adequate coronary perfusion.**

      b. Increased LV systolic and diastolic pressures increase wall tension and so increase myocardial oxygen demand.

      c. Tachycardia or supraventricular dysrhythmias may decrease stroke volume and so cause ischemia. Atrial contraction normally contributes 20% to 25% of the total stroke volume. In severe AS, the atrial contribution increases to 30% to 40%. Thus, normal atrial contraction is essential for optimal cardiac function in patients with AS.

      d. Reduction in systemic vascular resistance (SVR) can result in hypotension that can be difficult to treat due to the inability of the heart to compensate through a fixed stenotic valve and the onset of ischemia. Yet, perhaps counterintuitively, carefully titrated nitroprusside sometimes improves cardiac output.

   B. **Signs, symptoms, and diagnosis**

   1. AS may be asymptomatic for years. Onset of symptoms indicates severe disease. The triad of angina pectoris, syncope, and congestive heart failure indicates a life expectancy of less than 5 years in untreated AS.

2. **Angina** can result from coexisting atherosclerotic coronary artery disease or from AS in isolation.
3. **Physical findings** indicative of AS include the following:
   a. A loud systolic murmur that is best heard at the base of the heart and radiates to the neck.
   b. A strong apical impulse.
   c. A slow-rising carotid upstroke.
4. The **degree of AS** is measured by echocardiography or by cardiac catheterization. **Stenosis** is graded as trace, mild, moderate, or severe. The **normal adult aortic valve area** (AVA) is 2.5 to 3.5 cm^2. Severe stenosis occurs when the AVA is less then 0.7 cm^2 or the mean systolic pressure gradient is more than 50 mm Hg.

C. **Hemodynamic changes**
1. The **systemic arterial pressure wave** typically shows a slow upstroke. The anacrotic notch occurs low in the pressure wave and the dicrotic notch is often absent.
2. The **pulmonary artery occlusion pressure (PAOP)** is increased in AS because of the elevated left ventricular end-diastolic pressure. As the disease progresses, atrial hypertrophy ensues and the mitral valve annulus widens, resulting in a prominent v-wave of mitral regurgitation.

D. **Management**
1. **Hypotension** must be treated promptly. Ischemia resulting from aortic root pressure falling below the subendocardial pressure may initiate a downward spiral of further ischemia, dysrhythmias, and hemodynamic instability. Cardiopulmonary resuscitation efforts may prove ineffective because of thickened myocardium and small valvular area.
2. **Dysrhythmias** can quickly result in unstable hemodynamics that may be refractory to pharmacologic treatment. The hypertrophic LV is highly dependent on atrial kick for adequate filling. Both **tachycardia and bradycardia** are poorly tolerated. Tachycardia may not allow enough time for proper diastolic filling. Bradycardia may overdistend the heart or not provide sufficient flow for proper perfusion. Cardiac depressants (beta-blockers, calcium-channel blockers) and cardiac stimulants (atropine, dopamine) should be used with caution. **Nodal rhythms** are poorly tolerated. Atropine (0.4 mg) may convert a slow nodal rhythm into a normal sinus rhythm. Atrial pacing may be needed.
3. **Nitroglycerin,** if needed, should be administered cautiously because high venous pressure may be required to maintain stroke volume.
4. **Pulmonary artery catheters** (PACs) can help to guide fluid balance and monitor cardiac performance. Insertion of a PAC may precipitate

dysrhythmias. A PAC with **pacing** capabilities can prove useful.

5. **Inotropic support** may be needed in severe AS. **Norepinephrine** can be helpful because of its combined intropic and vasoconstrictive effects. Milrinone and dobutamine may be useful, but they decrease systemic vascular resistance (SVR) and may decrease the aortic root pressure more than is desired. Beta-agonists carry a risk of tachydysrhythmias.

E. **Postoperative care after aortic valve replacement or commissurotomy.** Although stroke volume increases and LV end-diastolic pressure decreases following aortic valve replacement or repair, the left ventricle remains **hypertrophied** for months. Maintaining adequate coronary artery perfusion is essential, along with maintenance of sinus rhythm. After the hypertrophied myocardium has returned to a near-normal state, increased subendocardial pressures are less problematic.

F. **Hypertrophic obstructive cardiomyopathy (HOCM).** Unlike valvular AS, HOCM causes a dynamic obstruction to the forward flow of blood from the left ventricle (LV). The large muscle mass of the subaortic region causes obstruction of the LV outflow tract. The dynamic obstruction of the outflow tract is worsened by tachycardia and by low filling volumes. Management includes maintenance of a slow heart rate to allow for longer diastolic filling, adequate intravascular volume repletion, and maintenance of adequate aortic root pressure. Patients with HOCM are prone to lethal ventricular dysrhythmias.

II. **Aortic regurgitation (AR)** can be acute or chronic. Causes include rheumatic fever, syphilitic aortitis, bacterial endocarditis, aortic dissection, trauma (often blunt chest trauma), and congenital abnormalities.

A. **Pathophysiology**

1. The compensatory response to AR is increased sympathetic tone, resulting in tachycardia and increased inotropy. If this response is inadequate, congestive heart failure (CHF) ensues. In acute AR, the LV has not had time to remodel through eccentric hypertrophy (an increase in the size of the ventricular cavity and the thickness of the myocardium). Both LV end-diastolic pressure and volume (LVEDP and LVEDV) increase acutely. In addition, a reduction in systemic arterial diastolic pressure can decrease coronary perfusion pressure and so result in ischemia.

2. In **chronic AR,** elevated LVEDV results in an eccentric myocardial hypertrophy. Although the LVEDV increases, there is little change in LVEDP because of compensatory changes in LV size and muscle mass. Thus, the heart may function normally for years. In general, function remains near normal if the regurgitant fraction remains less then 40%. Symptoms often

result when the regurgitant fraction exceeds 60%. An LVEDP of greater then 20 mm Hg is a sign of poor compensation.

B. Signs, symptoms, and diagnosis

1. **Acute AR** often presents with CHF, angina, and tachycardia. **Chronic AR** may be asymptomatic for years. When symptoms (shortness of breath, palpitations, fatigue, or angina) develop, average survival without valve replacement is about 5 years.

2. **Physical findings** that are indicative of AR include the following:

   a. Widened arterial pulse pressure.

   b. Bounding peripheral pulses.

   c. Quincke's pulses (visible capillary pulsations with compression of the nail bed).

   d. Decrescendo diastolic murmur along the left sternal border.

   e. Austin-Flint murmur (an apical diastolic rumble caused by regurgitant flow impinging on the anterior mitral leaflet).

   f. Maximal cardiac impulse shifted downward and to the left.

3. The **degree of AR** depends upon the hemodynamic state (i.e., afterload, heart rate, inotropy). The echocardiographic grading system distinguishes severe, moderate, mild, and trace categories, depending on the width and height of the regurgitant jet. Jets of fluid passing through a narrow orifice exhibit a hydraulic constriction occurring just past the orifice. The width of this constriction, termed the **vena contracta** by Newton, is more than 6 mm in severe AR. In severe AR, Doppler examination shows holodiastolic flow reversal in the descending aorta.

C. Hemodynamic changes

1. The systemic arterial pulse pressure often is widened, with a very rapid upstroke due to the large stroke volume.

2. A rapid descent of the arterial pressure waveform results from the rapid flow of blood back into the LV.

3. The PAOP may exhibit prominent v-waves because of LV volume overload and accompanying mitral regurgitation. The PAOP may underestimate the LVEDP because the aortic regurgitant jet causes premature closure of the mitral valve.

D. Management

1. **Afterload reduction,** an **increased heart rate** (to decrease filling time and thus decrease LVEDV) and **inotropic support** are keys to acute management. Urgent surgical intervention may be necessary.

2. Echocardiography can be useful in guiding therapy. Echo imaging reveals dynamic changes in the regurgitant jet, inotropic state, and LV filling.

3. **Dobutamine** often is the inotrope of choice for patients with AR. It increases contractility, reduces peripheral resistance, and maintains a relatively

rapid heart rate. Milrinone also provides inotropic support and afterload reduction, but with less increase in heart rate.

E. **Postoperative care after aortic valve repair or replacement for AR**
   1. Because of persistent cardiomegaly in patients with longstanding AR, adequate ventricular filling remains essential for good cardiac function.
   2. Inotropic support may be required postoperatively.
   3. An intraaortic balloon pump (IABP) is contraindicated in patients with AR prior to valve replacement. The IABP augments aortic diastolic pressure and therefore worsens the regurgitation. However, the device may provide support after valve replacement.

III. **Mitral stenosis (MS)**
   A. **Pathophysiology. Rheumatic fever** results in scarring and calcification of the edges of the valve leaflets, with eventual fibrosis of the commissures. Patients with rheumatic heart disease can remain asymptomatic for years. When symptoms appear, there is a 20% chance of death within the first year. **Senile calcification** is another mechanism of MS and may begin with calcification of the valvular annulus.
   B. **Signs, symptoms, and diagnosis**
      1. **Symptoms** usually first present during exercise or other high-output states. Inactive patients may present upon the onset of atrial fibrillation or flutter caused by atrial distention.
      2. Patients complain of dyspnea, palpitations, fatigue, chest pain, and paroxysmal nocturnal dyspnea. Some patients develop hoarseness due to the compression of the left recurrent laryngeal nerve by the dilated left pulmonary artery or left atrium. Patients can also present with hemoptysis because of high pulmonary venous pressures.
      3. **Atrial fibrillation** may trigger CHF due to decreased diastolic filling time and increased left arterial pressure (LAP).
      4. An **echocardiogram** confirms the diagnosis of MS. The mitral valve area (MVA) is inversely proportional to the pressure half-time (PHT), where PHT is the time for the Doppler peak velocity across the valve to decline by 30%. MVA (cm^2) equals 220 divided by PHT (msec). A PHT longer than 220 msec indicates severe stenosis (MVA <1 cm^2).
      5. **Physical findings** that are indicative of MS include the following:
         a. A loud S_1 heart sound on auscultation.
         b. A presystolic or mid-diastolic rumble.
         c. A prominent jugular a-wave.
   C. The **degree of MS** can be assessed by echocardiography or angiography.
      1. The area of the normal mitral valve is 4.0 to 6.0 cm^2.
      2. Patients with **moderate MS** (1.5–2.5 cm^2) often only show symptoms with increased cardiac demand.

Symptoms (dyspnea, fatigue) are related to increased LAP.

3. Critical MS is defined as a valve area of less than 1.0 cm^2. Patients with critical MS are often asymptomatic at rest but tolerate exercise poorly. Increased pulmonary vascular pressures can precipitate pulmonary edema.

D. Hemodynamic changes

1. The PAOP is increased and may not accurately reflect LVEDP.

2. The PAOP waveform can exhibit a large a-wave if normal sinus rhythm is present. Because MS often is associated with some degree of mitral regurgitation, large v-waves may also be present.

3. **Pulmonary hypertension** is common. Because of the increased PA pressures and decreased PA compliance, there is increased risk of PA rupture with inflation of the balloon of a PAC. Severe pulmonary hypertension can lead to RV failure (cor pulmonale).

E. Management

1. **Adequate preload** is essential for good cardiac function. Flow across the mitral valve is dependent on elevated left atrial pressures. This requirement must be balanced with the propensity of patients with MS to develop CHF. No specific PAOP is universally correct. Parameters used to gauge optimum preload for a given patient include signs and symptoms of organ perfusion, oxygenation, and CHF.

2. A **slow heart rate** facilitates LV filling. Because blood flow across the MV occurs during diastole, a heart rate that is too fast does not allow enough time for proper filling. This consideration must be balanced with the fact that too slow a heart rate will reduce cardiac output. The goal is a heart rate that maintains adequate organ perfusion in the absence of CHF.

3. If AV pacing is required, a long PR interval (0.2 seconds) will allow more time for blood to flow across the mitral valve.

4. Patients with MS may need **inotropic support.** Digoxin is commonly used in these patients because it has both negative chronotropic and positive inotropic effects. If more aggressive inotropic support is needed, drugs without positive chronotropy (such as milrinone) may be useful.

5. **Supraventricular dysrhythmias** that are hemodynamically significant (i.e., cause a decrease in blood pressure) must be treated aggressively, usually with electrocardioversion. Many clinicians suggest starting with high energy (i.e., 200 J monophasic or equivalent biphasic). Cardiopulmonary resuscitation is often ineffective in the setting of a stenotic mitral valve.

6. **Percutaneous balloon valvuloplasty** can greatly relieve stenosis without need for postoperative

anticoagulation. The best candidates have no left atrial thrombus, mild or no mitral regurgitation (MR), and low echocardiographic scores for leaflet immobility, valvular thickening, subvalvular thickening, and valvular calcification. MR is not improved, and there is an increased risk of severe MR after balloon valvuloplasty.

F. **Postoperative care after mitral valve replacement or commissurotomy**
   1. **Preload augmentation** is often needed in the postoperative period. Stroke volume, PAOP, and TEE can guide proper fluid replacement.
   2. **Afterload reduction** can improve hemodynamics postoperatively, although preoperatively it has little effect due to the fixed stenosis.
   3. **Inotropic support** may be required following valve repair or replacement because of an underlying decrease in LV function caused by chronic underfilling of the ventricle.
   4. **Chronic atrial fibrillation** is common in patients with long-standing MS. The use of amiodarone, procainamide, or overdrive pacing may be necessary.
   5. If there is a sudden decrease in blood pressure following MV repair or replacement, one should consider the very rare possibilities of atrioventricular disruption or (in the case of valve replacement) a valve that is caught in the closed position. Both processes are emergencies that often require surgery at the bedside.

IV. **Mitral regurgitation**
   A. **Pathophysiology.** The etiology of MR can be rheumatic or nonrheumatic.
      1. **Rheumatic MR** often occurs concomitantly with MS. Like MS, the asymptomatic period can last for years.
      2. **Nonrheumatic MR** can be caused by papillary muscle dysfunction (often seen in patients with posterior septal or anterior septal ischemia or infarction), bacterial endocarditis, or ruptured cordae tendinae.
      3. **Acute MR** occurs when there is a sudden backflow of blood across the mitral valve into the left atrium. This results in a sudden volume overload of the atrium, causing increased pulmonary vascular pressures and often CHF. The compensatory response of increased sympathetic output results in tachycardia and increased inotropy. The increased LV volume can lead to annular dilation of the MV and worsen the amount of regurgitation. **Myocardial ischemia** may occur because of increased myocardial oxygen demand (due to increased sympathetic output) and increased LVEDP.
      4. **Chronic MR** differs from acute MR in that there is time for the LV to compensate for the increased

volume load. Adaptations include eccentric hypertrophy of the LV, which causes the heart to dilate and allows a relatively constant LVEDP despite a greatly increased LVEDV. The left atrium enlarges and may maintain a normal pressure. In the late stage of the compensatory process, the dilation of the LV may lead to dilation of the mitral annulus and thus increased MR. The LV ejection fraction often remains normal, but forward flow may decrease. When the regurgitant fraction exceeds 60%, the likelihood of congestive heart failure increases dramatically. A decreasing ejection fraction (<50%) indicates failing LV function. In the final stages of chronic MR, the increased pulmonary pressures can precipitate right ventricular (RV) failure (cor pulmonale).

B. Signs, symptoms, and diagnosis

1. **Acute MR** often presents as sudden dyspnea, fatigue, or acute CHF. Patients may suffer palpitations because of atrial fibrillation. Some develop chest pain. **Chronic MR** may remain asymptomatic for years, but the onset of symptoms usually indicates a rapid downward course. Patients may present with dyspnea, fatigue, CHF, or atrial fibrillation.

2. The **physical examination** can aid in the diagnosis of MR. Physical findings that are indicative of MR include the following:

   a. A hyperdynamic apex with or without an apical lift or thrill.

   b. A holosystolic murmur best heard at the apex (that may radiate to the left axilla).

   c. Rarely, a mid-systolic rumble.

3. The grade of MR depends on the hemodynamic state (i.e., afterload, heart rate, and inotropy). When evaluating MR with echocardiography, many physicians use the grading system of severe, moderate, mild, and trace, depending on the width and height of the regurgitant jet.

4. **Echocardiography.** Two-dimensional echocardiography may visualize flail leaflet or ruptured papillary muscle. In severe MR, Doppler can reveal systolic flow reversal in pulmonary veins. The flow reversal may not be observed if the jet of MR is not directed toward the pulmonary vein under examination. A color jet reaching the posterior wall of the left atrium or comprising more than 40% of the LA indicates severe MR. The narrow portion of the base of the jet is the vena contracta. A vena contracta width of more than 6.5 mm indicates severe regurgitation. The LA may be enlarged to a diameter of more than 5.5 cm.

C. Hemodynamic changes

1. The PAOP waveform is characterized by giant v-waves. The size of the v-wave depends on the compliance of the LA and pulmonary vasculature and may not reflect the amount of regurgitation.

2. The giant *v*-waves can make the PAOP difficult to differentiate from the PAP waveform. A helpful sign is that the peak of the pressure waveform shifts to the right, compared to the systemic arterial waveform, when the PA balloon is inflated and a PAOP tracing is obtained.

D. Management

1. The **heart rate** should be kept in a normal to high-normal range. A slow heart rate can cause volume overload of the LV.

2. **Maintenance of adequate LV preload** must be weighed against the possibility that excess LV volume may dilate the mitral annulus and make the severity of the regurgitation worse.

3. **Afterload reduction** is often necessary. A decreased peripheral resistance increases the forward ejection of the stroke volume. In patients with coronary artery disease and MR, nitroglycerin may be a reasonable intervention, achieving coronary vasodilation and some afterload reduction. Calcium-channel blockers have also been used.

4. **Inotropic agents** can increase forward flow. Dobutamine and milrinone increase contractility and can beneficially decrease afterload.

5. **Pulmonary hypertension** develops in severe cases of MR and can lead to right heart failure. In fragile patients, it is prudent to avoid further increasing PA pressures (i.e., avoid hypoxia, hypercarbia, and acidosis). Prostaglandin E_1, prostacyclin, or inhaled nitric oxide may be beneficial in patients with right heart failure. Intraaortic balloon counterpulsation may be life saving.

E. Postoperative care after mitral valve repair or replacement for mitral regurgitation

1. After repair of MR, the entire stroke volume is ejected into the aorta. The LV may fail because of the increased afterload.

2. **Inotropic support** is often needed. In severe cases, intraaortic balloon counterpulsation may be necessary to augment forward flow and coronary perfusion.

3. **Atrial fibrillation** is not well tolerated postoperatively. Every attempt should be made to maintain normal sinus rhythm. Antidysrhythmics (such as procainamide or amiodarone) or overdrive atrial pacing may be necessary.

4. **Transesophageal echocardiography** can be useful for determining valvular function and LV performance.

V. Tricuspid stenosis

A. Pathophysiology. The occurrence of tricuspid stenosis (TS) is rare compared to the previously mentioned valvular lesions. Patients with TS often have associated MS. Tricuspid stenosis is most often caused by rheumatic fever, carcinoid syndrome, systemic lupus erythematosus, or endomyocardial fibroelastosis. There is generally a long asymptomatic period. As TS worsens, flow across the valve decreases, and right atrial size and pressures increase. Atrial tachydysrhythmias are common.

B. Signs, symptoms, and diagnosis

1. TS can cause peripheral edema, jugular venous distention, ascites, hepatomegaly, and hepatic dysfunction, all secondary to elevated right atrial pressures. As is the case with MS and AS, symptoms of fatigue with exercise may be the presenting complaint. In addition, patients may first present with palpitations caused by supraventricular dysrhythmias.

2. Physical findings indicative of TS include the following:

   a. A holosystolic murmur that is best heard at the left sternal border. The murmur often becomes louder during inspiration.

   b. A right ventricular heave.

   c. Associated murmurs of other valvular abnormalities.

   d. Hepatic pulsations, ascites, and peripheral cyanosis in severe cases.

3. The normal area of the tricuspid valve is 7 to 9 cm^2. Tricuspid stenosis is considered significant when the valve area decreases to 1.5 cm^2. The normal tricuspid gradient is 1 mm Hg. A gradient as small as 3 mm Hg indicates a moderate stenosis, whereas a gradient of 5 mm Hg is severe.

C. Hemodynamic changes

1. A large a-wave is evident on the central venous pressure (CVP) waveform. This corresponds to the right atrium contracting against a high-resistance orifice.

2. Central venous pressure may be increased due to systemic volume overload.

D. Management

1. A **slow normal heart rate** is essential to allow sufficient diastolic filling of the RV.

2. **Tachydysrhythmias** can decrease cardiac output and increase central venous pressure.

3. **Adequate preload** is essential for forward flow. However, care must be taken not to overfill the right atrium because this will stretch the right atrium and predispose to supraventricular tachydysrhythmias.

4. Although reducing RV afterload and increasing contractility will not directly affect the degree of TS, these maneuvers may help to maintain cardiac output.

E. Postoperative care after tricuspid valve replacement or repair for stenosis

1. The patient may have right-sided dysfunction because of the chronically underfilled RV. Afterload reduction and inotropic support may be needed.

2. Avoiding increased pulmonary artery pressures is essential. Prostacyclin, prostaglandin E_1, or inhaled nitric oxide may reduce PA pressure, thereby reducing RV afterload.

3. **Tachydysrhythmias** should be avoided. Antidysrhythmics such as procainamide or amiodarone may be necessary.

4. Because of the prosthetic valve, the patients are often managed without a PA line. If a PAC is deemed necessary, then it must be placed surgically when a nontissue prosthesis is implanted. Alternatively, a surgically placed LA line may be used.

VI. Tricuspid regurgitation (TR)

A. Pathophysiology

1. TR usually accompanies other valvular lesions such as MS or AS. Rarely, isolated TR may be caused by endocarditis, chest trauma, or carcinoid syndrome.

2. TR results in volume overload of the atrium and increased pressure within the systemic venous system. Isolated TR can be well tolerated. When TR is due to pulmonary hypertension from valvular abnormalities or LV dysfunction, the ability to compensate is poor.

B. Signs, symptoms and diagnosis

1. The increased volume load in the RA can distend the atrium and cause **atrial fibrillation.**

2. **Physical findings** that are indicative of TR include the following:
   a. An S_3 gallop (accentuated by inspiration).
   b. A systolic murmur that increases during inspiration.
   c. An accentuated P_2 heart sound.

3. Doppler evidence of systolic flow reversal in hepatic veins is evidence of severe TR. Echocardiography may reveal an annulus diameter of greater than 4 cm or a regurgitant jet covering more than 30% of the right atrial area.

C. Hemodynamic changes

1. The **central venous pressure** may be normal or increased in TR.

2. The CVP waveform may exhibit giant *v*-waves, corresponding to the large regurgitant jet during right ventricular systole. The size of the *v*-wave depends in part on the compliance of the right atrium and does not simply correspond to the size of the regurgitant volume.

D. Management

1. **A high heart rate** helps to minimize peripheral congestion and RV volume overload while increasing forward flow from the RV.

2. **Atrial fibrillation** is common. Hemodynamic parameters nearly always improve if a sinus rhythm can be achieved.

3. **Adequate preload** is essential for forward flow. Decreased RV filling can severely limit cardiac output.
4. **Minimizing pulmonary vascular resistance** (i.e., avoiding hypoxemia, hypertension, and acidosis) will aid forward flow.
5. **Inotropic support** of the failing RV can be useful in TR. Dobutamine and milrinone are examples of drugs that provide increased inotropy but do not greatly increase PA pressures. Agents that decrease PA pressures (e.g., prostaglandin E_1, prostacyclin, and inhaled nitric oxide) may be helpful when used in conjunction with inotropic medications.

E. **Postoperative care after tricuspid valve replacement or repair of TR**
1. Because the TR is no longer present to provide a "pop off" and limit RV pressure, the pressure load of the RV can be acutely increased after tricuspid valve repair. RV dysfunction may occur, and inotropic support may be necessary.

VII. **Pulmonic valve disease**
A. **Congenital pulmonic stenosis** presents as right heart failure. **Acquired pulmonic stenosis** is rare.
B. **Pulmonic regurgitation** is well tolerated as long as right ventricular function is adequate. Acquired pulmonic regurgitation can result from infective endocarditis or rheumatic heart disease. Operative intervention in pulmonic regurgitation due to endocarditis generally consists in excision of the affected valve without replacement by a prosthetic device.

VIII. **Endocarditis.** Bacteremia can seed both native and prosthetic valves. Bacterial endocarditis induces metaplasia of the endothelial cells, which then lose contact with each other. Collagen fibers are removed, resulting in large cavities. Localized hyperplasia results in the development of valvular vegetations that can often be visualized by echocardiography. The vegetations may result in regurgitant valvular pathology. Endocarditis can lead to papillary muscle rupture, the result of which is abrupt severe mitral valve incompetence. The microbiology, manifestations, complications, diagnosis, and management of infective endocarditis are reviewed in detail in Chapter 28.

IX. **Antibiotic prophylaxis against bacterial endocarditis.** Transient bacteremia following invasive procedures, surgery, and dental procedures can lead to valvular endocarditis. Blood-borne bacteria lodge on damaged or abnormal tissues. Antibiotic prophylaxis is recommended for patients with prosthetic cardiac valves, a previous history of endocarditis, most congenital malformations, rheumatic heart disease, hypertrophic cardiomyopathy, and mitral regurgitation. Prophylaxis is not prompted by permanent pacemakers, implantable defibrillators, or mitral valve prolapse without regurgitation. Transesophageal echo studies are not associated with bacteremia. The American Heart Association recommendations for antibiotic prophylaxis vary according to the procedure being performed. Dental, oral, respiratory tract, or esophageal procedures should be covered with oral amoxicillin or intravenous ampicillin. Clindamycin is a good alternative for penicillin-allergic patients. Endocarditis prophylaxis for genitourinary or gastrointestinal procedures includes ampicillin plus gentamicin. Vancomycin can be substituted for ampicillin in penicillin-allergic patients.

SELECTED REFERENCES

Abaci A, Oguzhan A, Unal S, et al. Application of the vena contracta method for the calculation of the mitral valve area in mitral stenosis. *Cardiology* 2002;98:50–59.

Buffington CW, Nystrom EUM. Neither the accuracy nor the precision of thermal dilution cardiac output measurements is altered by acute tricuspid regurgitation in pigs. *Anesth Analg* 2004;98: 884–890.

Dajani AS, Taubert KA, Wilson W, et al. Prevention of bacterial endocarditis: recommendations by the American Heart Association. *Circulation* 1997;96:358–366.

Khot UN, Novaro GM, Popovic GC, et al. Nitroprusside in critically ill patients with left ventricular dysfunction and aortic stenosis. *N Engl J Med* 2003;348:1756–1763.

Krishnagopalan S, Kumar A, Parrillo JE, et al. Myocardial dysfunction in the patient with sepsis. *Curr Opin Crit Care* 2002;8:376–388.

Levine RA, Vlahakes GJ, Lefebvre X, et al. Papillary muscle displacement causes systolic anterior motion of the mitral valve. Experimental validation and insights into the mechanism of subaortic obstruction. *Circulation* 1995;91:1189–1195.

Oh JK, Seward JB, Tajik AJ. *The echo manual,* 2nd ed. Philadelphia: Lippincott Williams & Wilkins, 1999.

Palacios IF, Sanchez PL, Harrell LC, et al. Which patients benefit from percutaneous mitral balloon valvuloplasty? Prevalvuloplasty and postvalvuloplasty variables that predict long-term outcome. *Circulation* 2002;105:1465–1471.

Quere JP, Tribouilloy C, Enriquez-Sarano M. Vena contracta width measurement: theoretic basis and usefulness in the assessment of valvular regurgitation severity. *Curr Cardiol Rep* 2003;5:110–115.

Yoerger DM, Weyman AE. Hypertrophic obstructive cardiomyopathy: mechanism of obstruction and response to therapy. *Rev Cardiovasc Med* 2003;4:199–215.

Cardiac Dysrhythmias

Harish Lecamwasam and Jagmeet Singh

I. **Epidemiology**
   A. Dysrhythmias of both supraventricular and ventricular origin are common in critically ill patients. Of the two, supraventricular dysrhythmias occur more frequently.
   B. Of all perioperative dysrhythmias, postoperative **atrial fibrillation (AF)** is the most intensely studied, given its high incidence (10%–65%) and associated morbidity.

II. **Clinical significance**
   Perioperative dysrhythmias are associated with increased mortality, cardiac and noncardiac morbidity (primarily neurologic and pulmonary), and utilization of resources in terms of increases in intensive care unit (ICU) days, ICU readmissions, and hospital stay.

III. **Classification.** Types of dysrhythmia can be essentially divided into **stable** and **unstable.**
   A. **Unstable dysrhythmias** are defined by the presence of hemodynamic instability (hypotension, myocardial ischemia, congestive failure, etc.) or cerebral hypoperfusion (syncope, altered mental status) in conjunction with dysrhythmia.
   B. **Stable dysrhythmias** can be subclassified by considering the following factors:
      1. Rate (bradydysrhythmias vs. tachydysrhythmias).
      2. Presence or absence of P waves.
      3. Relationship of P waves to the QRS complex.
      4. Width of the QRS complex (narrow vs. wide).
      5. Regularity of the QRS complex (regular vs. irregular).

IV. **Bradydysrhythmias**
   A. **Classification**
      1. **Sinus node dysfunction**
         a. Describes a host of bradycardic dysrhythmias involving the sinus node, including sinus bradycardia, sinus pauses, and the tachycardia-bradycardia syndrome.
         b. Risk factors include advanced age and structural heart disease.
         c. Frequently associated with a malignant course involving progressive nodal dysfunction.
         d. One of the most common causes of permanent pacemaker placement in the United States.
      2. **Atrioventricular (AV) nodal dysfunction**
         a. **First-degree AV block**
            (1) Characterized by a PR interval exceeding 200 msec (normal 120–200 msec).
            (2) Typically a benign condition unless associated with another form of conduction disease or problems with AV synchrony.

b. Second-degree AV block
  (1) Mobitz type 1 (Wenckebach)
    i. Characterized by a progressive widening of the PR interval with a subsequently non-conducted P wave (i.e., nonconducted atrial contraction).
    ii. Disease is typically high in the AV node.
  (2) Mobitz type 2
    i. Characterized by a fixed, normal PR interval with episodic nonconducted P waves.
    ii. Disease is typically lower in the AV node or bundle of His.
  (3) Differentiation between Mobitz types 1 and 2 cannot be made if AV block is 2:1. This is important because the risk of proceeding to a complete heart block is higher with a Mobitz type 2 block.
c. Third-degree AV block (complete heart block):
  (1) Nonconductance of P waves across the AV node and complete AV dissociation.
  (2) Can be associated with a junctional or ventricular escape.
  (3) Presence of a junctional escape (typical rate 40–50 beats per minute [bpm]) suggests disease high up in the AV node. Presence of a ventricular escape (typical rate 30–40 bpm) suggests disease is lower down in the conduction pathway.
d. Fascicular blocks
  (1) The conduction system is comprised of the sinoatrial (SA) node, the AV node, the bundle of His, and the left and right bundle branches. The left bundle branch divides into the anterior and posterior fascicles.
  (2) A bifascicular block is defined as a right-bundle-branch block (RBBB) in conjunction with either a left anterior or a left posterior hemiblock.
  (3) A trifascicular block is defined as a bifascicular block in conjunction with a first-degree AV block.
B. Etiopathogenesis of bradydysrhythmias can be divided into intrinsic and extrinsic causes.
  1. Common intrinsic causes seen in the critically ill patient include degenerative (sinus node dysfunction) and ischemia/infarction.
    a. The SA node and AV node are predominantly supplied by the right coronary circulation.
    b. The His-Purkinje system is predominantly supplied by the left coronary circulation.
    c. Therefore, right coronary disease is more commonly associated with SA or AV nodal aberrancies, whereas left coronary disease is more commonly associated with bundle-branch blocks.

2. Common extrinsic causes seen in critically ill patients include neurocardiogenic causes (e.g., vagal response to intubation or tracheal suctioning, imbalance of sympathetic/parasympathetic tone postoperatively or related to sepsis or the systemic inflammatory response), medications, hypothermia, electrolyte imbalances, infection (endocarditis/myocarditis), and trauma (e.g., iatrogenic due to valvular surgery or central venous catheter placement). The incidence of causing a RBBB while placing a pulmonary artery catheter has been estimated at 3%. Therefore, it is recommended that back-up ventricular pacing be available when placing a pulmonary artery catheter in a patient with a preexisting left-bundle-branch block (LBBB).

C. Treatment options include:
   1. Correction of an underlying disorder.
   2. Observation, if the patient is "stable."
   3. Temporary or permanent pacing.
      a. Pacing modalities include epicardial, transvenous (directly or through a pulmonary artery catheter), transesophageal, and transcutaneous. Transvenous approaches are preferred and most practical.
      b. Transesophageal pacing typically enables only atrial capture. Therefore, this modality should not be used in patients with AV conduction aberrancies.
      c. Transcutaneous pacing enables ventricular capture. Loss of AV synchrony can be associated with hypotension. This modality is also associated with significant discomfort in an awake patient.
      d. Thresholds can be affected by multiple factors in the critically ill including myocardial ischemia or infarction, hypothermia, electrolyte imbalances, medications, and defibrillation/cardioversion events.
      e. There has been some debate over whether ventricular pacing or dual chamber (physiologic AV) pacing is preferable in patients with sinus nodal dysfunction. The most recent evidence suggests that physiologic pacing is superior by lowering risk of progression to atrial fibrillation, reducing hospital admissions for congestive failure, and improving quality-of-life scores.

V. Tachydysrhythmias
   A. Etiopathogenesis is related to a complex interaction between preexisting pathology (ischemia, scar, etc.), triggering factors (premature beats, high sympathetic tone, etc.), and aggravating factors (atrial stretch, trauma, etc.).
   B. Classification
      1. Narrow QRS complex, regular rhythm
         a. Sinus tachycardia.

b. Sinus nodal reentry
   (1) P-wave morphology is similar to sinus origin with heart rates usually not greater than 160 beats per minute (bpm).
   (2) Can be differentiated from sinus tachycardia by abrupt onset and termination, suggestive of a reentrant circuit. It is frequently set off by atrial extra stimuli.
   (3) Responsive to calcium-channel blockers.
c. Ectopic atrial tachycardia (AT)
   (1) Consequence of an ectopic atrial focus with enhanced automaticity that overdrives the sinus node. The atrial rate is regular and typically is between 100 and 200 bpm. The ventricular rate may vary depending on the presence of a concomitant AV nodal block.
   (2) P-wave morphology is dependent on the origin of the ectopic focus. The PR interval is dependent on the rate, and the QRS morphology is dictated by normal conduction or aberrancy.
   (3) Common causes of atrial tachycardia include increased sympathetic tone, pulmonary disease, coronary artery disease, hypoxia, and electrolyte imbalances. One of the most common causes of paroxysmal atrial tachycardia with block is **digoxin toxicity.**
   (4) **Treatment is** directed at the etiology. **Heart-rate-controlling agents** such as β-blockers and **calcium-channel antagonists** may be used to slow the ventricular rate. **Digoxin** is typically less efficacious in settings associated with high sympathetic tone as frequently seen in the critically ill. Alternate agents such as **procainamide, sotalol,** and **amiodarone** may be used for resistant tachycardias. Catheter ablation can be employed in situations where medical treatment is ineffective, contraindicated, or refused.
d. Atrial flutter
   (1) The most common form is classified as type I atrial flutter and involves a reentrant loop within the right atrium, moving in a counterclockwise direction.
   (2) It is classically associated with an atrial rate of 300 bpm with 2:1 AV block, producing a ventricular rate of 150 bpm. A saw-toothed pattern is characteristic of typical atrial flutter (see Fig. 19-1).
   (3) **Therapy** is similar to that for atrial fibrillation (section **V.2.b(9)**). Direct current (DC) cardioversion should be attempted in the setting of clinical instability.
      i. A clear role for anticoagulation with atrial flutter is not established. However,

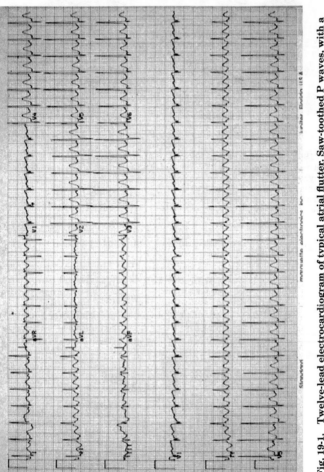

Fig. 19-1. Twelve-lead electrocardiogram of typical atrial flutter. Saw-toothed P waves, with a ventricular rate of 150 beats/min.

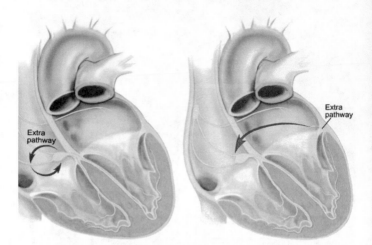

Fig. 19-2. Schematic representation of (A) atrioventricular nodal reentrant tachycardia (AVNRT) and (B) atrioventricular reentrant tachycardia (AVRT). Panel B shows the presence of an accessory pathway along the left lateral wall. (From Wang PJ and Estes M. Supraventricular tachycardia. *Circulation* 2002;106:e206–e208. With permission.)

given the frequent coexistence of atrial fibrillation, anticoagulation should be considered.

    ii. In certain circumstances (e.g., in patients with implanted pacemakers), overdrive pacetermination may be attempted. Radiofrequency catheter ablation can also be attempted as a definitive cure for both typical and atypical forms of atrial flutter.

e. AV nodal reentrant tachycardia (AVNRT)

    (1) Typical

        i. Associated with conduction down a slow anterograde limb and up the fast retrograde limb (see Fig. 19-2A).

        ii. Resulting atrial and ventricular activation times are such that P waves are typically buried within the QRS complex (see Fig. 19-3). Often the retrograde P waves can produce a "pseudo R-wave" pattern in lead V1.

    (2) Atypical

        i. Associated with conduction down the fast anterograde limb and up the slow retrograde limb.

        ii. Resulting atrial and ventricular activation times are such that P waves typically precede each QRS complex. However, because the atria are depolarized from the AV node upward (as opposed to the normal SA node downward), atypical AVNRT

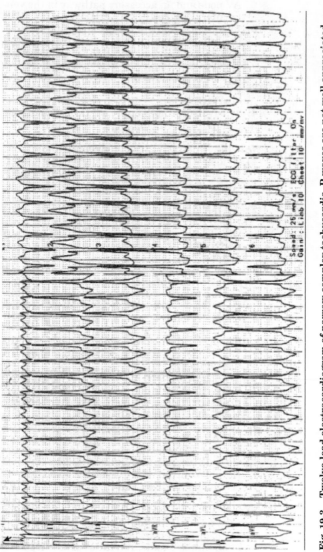
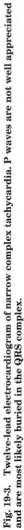

Speed : 25 mm/s ECG filter : On
Gain : Limb 10 Chest 10 mm/mv

Fig. 19-3. Twelve-lead electrocardiogram of narrow complex tachycardia. P waves are not well appreciated and are most likely buried in the QRS complex.

is associated with inverted P waves in the inferior leads.

f. **Orthodromic AV reentrant rhythm (AVRT)**

  (1) Associated with a reentrant loop involving the AV node and an accessory pathway in the ventricular wall (see Fig. 19-2B).

  (2) Results in a narrow complex rhythm because the anterograde limb of the reentrant loop involves the AV node and His-Purkinje system (as opposed to an *antidromic* AVRT described in section **V.B.3.b**).

  (3) Abrupt onset is usually suggestive of AVNRT or AVRT.

  (4) The Valsalva maneuver or carotid massage can be used to diagnose (and/or treat) AV nodal-dependent tachycardias.

g. **Wolf-Parkinson-White (WPW) syndrome**

  (1) Evidence of preexcitation (shortened PR interval and delta wave) on the electrocardiogram (ECG) may indicate the presence of an accessory pathway (see Fig. 19-4).

  (2) AV nodal blockade with WPW may facilitate rapid conduction down the accessory pathway. Therefore, cardioversion/defibrillation capability should be available whenever a nodal agent is used in the treatment of a tachycardia with a possible preexcitation syndrome.

h. **AV junctional tachycardia**

  (1) Occurs from increased automaticity of the AV node, and is characterized by heart rates of 60 to 120 bpm.

  (2) Inciting factors include digoxin toxicity, increased catecholamine levels, myocarditis, electrolyte imbalances, and trauma (post cardiac surgery).

  (3) The characteristic ECG shows retrograde P waves in the inferior leads. The QRS complex, although typically narrow, may occasionally be wide from concomitant aberrancy.

  (4) In certain circumstances, as with the isorhythmic AV dissociation seen with inhalation anesthesia, a junctional tachycardia may coexist with AV dissociation from competitive activation of both SA and AV nodes. Here the relationship between the P waves and the QRS complex may vary.

  (5) Typically, AV junctional tachycardias are benign and self-limited. Therapy involves treatment of triggering factors and/or withdrawal of offending agents. **Atrial overdrive** pacing may suppress a junctional focus, and allow the sinus node to regain control of conduction and normalize AV synchrony. **Phenytoin, lidocaine,** and **β-adrenergic antagonists** may also be of benefit.

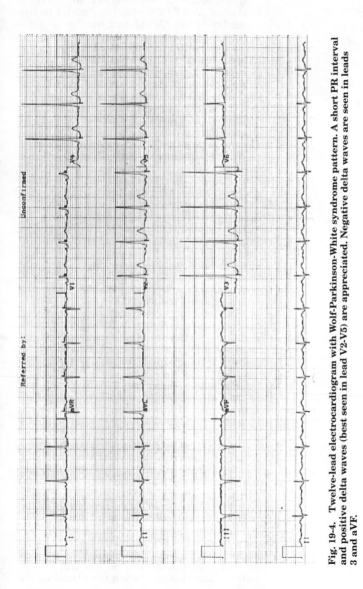

Fig. 19-4. Twelve-lead electrocardiogram with Wolf-Parkinson-White syndrome pattern. A short PR interval and positive delta waves (best seen in lead V2-V5) are appreciated. Negative delta waves are seen in leads 3 and aVF.

       i. Incidence. Among supraventricular tachycardias in the general population, the incidence of AVNRT (50%–60%) is higher than that of AVRT (30%–40%) and atrial tachycardia (10%). Atrial tachycardia is relatively more common in the critically ill.

2. Narrow QRS complex, irregular rhythm

  a. Multifocal atrial tachycardia (MAT)

    (1) Narrow complex, irregular tachycardia exhibiting at least three separate P waveforms and associated PR intervals.

    (2) A similar rhythm with heart rate less than 100 bpm is termed a **wandering atrial pacemaker.**

    (3) Commonly seen in patients with chronic obstructive pulmonary disease or congestive failure.

    (4) **Treatment** is similar to that for ectopic atrial tachycardia (section **V.B.1.c**).

  b. AF

    (1) The reported incidence of postoperative AF varies between 10% and 65%, with a recent large meta-analysis describing an incidence of 26.5%.

    (2) Risk factors include male gender, old age, history of prior AF, structural heart disease, hypertension, chronic obstructive lung disease, type of surgery (i.e., surgery involving cardiac valves, coronary bypass surgery, thoracic surgery, etc.), withdrawal of medications (β-blockers, angiotensin-converting-enzyme inhibitors, nonsteroidal antiinflammatory agents), and prolonged mechanical ventilation.

    (3) Postoperative AF can result from alteration in the atrial myocyte conduction velocity or refractory period due to atrial trauma, stretch, or ischemia. Hypoxia, electrolyte imbalances, or increased sympathetic nervous system activity may trigger AF.

    (4) Recent evidence also supports the activation of foci within the pulmonary veins or, less commonly, in the right atrium as playing a pivotal role in the genesis of AF.

    (5) Regardless, the final common pathway in the pathogenesis of AF is the formation of multicircuit reentrant loops within the atria.

    (6) Significant (50%–75%) reductions in the rate of postoperative AF have been demonstrated by using β-blockers, sotalol, and oral or parenteral amiodarone during the perioperative period.

    (7) Classification

       i. Lone AF is AF without structural heart disease or hypertension. In patients of age less than 60 years, lone AF is associated with a benign prognosis.

ii. Recurrent or paroxysmal AF.

iii. Persistent AF is characterized as AF persisting for greater than 1 week.

(8) Greater than 50% of AF episodes will spontaneously convert to sinus rhythm within 24 hours. After 24 hours, the incidence of spontaneous conversion to sinus rhythm declines precipitously. The rate of spontaneous conversion of persistent AF is negligible.

(9) Treatment options include electrical or pharmacologic therapy.

   i. Electrical

   (a) Synchronized cardioversion is indicated if a patient is unstable.

   (b) Cardioversion can begin at 50 J and escalate as needed (maximum 360 J with monophasic devices or 150 J with biphasic devices). The lowest possible energy is preferred to minimize myocardial injury.

   (c) Risk factors for poor response to cardioversion include presence of high sympathetic tone, critical illness, a large left atrium, and history of chronic dysrhythmia.

   ii. Pharmacologic therapy specific to AF can be divided into three components.

   (a) Anticoagulation.

   (b) Heart rate control.

   (c) Rhythm control.

   iii. Cardioversion without anticoagulation for rhythm control can be performed in a stable patient if the duration of AF is less than 48 hours.

   iv. Cardioversion without anticoagulation for AF exceeding 48 hours is associated with an increased risk of thromboembolic complications.

   v. If elective cardioversion is planned in a patient with AF of unknown or greater than 48-hour duration, evidence supports either:

   (a) Ruling out the presence of atrial thromboses by transesophageal echocardiography, systemic heparin therapy with target activated partial thromboplastin time (aPTT) 1.5 to 2.5 times control, and post-cardioversion warfarin therapy with target International Normalized Ratio (INR) 2 to 3 for 3 to 4 weeks.

   (b) Pre-cardioversion warfarin therapy with target INR 2 to 3 for

3 to 4 weeks followed by post-cardioversion warfarin therapy with similar INR target for 3 to 4 weeks.

vi. Controversy exists regarding the relative benefit or rhythm control over heart rate control in specific populations.

(a) Rate control appears to *not be inferior* to rhythm control in elderly patients with recurrent or persistent AF. Recent controlled trials suggest that rate control may be superior to rhythm control in elderly patients with recurrent or paroxysmal AF. New-onset AF in the critical care setting is often secondary to a trigger, and the approach to treatment should be individualized. The need for rate or rhythm control in this situation is often decided based on the underlying clinical scenario and cardiac substrate.

vii. Current evidence indicates that cerebral thromboembolic complications occur in patients with persistent or recurrent AF in the presence of inadequate (INR <2) or discontinued anticoagulation.

viii. Heart rate control can be attempted using nodal agents that decrease AV conduction. Commonly used agents include **calcium-channel blockers, β-blockers,** and **digoxin** (see Table 19-1).

ix. Acute pharmacologic conversion:

(a) Timing of chemical conversion with respect to thromboembolic risk is similar to that with electrical cardioversion.

(b) Pharmacologic agents from most classes of antiarrhythmics can be used for acute conversion where electrical conversion is not warranted. With most antiarrhythmics, patients should be closely monitored for QT-interval prolongation and drug-induced proarrhythmia such as torsades de pointes. Most antiarrhythmic agents also have a negative inotropic effect, and, thus, monitoring for hypotension and heart failure is warranted.

x. Drugs commonly used include the following:

(a) **Amiodarone.** Intravenous (IV) loading dose of 150 mg over 10 minutes, followed by a 1-mg/min infusion for 6 hours and then 0.5 mg/min

**Table 19-1. Common nodal agents
used for rate control in atrial fibrillation**

Agent	Class	Dose
Metoprolol	β-blocker	5 mg IV over 2 min; may be repeated as necessary
Propranolol	β-blocker	1 mg IV over 2 min
Verapamil	Calcium-channel blocker	5–10 mg over 2 min; may repeat in 30 min
Diltiazem	Calcium-channel blocker	Bolus: 0.25 mg/kg (or 20 mg) IV over 2 min; may repeat after 15 min, with 0.35 mg/kg (25 mg). Continuous infusion: 5–10 mg/h; increase in 5-mg/h increments up to 15 mg/h maintained for up to 24 h
Digoxin	NaK-ATPase pump inhibitor	0.5 mg IV, then may give 0.25 mg every 6 h for two doses to a maximum of 1 mg as an initial load.

for another 18 hours. A repeat load of 150 mg can be considered for recurrent dysrhythmias.

(b) **Procainamide.** Dose 15 mg/kg IV at a rate less than 50 mg/min. Alternatively 500 to 750 mg enterally, followed by a four-time-daily regimen.

(c) **Ibutilide.** Dose 1 mg IV over 10 min, repeated once if necessary. Pretreatment with magnesium sulfate is recommended.

(d) **Flecainide.** Loading dose of 300 mg enterally, followed by a twice-daily regimen of 50 to 150 mg. Contraindicated in patients with coronary disease.

(e) **Propafenone:** Loading dose of 600 mg enterally, followed by a thrice-daily regimen of 150 to 300 mg.

(f) **Sotalol:** Enteral dose of 80 to 240 mg twice daily.

(g) **Dofetilide:** Enteral dose of 125 to 500 micrograms twice daily depending on QT-interval duration and renal function.

xi. Long-term treatment

(a) Rate control may be attempted using calcium-channel blockers, beta-blockers, or digoxin.

> > (b) Rhythm control may be attempted using one of the agents discussed previously.

3. Wide complex, regular rhythm
   a. **Ventricular tachycardia (VT)**
      (1) VT is defined as three or more consecutive complexes of ventricular origin with a rate greater than 110 bpm.
      (2) VT may be nonsustained (<30-seconds' duration) or sustained (>30 seconds' duration). Morphologically, VT is classified as monomorphic when the QRS morphology is uniform and polymorphic when the QRS morphology is variable. In general, polymorphic VT is more ominous than monomorphic VT. In the structurally normal heart, monomorphic VT, originating from the right or left ventricular outflow tract (see Fig. 19-5), is usually well tolerated and often may be treated conservatively.
      (3) Hemodynamic consequences are related to the underlying cardiac function, comorbidities, the chamber of origin, and rate of the VT.

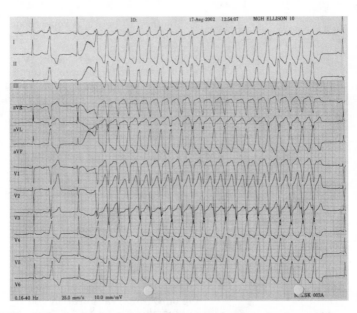

Fig. 19-5.   Twelve-lead electrocardiogram showing a monomorphic ventricular tachycardia originating from the right ventricular outflow tract. Classic features are a left-bundle-branch–like morphology, evidence of atrioventricular dissociation, and inferior axis in the inferior leads (2, 3, and aVF).

(4) Risk factors include coronary artery disease with previous scar, acute ischemia, nonischemic cardiomyopathy, myocarditis, drug-induced proarrhythmias, infiltrative disorders, electrolyte abnormalities, and myocardial toxins.

(5) Treatment

i. Unstable VT should be immediately treated with synchronized DC cardioversion (see Chapter 14).

ii. Stable forms can be treated pharmacologically.

(a) The choice of the antiarrhythmic agent should be determined by the underlying left ventricular function.

(b) Patients with preserved function may be treated with lidocaine, procainamide, or amiodarone (doses as in section **V.B.2.c.**). **Lidocaine** may be initially administered as a bolus of 50 to 100 mg followed by a maintenance drip at 1 to 4 mg/min.

(c) Patients with depressed function may be treated with lidocaine and **amiodarone.** Alternately, urgent cardioversion can be attempted.

(d) In some patients with recurrent VT, autonomic blockade using incremental doses of β-blockers can be attempted.

(e) Repetitive nonsustained MMVT (see Fig. 19-4) can be treated with beta-blockade and calcium-channel blockers. Refractory cases may require a more definitive approach such as catheter ablation (see Table 19-2).

iii. Long-term strategies and selection of antiarrhythmic agents depend on the cardiac substrate (ischemic vs. nonischemic), precipitating factors, renal function, exercise testing, cardiac function, and ambulatory electrocardiographic monitoring.

b. Antidromic AV reentrant tachycardia (AVRT)

(1) Involves a reentrant pathway with an anterograde limb involving a ventricular accessory pathway and a retrograde limb involving the His-Purkinje system (contrast with an orthodromic AVRT described in section **V.B.1.f**).

(2) Typically occurs with an underlying preexcitation syndrome such as WPW.

(3) Caution must be exercised in the use of AV nodal agents to treat AF in patients with preexcitation with AV nodal agents. AV nodal

Table 19-2. Success rates for catheter ablation of arrhythmias

Arrhythmia	Success (%)
WPW or AVRT	90+
Atrioventicular node reentry	95+
Atrial fibrillation	
Atrioventricular node ablation	95+
Pulmonary vein isolation	75
Typical atrial flutter	90
Atrial tachycardia	80
Ventricular tachycardia	
Normal heart	95
Structural heart disease	70

WPW, Wolf-Parkinson-White syndrome; AVRT, atrioventricular reentrant tachycardia.

blockade may paradoxically increase ventricular rate by promoting conduction down the accessory pathway.

c. Accelerated idioventricular rhythm (AIVR)
  (1) AIVR is an abnormal automatic rhythm originating from the terminal His-Purkinje system.
  (2) Risk factors include acute ischemia, digitalis toxicity, and myocarditis.
  (3) There is a monomorphic, wide-complex rhythm with a heart rate between 60 and 110 bpm on ECG. Retrograde P waves with AV dissociation and sinus capture beats can be seen.
  (4) Typically a benign, self-limited rhythm except when patients are dependent on AV synchrony for adequate cardiac output. In symptomatic patients, therapy (atrial overdrive pacing, isoproterenol or atropine) is directed at increasing the sinus nodal rate to overdrive and suppress the ectopic ventricular focus.

d. SVT with aberrancy
  (1) A preexisting bundle-branch block or rate-dependent aberrancy can cause confusion regarding whether a wide-complex tachycardia is supraventricular or ventricular in origin.
  (2) The presence of VT is favored by:
    i. History of structural heart disease.
    ii. Old electrocardiogram without evidence of conduction disease.
    iii. Evidence of AV dissociation: canon *a*-waves on a central venous pressure tracing, fusion beats or capture beats on ECG, evidence of organized yet dissociated

atrial activity on an esophageal electrocardiogram.

    iv. Other electrocardiographic evidence of ventricular tachycardia includes the following:

        (a) Positive concordance of the QRS complex across the precordial leads.

        (b) LBBB with right-axis deviation, QRS axis less than −90 or greater than 180 degrees.

        (c) QRS duration greater than 140 msec with a RBBB or QRS duration greater than 160 msec with a LBBB.

  (3) In the critically ill patient, when in doubt, it is typically more prudent to treat a wide-complex tachycardia as if it were ventricular in origin.

4. Wide-complex, irregular rhythm

  a. Ventricular fibrillation (VF)

    (1) Pharmacologic treatment

      i. Epinephrine remains the mainstay of pharmacologic therapy. Current evidence does not support the use of high-dose epinephrine therapy.

      ii. Limited evidence exists for a single bolus dose of **vasopressin** 40 U IV.

      iii. Data from out-of-hospital arrest trials support a single bolus dose of **amiodarone** 300 mg IV.

      iv. Current evidence and recommendations do not support routine use of lidocaine.

    (2) Electrical treatment

      i. Defibrillation: 300 J, 360 J, and 360 J using monophasic machines and three defibrillations at 150 J using **biphasic** machines.

      ii. Automated implantable cardiac defibrillators (AICD)

        (a) Current evidence supports use of AICDs for both primary and secondary prevention of sudden death in patients with ischemic cardiomyopathy (left ventricular ejection fraction <35%–40%).

        (b) Patients with hypertrophic obstructive cardiomyopathy at risk for sudden death may benefit from placement of AICDs.

        (c) Recent evidence supports prophylactic use of AICD with nonischemic dilated cardiomyopathy and heart failure.

  b. Torsades de pointes (TDP)

    (1) Classically associated with a prolonged QT interval.

      i. Although an absolute threshold for TDP is not defined, almost all cases of TDP are reported with a corrected QT value exceeding 500 msec.

      ii. QT prolongation can be produced by medications (e.g., antidysrhythmics, antipsychotics, antimicrobials), electrolyte imbalances (hypomagnesemia, hypocalcemia), and ischemia.

      iii. Onset of TDP is typically associated with short-long-short sequences of the ventricular cycle length (measured by the RR interval).

      iv. Occasionally, TDP can develop without marked prolongation of the QT interval. The duration of the QT interval in these patients does not predict the occurrence of the arrhythmia.

    (2) Characteristic appearance on ECG, where the undulating peaks of sequential QRS complexes and T waves give it an appearance of twisting about an axis (see Fig. 19-6).

    (3) Treatment

      i. Cardioversion/defibrillation.

      ii. Treatment of any concurrent myocardial ischemia.

      iii. Magnesium sulfate 1 to 2 g IV in setting of hypomagnesemia.

      iv. Overdrive pacing using either temporary pacing or isoproterenol infusion which acts to shorten the QT interval and decrease the likelihood of short-long-short sequences.

      v. Patients at increased risk for recurrences without clearly reversible causes may benefit from prophylactic AICD implantation.

VI. Thoracic epidural anesthesia

    A. High thoracic epidural anesthesia (T1–T5 level) with local anesthetics can reduce activity of the cardiac sympathetic axis.

    B. Experimental models have shown that high thoracic epidural anesthesia with local anesthetics can increase the threshold dose of parenteral epinephrine required to generate sustained premature ventricular complexes independent of the plasma concentration of local anesthetic, consistent with an antiarrhythmic effect.

    C. Animal models have also shown that high thoracic epidurals with local anesthetics can attenuate ventricular ectopy in the setting of acute coronary occlusion.

    D. Clinical evidence indicates that high thoracic epidural anesthesia with local anesthetic agents is associated with a decreased incidence of supraventricular dysrhythmias in the postoperative setting.

    E. Some controversy exists on the ability of high thoracic epidural anesthesia to specifically reduce the incidence

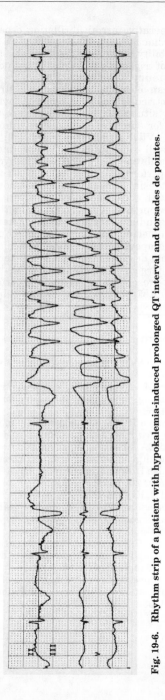

Fig. 19-6. Rhythm strip of a patient with hypokalemia-induced prolonged QT interval and torsades de pointes.

of postoperative atrial fibrillation especially following open cardiac surgery. Whether this is a result of an impaired ability of thoracic epidural anesthesia to inhibit activity of triggering atrial foci is unknown.

VII. Radiofrequency ablation (RFA)

    A. RFA is an elective and definitive strategy for most supraventricular and ventricular arrhythmias.

    B. In many situations, RFA has become the first line of therapy for supraventricular arrhythmias inclusive of AVNRT, AVRT, atrial flutter, and focal atrial tachycardias. It still constitutes the second line of therapy for atrial fibrillation and ventricular tachycardias.

    C. RFA is performed under conscious sedation with local anesthesia. Three to five transvenous catheters are placed, with occasional need for arterial or transseptal catheter approach. A diagnostic evaluation is performed, including induction of arrhythmia, determination of the potential mechanism, and assessment of the activation map. Therapeutic intervention immediately follows using current delivered through a catheter electrode to ablate the target. To conclude the procedure, a reassessment for presence of arrhythmia is performed.

    D. Success rates for RFA are shown in Table 19-2.

REFERENCES

Amar D. Perioperative atrial tachyarrhythmias. *Anesthesiology* 2002;97:1618–1623.

Dimarco JP. Implantable cardioverter-defibrillators. *N Engl J Med* 2003;349:1836–1847.

Lamas GA, Kerry LL, Sweeny MO, et al. Ventricular pacing or dual-chamber pacing for sinus-node dysfunction. *N Engl J Med* 2002;346:1854–1862.

Mangrum JM, Dimarco JP. The evaluation and management of bradycardia. *N Engl J Med* 2000;342:703–709.

Opolski A, Torbicki DA, Kosior M, et al. Rate control vs rhythm control in patients with nonvalvular persistent atrial fibrillation: the results of the Polish How to Treat Chronic Atrial Fibrillation (HOT CAFE) Study. *Chest* 2004;126:476–486.

Scott NB, Turfrey DJ, Ray DA, et al. A prospective randomized study of the potential benefits of thoracic epidural anesthesia and analgesia in patients undergoing coronary bypass artery grafting. *Anesth Analg* 2001;93:528–535.

Stone KR, McPherson CA. Assessment and management of patients with pacemakers and implantable cardioverter defibrillators. *Crit Care Med* 2004;(4 Suppl):S155–S165.

The AFFIRM Trial Investigators. A comparison of rate control and rhythm control in patients with atrial fibrillation. *N Engl J Med* 2002;347:1825–1833.

The Acute Respiratory Distress Syndrome

Luca M. Bigatello, Sascha Beutler, and
Kristopher Davignon

I. **The acute respiratory distress syndrome (ARDS)** remains a tremendous challenge to the intensivist. Although great progress has been made in understanding its pathophysiology, treatment remains largely supportive. However, recent randomized trials that tested therapeutic interventions for critically ill patients have provided the intensivist with tools of proven benefit that may increase survival of patients with ARDS.

II. **Epidemiology**

   A. **Definition** (see Table 20-1). ARDS defines a syndrome of acute respiratory failure of diverse etiology, characterized by noncardiogenic pulmonary edema, hypoxemia, and diffuse lung parenchymal consolidations. **Acute lung injury** (ALI) defines an early clinical stage of the same syndrome, with a milder degree of hypoxemia. The reason we identify an early stage of the syndrome is so we can apply and test therapeutic measures in a larger patient population and before substantial damage to the lung has occurred.

   B. **Etiology.** Table 20-2 lists common causes of ALI/ARDS. Infectious pneumonia, aspiration pneumonitis, and lung contusion are frequent **pulmonary** etiologies. Abdominal sepsis, acute pancreatitis, and multiple trauma are **extrapulmonary** etiologies. Regardless of the anatomic origin, the lung is the target organ, but the radiographic pattern of injury may be quite variable. Figure 20-1 shows representative computed tomography (CT) scans of two patients. ARDS secondary to acute pancreatitis (Fig. 20-1A) shows a diffuse, almost homogeneous pattern of consolidation. ARDS secondary to bronchopneumonia (Fig. 20-1B) shows dense consolidations localized preferentially to the lower lung fields. Although there is no evidence that these are two separate syndromes from a pathophysiologic standpoint, they present different mechanical characteristics that may affect the choice of therapeutic strategies (see sections **VI.B** and **VI.C**).

   C. The **incidence** of ARDS in the United States is estimated to be between 5 and 75 cases per 100,000 population. Despite this relatively small occurrence, the impact of ARDS on resource utilization in tertiary care referral centers is significant because these patients suffer from multiple acute medical problems and may receive intensive care and subsequent rehabilitation for prolonged periods of time.

Table 20-1.   Definition of acute lung injury and acute respiratory distress syndrome according to the American-European Consensus Conference on ARDS, 1994

Acute onset of respiratory distress
Hypoxemia
    ALI: PaO_2/FiO_2 $\leq$300 mm Hg
    ARDS: PaO_2/FiO_2 $\leq$200 mm Hg
Bilateral consolidation of chest radiograph
Absence of clinical findings of cardiogenic pulmonary edema

ALI, acute lung injury; ARDS, acute respiratory distress syndrome; FiO_2, inspired oxygen; PaO_2, partial arterial oxygen pressure.

    D. Prognosis. Survival from ARDS depends on a number of factors such as its etiology, the patient's age, and the presence of comorbid factors. Young and previously healthy trauma victims with isolated ARDS have a more than 90% chance of survival. Elderly ARDS patients with chronic disease, multiple organ dysfunction syndrome (MODS), and sepsis have a significantly poorer prognosis. Overall, in a mixed population of ALI/ARDS of various etiologies, a mortality rate of 30% to 40% can be expected.

    E. Recovery. The same categories of patients who enjoy higher survival rates—young patients with low comorbidity—also have the best chance of recovery from ARDS. Over the first 3 to 6 months following discharge from the intensive care unit (ICU), lung function steadily improves, reaching a level of approximately 70% of normal, allowing these patients to lead a productive life. However, consequences of ARDS are not limited to the respiratory system. Patients who undergo extended periods of mechanical ventilation in the ICU are susceptible to prolonged muscle wasting and weakness, a lower health-related quality of life, and some degree of impairment of memory, cognition, and ability to concentrate.

Table 20-2.   Common etiologies of the acute respiratory distress syndrome

Direct lung injury	Aspiration and other chemical pneumonitis
	Infectious pneumonia
	Lung contusion, penetrating chest injury
	Near-drowning
Distant injury	Inflammation, necrosis, sepsis
	Multiple trauma, burns
	Shock, hypoperfusion
	Acute pancreatitis

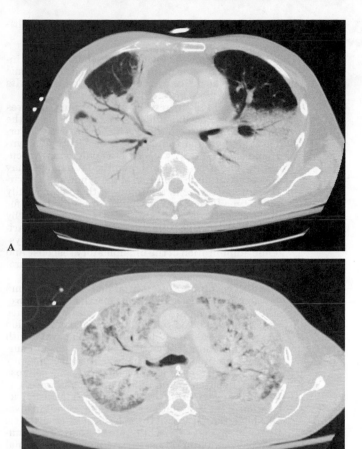

Fig. 20-1. Computed tomography (CT) scans of two patients.
A. ARDS secondary to acute pancreatitis shows a diffuse, almost
homogeneous pattern of consolidation. B. Acute respiratory distress
syndrome (ARDS) secondary to bronchopneumonia shows dense
consolidations localized preferentially to the lower lung fields.

III. Pathogenesis. ARDS is primarily an inflammatory phenomenon. Regardless of the site of origin, the original insult
triggers a systemic inflammatory response that injures the
lungs as well as other organs. It is possible that the lung
itself is a site where the inflammatory response is ampli-
fied by a combination of factors, included the mechanical
stress induced by positive-pressure ventilation (ventilator-
induced lung injury; see later discussion). Activated leukocytes release mediators that further amplify local and

systemic injury and may contribute to the onset of multiple organ system failures.

IV. **Anatomy**

A. The lung tends to respond to acute, nonneoplastic injuries in a reproducible manner, generating an anatomic picture known as **diffuse alveolar damage (DAD).** Its main characteristics are as follows:

1. **Acute alveolar injury.** The initial injury involves both the endothelial and the epithelial side of the alveolocapillary membrane. This is important in order to understand the evolution of ARDS as a syndrome of both the airways and the pulmonary vasculature. The degree of initial epithelial damage may affect the ultimate evolution of the syndrome. Of particular importance is the injury of the metabolically active type II alveolar cells, which are responsible for the production of surfactant, clearance of edema by fluid transport, and differentiation into the flat, parietal type I cells. Damage to type II cells fosters systemic amplification of the inflammatory response and affects the degree of subsequent high-grade fibroproliferative response.

2. **Exudative phase.** Interstitial and alveolar edema develop from endothelial damage rather than hydrostatic forces. The exudate contains plasma proteins, white and red blood cells, platelets, and coagulation factors, and eventually lines the alveolar walls with hyaline membranes. Inactivation of the existent surfactant and production of abnormal surfactant may occur. Alveolar edema, consolidation, and collapse produce hypoxemia and reduce lung compliance.

3. **Pulmonary vascular lesions.** Tissue injury and activation of the coagulation cascade may result in alveolar hemorrhage and in thrombosis of small arteries. Remodeling may later obliterate sections of the pulmonary vasculature. Loss of vascular cross-sectional area, vasoconstrictive mediators, and **hypoxic pulmonary vasoconstriction (HPV)** may contribute to the onset of moderate **pulmonary artery hypertension,** which fosters the formation of pulmonary edema.

4. **Fibroproliferative phase.** Within approximately 7 to 10 days, the inflammatory infiltrate acquires chronic characteristics, with a predominance of macrophages, monocytes, and eventually fibroblasts. The initial lesions heal by collagen deposition, leading to obliteration of air spaces and interstitial fibrosis. The intensity of fibroproliferative phenomena is variable and may be related to the severity of the initial injury (see section **IV.A.1**).

B. **Anatomic diagnosis.** The time course of the described phenomena varies among patients and among adjacent areas of the lung within the same patient. The presence of **infection,** either as a cause or a result of ARDS, adds to the complexity of this picture. Estimating the anatomic stage of ARDS may affect therapeutic options. For example, alveolar recruitment with positive pressure may be effective in the early phase of lung injury when alveolar edema and collapse predominate; on the other hand, corticosteroid therapy may be indicated later to treat fibroproliferative changes. Hence, an anatomic diagnosis is often desirable to pursue the etiology, evaluate the degree of fibrosis, and rule out infection. Such diagnosis can be attempted with different degrees of invasiveness:

1. **Bronchoalveolar lavage** (BAL) is performed during fiberoptic bronchoscopy. The diagnostic yield of a BAL is highly dependent on its proper execution and should be performed by experienced clinicians. Briefly, one or more areas of the lung are lavaged with saline solution to retrieve 30 to 60 ml of fluid, which is sent for cytologic and bacteriologic analysis as well as selected immunologic studies. The indication for a BAL must be weighed against the patient's clinical condition because a prolonged procedure, the saline lavage, and the loss of positive airway pressure may lead to hypoxemia and instability.

2. **Open lung biopsy** carries the higher risk of a surgical procedure. The widespread availability of video-assisted thoracoscopy has substantially reduced the invasiveness of this procedure, but complications such as hemorrhage and bronchopleural fistula can still occur.

V. **Physiology.** Hypoxemia and low lung compliance are hallmarks of ARDS.

    A. **Hypoxemia** in ALI/ARDS is caused by alveolar edema, consolidation, and collapse. As ventilation decreases or completely ceases in different areas of the lung, partially or fully desaturated blood mixes with oxygenated blood. When true shunt (i.e., no ventilation) rather than ventilation/perfusion (V/Q) mismatch (i.e., low ventilation) is the main determinant of hypoxemia, as it is in ARDS, the arterial partial oxygen pressure (PaO_2) can be increased only through the recruitment of nonventilated alveoli. Hypoxemia in ARDS is in part attenuated by the physiologic response of **HPV,** which diverts pulmonary blood flow away from hypoventilated alveoli. HPV may be inhibited by local production of vasodilator substances such as prostanoids and nitric oxide (NO) during inflammation. It may also be blunted by the administration of vasodilators such as nitroglycerin and sodium nitroprusside.

    B. **Vascular occlusion,** airways overdistention, and hypovolemia create areas of high V/Q and true **dead space** (i.e., no perfusion). An increased ratio of dead space to tidal volume hinders CO_2 elimination, increases ventilatory requirements, and may be an early independent predictor of mortality in ALI/ARDS.

C. **Low lung compliance.** In the early phase of ARDS, lung compliance decreases because of diffuse alveolar edema, consolidation, and collapse. Because this injury is not homogeneous, the low compliance of early ARDS is really the average of the various mechanical characteristics of individual lung regions. The two CT scans in Fig. 20-1 illustrate how a certain value of compliance measured in patients with ALI/ARDS may be determined by very different distributions of the lesions, which have implications in the choice of ventilatory management (see section **VI**).

D. **Low chest wall compliance** may occur as a result of abdominal distention, massive trunk edema, circumferential burns, and tight chest bandages. Abdominal distention is frequent in surgical patients, who may require higher pressure applied at the airway to achieve a desired change in lung volume. Intrathoracic pressure can be estimated by means of an **esophageal balloon;** the (approximate) knowledge of the intrathoracic pressure makes it possible to separate the mechanics of the lung and the chest wall. **Measuring respiratory compliance** is useful for following the evolution of the syndrome and testing the effect of changes of ventilatory settings. Bedside methods for estimating lung and chest wall compliance are described in Chapter 3.

VI. **Treatment of ARDS**

A. **General measures.** ALI/ARDS must be viewed as part of a systemic inflammatory injury that has a specific etiology and is commonly associated with the failure of other vital organs.

1. **Diagnosis and treatment** of the underlying condition must be sought, even when respiratory failure dominates the clinical picture. Important early interventions in surgical patients include the drainage of abscesses, debridement of devitalized tissue, fixation of fractures, and grafting of burned tissue.

2. **Hemodynamic management.** Judicious fluid restriction limits the formation of pulmonary edema, improving gas exchange and respiratory mechanics. However, an excessive fluid-restrictive strategy may result in hypoperfusion and damage of vital organs. It seems reasonable to guide hemodynamic management based on each patient's physiology, which may be complex and require invasive monitoring.

3. **Treatment of infections.** Antimicrobial therapy should be targeted to cultured organisms whenever possible. The appeal of broad-spectrum antibiotic prophylaxis and coverage must be weighed against the potential for toxicity and selection of resistant microbial flora (Chapters 11 and 28). **Nosocomial pneumonia** (Chapters 12 and 28) is frequent in patients with acute respiratory failure and is associated with an increased mortality. Skillful airway management and measures for reducing the risks of aspiration (infection control measures, head-up position, oral

hygiene, gastric decompression) decrease the incidence of nosocomial pneumonia.

4. **Nutrition** should be started early because a prolonged ICU course is likely. Enteral feeding is generally preferred (see Chapter 9).

5. **Avoiding iatrogenic complications.** All diagnostic and therapeutic decisions in critically ill patients must be weighed in terms of benefits and risks. Iatrogenic complications during acute respiratory failure include complications of line and tube insertions, ventilator-induced lung injury, oxygen toxicity, fluid overload, tissue hypoperfusion, and the induction of microbial overgrowth through indiscriminate use of antimicrobial agents.

6. **Support of other organ system functions** is an integral part of the treatment of ALI/ARDS. Hemodynamic instability, acute renal failure, gastrointestinal hemorrhage, coagulation abnormalities, and neuromuscular changes may complicate the course of these critically ill patients. We refer to the relevant specific chapters for their management.

B. **Mechanical ventilation**

1. **The traditional approach to mechanical ventilation** of patients with severe acute respiratory failure was based on the use of large tidal volumes (V_T) and high positive end-expiratory pressure (PEEP) to ensure adequate gas exchange and limit oxygen toxicity.

2. **The current approach to mechanical ventilation** of patients with ALI/ARDS challenges the aforementioned principles, for the following reasons:

   a. Mechanical ventilation with large V_T and high alveolar pressure damages the lung. This **ventilator-induced lung injury** compounds the original alveolar injury and may adversely affect the outcome of patients with ALI/ARDS. Figure 20-2 shows the portable chest radiogram (Panel A) and the CT scan (Panel B) of a patient who developed **ventilator-induced lung injury** in our ICU.

   b. A recent multicenter clinical trial (the ARDS-Net study) showed that ventilating ALI/ARDS patients with a **lung-protective strategy** of low V_T (6 ml/kg of ideal body weight) and low airway pressure (inspiratory plateau pressure <30 cm H_2O) might improve survival.

3. **Based on the current evidence, we suggest** the following procedures:

   a. Limit the size of V_T, ideally to 6 ml/kg. We may allow for a slightly higher V_T if the **end-inspiratory plateau airway pressure** measured in a relaxed patient (see Chapter 3) is lower than 25 to 30 cm H_2O, if the patient is dyssynchronous with the ventilator or is acidemic. If the use of low V_T causes significant acidemia, we first increase the respiratory rate, aiming at an arterial

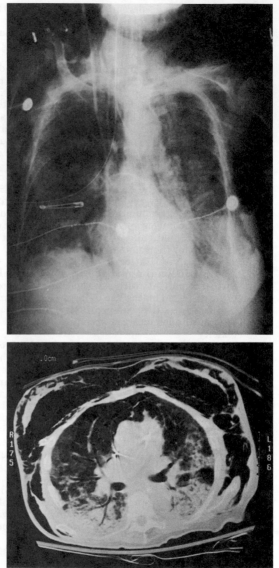

Fig. 20-2. Portable chest radiogram (A) and chest computed tomography (CT) scan (B) of a patient with early acute respiratory distress syndrome and ventilator-induced lung injury. Note the striking difference in the morphologic information provided by the two techniques. In the CT image, one can distinguish inhomogeneous areas of consolidation, preferentially located in the dependent regions of the lungs, the massive subcutaneous emphysema, the peribronchial and pericardial air, and the subpleural loculated pneumothoraces.

pH value (admittedly arbitrary) close to 7.30 (see also section **VI.B.3.d**).

b. Apply a **level of PEEP** aimed at optimizing respiratory mechanics, that is, at preventing alveolar collapse at end-expiration. Ideally, static volume–pressure curves of the respiratory system (see Chapter 3) may identify such a pressure. However, they are cumbersome and often unreliable. A simpler way to test the effect of a change in PEEP on lung volume is to apply a stepwise increase in PEEP while maintaining a set level of pressure above PEEP **("PEEP trial")**. If the V_T increases or stays the same, this is an indication that the new level of PEEP has recruited or prevented collapse of lung tissue and has not overdistended previously recruited lung. PEEP is an expiratory phenomenon, and the levels commonly used (5–15 cm H_2O) mainly avoid de-recruitment rather than provide full recruitment. Hence, changes in PEEP should be made while being cognizant of the state of recruitment of the lung (see next section).

c. **Further recruitment of the lung.** The pressure necessary to open collapsed alveoli may be several times higher than the levels of PEEP commonly used. Furthermore, ventilating with a low V_T tends to promote alveolar collapse. Therefore, lung-protective strategies of low V_T and airway pressure tend to include additional means to recruit the lung **(recruitment maneuvers)** by applying higher pressures at the airway for limited periods of time. Recruitment maneuvers are of two main varieties:

(1) A **sustained inflation** of 30 to 60 seconds at a pressure higher than the inflating pressure; for example, 40 to 60 cm H_2O, increases the PaO_2 in more than 50% of patients with ALI/ARDS. However, its effect is transient and generally regresses within 20 minutes. Combining a sustained inflation with an increase in PEEP tends to stabilize the lung at a higher level of recruitment. Similarly, performing a sustained inflation before a PEEP trial (see preceding section) optimizes the effect of PEEP. However, sustained inflations may cause **hemodynamic instability** and **lung damage.** If high airway pressures are applied to lungs with normal compliance, a significant fraction is transmitted to the pleural space, impeding venous return and decreasing cardiac output. In addition, they can induce a traumatic pneumothorax. Hence, they should be carried out by experienced clinicians with **continuous monitoring** of the arterial blood pressure and only in patients whose

hypoxemia is suspected to be due to alveolar collapse.

(2) A **sigh** is a large breath interspersed among the breaths of a set V_T or pressure. Although not a new concept, current ventilators may provide higher versatility to set the parameters of a sigh. A simple way to deliver a sigh is to have the patient breathe on pressure-support ventilation and add a single pressure-control breath of the desired pressure and duration.

(3) Despite their apparent immediate benefits, recruitment maneuvers have not been proven beneficial beyond their transient effect on gas exchange. Furthermore, studies aimed at confirming the long-term safety of the high-volume/pressure settings (albeit transient) on lung integrity are not available. Therefore, we recommend carefully evaluating the benefits and risks of these maneuvers and considering that the ARDS lung may not need to be fully recruited at all times. In the same vein, it is important to note that the use of different levels of PEEP has not been associated with any change in survival, that is, **a higher PEEP is likely to improve the PaO_2 but not necessarily the outcome** of patients with ALI/ARDS.

d. **Arterial carbon dioxide tension ($PaCO_2$) control.** Using low V_T values may cause hypoventilation. Acute acidemia is avoided by increasing the respiratory rate and/or by temporarily administering a buffer such as sodium bicarbonate or tromethamine. A slow rise of the $PaCO_2$, on the other hand, may not be harmful as long as pH compensation is allowed to occur. This approach, called **permissive hypercapnia,** has been advocated as a way to limit ventilator-associated acute lung injury. Despite its widespread use, however, there is no evidence of its efficacy. Contraindications to permissive hypercapnia include increased intracranial pressure, right ventricular failure, and ongoing acidemia.

4. **Modes of ventilation.** The basic concepts of mechanical ventilation are discussed in Chapter 5. Here we will review their application to the treatment of patients with ALI/ARDS.

a. **Pressure versus volume-control ventilation.** **Pressure-control** ventilation has often been recommended in ARDS. Its potential advantages include a **high and variable inspiratory flow rate,** which may enhance synchrony during patient-triggered breaths, and the ability to reach **the set airway pressure early in inspiration,** providing a higher mean airway pressure than an equivalent setting in the volume-control mode. The higher mean airway pressure may promote alveolar recruitment and increase the PaO_2. However, current mechanical ventilators can deliver volume-control ventilation with airflow patterns similar to what we just described for pressure control. In addition, volume control always **assures the set minute ventilation,** which may be desirable in some patients. Hence, the choice between pressure and volume ventilation when using a modern ventilator is not a factor that affects patient outcome, but rather an individual preference.

b. **Mandatory versus spontaneous ventilation**

(1) **Mandatory ventilation** makes it possible to deliver high levels of alveolar pressure with complex and often "unphysiologic" flow waveforms that may improve gas exchange. For example, a prolonged inspiratory time may recruit alveoli and improve PaO_2, but is not generally tolerated by a spontaneously breathing patient. Hence, ventilation with high levels of support may require heavy sedation and neuromuscular blockade (see section **VI.B.5.a**).

(2) Conversely, maintaining some degree of spontaneous breathing activity may have beneficial effects. It may improve **gas exchange** due to the prevailing role of the diaphragm during spontaneous breathing, which applies inflating pressure to the lung bases, a larger and less expanded lung field. In addition, the **maintenance of respiratory muscle activity** may reduce the degree of weakness and atrophy of the respiratory muscles that is common after a prolonged course of acute respiratory failure (see section **II.E**).

c. **"Bilevel" modes.** Under this term we include a group of ventilatory modes that deliver two levels of airway pressure ("high" and "low") and allow spontaneous breathing. Despite a rich nomenclature, these modes operate in similar ways. We refer to Chapter 5 for a more detailed description.

d. **High-frequency ventilation (HFV)** and **high-frequency oscillation (HFO)** deliver very small V_T values at high rates and a set mean airway pressure. The V_T can be so low that only the anatomic dead space is ventilated. The mechanism of gas exchange is complex, related in part to apneic oxygenation and to air mixing within the large airways. The appeal of this type of ventilation lies in the ability to provide gas exchange at low measurable pressures, thus presumably limiting ventilator-induced lung injury. However, expiratory flow limitation may occur, causing high levels of auto-PEEP. The use of HFV and HFO in adults is limited while waiting for the results of ongoing clinical trials.

5. **Additional strategies**

a. **Sedation and neuromuscular blockade** may improve gas exchange by enhancing synchrony with the ventilator and allowing the delivery of high levels of ventilatory support. Most clinicians titrate sedation to comfort and limit the use of neuromuscular blockade to the most difficult cases to ventilate (see Chapter 6). The use of neuromuscular blocking agents, particularly of the steroid group, has been associated with prolonged weakness and polyneuropathy of critical illness (see Chapter 30).

b. **Prone ventilation.** A significant increase in PaO_2 occurs in more than half of ARDS patients who are turned prone, tends to last throughout the period of prone ventilation, and fades at variable rates as the supine position is resumed. Patients can be kept prone for several hours at a time and turned supine for nursing care, physical exam, and relief of skin pressure. Complications of prone ventilation are rare in experienced hands, and are mostly related to the loss of lines, tubes (endotracheal tube!), and monitoring devices during the turning procedure. Rarely, skin pressure sores and nerve damage from incorrect positioning may occur. Transient hemodynamic instability may also occur, which makes proning a **high-risk maneuver in unstable patients.** We prefer to fully sedate patients who are ventilated prone and often use neuromuscular blockade to facilitate this practice. **The mechanism** of the effect of prone ventilation on gas exchange in ARDS is not fully understood. Although gravitational factors redistribute ventilation to the previously collapsed dorsal areas of the lung, they do not explain the persistence of the effect of the prone position over time. It is also possible that changes in the geometry and mechanical properties of the chest wall may redirect airflow away from inflated ventral lung areas to previously collapsed, dorsal areas. If this last concept is correct, simply compressing the anterior portion of the chest with **sand bags** during supine ventilation should improve gas exchange. Occasionally, the effects of using sand bags on gas exchange are obvious and reproducible. We use two sand bags of 2.5 pounds each placed on each hemithorax particularly in patients who are deemed at increased risk for prone ventilation (see prior discussion).

C. **Additional therapeutic options**

1. **Inhaled nitric oxide** (NO) reduces pulmonary hypertension and increases PaO_2 in the majority of

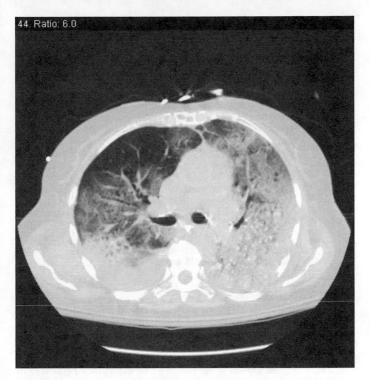

Fig. 20-3. Chest computed tomography scan of a patient with late acute respiratory distress syndrome, 10 to14 days from the onset. The radiographic findings had always predominated in the left lung, which had been the "down lung" during a right-side pleural decortication. Here, the left lung is the site of an intense fibrotic reaction.

patients with ARDS. Unfortunately, this beneficial effect is transient, and most of the time it does not result in an appreciable change in ventilatory management. Currently, the best indication for inhaled NO in ARDS seems to be as a bridge to more complex therapies during the initial stabilization of severely hypoxemic patients.

2. **Exogenous surfactant.** Alveolar surfactant is diminished or dysfunctional in patients with ALI/ARDS due to the damage to the type II alveolar cells (see section **IV.8.1**). Surfactant replacement is effective in premature newborns with respiratory distress syndrome, where the lack of surfactant is the primary etiology. In adults, it has not been as successful. Newer formulations and improved delivery systems may renew interest in the use of surfactant for ALI/ARDS.

3. **Extracorporeal membrane oxygenation (ECMO)**
   provides a temporary substitute for transpulmonary
   respiration while severely injured lungs are allowed
   to rest and recover. Extracorporeal gas exchange
   techniques in adults are confined to a few, highly
   specialized centers for limited indications.

4. **Corticosteroids** may improve the course of "late"
   ARDS, that is, the fibroproliferative phase that starts
   approximately 7 to 10 days from the onset of the syndrome (see section **IV.3**). Based on the results of a
   small controlled trial, a course of 0.5 mg/kg of methylprednisolone every 6 hours is conducted for up to
   3 weeks, followed by a fast taper. The main risk of this
   therapy is **infection.** Careful search for infectious focuses, which is particularly challenging after a prolonged ICU course, must be carried out throughout
   the course of corticosteroid therapy. Figure 20-3
   shows the CT scan of a patient with ARDS of 12 to
   14 days' duration, where the entire left lung showed a
   marked fibrotic reaction. This patient responded very
   well to corticosteroid treatment.

SELECTED REFERENCES

ARDS Clinical Trials Network (National Heart, Lung and Blood In-
stitute). Ventilation with lower tidal volumes as compared with
traditional tidal volumes for acute lung injury and the acute respiratory distress syndrome. *N Engl J Med* 2000;342:1301–1308.

ARDS Clinical Trials Network (National Heart, Lung and Blood In-
stitute). Higher versus lower positive end-expiratory pressures in
patients with the acute respiratory distress syndrome. *N Engl J
Med* 2004;351:1327–1336.

Artigas A, Bernard G, Claret J, et al. The American-European consensus conference on ARDS, Part 2. *Am J Respir Crit Care Med*
1998;157:1332–1347.

Ashbaugh DG, Bigelow DB, Petty TL, et al. Acute respiratory distress
in adults. *Lancet* 1967;2:319–323.

Bernard GR, Artigas A, Brigham KL, et al. The American-European
consensus conference on ARDS, Part 1. *Am J Respir Crit Care Med*
1994;149:818–824.

Dreyfuss D, Saumon G. Ventilator-induced lung injury. *Am J Respir
Crit Care Med* 1998;157:294–323.

Herridge MS, Cheung AM, Tansey CM, et al. One-year outcomes of
survivors of the acute respiratory distress syndrome. *N Engl J Med*
2003;348:683–693.

Katzenstein A, Asken FB. Acute lung injury patterns: diffuse alveolar damage, acute interstitial pneumonia, bronchiolitis obliterans-
organizing pneumonia. In: Katzenstein A, Asken FB, eds. *Surgical
pathology of the non neoplastic lung diseases*, 2nd ed. Philadelphia:
WB Saunders, 1990:9–56.

Ware LB, Matthay MA. The acute respiratory distress syndrome.
N Engl J Med 2000;342:1334–1349.

West JB. Ventilation-perfusion relationships. In: *Respiratory physiology—the essentials*, 5th ed. Baltimore: Williams & Wilkins,
1995:51–69.

Chronic Obstructive Pulmonary Disease and Asthma

Joseph S. Meltzer and Kenneth E. Shepherd

I. Patients with **chronic obstructive pulmonary disease (COPD) and asthma** have a wide spectrum of disease severity. This chapter provides a guide to the care of patients having moderate to severe stable or unstable obstructive lung disease requiring care in an intensive care unit (ICU). A clinical guide to patients with less severe lung dysfunction is also provided.

II. The following **definitions** consider each disease process as an isolated entity. Although relatively pure forms of these processes occur, there is generally some degree of overlap. Thus, many of the clinical findings and treatment modalities are similar. Nonetheless, the individual processes often differ sufficiently in certain respects (e.g., cellular and inflammatory mediators, degree of reversibility) to warrant individual discussion.

   A. **COPD** is a disease due to emphysema or chronic bronchitis, characterized by airflow limitation that is not fully reversible. This airflow limitation is usually progressive and is associated with an abnormal inflammatory response of the lungs to noxious gases or particles.

      1. **Emphysema** is anatomically defined as permanent, destructive enlargement of the air spaces distal to the terminal bronchioles with accompanying destruction of the air space walls (without obvious fibrosis).

      2. **Chronic bronchitis** is clinically defined as the presence of productive cough for at least 3 months in at least two successive years in a patient in whom other causes of chronic cough have been ruled out.

   B. **Asthma** is an inflammatory condition in which complex cellular, chemical, and nervous system (sympathetic, cholinergic, and nonadrenergic-noncholinergic) mediators lead to heightened bronchial responsiveness and episodic, variable, and reversible airway obstruction.

III. **ICU evaluation**

   A. **History**

      1. The general respiratory history should elicit specific symptoms about cough, sputum, hemoptysis, dyspnea, chest tightness or pain, wheezing, and exercise tolerance. Information on cigarette smoke, occupational, environmental, and infectious exposures, previous diagnostic tests and diagnoses, symptoms of sleep-disordered breathing, current medications,

allergies (e.g., drug, environmental, food), and stability of clinical status should be obtained.

2. The most important historical information to obtain from patients with COPD is exposure to cigarette smoke and environmental or occupational pollutants. Symptoms to elicit are coughing, sputum production, and wheezing.

3. The most important background information in patients with asthma is cough, sputum, and wheezing. Also important are the presence of nocturnal and/or exercise-induced dyspnea/cough/wheezing, diurnal or seasonal variability of symptoms, and hospitalizations (and treatments) for asthma.

B. **Physical examination and vital signs**

1. **Inspection.** Especially in patients with asthma, the upper respiratory tract should be assessed for **nasal polyps.** Polyps suggest that aspirin and other nonsteroidal antiinflammatory drugs may induce bronchospasm in the patient. Nasal polyps can complicate nasal intubation. Inflammation of the pharynx is suggestive of aspiration, postnasal drainage, or infection. One should assess the mobility of the trachea and assess the skin for evidence of a previous tracheostomy that can cause upper airway obstruction or difficulty with translaryngeal intubation. The neck veins and use of accessory respiratory muscles should be assessed. In COPD, neck vein distention combined with upper extremity venous distention suggests superior vena cava obstruction (e.g., from lung cancer). The chest should be inspected for signs of previous/current surgery or trauma, kyphoscoliosis, and anterior-posterior diameter ("barrel chest"). The extremities should be assessed for clubbing, cyanosis, and edema.

2. **Palpation.** When the chest is hyperinflated, the cardiac apical impulse (normally in the left midclavicular line) may be displaced toward the xiphoid process. Simultaneous palpation of the chest and abdomen reveals the presence of thoracoabdominal dyssynchrony that may occur with respiratory failure.

3. **Percussion.** Bilateral hyperresonance may indicate the presence of hyperinflation. Unilateral hyperresonance suggests pneumothorax.

4. **Auscultation.** One should compare breath sounds bilaterally for uniformity, intensity, and presence or absence of adventitious sounds. **Rhonchi** in the spontaneously breathing patient suggest large airway secretions, a frequent finding in chronic bronchitis. **Crackles** that begin in early inspiration, a forced expiratory time greater than 4 seconds, and **wheezing** during expiration suggest airway obstruction and/or bronchospasm. **Inspiratory stridor** suggests the presence of upper airway obstruction.

5. **Vital signs.** Tachycardia, tachypnea, and **pulsus paradoxus** (i.e., a difference in systolic blood

pressure between expiration and inspiration greater than 15 mm Hg when breathing spontaneously) suggest bronchospasm.

C. Radiographic and laboratory studies suggestive of COPD or asthma

1. **Chest x-ray**
   a. Hyperinflation of the lungs (flattened diaphragms with increased retrosternal air) with decreased vascular markings is characteristic of emphysema.
   b. With asthma, the chest x-ray may be normal or there may be increased vascularity.
   c. Blebs and bullae are consistent with COPD.
   d. Other findings, such as tracheal narrowing, pulmonary edema, pneumothorax, or pleural effusions, may be present, and, although not necessarily due to asthma or COPD, may complicate these diseases in the ICU.

2. **Electrocardiogram**
   a. Hyperinflation can cause low-voltage and poor R-wave progression.
   b. **Cor pulmonale** can manifest as right-axis deviation, right ventricular hypertrophy, and/or right-bundle-branch block.

3. **Arterial blood gas and pH analysis** is helpful for assessing clinical status and guiding respiratory therapies.
   a. A **partial pressure of oxygen (PaO_2)** less than 60 mm Hg while breathing room air indicates a severe asthma attack and the need for supplemental oxygen therapy. The PaO_2 is usually low in stable COPD and falls further with exacerbation.
   b. The **partial pressure of carbon dioxide (PaCO_2)** is normal in controlled asthma and emphysema, less than 45 mm Hg in mild or moderate asthma attacks, elevated in chronic bronchitis, and elevated further in acute exacerbations of COPD and in severe asthma attacks (Table 21-1).
   c. **Assessment of pH** in conjunction with the PaCO_2 allows one to assess the acuteness and severity of the acid-base status.

4. **Pulmonary function tests** give an indication of functional reserve and airway responsiveness and may help to guide management. **Peak expiratory flow** measured with an inexpensive peak flowmeter is commonly used to guide the management of asthma. A peak flow of 60% or less of the predicted value indicates severe persistent asthma.

IV. ICU management

A. Individual factors act in various combinations to produce respiratory failure in COPD and asthma. In asthma, the primary derangement is often an increased airway inflammation and tone.

1. **Increased resistive and elastic load**
   a. Upper airway obstruction due to tracheal stenosis or edema.

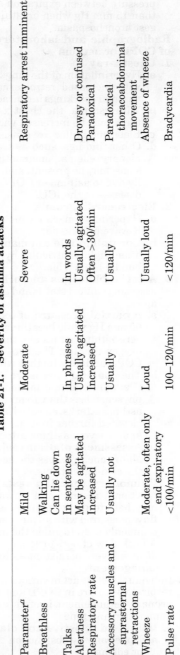

Table 21-1. Severity of asthma attacks

Parameter[a]	Mild	Moderate	Severe	Respiratory arrest imminent
Breathless	Walking Can lie down			
Talks	In sentences	In phrases	In words	
Alertness	May be agitated	Usually agitated	Usually agitated	Drowsy or confused
Respiratory rate	Increased	Increased	Often >30/min	Paradoxical
Accessory muscles and suprasternal retractions	Usually not	Usually	Usually	Paradoxical thoracoabdominal movement
Wheeze	Moderate, often only end expiratory	Loud	Usually loud	Absence of wheeze
Pulse rate	<100/min	100–120/min	<120/min	Bradycardia

PEF after initial bronchodilator (% predicted or % personal best)	>80%	60%–80%	<60% or response lasts <2 h
Pao_2 (on air)	Normal (not usually necessary)	>60 mm Hg	<60 mm Hg
$PaCO_2$	<45 mm Hg	<45 mm Hg	>45 mm Hg
Spo_2 (on air)	>95%	91%–95%	<90%

$PaCO_2$, partial pressure of carbon dioxide; Pao_2, partial pressure of oxygen; PEF, peak expiratory flow; Spo_2, oxygen saturation measured by pulse oximetry.

[a]The presence of several parameters, but not necessarily all, indicates the general classification of the attack.

Adapted from the Global Initiative for Asthma (GINA) *Pocket guide for asthma management and prevention* and *Pocket guide for asthma management and prevention in children*, available at http://www.ginasthma.com.

   b. Bronchospasm.
   c. Airway edema and secretions.
   d. Increased functional residual capacity and dynamic airway collapse.
   e. Intrinsic positive end-expiratory pressure (intrinsic PEEP) or **auto-PEEP** leads to dynamic hyperinflation. In patients with flow limitation, expiratory airflow may continue to the beginning of the next inspiration. Alveolar pressure fails to return to zero at the end of expiratory phase (intrinsic PEEP) and lung volume fails to return to its normal functional residual capacity (dynamic hyperinflation). The increased lung volume places an excessive demand on the inspiratory muscles, which are already at a mechanical disadvantage from COPD.
2. **Increased chest wall load**
   a. Preexisting kyphoscoliosis or obesity.
   b. Splinting caused by surgical pain.
3. **Decreased respiratory muscle strength and endurance**
   a. COPD places the diaphragm at a mechanical disadvantage.
   b. Preexisting (e.g., myasthenia gravis) or acquired (e.g., critical illness polyneuromyopathy) neuromuscular disease.
   c. Neuromuscular blockade from drugs.
   d. Decreased substrate delivery (e.g., shock, anemia).
   e. Respiratory muscle metabolic abnormalities due to decreased levels of magnesium, potassium, phosphate, calcium, and/or malnutrition.
   f. Acute hypoxemia, hypercarbia, and acidosis with depressant actions on the diaphragm and heart.
4. **Depressed respiratory drive**
   a. Narcotics.
   b. Anesthetic agents.
B. Hypoxemia
1. The primary gas exchange abnormality in patients with COPD is ventilation-perfusion ($\dot{V}/\dot{Q}$) mismatching. The hypoxemia due to $\dot{V}/\dot{Q}$ inequality responds well to supplemental oxygen. Careful oxygen administration seldom leads to loss of respiratory drive. However, patients with simultaneous hypercarbia and hypoxemia are at greatest of developing respiratory failure. Oxygen is essential to prevent end-organ dysfunction. Reversal of hypoxemia can improve respiratory muscle function and reverse pulmonary hypertension that could otherwise cause right ventricular failure.
2. **Oxygen** may be administered by nasal cannula or air entrainment mask. Most commonly, oxygen is administered by nasal cannula at 1 to 2 L/min. The response to oxygen administration is evaluated by arterial blood gas analysis. Although pulse oximetry is

useful, it must be remembered that it provides little information about carbon dioxide retention. The target PaO_2 is 55 to 60 mm Hg, which usually has little effect on carbon dioxide retention.

C. Wheezing

1. Some patients with COPD gain dramatic improvements with treatment of airway obstruction. Because even small improvements in airway resistance may be of significant benefit, many patients with COPD and wheezing are treated with bronchodilators, antibiotics, and corticosteroids. Chest physiotherapy has a limited role, except in selected patients who have difficulty with secretion clearance.

2. **Anticholinergics.** Parasympatholytics have a direct bronchodilating effect by blocking formation of cyclic guanine monophosphate. Because the site of bronchospasm in COPD is often in central airways corresponding to the parasympathetic innervation, these drugs, when administered by inhalation, are quite often effective in patients with COPD. Anticholinergics can also be useful in the management of asthma. Short-acting agents include ipratropium bromide and **glycopyrrolate** (see Table 21-2). The long-acting anticholinergic agent **tiotropium** is useful for management of stable COPD, but its role in management of an exacerbation is limited.

3. **Sympathomimetics.** β_2-adrenergic receptor agonists cause bronchodilation via cyclic adenosine monophosphate (cAMP)–mediated relaxation of bronchial smooth muscle. Only short-acting agents such as **albuterol** are indicated in the acute situation (see Table 21-3). Long-acting drugs in this class (e.g., **salmeterol** and **formoterol**) are never indicated for acute bronchospasm. The beta agonists are generally

Table 21-2. Commonly inhaled anticholinergic drugs

Drug	Brand Name	Administration	Initial Adult Dose	Interval (h)
Ipratropium bromide	Atrovent	MDI (18 μg)	2–3 puffs	4–6
		Nebulizer (0.2 mg/ml)	500 μg (2.5 ml)	6–8
Tiotropium	Spiriva	DPI (18 μg/ capsule)	1 capsule	24
Glycopyrrolate methylbromide	Robinul	Nebulizer (0.2 mg/ml)	2–4 ml	4–6

Initial adult doses are for spontaneously breathing adults. Increased doses may be required for patients who are tracheally intubated.
MDI, metered-dose inhaler; DPI, dry-powder inhaler.

Table 21-3. Some common inhaled beta$_2$-adrenergic drugs

Drug	Brand Name	Administration	Initial Adult Dose	Interval (h)
Albuterol	Proventil, Ventolin	MDI (90 μg)	2 puffs	4–6
		Nebulizer (5 mg/mL)	0.5 ml	
Terbutaline	Brethaire	MDI (200 μg)	2–3 puffs	4–6
Metaproterenol	Alupent, Metaprel	MDI (650 μg)	2–3 puffs	3–4
		Nebulizer (50 mg/ml)	0.2–0.3 ml	
Isoetharine mesylate	Bronkosol	MDI (340 μg)	1–2 puffs	4–6
		Nebulizer (10 mg/ml)	0.25–0.5 ml	
Pirbuterol	Maxair	MDI (200 μg)	2 puffs	4–6
Salmeterol	Serevent	DPI (50 μg)	1 inhalation	12
Formoterol	Foradil	DPI (12 μg)	1 inhalation	12
Racemic epinephrine	VapoNefrin, MicroNefrin	Nebulizer (22.5 mg/ml)	0.25–0.5 ml	1–2

Initial adult doses are for spontaneously breathing adults. Increased doses may be required for patients who are tracheally intubated.
MDI, metered-dose inhaler; DPI, dry-powder inhaler.

administered by inhalation but can be given intravenously. **Epinephrine** (0.25–2 μg/min by continuous infusion in the adult) is used when other measures have failed. Epinephrine in these doses by the parenteral (intravenous) route can be used safely, but the clinician should recognize the higher likelihood of dysrhythmias and other undesirable side effects in older patients.

4. **Corticosteroids.** These drugs act via complex and incompletely understood mechanisms to reduce airway inflammation, airway responsiveness, mucus secretions, and edema. Steroids enhance beta-adrenergic responsiveness and relax bronchial smooth muscle. Their use in the ICU has not been adequately studied.

   a. Inhaled corticosteroids may be useful for controlling airway inflammation and responsiveness in asthmatics to prevent exacerbation (see Table 21-4). The role of inhaled steroids in COPD is controversial, and they are usually limited to patients with severe disease. The inhaled route avoids some untoward metabolic, wound healing, and infectious events that are possible with systemic administration.

   b. In exacerbations of asthma, systemic administration is often necessary. From 120 to 180 mg/d of intravenous methylprednisolone is recommended in acute, severe asthma attacks, divided into three or four doses per day for 48 hours. This is followed by 60 to 80 mg of intravenous methylprednisolone per day until the peak flow reaches 70% of normal. Then 20 mg of prednisone for 3 to 10 days is recommended to complete therapy.

   c. In COPD exacerbations, various regimens have been recommended. From 30 to 40 mg of oral prednisone (or intravenous methylprednisolone) daily for 10 to 14 days may be a reasonable regimen balancing efficacy and safety.

   d. The use of corticosteroids should be based on individual clinical circumstances because the doses to employ to initiate therapy, when to start tapering, the rate of dose reductions, and the total length of corticosteroid course remain open questions in both asthma and COPD. In COPD, a 2-week course of steroids has been shown to be equally efficacious to a 6-week course and has fewer side effects.

   e. Replacement corticosteroid therapy may be needed in patients with a history of recent corticosteroid use who are not currently receiving intravenous methylprednisolone in sufficient doses to prevent acute adrenal insufficiency. The need for replacement therapy may be guided by laboratory tests (e.g., cosyntropin stimulation testing) and is influenced by patient characteristics, preoperative dose, duration and route of therapy,

Table 21-4. Common inhaled steroids

Drug	Brand Name	Administration	Initial Adult Dose	Interval (h)
Dexamethasone	Decadron Respihaler	MDI (100 μg)	3 puffs	6–8
Beclomethasone	Beclovent, Vanceril	MDI (42 μg)	2 puffs	6–8
Fluticasone	Flovent	MDI (44, 110, 220 μg)	2–4 puffs	12
Salmeterol and fluticasone	Advair	DPI (50 μg salmeterol + 100, 250, or 500 μg fluticasone)	1 inhalation	12
Triamcinolone	Azmacort	MDI (100 μg)	2 puffs	6–8
Flunisolide	Aerobid	MDI (250 μg)	2 puffs	12
Budesonide	Pulmicort	MDI (200 μg)	2 puffs	12

Initial adult doses are for spontaneously breathing adults. Increased doses may be required for patients who are tracheally intubated.
MDI, metered-dose inhaler; DPI, dry-powder inhaler.

as well as the type of surgical procedure and the presence or absence of postoperative complications.

5. **Nebulizer versus inhaler.** The use of a nebulizer or an inhaler for the delivery of aerosolized medications is controversial. Both methods have been used effectively. During acute exacerbations, many patients have difficulty using the inhaler effectively. It is also difficult to deliver high doses with the inhaler. For severe asthma, continuous nebulization of beta-agonists may be required. The use of a holding chamber improves the performance of the inhaler in patients with poor hand–breath coordination. The holding chamber also decreases pharyngeal deposition, which is important when inhaled steroids are used. Dry-powder inhalers (DPI) are increasingly becoming available. As with the metered dose inhaler (MDI), patients must be instructed in the proper technique for use of a DPI. The use of inhaler or nebulizer during mechanical ventilation is also controversial, and the choice of method is determined by clinician bias or institutional preference. A dry-powder inhaler cannot be used during mechanical ventilation.

6. **Methylxanthines** are weak bronchodilators. Specific agents include **theophylline** and **aminophylline** (80% theophylline by weight). These agents may improve respiratory drive and muscle function, but this is controversial and their effect is small. These agents are not recommended for asthma attacks when high doses of β_2-agonists are used. The mechanisms of action for these agents are complex, multiple, and incompletely understood. These include nonspecific inhibition of phosphodiesterase to increase intracellular cAMP, blockade of adenosine, direct activation of histone deacetylases, and release of endogenous catecholamines. When used for asthma or COPD, methylxanthines are administered intravenously (with or without a loading bolus) in the ICU and have a half-life of 3 to 4 hours, which is prolonged unpredictably in patients with right heart failure and with certain concomitant drugs. Methylxanthines can cause gastrointestinal symptoms such as nausea and more serious toxic reactions such as dysrhythmias and seizures. Thus, these agents have limited use. The clinical effectiveness of intravenous epinephrine is greater and the toxicity less than theophylline. Given the shorter half-life of epinephrine, we favor the careful infusion of epinephrine. When methylxanthines are used, clinical findings and serum levels should be followed closely with dose adjusted accordingly, keeping serum theophylline levels less than 20 μg/dl.

7. **Mucolytics** such as nebulized acetylcysteine or hypertonic saline may be indicated in selected patients to decrease the viscosity of mucus, but are generally

Table 21-5.   Leukotriene-receptor antagonists and synthesis inhibitors

Drug	Brand Name	Administration	Initial Adult Dose	Interval
Zafirlukast	Accolate	Oral	20 mg	Twice daily
Montelukast	Singulair	Oral	10 mg	Once daily, in the evening
Zileuton	Zyflo	Oral	600 mg	Four times daily with meals

not recommended in treating asthma attacks or COPD exacerbations. Because they induce bronchospasm, they should be administered with caution and in combination with inhaled β_2-adrenergic agonists. **Dornase alfa (Pulmozyme)** may have a role in selected patients with cystic fibrosis, but it is not indicated in patients with COPD or asthma.

8. **Leukotriene receptor antagonists (zafirlukast and montelukast) and synthesis inhibitors (zileuton)** (see Table 21-5) are modestly effective for maintenance treatment of chronic asthma. These are inadequately studied in patients with either COPD or asthma in the ICU, although recent studies suggest efficacy.

9. **Cromolyn** stabilizes mast cells and may modulate the nonadrenergic, noncholinergic nervous system. It is not indicated in acute bronchospasm and thus is not indicated in the ICU.

10. **Magnesium, cyclosporine, and methotrexate** are occasionally used in patients with asthma or COPD whose disease is not adequately controlled with the medications just outlined, with tolerable side effects.

11. **Helium–oxygen ("heliox")** is a gas mixture that is used successfully on occasion to decrease upper airway obstruction due to postextubation edema in patients with COPD and asthma. Heliox is also effective in reducing the work of breathing in some patients with acute exacerbation of asthma.

12. **Anesthetic agents** (e.g., intravenous propofol, dexmedetomidine, or ketamine) and inhaled volatile anesthetics (e.g., sevoflurane) are used on occasion as bronchodilators and to facilitate patient–ventilator interactions when the patient is intubated. Sedatives must be used cautiously, if at all, when the patient is breathing spontaneously.

D. **Surgical therapies for severe COPD**

1. **Lung volume reduction surgery** is performed in selected patients with COPD either as a primary

therapy or as a bridge to lung transplantation. Common postoperative problems include air trapping (dynamic hyperinflation), secretion retention, persistent air leaks, pain, hypercapneic respiratory failure, and anxiety. Postoperative invasive mechanical ventilation carries risks of infection, causing or enlarging airway leaks. Adequate pain control, often provided by epidural infusion, is essential to allow adequate postoperative pulmonary function. Detailed postoperative considerations are discussed in Chapter 37.

2. **Lung transplantation** is a treatment for a subset of patients with COPD. The patient remains sedated and intubated and mechanically ventilated in the immediate postoperative period until the transplanted lung(s) begin(s) to function well and symptoms of reperfusion injury, pulmonary hypertension/cor pulmonale, and acute rejection are controlled. Serial measurements of arterial blood gases help to document function of the transplanted lung(s) and are used to assess acute rejection. Monitoring for signs of toxicity from the immunosuppressive regimen is undertaken. Patients may present with subacute or chronic complications following transplantation. One should focus on detecting surgical airway complications, respiratory insufficiency, and rejection, including development of obliterating bronchiolitis. Complications relating to immunosuppressive medications can occur leading to infection, development of neoplasms, renal insufficiency, hematologic impairment, Cushing's syndrome, or osteoporosis. Specifics of the evaluation and management of the postoperative complications are discussed in Chapters 37 and 39.

E. **Infectious processes**

1. The airways of patients with COPD are often colonized with potential pathogens. In the ICU, patients with COPD are at increased risk of acute respiratory failure due to worsening of airway colonization, which can lead to more severe purulent bronchitis and possibly pneumonia. It sometimes may be appropriate to treat patients with acute COPD with antibiotics, despite having no evidence of parenchymal lung infection. Unless acute respiratory failure is clearly due to the worsening bacterial colonization (e.g., excessive mucus secretions), the patient is often not treated with antibiotics. Attention is more properly directed to aspects of care such as pain relief and secretion clearance. The presence of a parenchymal infiltrate represents a different problem. The diagnosis of pneumonia versus bronchitis (often with edema or atelectasis) in the intubated, mechanically ventilated patient with COPD is not straightforward. Pneumonia is poorly tolerated in patients with advanced COPD. Early or preemptive antibiotic therapy is often the

most prudent course for the critically ill patient with COPD.

2. Patients with asthma generally do not have chronic bacterial colonization of their airway. In the asthmatic patient with bronchospasm, mucus production, but without infiltrates on chest radiography, performing both a Gram's and a Wright stain of sputum may differentiate acute infection from a noninfectious exacerbation of asthma.

F. Pulmonary embolism

1. Patients with COPD often have a hypercoagulopathy from bed rest and possibly hypoxemia and are at risk of pulmonary embolism. History, physical findings, laboratory findings (e.g., D-dimers), arterial blood gas measurements, electrocardiogram, chest radiograph, ventilation/perfusion scintigraphy, and helical computed tomography may help to exclude or rule in this diagnosis. If these are nondiagnostic, pulmonary angiography may be indicated. Therapy must be individualized (Chapter 22).

G. Other causes of respiratory failure in patients with obstructive lung disease include cardiac disease (e.g., ischemia, infarction, failure, dysrhythmia), pneumothorax, pleural effusion, and upper airway obstruction (e.g., edema, inflammation, infection, tracheal stenosis).

1. Patients with COPD and some with asthma often have coexisting cardiac diseases. Cardioselective beta-blockers do not produce clinically significant adverse respiratory effects in asthmatic and COPD patients with chronic airways obstruction and/or mild to moderate reactive airway disease. Given their demonstrated benefit in the perioperative period in reducing cardiovascular morbidity and mortality and in chronic conditions such as congestive heart failure, cardiac arrhythmias, and hypertension, cardioselective beta-blockers should not be withheld from patients with chronic airways disease or mild to moderate reactive airways disease when indicated in the postoperative ICU setting. In patients at risk for adverse perioperative coronary artery events that have greater degrees of reactive airways disease and in whom beta-blockers would be contraindicated, clonidine may be effective in reducing the incidence of cardiovascular morbidity and mortality.

V. Mechanical ventilation (see also Chapter 5)

A. Specific conditions requiring mechanical ventilation include respiratory acidosis, severe hypoxemia, retained secretions, atelectasis, pneumonia, laryngospasm, and upper airway edema.

B. Noninvasive positive-pressure ventilation (NPPV)

1. Compared to conventional therapy, controlled studies have reported reduced intubation rates and increased survival with NPPV, and the greatest benefit

for NPPV has been shown in patients with exacerbations of COPD.

2. NPPV should not be used if the patient requires an artificial airway for airway protection or secretion clearance.

3. Either **nasal or oronasal masks** can be used, but oronasal masks are preferred to avoid problems with mouth leak during acute respiratory failure.

4. Either critical care ventilators or BiPAP machines can be used to provide NPPV. Carbon dioxide rebreathing and supplemental oxygen administrations are potential problems with BiPAP machines.

C. A suggested approach to invasive mechanical ventilation of the patient with obstructive lung disease is shown in Fig. 21-1.

D. **Pressure versus volume ventilation**

1. **Volume ventilation** maintains a constant tidal volume during changes in airways resistance and lung compliance. The fixed inspiratory flow during volume-controlled ventilation may produce patient–ventilator dyssynchrony. The fixed tidal volume during volume ventilation may produce hyperinflation if auto-PEEP is present.

2. **Pressure-controlled ventilation** may improve patient–ventilator synchrony because flow varies with patient demand. Pressure ventilation also prevents hyperinflation if auto-PEEP occurs. The tidal volume will change with changes in airways resistance, respiratory system compliance, auto-PEEP, and patient effort.

3. **Pressure support ventilation** can produce an excessive inspiratory time in the patient with COPD because a low inspiratory flow rate may be required to cycle the ventilator to the expiratory phase (Chapter 5). The patient may need to exhale actively against the ventilator breath to reduce the inspiratory flow rate and cycle the ventilator to exhalation. A simple way to correct this problem is to use pressure-controlled ventilation with a defined inspiratory time setting (e.g., 0.8 to 1.2 seconds). Another way to correct this is to adjust the flow cycle criteria on the ventilator if the ventilator has this capability.

E. **Mode**

1. **Synchronized intermittent mandatory ventilation (SIMV)** fails to completely relieve the patient's inspiratory efforts during both the mandatory breaths and the intervening unsupported breaths, and, therefore, this mode is not preferred.

2. **Continuous mandatory ventilation (assist/control)** is preferred when respiratory muscle unloading is desired.

F. **Auto-PEEP**

1. **Auto-PEEP** is common during mechanical ventilation of patients with COPD and asthma.

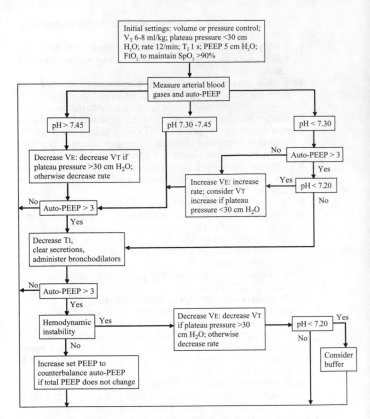

Fig. 21-1. Suggested approach to mechanical ventilation of the patient with obstructive lung disease. FIO_2, inspired oxygen; PEEP, positive end-expiratory pressure; V_E, minute ventilation; V_T, tidal volume; T_I, inspiratory time (Adapted from Hess D, Medoff BD. Mechanical ventilation of the patient with chronic obstructive pulmonary disease. *Respir Clin North Am* 1998;4:439–473.)

2. **Auto-PEEP** is corrected by decreasing airways resistance (e.g., bronchodilator administration) or decreasing minute ventilation (e.g., permissive hypercapnia).
3. In patients with COPD, the addition of PEEP may counterbalance auto-PEEP and improve the patient's ability to trigger the ventilator.
   a. When this approach is used, care must be exercised to avoid further hyperinflation.
   b. PEEP often counterbalances auto-PEEP in patients with dynamic airway closure (e.g., COPD), but its effects on other causes of auto-PEEP (e.g., asthma, high minute ventilation) are less

predictable and more likely to exacerbate hyperinflation.
G. **Discontinuation of mechanical ventilation** (see Chapter 23)
   1. Patients should be regularly screened for weaning readiness: resolution of exacerbation, gas exchange, hemodynamic stability, need for sedation.
   2. The best approach to determining readiness for ventilator discontinuation is a spontaneous breathing trial.
   3. Several controlled studies have reported lower rates of successful weaning using SIMV compared with gradually tapering pressure support ventilation or trials of spontaneous breathing.
   4. If the patient tolerates 30 to 60 minutes of spontaneous breathing without signs of fatigue (e.g., tachypnea, tachycardia, increased accessory muscle use, diaphoresis), extubation should be considered.
   5. In selected patients who fail a spontaneous breathing trial, extubation to noninvasive ventilation should be considered.

SELECTED REFERENCES

Crossley DJ, McGuire GP, Barrow PM, et al. Influence of inspired oxygen concentration on deadspace, respiratory drive, and $Paco_2$ in intubated patients with chronic obstructive pulmonary disease. *Crit Care Med* 1997;25:1522–1526.

DeMeo DL, Ginns LC. Clinical status of lung transplantation. *Transplantation* 2001;72:1713–1724.

Felix SF, Wright J, Brocklbank D, et al. Systematic review of clinical effectiveness of pressurized metered dose inhalers versus other hand held inhaler devices for delivering B2 agonists bronchodilators in asthma. *BMJ* 2001;323:1–7.

Fink JB, Tobin MJ, Dhand R. Bronchodilator therapy in mechanically ventilated patients. *Respir Care* 1999;44:53–72.

GINA (Global Initiative for Asthma), Global Strategy for Asthma Management and Prevention, 2004. www.ginasthma.com.

Gold Scientific Committee. Global strategy for the diagnosis, management, and prevention of chronic obstructive pulmonary disease. *Am J Respir Crit Care Med* 2001;163:1256–1276.

Hess D, Medoff BD. Mechanical ventilation of the patient with chronic obstructive pulmonary disease. *Respir Clin North Am* 1998;4:439–473.

Ho AM, Lee A, Karmakar MK, et al. Heliox vs air–oxygen mixtures for the treatment of patients with acute asthma: a systematic overview. *Chest* 2003;123:882–890.

Jaber S, Carlucci A, Boussarsar M, et al. Helium–oxygen in the postextubation period decreases inspiratory effort. *Am J Respir Crit Care Med* 2001;164:633–637.

Lightowler JV, Wedzicha JA, et al. Non-invasive positive pressure ventilation to treat respiratory failure resulting from exacerbations of chronic obstructive pulmonary disease: Cochrane systematic review and meta-analysis. *BMJ* 2003;326:185–189.

McCrory DC, Brown C, Gelfand SE, et al. Management of acute exacerbations of COPD: a summary and appraisal of published evidence. *Chest* 2001;119:1190–1209.

McFadden ER Jr. Acute severe asthma. *Am J Respir Crit Care Med* 2003;168:740–759.

Mehta S, Hill NS. Noninvasive ventilation. *Am J Respir Crit Care Med* 2001;163:540–577.

Rello J, Diaz E. Pneumonia in the intensive care unit. *Crit Care Med* 2003;31:2544–2551.

Rodrigo GJ, Rodrigo C, Pollack CV, et al. Use of helium–oxygen mixtures in the treatment of acute asthma: a systematic review. *Chest* 2003;123:891–896.

Salpeter SR, Ormiston TM, Salpeter EE. Cardioselective beta-blockers in patients with reactive airway disease: a meta-analysis. *Ann Intern Med* 2002;137:715–725.

Smith D, Riel J, Tiles I, et al. Intravenous epinephrine in life-threatening asthma. *Ann Emerg Med* 2003;41:706–711.

Wallace AR, Galindez D, Salahieh A, et al. Effect of clonidine on cardiovascular morbidity and mortality after noncardiac surgery. *Anesthesiology* 2004;101:284–293.

Warner DO, Warner MA, Barnes RD, et al. Perioperative respiratory complications in patients with asthma. *Anesthesiology* 1996;85:460–467.

Pulmonary Embolism and Deep Venous Thrombosis

Deborah A. Quinn and B. Taylor Thompson

I. **Overview.** Embolization of thrombus from the deep venous system to the pulmonary vascular bed results in a nonspecific clinical presentation that is frequently unrecognized. The estimated annual incidence of pulmonary embolism in the United States is 500,000, and the prevalence for nonfatal pulmonary embolism approaches 20 per 1,000 inpatients. Treatment with anticoagulants reduces mortality from between 30% and 40% to between 2% and 8%, primarily by preventing further emboli. Pulmonary embolism and deep venous thrombosis have been less well studied in critically ill patients, but studies indicate that approximately 13% of critically ill patients may develop deep venous thrombosis even with prophylaxis. A high level of surveillance is needed in critically ill patients.

II. **Natural history**

   A. **Deep venous thrombosis (DVT)** usually begins in the lower extremities, although occasional thrombi form in pelvic veins, renal veins, upper extremity veins, and the right heart. Most thrombi originate in the soleal veins of the calf near valve cusps or bifurcations. Calf thrombi may resolve spontaneously, and embolization to the lung is uncommon. About 20% to 30% of clots propagate to the popliteal, femoral, or iliac veins (so-called proximal DVT), and an additional 10% to 20% of all DVT begin in the thigh without prior calf involvement.

   B. **Pulmonary emboli (PE).** Once in the pulmonary circulation, large emboli may lodge at the bifurcation of the pulmonary and lobar arteries, causing hemodynamic instability. Smaller emboli continue distally into small arteries or arterioles. The lower lobes are more often involved than the upper lobes, and multiple emboli are usually present at the time of diagnosis. Only 10% to 20% of emboli cause infarction, usually in patients with preexisting cardiopulmonary disease.

III. **Risk factors for DVT and PE**

   A. Prior venous thromboembolism.

   B. Factors promoting stasis such as bed rest, congestive heart failure, or inactivity.

   C. Endothelial damage such as lower extremity surgery or trauma.

   D. Hypercoagulable states such factor Leiden, prothrombin mutation, anti–thrombin III deficiency, lupus anticoagulant, and antiphospholipid antibody.

   E. Malignancy. Approximately 15% of patients with venous thromboembolic disease who have no known risk factors for DVT or PE will have an occult malignancy diagnosed within 2 years.

F. Spinal cord injury. DVT occurs in 38% of these patients within 3 months of paralysis, with a corresponding frequency of PE of approximately 5%.

G. Heparin-induced thrombocytopenia (HIT). In patients who develop HIT and have heparin therapy discontinued, 38% to 76% subsequently develop DVT and/or PE.

H. Airline travel greater than 3,100 miles.

IV. Clinical manifestations

A. Symptoms and signs

1. DVT. Many lower extremity venous thrombi are asymptomatic, probably because they remain nonocclusive or because of the development of collaterals. Symptomatic thrombi produce calf pain, edema, venous distention, and pain on passive dorsiflexion of the foot (Homan's sign). These symptoms and signs are nonspecific. Prospective studies of outpatients with symptoms suggestive of DVT actually find DVT by objective testing in only one-third of patients. In patients with leg symptoms suggesting DVT but in whom venography is normal, musculoskeletal injuries, Baker's cysts, and chronic lymphatic or venous insufficiency are the usual explanations.

2. PE. Autopsy series suggest that many PE are silent. When clinically apparent, symptoms and signs depend on the size of the embolus. Symptoms of small to medium emboli include dyspnea, chest pain, and cough. Tachypnea and tachycardia are present in the majority of patients. Mild fever below 39°C is common, and wheezing occurs in less than 5% of patients. If infarction occurs, hemoptysis, pleuritic pain, and pleural rub are present. Massive emboli often produce cardiovascular findings. Symptoms include syncope, chest pain, and dyspnea along with signs of right ventricular dysfunction such as a right ventricular heave, a right ventricular S3, jugular venous distention, or a murmur of tricuspid regurgitation.

B. Hemodynamic findings. After PE, cardiac output is usually normal, but in hypotensive patients with massive PE the cardiac output is low. In this setting, right ventricular diastolic and right atrial mean pressures are always elevated. Pulmonary artery pressure tends to be increased but correlates poorly with the size of the embolus and may be normal even in massive PE.

C. Differential diagnosis. Smaller PE may mimic pneumothorax, hyperventilation, asthma, myocardial infarction, congestive heart failure, pleurodynia, or serositis. If infarction is present, clinical findings may resemble pneumonia, bronchial obstruction by mucus or tumor, or pleural effusion. The differential diagnosis for massive PE includes right ventricular infarction, pericardial tamponade, and venous air embolism.

V. Laboratory evaluation

A. **The electrocardiogram (ECG)** is often abnormal in small to medium PE, but findings are nonspecific. The ECG is normal in 23% of patients with submassive embolism and in 6% of patients with massive PE.

B. **Chest radiography.** Even without infarction, radiographic abnormalities occur in the majority of patients with pulmonary emboli and include elevation of a hemidiaphgram, atelectasis, and effusion. An infarct appears as a pleural-based infiltrate with a convex margin directed toward the hilum.

C. **Noninvasive studies** for DVT. **Color-flow Doppler** with compression ultrasound (referred to as **venous ultrasound**) has high sensitivity (89%–100%) and specificity (89%–100%) in comparison with venography for the detection of proximal DVT and slightly less sensitivity and specificity for calf vein thrombi. Venous ultrasound is also useful for the detection of a Baker's cyst. Sensitivity falls dramatically when venous ultrasonography is used for asymptomatic, high-risk patients (33%). **Impedance plethysmography (IPG)** also offers high sensitivity, slightly less specificity, and lower cost in comparison to venous ultrasound. IPG is not accurate for the detection of calf vein thrombi. **Computed tomography (CT) venography** has not undergone rigorous testing, but offers the convenience of allowing assessment of both pelvic and leg veins. The results of the Prospective Investigation of Pulmonary Embolism Diagnosis (PIOPED) II study offer more data on CT venography (see section **V.J**).

D. **D-dimers** are usually present in the serum of patients with pulmonary emboli, but are nondiagnostic. However, a level below 500 u/ml has a high negative predictive value of 91% (95% confidence interval [CI] 77%–98%). Because the rapidly available and inexpensive red cell agglutination assay is negative below a level of 500 D-dimer units/ml, a negative test makes DVT or PE unlikely, particularly in patients with low pretest probabilities for PE.

E. **HIT Antibodies.** HIT testing should be performed in all patients being treated with any form of heparin treatment when there is a platelet count decrease of greater than 50% from baseline or to below 100,000/μl. Heparin should be discontinued while awaiting results of HIT testing.

F. **Lung scintigraphy.** Perfusion lung scans are performed by injection of radiolabeled albumin macroaggregates or microspheres. Scans are sensitive; a negative perfusion scan virtually excludes PE. Results are also nonspecific. Because pulmonary arterioles constrict in response to hypoxia, perfusion defects, especially if nonsegmental, may be secondary to a ventilatory abnormality and not to obstruction of flow by an embolism. Perfusion scans may be abnormal in atelectasis, asthma, chronic airway obstruction, and other causes of regional hypoventilation. A large multicenter study (PIOPED) of the accuracy of ventilation perfusion scans compared with pulmonary angiography suggested that multiple segmental or larger perfusion defects, not matched by ventilation defects, are fairly consistent with the presence of PE and have a false-positive rate of about 14%. Most patients with a high-probability lung scan and a negative angiogram have either chronic pulmonary emboli or cancer with vascular involvement. Multiple subsegmental perfusion defects that are matched by ventilation defects are uncommonly associated with PE with a false-negative rate of 15%. Clinical probability assessments and lung scan probability assessments are complimentary. The value of lung scintigraphy in intubated patients or unconscious patients is limited due to poor image quality.

G. **Noninvasive diagnostic approach.** Unfortunately, many of the clinical and scan probabilities fall in the nondiagnostic zone (low or intermediate). In such patients, noninvasive assessment for DVT may be helpful. If venous ultrasound is positive for DVT, then the indication and rationale for anticoagulation are the same as for confirmed PE. More than one-third of patients with angiographic evidence of PE have negative leg studies for DVT. Such patients either have false-negative leg studies, thrombi that originated from calf vein thrombi that were missed by noninvasive leg studies, or a source of emboli other than the legs, or such patients embolized their entire lower extremity clot burden in one clinical event.

H. **Outcome studies.** The safety of withholding anticoagulation in patients with suspected PE (low or moderate suspicion), nondiagnostic lung scans, and negative serial leg studies (over 2 weeks) has recently been shown in a large, five-hospital outcome study. Substituting a single negative D-dimer for serial leg studies in this approach was supported in a parallel study of the same cohort.

I. **Pulmonary angiography.** Despite the advantages of noninvasive techniques, a significant proportion of patients require angiography to confirm or exclude pulmonary embolism with certainty. Angiography is the definitive diagnostic technique in this disease, and is performed by injecting radiocontrast dye into a pulmonary artery branch after percutaneous catheterization, usually transfemorally. The injection catheter should be advanced at least into the right or left pulmonary artery to achieve good dye concentration in the pulmonary vessels. A positive result consists of a filling defect or sharp cutoff of small vessels. Mortality of the procedure is less than 0.5%. Morbidity occurs in about 5%, usually related to catheter insertion and contrast reactions.

J. **Contrast spiral CT** appears to have 60% to 80% sensitivity for PE lodged in segmental or larger vessels and

80% to 95% specificity. High specificity requires reader expertise, and emboli in smaller vessels are not reliably detected with this technique. In critically ill patients the sensitivity and specificity have been reported to be as low as 45% and 82%, respectively, though further study is needed. The use of the newer 16- and 64-slice CT scanners decreases the time needed for breath hold and may increase the sensitivity, specificity, and quality of the CT scan in critically ill patients. Contrast CT chest can also be performed with imaging of the pelvic and leg veins.

K. Magnetic resonance angiography (MRA) has high sensitivity and specificity. Emergency availability of MRA and the appropriate monitoring of unstable patients in the scanner are potential limitations.

VI. Prophylaxis for DVT and PE

A. High-risk patients include those immobilized or at bed rest and who have severe head injury (Glasgow Coma Score ≤8), severe blunt chest or abdominal injury, pelvic fractures, severe lower extremity injuries, and selected burns, especially electrical burns.

B. Relatively immobile patients should receive prophylaxis, if possible, if they have additional risk factors such as previous history of DVT or PE, obesity, age older than 60 years, presence of femoral venous catheter, pregnancy, cancer, and marginal cardiopulmonary reserve.

C. Critically ill patients. All critically ill patients require prophylaxis.

D. Prophylaxis includes nonpharmacologic and pharmacologic measures.

  1. **Elastic stockings and sequential compression boots** are routine, but their efficacy appears to be marginal. Increasing patient mobility reduces venous stasis and the formation of DVT. These measures should usually be supplemented by pharmacologic prophylaxis, especially in critically ill patients, though the efficacy of combined therapy has not been evaluated. Critically ill patients at high risk of bleeding should receive sequential compression boots.

  2. **If a mild to moderate risk of bleeding exists, subcutaneous heparin** (in the adult, 5,000 units every 12 hours, or every 8 hours for patients > 100 kg) or **dalteparin** (Fragmin; 5,000 units subcutaneously, once daily) can be administered.

  3. **If anticoagulation is contraindicated,** periodic systematic screening for deep venous thrombosis with venous ultrasound (see section **V.C**) should be conducted. In high-risk patients, this is usually performed twice per week.

  4. If surveillance cannot be adequately performed, prophylactic placement of an **inferior vena caval filter** can be considered in high-risk patients (see section **VII.F**).

  5. For patients who present with thrombocytopenia associated with HIT, **lepirudin** or **argatroban** can be

used for prophylaxis. Because argatroban is eliminated by hepatic metabolism and lepirudin is cleared
by renal excretion, argatroban should be used in patients with hepatic dysfunction and lepirudin should
be used in patients with renal impairment.

6. For patients receiving activated protein C for severe
sepsis the best method for prophylaxis without increasing the risk of bleeding is unknown.

VII. Treatment

A. Unfractionated heparin

1. **Dose.** The constant intravenous infusion of unfractionated heparin is the current standard of care for
most patients with DVT or PE. A bolus of 75 u/kg
should be followed by approximately 18 u/kg/h in most
patients. An activated partial thromboplastin time
(aPTT) of 1.5 to 2.5 times the mean laboratory control
should be achieved within 24 hours, and this should
correspond to a heparin level of 0.2 to 0.4 u/ml in
plasma. Fatal recurrences on anticoagulant therapy
usually occur within the first week after diagnosis,
and failure to reach a therapeutic aPTT increases the
risk for recurrence or extension of DVT 10-fold.

2. **The duration** of heparin therapy should be 5 to
7 days, with 5 days of overlap with **Coumadin.** For
massive PE and ileofemoral thrombosis, a longer period of heparin may be considered.

3. **Complications.** Hemorrhage is the major complication of heparin therapy, occurring in about 1% of
patients per day after the first day. Heparin may
also cause thrombocytopenia (3%–4%) with or without thrombosis.

4. **Contraindications.** Absolute contraindications to
heparin are intracranial bleed or tumor, active gastrointestinal (GI bleeding), retroperitoneal hemorrhage, proliferative retinopathy with hemorrhage,
heparin-associated thrombocytopenia, and malignant
pericarditis. A known bleeding diathesis and recent
surgery are relative contraindications.

B. Fractionated or low-molecular-weight (LMW) hep-
arins such as **dalteparin** are derived from unfractionated heparin. They are typically administered by subcutaneous injection, have more predictable dose–response
characteristics than unfractionated heparin, and can be
given without the need for monitoring of an anticoagulant effect. They are equally effective and possibly safer
than unfractionated heparins. LMW heparin is the preferred prophylaxis for spinal cord injuries. It is important to note that **spinal or epidural hematomas** have
been associated with spinal or epidural anesthesia and
lumbar punctures in patients receiving fractionated heparins or heparinoids. The risk of epidural hematoma
formation is increased in patients who have indwelling
epidural catheters or are also receiving other drugs that
may adversely affect hemostasis.

C. **Direct thrombin inhibitors. Lepirudin** and **arga-troban** are direct thrombin inhibitors that can be used for treatment of thrombosis associated with HIT. Argatroban is given at 0.5 μg/kg/min intravenously and adjusted until steady-state aPTT is 1.5 to 3 times the initial baseline value (not to exceed 100 seconds). Because argatroban artificially elevates the International Normalized Ratio (INR), when starting warfarin, discontinue argatroban when INR reaches 4.0. Recheck INR in 4 hours to confirm therapeutic range has been achieved with warfarin. Lepirudin is given intravenously with a loading dose of 0.4 mg/kg followed by 0.15 mg/kg/h until steady-state aPTT is 1.5 to 3 times the initial baseline value. Lepirudin does not artificially elevate the INR.

D. **Oral anticoagulants**

1. **Onset of action.** Because the antithrombotic effect of Coumadin is due to prothrombin (factor II) depletion and because it takes roughly 5 days for prothrombin to fall to an effective antithrombotic level (roughly 20% of normal), Coumadin should not be used alone in the acute setting.

2. **Monitoring.** An INR of 2.5 should be targeted for most patients.

3. **Duration of treatment.** Six weeks of Coumadin is sufficient for calf vein thrombosis. Three to 6 months is recommended for patients with proximal DVT and for patients with PE. Patients with idiopathic venous thrombosis are likely to exhibit recurrence even after 6 months of Coumadin (2-year incidence up to 27%), and 6 to 12 months of anticoagulation is reasonable in this setting. Lifelong anticoagulation is considered for recurrent episodes or a first event with a nonreversible risk factor such as cancer, homozygous factor V Leiden carriers, or antiphospholipid antibody syndrome.

4. **New oral anticoagulants.** Oral direct thrombin inhibitors such as **ximelagartan** are under investigation for both prophylaxis and treatment of PE/DVT.

E. **Thrombolytic therapy**

1. **Indications.** Thrombolytic therapy is approved for proximal DVT and massive PE (filling defects in two or more lobar vessels or emboli causing hemodynamic instability). Some authors recommend lytic therapy for those with echocardiographic evidence of right ventricular dysfunction during acute embolization. Because mortality is similar and complications are less with heparin, we favor the use of thrombolytic therapy only for acute massive PE with hemodynamic compromise. Others have suggested that the use of alteplase should be considered for hemodynamically stable patients with evidence of right ventricular dysfunction.

2. **The objective** of thrombolysis for DVT is complete and rapid removal of thrombus and preservation of venous valvular function, leading to a reduction in postphlebitic complications. Severe postphlebitic complications (e.g., edema, pain, and ulceration) are probably reduced with streptokinase compared to heparin, but the effect is small. The objective of thrombolytic agents for PE is to accelerate clot lysis, reduce pulmonary artery pressure, improve right ventricular function, and improve survival. Although no reduction in mortality has been shown in comparison with heparin in large prospective series, a recent, smaller study of tissue plasminogen activator (tPA) hinted at a survival advantage with lysis, though the heparin dosing schedule was suboptimal. Thrombolytic therapy may allow improved pulmonary function after recovery, and a recent long-term follow-up study suggested improved exercise tolerance 7 years after thrombolysis.

3. **Contraindications.** Absolute contraindications include intracranial bleeding or a strong possibility thereof, or other major bleeding. Relative contraindications are recent (10 days) surgery or trauma.

4. **Choice of thrombolytic agent.** The three thrombolytic agents approved for the treatment of pulmonary embolism and their recommended doses and costs are shown in Table 22-1. There are no conclusive data to suggest that any one of these agents is either more effective or safer than another. Urokinase and tPA are expensive. Streptokinase is antigenic in humans and reacts with antistreptococcal antibodies. tPA appears to be as effective as other thrombolytic agents in the treatment of PE, but is not necessarily safer at the currently recommended doses. Three studies of weight-adjusted bolus dosing of tPA (0.6 mg/kg over 3–15 minutes) show similar efficacy but no reduction in bleeding complications.

Table 22-1.   Choice of thrombolytic agents for pulmonary embolism

Drug	FDA-Approved Dose	Alternative Dose	Cost ($)
Streptokinase	250,000 U× 20 min, 100,000 U/h × 24–72 h	1,500,000 U × 1 h	350
Urokinase	4,400-U/kg bolus, 4,400 U/kg/h × 12 h	3,000,000 U × 2 h	2,000–2,700
tPA	100 mg × 2 h	0.6 mg/kg × 3–15 min	2,000–4,200

FDA, Food and Drug Administration; tPA, tissue plasminogen activator.

5. Complications. Bleeding complications correlate poorly with coagulation parameters but are increased by performing invasive procedures. Patients in whom thrombolytic therapy is considered should have procedures performed in distal vessels, if possible. As many as one-third of patients treated with streptokinase develop mild fever, and a smaller number have allergic reactions, usually manifested by urticaria, itching, or flushing. Hypotension may occur in approximately 10% and limits the use of this agent in unstable patients.

F. Inferior vena caval filters. If anticoagulation is strongly contraindicated or if emboli recur despite adequate anticoagulation, an inferior vena cava interruption procedure should be performed to prevent further embolization from leg or pelvic veins. Removable inferior vena caval filters are now available. These offer an attractive alternative because there is increased risk of new or recurrent DVT post–vena caval filter placement. Depending on the type, filters can be removed 2 weeks to 3 months after placement. More data are needed on their efficacy and long-term outcomes.

G. Pulmonary embolectomy. The utility of emergency pulmonary embolectomy for massive PE is uncertain. Eighty percent of those who die from emboli do so in the first hour. Only rarely can an embolectomy be accomplished in this time frame. Mortality during thromboembolectomy is extremely high (57% in emergency procedures and 25% in semiurgent procedures). Randomized comparison with thrombolytic therapy has not been performed. Transvenous catheter embolectomy or catheter fragmentation can be considered as an alternative to operative embolectomy in nonsurgical candidates. The use of newer techniques of pulmonary embolectomy in patients with large clot burden and right ventricular dysfunction has been evaluated in a small number of patients, with only 11% mortality, but the use of these techniques in the critically ill patient needs further investigation.

SELECTED REFERENCES

Aklog L, Williams CS, Byrne JG, et al. Acute pulmonary embolectomy: a contemporary approach. *Circulation* 2002;105:1416–1419.

Anderson FA, Spender FA. Risk factors for venous thromboembolism. *Circulation* 2003;107:9–16.

Decousus H, Leizorovicz A, Parent F, et al. A clinical trial of vena caval filters in the prevention of pulmonary embolism in patients with proximal deep-vein thrombosis. *N Engl J Med* 1998;338:409–415.

de Gregorio MA, Gamboa P, Gimeno MJ, et al. The Gunther Tulip retrievable filter: prolonged temporary filtration by repositioning within the inferior vena cava. *J Vasc Interv Radiol* 2003;14:1259–1265.

Geerts W, Selby R. Prevention of venous thromboembolism in the ICU. *Chest* 2003;124:357S–363S.

Goldhaber SZ. Thrombolysis for pulmonary embolism. *N Engl J Med* 2002;347:1131–1132.

Gulba DC, Schmid C, Borst HG, et al. Medical compared with surgical treatment for massive pulmonary embolism. *Lancet* 1994;343:576–577.

Hirsh J, Heddle N, Kelton JG, et al. Treatment of heparin-induced thrombocytopenia: a critical review. *Arch Intern Med* 2004;164: 361–369.

Hyers TM. Management of venous thromboembolism: past, present and future. *Arch Intern Med* 2003;163:759–768.

Kanne JP, Lalani TA, et al. Role of computed tomography and magnetic resonance imaging for deep venous thrombosis and pulmonary embolism. *Circulation* 2004;109:I15–21.

Kearon C, Ginsberg JS, Hirsh J. The role of venous ultrasonography in the diagnosis of suspected deep venous thrombosis and pulmonary embolism. *Ann Intern Med* 1998;129:1044–1049.

Kearon C, Julian JA, Math M, et al. Noninvasive diagnosis of deep venous thrombosis. *Ann Intern Med* 1998;128:663–677.

Koning R, Cribier A, Gerber L, et al. A new treatment for severe pulmonary embolism: percutaneous rheolytic thrombectomy. *Circulation* 1997;96:2498–2500.

Kostantinides S, Geibel A, Heusel G, et al. Heparin plus alteplase compared with heparin alone in patients with submassive pulmonary embolism. *N Engl J Med* 2002;347:1143–1150.

Lapostolle F, Surget V, Borron SW, et al. Severe pulmonary embolism associated with air travel. *N Engl J Med* 2001;345:779–783.

Meyer G, Tamisier D, Sors H, et al. Pulmonary embolectomy: a 20-year experience at one center. *Ann Thorac Surg* 1991;51:232–236.

Rocha AT, Tapson VF. Venous thromboembolism in intensive care. *Clin Chest Med* 2003;24:103–122.

Stein PD, Terrin ML, Hales CA, et al. Clinical, laboratory, roentgenographic and electro-cardiographic findings in patients with acute pulmonary embolism and no pre-existing cardiac or pulmonary disease. *Chest* 1991;100:598–603.

Tapson VF, Carroll BA, Davidson BL, et al. The diagnostic approach to acute venous thromboembolism: a clinical practice guideline. *Am J Respir Crit Care Med* 1999;160:1043–1066.

The PIOPED Investigators. Value of the ventilation/perfusion scan in acute pulmonary embolism. Results of the Prospective Investigation of Pulmonary Embolism Diagnosis (PIOPED). *JAMA* 1990;263:2753–2759.

Velmahos GC, Nigro J, Tatevossian R, et al. Inability of an aggressive policy of thromboprophylaxis to prevent deep venous thrombosis (DVT) in critically injured patients: are current methods of DVT prophylaxis insufficient? *J Am Coll Surg* 1998;187:529–533.

Velmahos GC, Vassiliu P, Wilcox A, et al. Spiral computed tomography for the diagnosis of pulmonary embolism in critically ill surgical patients: a comparison with pulmonary angiography. *Arch Surg* 2001;136:505–511.

Wells PS, Anderson DR, Rodger M, et al. Evaluation of D-dimer in the diagnosis of suspected deep-vein thrombosis. *N Engl J Med* 2003;349:1227–1235.

Wells PS, Ginsberg JS, Anderson DR, et al. Use of a clinical model for safe management of patients with suspected pulmonary embolism. *Ann Intern Med* 1998;129:997–1005.

Wood KE. Major pulmonary embolism: review of a pathophysiologic approach to the golden hour of hemodynamically significant pulmonary embolism. *Chest* 2002;121:877–905.

Discontinuation of Mechanical Ventilation

Jean Kwo and Dean Hess

Due to complications associated with its use, the ventilator should be discontinued as soon as the conditions that caused the patient to be placed on mechanical ventilation stabilize and begin to resolve.

I. **Definitions**
   A. **Weaning** is the gradual withdrawal of ventilator support.
   B. **Discontinuation** refers to the removal of ventilator support. Many patients can be successfully liberated from mechanical ventilation without weaning.
   C. **Extubation** is the removal of the endotracheal tube.
   D. **Decannulation** is the removal of a tracheostomy tube.
II. **Evidence-based guidelines** for the discontinuation of mechanical ventilation were developed by a combined task force of the American College of Chest Physicians, American Association for Respiratory Care, and Society for Critical Care Medicine. They conducted a comprehensive review of the literature that addressed five issues:
   A. The pathophysiology of ventilator dependence.
   B. Criteria for identifying patients ready for discontinuation of mechanical ventilation.
   C. Strategies for ventilator management to maximize the potential for liberation from mechanical ventilation.
   D. The role of the tracheostomy.
   E. The role of long-term facilities.
III. **Ventilator dependence** is defined as a need for mechanical ventilation beyond 24 hours or a failure to respond to attempts at discontinuation of mechanical ventilation. Correcting the cause of ventilator dependence is the most important aspect of the ventilator discontinuation process.
   A. **Respiratory issues** leading to continued ventilator dependence can be due to respiratory pump insufficiency, an elevated respiratory muscle load, or a mismatch between these two factors. Patients with an imbalance between respiratory pump capacity and load often exhibit rapid shallow breathing during a **spontaneous breathing trial (SBT)**.
      1. **Respiratory load** depends on both respiratory system mechanics (resistance and compliance) and ventilatory drive (estimated by the minute ventilation).
         a. **Airways resistance** (R_{aw}) may be due to bronchoconstriction, airway inflammation, or secretions in the airway. Increased R_{aw} is treated with bronchodilators, airway clearance, and steroids.

(1) In patients with airways obstruction, the load imposed by **dynamic hyperinflation** (intrinsic positive end-expiratory pressure [PEEP] or auto-PEEP) can be an important contributor to ventilator dependence.

b. **Respiratory system compliance** (C_{RS}) determines the pressure needed to inflate the lungs and chest wall by a given volume. The compliance of the total respiratory system is determined by lung compliance and chest wall compliance.

(1) Decreased lung compliance may be due to pulmonary edema, lung consolidation, infection, or fibrosis.

(2) Decreased chest wall compliance (C_{CW}) may be due to either chest wall abnormalities or intraabdominal processes.

c. **Minute ventilation** ($\dot{V}_E$) is normally less than 10 L/min. An increase in carbon dioxide production ($\dot{V}CO_2$) or an increase in dead space ($\dot{V}_D$) requires $\dot{V}_E$ to increase to maintain a normal arterial partial pressure of carbon dioxide ($PaCO_2$).

(1) Although a high $\dot{V}_E$ (>15 L/min) may identify patients who are unlikely to be liberated from the ventilator, a normal $\dot{V}_E$ is not predictive of weaning success.

2. **Respiratory pump insufficiency**

a. **Metabolic factors** such as nutrition, electrolyte imbalances, and hormones may affect ventilatory muscle function (see Chapter 9).

(1) Adequate **nutritional support** is necessary to prevent respiratory muscle protein catabolism and loss of muscle performance.

  i. **Overfeeding,** particularly with carbohydrate, can lead to excess CO_2 production leading to an increased ventilatory load.

(2) **Electrolyte imbalances** can impair respiratory muscle function.

  i. Phosphate depletion has been associated with muscle weakness and failure of the patient to liberate from the ventilator.

  ii. Magnesium deficiency has also been associated with muscle weakness.

(3) **Hormonal factors** such as severe hypothyroidism can lead to diaphragm weakness and a decreased respiratory drive (i.e., decreased response to hypercapnia and hypoxia).

  i. Insulin, glucagon, and adrenal corticosteroids are necessary for optimal muscle function.

3. **Sedative** drugs are often used to treat anxiety, agitation, and patient–ventilator dyssynchrony. Sedatives are usually infused continuously to provide a constant level of sedation and improve patient comfort (see Chapter 6).

    a. The administration of sedatives by continuous infusion is an independent predictor of a longer duration of mechanical ventilation.

    b. Prior to starting an SBT, sedatives should be adjusted to allow sleep at night and maximum alertness and cooperation during the day.

    c. Protocols for the management of analgesia and sedation are associated with a reduction in the duration of mechanical ventilation.

4. Neurologic diseases such as brainstem stroke, central apnea, or occult seizures can decrease central respiratory drive from the ventilatory pump controller in the brainstem.

5. Critical illness polyneuropathy (CIP) often becomes apparent when patients have difficulty liberating from the ventilator (see Chapter 30).

    a. CIP occurs in patients with a history of sepsis, multiorgan failure, respiratory failure, or systemic inflammatory response syndrome (SIRS).

    b. Neuromuscular blocking agents, steroids, or prolonged immobility may contribute to CIP.

6. Cardiovascular issues may play a role in patients with limited cardiac reserve.

    a. With the transition from positive-pressure ventilation to spontaneous ventilation, there are increased metabolic demands and thus increased circulatory demands as well.

    b. The withdrawal of positive-pressure ventilation increases venous return.

    c. Increases in heart rate, blood pressure, and arrhythmias may occur during weaning. This may induce ischemia or congestive heart failure in patients with coronary artery disease.

7. Psychological factors such as fear of the loss of a life support system may be an important factor in ventilator dependence. Frequent communication and reassurance for the patient and family can minimize stress.

IV. Assessment for ventilator discontinuation potential

  A. A few simple criteria should be evaluated before the patient undergoes an assessment of discontinuation potential.

    1. There should be some evidence of **resolution of underlying disease** that led to respiratory failure and the need for mechanical ventilation.

    2. There should be **adequate gas exchange** as evidenced by adequate oxygenation (arterial oxygen partial pressure [PaO_2] >60 mm Hg on PEEP <8 cm H_2O and inspired oxygen [FiO_2] <50%) and adequate ventilation (pH ≥ 7.25).

    3. The patient should be **hemodynamically stable** with no evidence of active myocardial ischemia and clinically significant hypotension requiring vasopressor support.

4. The patient should be able to initiate an **inspiratory effort.**
   a. **Sedation** should be adjusted so the patient is awake and able to cooperative with the weaning process.
B. **Weaning parameters** are objective measures used to assess a patient's readiness to successfully maintain spontaneous ventilation.
   1. Most of these parameters reflect only a single component of the respiratory system and thus are limited predictors of weaning outcome.
   2. The **rapid shallow breathing index (RSBI)** is obtained by dividing the respiratory rate by the tidal volume.
      a. RSBI is measured during the first minute of spontaneous breathing.
      b. A low RSBI (<105) has been used to predict successful ventilator liberation, whereas a high RSBI (i.e., rapid, shallow breathing) has been used to predict the need for continued ventilator dependence.
      c. Although initial reports found this index useful, more recent studies have reported limited usefulness for this index.
   3. **Maximal inspiratory pressure** ($P_{i,max}$ or MIP), also called the negative inspiratory force (NIF):
      a. This is a measure of respiratory muscle strength.
      b. Because it measures the pressure generated against a prolonged airway occlusion, this maneuver requires no patient coordination and cooperation.
      c. A $P_{i,max}$ more negative than -30 cm H_2O has been used to predict successful ventilator liberation, but it is often of limited usefulness.
   4. The **$P_{0.1}$** is the **airway occlusion pressure** measured 0.1 second after initiation of inspiration against an occluded airway.
      a. This is an index of respiratory drive.
      b. A high respiratory drive ($P_{0.1}$ of -4 to -10 cm H_2O) has been used to predict patients with continued ventilator dependence.
      c. Measurement of the $P_{0.1}$ usually requires specialized equipment, but it can be measured directly by some ventilators.
   5. Because respiratory failure is often multifactorial, indices that combine several different variables may be more predictive of weaning outcome.
      a. The **CROP index** includes variables reflecting gas exchange, respiratory load, and respiratory muscle strength: CROP = $C_{dyn} \times P_{i,max} \times (PaO_2/PAO_2)/f$, where PAO_2 is the alveolar oxygen partial pressure and C_{dyn} is the dynamic compliance, equal to $V_T/(peak inspiratory pressure - PEEP)$.

        (1) A CROP greater than 13 is predictive of ventilator liberation.

        (2) This complicated calculation has not gained widespread use.

    b. Work-of-breathing indices have generally been limited to research applications and need further study before they can be applied to predict weaning outcome.

V. Ventilator modes and weaning

  A. There are no data that support gradual removal of ventilator support to "train" respiratory muscles.

  B. With **pressure support ventilation (PSV),** the level of inspiratory pressure assistance can be gradually decreased until the patient is able to breathe without assistance (usually a pressure support of <10 cm H_2O).

  C. With **synchronized intermittent mandatory ventilation (SIMV),** the mandatory rate is decreased gradually until the patient is able to breathe without assistance (usually when the patient receives fewer than four mandatory breaths per minute). Several studies suggest that SIMV weaning is inferior to other approaches and may prolong the duration of mechanical ventilation.

  D. A SBT is the best way to assess a patient's breathing without ventilator support.

    1. A SBT is more predictive of a patient's readiness to breathe without ventilator support than is any weaning parameter reported to date.

    2. Most patients who tolerate a SBT of 30 to 120 minutes can be discontinued from mechanical ventilation.

      a. The initial few minutes of a SBT should be closely monitored because the detrimental effects of ventilatory muscle overload usually occur early.

  E. Two randomized trials compared weaning methods.

    1. Three-fourths of the patients tolerated the first 2-hour SBT and were extubated.

    2. SIMV was associated with a longer duration of mechanical ventilation.

    3. One study found that PSV led to shorter weaning times, whereas the other found that repeated SBTs led to a shorter duration of mechanical ventilation.

  F. No new mode on the ventilator has been shown to produce better outcomes for discontinuation of mechanical ventilation than a spontaneous breathing trial.

VI. A **carefully monitored SBT** is the best clinical indicator of readiness to discontinue mechanical ventilation. Several technical approaches for the SBT can be used.

  A. A SBT performed with a **T-piece or tracheostomy collar** is the technique most commonly reported in the literature.

    1. With this approach, there is no additional work imposed on breathing from the ventilator, although this is generally not an issue with current-generation ventilators.

B. Several **on-ventilator approaches** to the SBT can be used.

1. With these approaches, the monitoring capabilities of the ventilator (tidal volume, respiratory rate, minute ventilation, apnea alarms) remain active.

2. If this patient does not tolerate the SBT, this approach allows rapid reinstitution of ventilator support.

3. The ϕ**PSV**/ϕ**PEEP** setting on the ventilator simulates a T-piece trial.

4. A **low-level of PSV** (5–7 cm H_2O) is acceptable and has been shown to have little effect on the outcome of the SBT.

   a. This approach may be useful if there is concern about the resistance through the endotracheal tube.

5. A **low-level continuous positive airway pressure (CPAP)** (5 cm H_2O) is acceptable in many patients.

   a. There is little evidence to support the belief that use of low-level CPAP provides "physiologic PEEP."

   b. A SBT with CPAP may facilitate breath triggering in patients with auto-PEEP. However, this may disguise the patient's inability to breathe adequately after extubation.

   c. A SBT with CPAP may decrease the preload and afterload in a patient with left ventricular dysfunction. In this case, the patient may develop acute cardiogenic pulmonary edema immediately following extubation.

6. **Tube compensation** is available on newer-generation ventilators.

   a. With this mode, the ventilator adds pressure to overcome resistance through the endotracheal tube or tracheostomy tube.

   b. The amount of pressure added to the airway is determined by the inspiratory flow and the resistance through the tube (tube size).

   c. No study has yet reported improved ventilator discontinuation using tube compensations.

   d. One study reported that the resistance through the endotracheal tube just prior to extubation is similar to the resistance through the upper airway after extubation; this suggests that tube compensation is unnecessary.

C. **SBT duration**

1. The duration of SBT most commonly reported in the literature is 120 minutes.

2. There is no benefit of a prolonged SBT (>120 minutes), and this may contribute to a greater likelihood of failure.

**Table 23-1. Criteria for determining
tolerance of a spontaneous breathing trial**

Objective criteria	
Gas exchange	pH >7.32; ↑$Paco_2$ ≤10 mm Hg; Pao_2 ≥50 to 60 mm Hg; Spo_2 ≥85% to 90%
Hemodynamics	HR <120 to 140/min or not changed >20%; SBP <180 to 200 mm Hg and >90 mm Hg; SBP not changed >20%
Ventilatory pattern	RR ≤30 to 35 breaths/min or not changed >50%
Subjective criteria	
Mental status	No new or excessive somnolence, anxiety, agitation
Discomfort	No new or worsened dyspnea
Diaphoresis	No diaphoresis
Increased work of breathing	No accessory respiratory muscle use, thoracoabdominal paradox

HR, heart rate; $Paco_2$, partial pressure of carbon dioxide; Pao_2, partial pressure of oxygen; RR, respiratory rate; SBP, systolic blood pressure; Spo_2, blood oxygen saturation.

3. One study suggested that a SBT of 30 minutes was as predictive of readiness for ventilator discontinuation as a SBT of 120 minutes. Because most patients who fail a SBT do so early after its initiation, a SBT of 30 to 60 minutes is usually sufficient.

D. How to recognize a **failed SBT**

1. The patient must be monitored closely during the SBT, and ventilator support should be promptly restored if there is clinical evidence of failure.

2. There is no single parameter to indicate whether a SBT is successful, but instead a constellation of physiologic and clinical parameters is used to judge tolerance of the SBT (Table 23-1).

3. Common objective measurements include acceptable gas exchange, hemodynamic stability, and stable ventilatory pattern.

4. Subjective parameters include mental status, degree of discomfort, diaphoresis, and signs of increased work of breathing.

E. **Ventilator settings after a failed SBT**

1. The ventilator should be set to a nonfatiguing, comfortable mode while a search for the cause of the failed SBT is underway.

2. The clinician should take into account patient effort, ease of triggering the ventilator, flow demand, and the presence of auto-PEEP when selecting the appropriate ventilator settings.

F. An approach to ventilator discontinuation using the SBT is shown in Fig. 23-1.

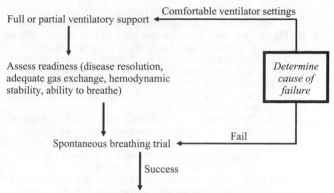

Fig. 23-1. A simple clinical approach to ventilator discontinuation that is independent of weaning parameters or ventilator mode.

VII. The cause of a failed SBT can be found in the same factors that led to the initiation of mechanical ventilation in the first place.
   A. Most often, further resolution of the underlying disease is needed.
   B. The possibility of **other contributory causes** such as dynamic hyperinflation, cardiac disease and myocardial ischemia, and critical illness neuropathy/myopathy should be thoroughly investigated.
   C. Other, less likely causes include malposition of the artificial airway (endotracheal tube or tracheostomy tube).
   D. Once the cause for the failed SBT is corrected, the SBT should be repeated.
   E. A SBT once per day is usually sufficient unless the cause of the failed SBT is rapidly resolved.
VIII. Extubation. Once a patient successfully completes a SBT, the clinician needs to assess whether there is a continued need for an artificial airway.
   A. Prior to extubation, patients should be evaluated for their ability **to protect the airway.**
      1. Patients with a poor cough or a large amount of secretions may fail extubation because the endotracheal tube allows easy suctioning of the airway.
      2. Assessment of a patient's ability to clear airway secretions includes noting the quality of cough during suctioning, the absence of excessive secretions, and the frequency of suctioning.
      3. The **white card test** assesses the ability of a patient to expel secretions onto a white card held 1 to 2 cm from the endotracheal tube. Patients who are unable to do so are more likely to fail extubation.

        4. Low **cough peak flows** (<60 L/min) has been associated with extubation failure and increased mortality.

  B. **Upper airway edema** can lead to extubation failure.

      1. This most commonly occurs with prolonged intubation, smaller airways (female gender, children), trauma, and repeated or traumatic intubation.

      2. A **leak test** performed with the cuff of the endotracheal tube deflated can identify patients at risk for upper airway obstruction.

         a. The presence of leak with cuff deflation suggests absence of significant upper airway swelling.

         b. Absence of a leak is affected by factors in addition to upper airway swelling, which limits its ability to predict postextubation stridor.

      3. Patients who develop postextubation stridor can be treated with nebulized epinephrine and/or steroids.

         a. Heliox (helium/oxygen mixture) may also be used to temporarily improve airflow through the upper airway.

         b. Mask CPAP may stent the airway open.

         c. Heliox and CPAP treat only the symptom of stridor and do not reduce upper airway swelling.

  C. **Patient cooperation** is a key component of a successful extubation.

      1. Ideally, the patient should be awake, comfortable, and able to follow instructions to cough.

      2. Judicious use of anxiolytics and pain medicines can help achieve that goal.

IX. The role of **noninvasive positive-pressure ventilation (NPPV)** periextubation

  A. **Extubation to NPPV**

      1. Selected patients, particularly those with chronic obstructive pulmonary disease (COPD), who fail a SBT may be considered for extubation to NPPV.

      2. Postextubation support with NPPV in carefully selected patients is associated with decreased duration of mechanical ventilation, decreased incidence of nosocomial pneumonia, decreased intensive care unit (ICU) stay, and increased survival.

  B. NPPV **following a failed extubation**

      1. The evidence does not support the use of NPPV in patients who develop respiratory failure following a planned extubation. One randomized clinical trial suggested potential for harm.

X. The role of **protocols**

  A. Protocols directing explicit management decisions that are executed by nurses and respiratory therapists have been shown to improve clinical outcomes and reduce costs for critically ill patients.

  B. Protocols should not be so rigid as to prevent the clinician deviating from the protocol after a careful assessment.

  C. Protocols should also be constantly reevaluated and take into account new data and new clinical practice patterns.

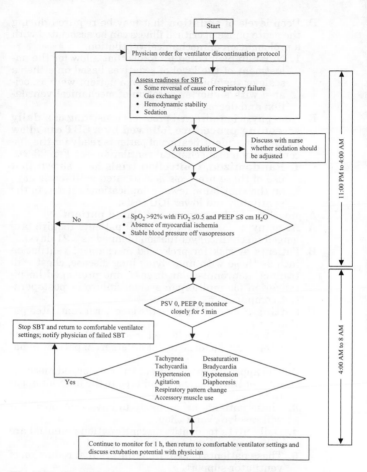

Fig. 23-2. Ventilator discontinuation protocol, adapted from that used in the medical ICU at the Massachusetts General Hospital. Note several characteristics (a) it emphasizes collaboration between respiratory therapist, nurse, and physician; (b) after receiving a physician order, it is implemented by nonphysicians; (c) it stresses bedside assessment and SBTs; and (d) it is completed before morning rounds, so a decision regarding extubation can be made at rounds. FiO₂, inspired oxygen fraction; PEEP, positive end-expiratory pressure; PSV, pressure support ventilation; SBT, spontaneous breathing trial; SpO₂, blood oxygen saturation.

   D. Deep levels of **sedation** that may be required during
        the acute phase of critical illness can be associated with
        a prolongation of mechanical ventilation.
     1. Nurse-implemented protocols that allow for the ad-
          justment of the level of sedatives based on either a
          scale or the ability to awaken a patient were associ-
          ated with a shorter duration of mechanical ventila-
          tion and decreased ICU stay.
   E. Non–physician-directed protocols consisting of a **daily
        screening procedure followed by a SBT** can allow
        for the early identification of patients ready for the dis-
        continuation of mechanical ventilation (see Fig. 23-2).
     1. Randomized, controlled trials have shown that
          use of these protocols is associated with fewer days
          on the ventilator, fewer complications related to the
          ventilator, and lower ICU costs.
XI. Approach to the **long-term ventilated patient**
   A. As many as 20% of medical ICU patients require pro-
        longed mechanical ventilation (defined as >21 days).
   B. Patients at risk for prolonged mechanical ventilation
        include those with underlying lung disease, chest wall
        trauma, neuromuscular disease, and prolonged hospi-
        talization for multiorgan system failure or postopera-
        tive complications.
   C. Setting the ventilator in the long-term ventilated pa-
        tient:
     1. The etiology of prolonged mechanical ventilation is
          often multifactorial and it differs from patient to pa-
          tient.
     2. The approach to the patient with prolonged mechan-
          ical ventilation must be tailored to the individual pa-
          tient.
     3. These patients are unlikely to have problems that
          will resolve over 24 hours.
     4. Daily SBTs to identify discontinuation potential are
          of limited utility in this patient population.
     5. These patients benefit from the gradual reduction of
          ventilator support.
       a. SBTs of increasing duration may be started
            once the patient is receiving partial ventilator
            support.
       b. A protocol approach may decrease the duration of
            mechanical ventilation.
   D. These patients have **problems that require special
        attention** because they are often debilitated after a
        long critical illness.
     1. Patients benefit from a multidisciplinary approach
          involving physicians, nurses, respiratory therapists,
          physical therapists, and speech therapists.
     2. Close attention to nutritional status with the ade-
          quate administration of calories and protein without
          overfeeding is needed.
     3. Physical therapy is needed for muscle strengthening
          and to prevent contractures and improves patients'
          functional status.

4. Speech therapy is needed because these patients often have swallowing dysfunction after a prolonged intubation.

E. **Long-term weaning units** that specialize in the care and weaning of patients on long-term mechanical ventilation have been shown to be safe and effective for weaning ICU patients from mechanical ventilation.

1. These units provide a structured program for the medically complex patient, with frequent physician monitoring and nurses skilled in the care of the ventilated patient.

2. Because they generally have less intensive staffing, these units are less costly. They can be free-standing long-term acute care hospitals and thus serve many hospitals in a geographic area, or they may be units within a host hospital.

F. Some patients may require **lifelong mechanical ventilation.**

1. A home-ventilator support program should be established.

2. Data from long-term weaning hospitals suggest that unless the patient has evidence for clearly irreversible disease (e.g., high spinal cord injury, amyotrophic lateral sclerosis), several months may be needed for a patient with respiratory failure to be discontinued from mechanical ventilation.

XII. **Decannulation** is the removal of a tracheostomy tube.

A. A tracheostomy improves patient comfort, facilitates talking, improves mouth care, and may decrease airways resistance. This may promote weaning from mechanical ventilation.

B. **Timing**

1. The tracheostomy may close within 48 to 72 hours of removal of the tracheostomy tube, leading to difficulty in replacement of the tube should respiratory difficulties arise.

2. A systematic assessment of a patient's readiness for decannulation is needed.

a. The patient should have a **stable respiratory status** after discontinuation of mechanical ventilation.

b. The patient should be able to **protect the airway.**

(1) This can be assessed by deflation of the tracheostomy cuff and observation for signs of aspiration.

(2) A small amount of blue dye can be introduced into the oral cavity and suctioning of the tracheostomy tube undertaken at regular intervals. The presence of any blue color at the tracheostomy site or within the suction catheter indicates that the patient is at risk for aspiration.

c. **Anatomic abnormalities** of the airway such as granulation tissue, strictures, and vocal cord injuries are a complication of long-term intubation.

d. Adequacy of the native airway can be assessed by deflating the tracheostomy cuff and capping the tube.

(1) Adults who can breathe around a capped 7 or 8 tracheostomy tube have adequate respiratory muscle function and a sufficiently preserved native airway to tolerate decannulation.

(2) Patients who fail breathing trials with capped tracheostomy tubes should be evaluated by **flexible fiberoptic bronchoscopy** above and below the tracheostomy tube for evidence of airway lesions.

e. Patients with limited ventilatory reserve due to neuromuscular disease or COPD may benefit from stepwise **downsizing and capping of the tracheostomy tube.**

(1) Patients who can breathe and clear secretions around a small, capped tube may be decannulated.

(2) Occasionally, the patient with moderate secretions may have difficulty because the presence of the tracheostomy impairs secretion clearance through the native airway. These patients may benefit from placement of a **tracheostomy button or minitracheostomy.**

SELECTED REFERENCES

Brochard L, Rauss A, Benito S, et al. Comparison of three methods of gradual withdrawal from ventilatory support during weaning from mechanical ventilation. *Am J Respir Crit Care Med* 1994;150(4):896–903.

Ely EW, Meade MO, Haponik EF, et al. Mechanical ventilator weaning protocols driven by nonphysician health-care professionals: evidence-based clinical practice guidelines. *Chest* 2001;120(6 Suppl):454S–463S.

Epstein SK. Decision to extubate. *Intensive Care Med* 2002;28(5): 535–546.

Esteban A, Alia I, Gordo F, et al. Extubation outcome after spontaneous breathing trials with T-tube or pressure support ventilation. *Am J Respir Crit Care Med* 1997;156(2 Pt 1):459–465.

Esteban A, Frutos F, Tobin MJ, et al. A comparison of four methods of weaning patients from mechanical ventilation. *N Engl J Med* 1995;332(6):345–350.

Esteban A, Frutos-Vivar F, Ferguson ND, et al. Noninvasive positive-pressure ventilation for respiratory failure after extubation. *N Engl J Med* 2004;350(24):2452–2460.

Ferrer M, Esquinas A, Arancibia F, et al. Noninvasive ventilation during persistent weaning failure: a randomized controlled trial. *Am J Respir Crit Care Med* 2003;168(1):70–76.

Hurford WE, Favorito F. Association of myocardial ischemia with failure to wean from mechanical ventilation. *Crit Care Med* 1995;23(9):1475–1480.

Keenan SP, Powers C, McCormack DG, et al. Noninvasive positive-pressure ventilation for postextubation respiratory distress: a randomized controlled trial. *JAMA* 2002;287(24):3238–3244.

MacIntyre NR, Cook DJ, Ely EW Jr, et al. Evidence-based guidelines for weaning and discontinuing ventilatory support. *Chest* 2001;120(6 Suppl):375S–395S.

Meade M, Guyatt G, Cook D, et al. Predicting success in weaning from mechanical ventilation. *Chest* 2001;120(6 Suppl):400S–424S.

Scheinhorn DJ, Chao DC, Hassenpflug MS, et al. Post-ICU weaning from mechanical ventilation: the role of long-term facilities. *Chest* 2001;120(6 Suppl):482S–484S.

Schweickert WD, Gehlbach BK, Pohlman AS, et al. Daily interruption of sedative infusions and complications of critical illness in mechanically ventilated patients. *Crit Care Med* 2004;32(6):1272–1276.

Smina M, Salam A, Khamiees M, et al. Cough peak flows and extubation outcomes. *Chest* 2003;124(1):262–268.

Acute Renal Failure

Harish Lecamwasam and Hasan Bazari

I. Definition

A. Acute renal failure (ARF) is a syndrome characterized by an acute decrease in glomerular filtration rate (GFR) in the setting of either previously normal renal function or stable chronic kidney disease.

B. Consensus on the definition of ARF using an elevation in serum creatinine (Cr) concentration does not exist. Most studies have used an absolute increase of 0.5 to 1.0 mg/dl or a relative increase of 25% to 100% in the Cr over 24 hours.

II. Epidemiology

A. The available epidemiologic data are confounded by variable definitions of ARF and the heterogeneous nature of the populations studied.

B. It is estimated that between 4% and 7% of all hospitalized patients and 20% of all critically ill patients develop ARF.

C. The most common cause of in-hospital ARF is decreased renal perfusion or nephrotoxic injury, with the more severe form occurring in the critically ill who have acute tubular necrosis.

D. ARF has been identified as an independent predictor of mortality. **In critically ill patients, the mortality associated with ARF is estimated at 30% to 50%.**

III. Manifestations

A. Accumulation of nitrogenous waste, primarily Cr and urea nitrogen (BUN).

1. Although **serum Cr** is typically used as a surrogate of GFR, the correlation between the Cr and GFR can be distorted for the following reasons:

a. Cr excretion depends on both filtration *and* tubular excretion (5%–20%).

b. Cr production depends on muscle mass and is relatively constant unless there is muscle damage as occurs in rhabdomyolysis.

c. Cr assays can be affected by the presence of chromophores (e.g., certain cephalosporin antibiotics and ketones).

2. The relationship between the GFR and BUN can be highly variable. For example, the BUN will be elevated with protein loading, steroid therapy, gastrointestinal bleeding, or a hypermetabolic state. Conversely, the BUN can be lowered with severe liver disease or malnutrition.

B. Oliguria (urine output less than 400–500 ml/24 h) may or may not be present.

Table 24-1.   Etiologies of prerenal acute renal failure

Intravascular volume depletion
  Gastrointestinal fluid loss
    Vomiting
    Diarrhea
    Enterocutaneous fistula
  Renal fluid loss
    Diuretics
    Osmotic diuresis
    Renal salt wasting
  Cutaneous losses
    Hyperthermia
    Burns
  Hemorrhage
  "Third-space" fluid loss
    Pancreatitis
    Severe hypoalbuminemia
    Capillary leak syndrome
Decreased effective arterial blood volume
  Congestive heart failure
  Cirrhosis
  Nephrotic syndrome
  Sepsis
  Anesthesia
Altered intrarenal hemodynamics
  Preglomerular (afferent) arteriolar vasoconstriction
    Prostaglandin inhibition
      Nonsteroidal antiinflammatory drugs
      Cyclooxygenase-2 inhibitors
    Hypercalcemia
    Hepatorenal syndrome
    Cyclosporine
    Tacrolimus
  Postglomerular (efferent) arteriolar vasodilation
    Angiotensin-converting-enzyme inhibition
    Angiotensin-receptor blockade
Abdominal compartment syndrome

From Acute renal failure. In: Glassock RJ, ed. *Nephrology self-assessment program (NephSAP)*, Vol. 2, No. 2. Philadelphia: Lippincott Williams & Wilkins, 2003:42.

IV. Classification

  A. ARF is traditionally divided into **prerenal** (Table 24-1), **postrenal** (Table 24-2), and **intrinsic renal** (Table 24-3) etiologies.

   1. **Prerenal ARF**
      a. Prerenal ARF is caused by **decreased renal perfusion** due to decreased effective circulating volume or altered renal hemodynamics.
      b. Renal hypoperfusion activates numerous neurohumoral responses that help to maintain renal perfusion pressure and GFR.

Table 24-2. Etiologies of postrenal acute renal failure

Upper urinary tract obstruction (bilateral obstruction or obstruction of a single functioning kidney)
  Intrinsic
    Stone
    Papillary necrosis
    Blood clot
    Transitional cell carcinoma
  Extrinsic
    Retroperitoneal fibrosis
    Aortic aneurysm
    Retroperitoneal or pelvic malignancy
Lower urinary tract obstruction
  Urethral stricture
  Benign prostatic hypertrophy
  Prostate cancer
  Transitional cell carcinoma of the bladder
  Bladder stones
  Blood clot
  Fungus ball
  Neurogenic bladder
  Malpositioned urethral catheter

From Acute renal failure. In: Glassock RJ, ed. *Nephrology self-assessment program (NephSAP)*, Vol. 2, No. 2. Philadelphia: Lippincott Williams & Wilkins, 2003:42.

  - (1) Efferent arteriolar vasoconstriction is produced by the activation of the sympathetic and renin–angiotensin system.
  - (2) Afferent arteriolar vasodilation is produced by activation of prostaglandins, the kallikrein system, nitric oxide, and direct myogenic influences.
  - c. ARF manifests when the reduction in renal perfusion pressure exceeds the compensatory ability of these autoregulatory mechanisms to maintain adequate GFR.
  - d. Prerenal azotemia is typically reversible, and renal function returns to baseline. However, with sustained hypoperfusion, prerenal azotemia can progress to acute tubular necrosis (ATN).
  2. **Postrenal ARF**
    - a. Postrenal ARF is caused by **obstruction** of urinary flow, either bilateral ureteral or below the level of the bladder with normal kidneys, or unilateral ureteral obstruction with a solitary kidney.
    - b. Complete obstruction results in anuria, whereas incomplete results in variable urine output.
    - c. GFR can be maintained by continued salt and water absorption, dilation of the collecting system

Table 24-3.   Etiologies of intrinsic acute renal failure

Acute tubular necrosis
  Ischemic
    Hypotension
    Hypovolemic shock
    Sepsis
    Cardiorespiratory arrest
    Cardiopulmonary bypass
  Nephrotoxic
    Drug-induced
      Aminoglycosides
      Radiocontrast agents
      Amphotericin
      Cisplatinum
      Acetaminophen
    Pigment nephropathy
      Intravascular hemolysis
      Rhabdomyolysis
Acute interstitial nephritis
  Drug induced
    Penicillins
    Cephalosporins
    Sulfonamides
    Rifampin
    Dilantin
    Furosemide
    Nonsteroidal antiinflammatory drugs
  Infection related
    Bacterial infection
    Viral infections
    Rickettsial disease
    Tuberculosis
  Systemic diseases
    Systemic lupus erythematosus
    Sarcoidosis
    Sjogren syndrome
    Tubulointerstitial nephritis and uveitis (TINU) syndrome
  Malignancy
    Malignant infiltration of interstitium
    Multiple myeloma
  Idiopathic
Acute glomerulonephritis
  Poststreptococcal glomerulonephritis
  Postinfectious glomerulonephritis
  Endocarditis-associated glomerulonephritis
  Systemic vasculitis
  Hemolytic uremic syndrome/thrombotic thrombocytopenic purpura
  Rapidly progressive glomerulonephritis (RPGN)
Acute vascular syndromes
  Renal artery thromboembolism
  Renal artery dissection
  Renal vein thrombosis
  Atheroembolic disease

From Acute renal failure. In: Glassock RJ, ed. *Nephrology self-assessment program (NephSAP),* Vol. 2, No. 2. Philadelphia: Lippincott Williams & Wilkins, 2003:43.

(and a resulting decrease in intratubular pressure), and changes in renal hemodynamics.

d. Diagnosis

   (1) Postrenal obstruction is usually diagnosed by **ultrasound,** which reveals **hydronephrosis.** False-negative results can arise in about 10% of cases, either early in the disease process (insufficient time for hydronephrosis to develop), with hypovolemia, or when obstruction is caused by retroperitoneal disease.

   (2) Abdominal computed tomography (CT) scan or **retrograde pyelography** are more sensitive and can be used when ultrasonography is indeterminate.

e. Treatment involves relief of obstruction. Following treatment, a postobstructive diuresis can ensue from the elimination of retained salt and water and from tubular defects incurred during the obstructive process.

f. Recovery of renal function is dependent on the duration of obstruction. It is estimated that complete recovery can be expected with an obstructive duration of less than 1 week, whereas minimal recovery is expected with obstructive duration exceeding 12 weeks.

3. Intrinsic ARF

   a. Intrinsic ARF is divided into tubular (ATN), interstitial, glomerular, and vascular disease.

   b. ATN (see section **V**) is the most common cause of intrinsic renal ARF.

   c. Interstitial disease most commonly presents as acute interstitial nephritis (AIN; see section **VIII.B.3).**

   d. Glomerular disease can be postinfectious (poststreptococcal, etc.), primary immune mediated, or vasculitic (lupus, Wegener's granulomatosis, etc.). **Rapidly progressing glomerulonephritis** (RPGN) is increasingly being identified as a cause of intrinsic ARF in the elderly.

   e. Vascular etiologies of intrinsic renal ARF include **large-vessel diseases** such as renovascular disease and aortic/renal artery dissection and **small-vessel diseases** including atheroembolic disease, antiphospholipid antibody, scleroderma, classical polyarteritis nodosa (PAN), hemolytic uremic syndrome (HUS), and thrombotic thrombocytopenic purpura (TTP). **Diagnosis** can be made using CT angiography, magnetic resonance angiography, or angiography for large-vessel involvement and a variety of diagnostic procedures for small-vessel disease. Treatment of acute renal artery thrombosis is rarely successful if revascularization is not performed within 3 hours of onset of the occlusion.

V. Acute tubular necrosis (ATN)

A. ATN is the most common cause of intrinsic ARF (>85% in the critically ill), with injury resulting from ischemia (50%), toxins (35%), or multifactorial causes.

B. Ischemic ATN results from prolonged renal hypoperfusion, including prolonged prerenal azotemia.

C. Nephrotoxic ATN can result from endogenous (e.g., myoglobin, hemoglobin) or exogenous (e.g., aminoglycoside, radiocontrast) toxins.

D. Risk factors for ATN include advanced age, trauma, hypotension, sepsis, and preexisting renal disease.

E. The **pathophysiology** of ATN involves multiple mechanisms including the following:

1. Intrarenal vasoconstriction leading to decreased blood flow to the renal cortex and outer medulla.
2. Tubular cell injury involving loss of the apical brush border, loss of polarity, and disruption of intercellular tight junctions.
3. Leukocyte infiltration.
4. Reperfusion injury.

F. Phases of ATN

1. **Initiation phase,** the period immediately following the renal insult, during which tubular injury has not occurred and ARF is potentially preventable.
2. **Maintenance phase,** which begins with the onset of tubular injury and defines the onset of a decrease in GFR and ARF. This phase can last from days to weeks and can manifest a variable urine output.
3. **Recovery phase,** in which cellular regeneration restores tubular integrity and function, with improvement in GFR and return of renal function to baseline or near baseline.

G. Epidemiologic data show that the presence of ATN, especially in the critically ill, is an independent predictor of short-term in-hospital mortality. Long-term outcomes of those who survive to hospital discharge are favorable (1-year survival of 69%, 5-year survival of 50%).

VI. Evaluation

A. History and physical examination: Determine volume status and identify baseline renal function, risk factors, and precipitating events.

B. Daily weights are poorly reproducible in the ICU setting, and total body water correlates poorly with intravascular volume of the critically ill patient.

C. Assessment of intravascular volume is made to evaluate for hypervolemia (e.g., jugular venous distention) or hypovolemia (e.g., tachycardia, hypotension). Because the physical signs of intravascular volume are unreliable for most but the best-trained physicians, invasive measurements such as the pulmonary artery occlusion pressure and stroke volume are often necessary (see Chapter 1).

D. Evaluation of the urine

1. **Urinalysis** and **determination of the urine indices** are simple and rapid and provide useful

diagnostic information. A summary is given in Table 24-4.

2. **Urine dipstick**

   a. **Proteinuria** is usually associated with glomerular lesions, but may also be seen with tubular injury. Glomerular injury permits large proteins to pass into the urine as indicated by a reading of 3 to 4+ on dipstick testing. Tubular injury of ATN may prevent the normal reabsorption of small, filtered proteins as indicated by mild proteinuria of 1 to 2+.

   b. **Heme-positive dipstick tests,** without red blood cells in the urinary sediment, suggest hemoglobinuria or myoglobinuria.

   c. Hemoglobin is poorly filtered at the glomerulus. The plasma of patients with hemoglobinemia, therefore, appears red-brown. Conversely, myoglobin is freely filtered. The plasma of patients with myoglobinemia, therefore, appears clear (unless renal failure has limited the excretion of myoglobin).

   d. **Microscopic examination** of the urine sediment provides insight into the pathogenesis of ARF. Tubular casts are an indirect indication of ongoing processes in the kidney.

      (1) **Hyaline casts** are acellular and are consistent with prerenal azotemia. They can often be seen in health.

      (2) **Granular casts** contain degenerating renal tubular epithelial cells and are seen in a process of ARF due to ischemic or nephrotoxic injuries. **Pigmented casts** can be seen in hemoglobin- and myoglobin-induced ARF.

      (3) **White blood cell casts** indicate an inflammatory process and may be seen in pyelonephritis and acute interstitial nephritis.

      (4) **Red blood cell casts** indicate glomerular pathology such as glomerulonephritis.

   e. **Diagnostic indices**

      (1) **Prerenal failure** has urine that reflects intact renal mechanisms of salt and water balance. This effort to augment intravascular volume results in elevation of the ratio of serum BUN to Cr concentration, high urine osmolality, and low fractional excretion of sodium (FENa). FENa reflects the ratio of urine to serum concentration of sodium (Na) and Cr:

      $$FENa = (urine\ Na/urine\ Cr)/(serum\ Na/serum\ Cr)\ \%$$

      (2) Disruption of tubular function with ATN usually produces a defect in urinary concentrating ability and the production of isotonic

Table 24-4. Diagnostic studies and indexes of urine

	Prerenal	Renal	Postrenal
Dipstick	0 or trace protein	Mild—moderate protein, hemoglobin, leukocytes	0 or trace protein, red and white cells
Sediment	Few hyaline casts	Granular and cellular casts[a]	Crystals and cellular casts possible
Urine osmolality	>500	<350	<350
Urine/serum plasma creatinine	>40	<20	<20
Urine/serum plasma urea	>8	<3	<3
FeNa	<1%	>1%	>1%

FENa, fractional excretion of sodium; FENa = (urine Na/urine Cr)/(serum Na/serum Cr) %, where Cr is creatinine.
[a]Composition of casts depends on cause of renal failure (see text).

urine. The associated FENa is typically greater than 1%.

  f. Specific limitations of urinary indices

    (1) **Preexisting renal disease** may affect salt and water homeostasis, making interpretation of urine electrolytes difficult. Patients with chronic kidney disease, adrenal insufficiency, and cerebral salt wasting may have a FENa of greater than 1% even when they are volume depleted.

    (2) **Diuretic** administration blocks tubular reabsorption of solute and can complicate data interpretation for up to 24 hours.

    (3) **Nonoliguric ATN** may present with a FENa greater than 1%, particularly in the early phase of the disease.

    (4) **Early urinary tract obstruction,** acute **glomerulonephritis,** or renal **emboli** may present with decreased GFR with normal tubular function. Highly concentrated urine is expected in these settings.

  g. Imaging techniques generally are used to exclude reversible causes of urinary tract obstruction or traumatic injury.

    (1) **Ultrasonography** is the most valuable tool for initial evaluation of obstruction and can be performed at the bedside in unstable patients (see section **IV**).

    (2) **Intravenous pyelography** is indicated only for the evaluation of renal trauma and has no role in the diagnosis of ARF.

    (3) **Antegrade** and **retrograde pyelography** may be used for exact localization of urinary tract obstruction and to accomplish drainage.

    (4) **Computed tomography** can provide useful detailed anatomic information on the kidneys, bladder, and urinary collecting system.

    (5) **Angiography, magnetic resonance angiography,** and **Doppler ultrasonography** can be used to assess the integrity of the renal arteries and veins.

  h. Renal biopsy is not indicated in most cases because history, physical examination, and noninvasive testing will indicate the cause of the renal failure. Biopsy may be indicated in cases of intrinsic ARF not caused by ischemia or toxins or for determining the cause of graft dysfunction after renal transplantation. The morbidity of renal biopsy is relatively low.

VII. Specific syndromes

  A. Syndromes related to **prerenal ARF**

    1. **ARF** induced by **angiotensin-converting-enzyme (ACE) inhibitors** and **angiotensin-receptor blockers (ARBs)**

a. Angiotensin-II (converted from angiotensin-I by ACE) is a potent constrictor of the efferent arteriole and maintains glomerular perfusion pressure and GFR during renal hypoperfusion.

b. Inhibition of the production of angiotensin-II by ACE inhibitors or blockade of the receptor by ARBs presents a risk for ARF. Patients with bilateral renal artery stenosis or stenosis of a single functioning kidney are particularly susceptible.

c. Other risk factors for ACE-inhibitor- or ARB-induced ARF include older age; depressed ventricular function; concurrent diuretic therapy, cirrhosis, cyclooxygenase inhibitor, cyclosporine or tacrolimus use; and chronic kidney disease.

d. Given that many of the patients who may benefit from ACE inhibitors/ARB therapy have risk factors for ARF, current guidelines suggest **continuing therapy if the increment in Cr** after a week **is less than 0.5 mg/dl with a baseline Cr of less than 2.0, or is less than 1.0 mg/dl with a baseline Cr of greater than 2.0.** Some patients who previously tolerated these drugs may develop ARF in the ICU setting. This does not preclude future use of these beneficial drugs.

2. **Nonsteroidal antiinflammatory drugs (NSAIDs)**

a. NSAIDs can be divided into nonselective (cyclooxygenase [COX]-1 and -2) or selective (COX-2) inhibitors of the enzyme cyclooxygenase, involved in the synthesis of prostaglandin precursors.

b. COX-1 and -2 are constitutively produced in the kidneys, where vasodilatory prostaglandins are important to the maintenance of normal intrarenal hemodynamics, especially in the face of hypoperfusion. Therefore, common nonselective COX inhibitors, such as ibuprofen and indomethacin, place patients at risk for abnormal renal perfusion and ARF. Whereas *selective* COX-2 inhibitors were initially thought to be "renal sparing," recent data suggest that their renal effects may be similar to their nonselective counterparts. Furthermore, these compounds are being closely scrutinized for their potential cardiovascular toxicity, and some have been taken off the market.

c. **Risk factors** for NSAID-induced ARF include the following:

(1) Old age.

(2) Congestive heart failure (CHF).

(3) Concurrent ACEI/ARB use.

(4) Advanced liver disease.

(5) Atherosclerotic vascular disease.

(6) Chronic kidney disease.

3. Abdominal compartment syndrome (ACS)

a. ACS is a multifactorial syndrome resulting from intraabdominal hypertension. Causes of ACS include trauma, pancreatitis, intraabdominal/retroperitoneal bleeding, and bowel ischemia.

b. Renal failure with ACS can result from a combination of hypoperfusion, aberrant intrarenal hemodynamics from the neurohumoral response to increased intraabdominal pressure, and increased renal venous pressure. Ureteral obstruction typically is not seen with ACS.

c. Intraabdominal pressure can be found by measuring intragastric or bladder pressure (see Chapter 4).

d. Oliguria typically occurs at bladder pressure above 15 mm Hg, whereas anuria typically occurs at bladder pressures exceeding 30 mm Hg.

e. Treatment of ACS is abdominal decompression. If the duration of insult was limited, renal function generally recovers shortly after decompression.

B. Syndromes related to **intrinsic ARF**

1. Radiocontrast nephropathy (RCN)

a. RCN is one of the most frequent etiologies of nephrotoxic ATN and has been identified as an independent predictor of morbidity and mortality.

b. Established risk factors for RCN are diabetes mellitus, chronic kidney disease, volume depletion, and dose of contrast administered.

c. The pathogenesis of RCN likely involves a combination of direct nephrotoxicity, intrarenal vasoconstriction, and free radical–mediated injury.

d. RCN is typically characterized by an acute elevation in the serum Cr at 24 to 48 hours following contrast administration, a peak in the Cr at 4 to 5 days following the onset of the Cr rise, and return of renal function to near baseline within 7 to 10 days. The ARF is most often associated with a FENa of less than 1% and can be oliguric or nonoliguric. Oliguria starts approximately 24 to 72 hours after contrast exposure, lasts for 24 to 72 hours, and is followed by a polyuric phase.

e. Prevention of RCN

(1) Discontinuation of medications with potential nephrotoxic effects, for example, NSAIDs.

(2) Hydration

i. Although hypovolemia is considered a risk factor for RCN, hydration has not been compared to no-fluid administration in preventing RCN.

ii. Isotonic (0.9%) saline infused at 1 ml/kg/h starting preprocedure and continuing postprocedure has been shown to reduce the risk of RCN compared to hypotonic

(0.45%) saline infused for the identical duration.

    iii. A dose of 150 mEq/L of sodium bicarbonate given at a rate of 3 ml/kg/h for 1 hour prior to contrast and 1 ml/kg/h for 6 hours after contrast was more effective than a similar infusion of 0.9% saline.

  (3) Use of nonionic, low-osmolality contrast agents. The major benefit of reducing the risk of RCN with these agents is seen in diabetic patients with baseline renal insufficiency.

  (4) *N*-Acetylcysteine (NAC)

    i. The incidence of RCN is reduced by pretreatment of patients at risk with NAC.

    ii. Evidence suggests that patients with moderate or greater renal insufficiency (creatinine clearance <60 ml/min), particularly those with diabetes mellitus, should receive pericontrast NAC in addition to hydration.

    iii. Although NAC has been shown to reduce the incidence of RCN, it has not been shown to decrease the progression to dialysis or affect mortality. Therefore, the clinical significance of NAC pretreatment remains ambiguous.

  (5) Diuretics. Mannitol and lasix have been shown to increase the incidence of RCN compared to 0.45% saline hydration. Therefore, there is no current role for diuretics in the prevention of RCN.

  (6) Vasodilators. Although there has been considerable interest in the use of renal vasodilators to prevent RCN, agents including dopamine, calcium-channel blockers, atrial natriuretic peptide, endothelin antagonists, and fenoldopam have not shown any conclusive benefit.

  (7) Renal replacement

    i. Trials have not shown a role for hemodialysis in the prevention of RCN.

    ii. In a recent trial, pre- and post-contrast continuous venovenous hemofiltration (CVVH) reduced the incidence of RCN and mortality in patients with renal insufficiency who underwent coronary interventions.

    iii. However, for a variety of reasons, the practice of pretreatment with CVVH has not been universally adopted pending confirmation of the study results.

2. Atheroembolic disease

  a. ARF secondary to atheroembolic disease is often seen in conjunction with RCN in patients undergoing angiographic or surgical manipulation of the aorta.

b. The pathophysiology of this syndrome involves the dislodgement of cholesterol crystals from atheromatous plaques and their subsequent lodging in small arteries and arterioles leading to inflammation, distal ischemia, and infarction.

c. Renal failure results from embolization into the renal arteries.

d. The **clinical signs and symptoms** of atheroembolic disease depend on the distribution of emboli. The classic syndrome includes livedo reticularis and manifestations of digital ischemia of the lower extremities, the "blue toe syndrome." Other manifestations can include neurologic deficits, coronary ischemia, intestinal ischemia, and rhabdomyolysis.

e. Disease onset is typically subacute, and can manifest with a staggered deterioration in renal function for up to 6 to 8 weeks after an inciting event. Unlike with RCN, **renal function rarely returns to baseline,** although it may improve after a period of deterioration.

f. Atheroembolic disease should be suspected with ARF following any angiographic or surgical manipulation of the aorta, especially if concurrent evidence of embolization is present. The pathognomonic finding is the identification of biconcave cholesterol crystals within blood vessels or skin lesions (most commonly) on biopsy. Although eosinophilia, eosinophiluria, and proteinuria have been described with this process, their sensitivity and specificity are poor.

g. Clinical distinction from RCN can be made based on onset of symptoms (subacute in atheroembolic disease vs. acute in contrast), recovery of renal function (residual dysfunction with atheroembolic ARF), and evidence of embolization to other organs.

h. Therapy is primarily supportive. Steroids have been associated with increased mortality. Mortality associated with atheroembolization has been estimated as high as 80% but is heavily weighted toward the most severe cases.

3. Acute interstitial nephritis (AIN)

a. AIN describes ARF associated with inflammation of the renal interstitium.

b. The majority of episodes can be attributed to drug hypersensitivity. Although an extensive list of agents has been implicated, the most common offenders include penicillins, cephalosporins, sulfonamides, fluoroquinolones, phenytoin, furosemide, thiazide diuretics, allopurinol, omeprazole, and NSAIDs (AIN with proteinuria).

   c. AIN can also develop as a complication following bacterial or viral infection or as a consequence of systemic diseases such as lupus or sarcoidosis.

   d. Onset of ARF is typically acute or subacute. Extrarenal signs can include fever, eosinophilia, rash, arthralgias, hematuria, and pyuria.

   e. Although the importance of **eosinophilia** in making the diagnosis of AIN is frequently emphasized, data suggest that it has a low sensitivity, albeit with a high specificity. The pathognomonic finding of AIN remains the identification of an inflammatory infiltrate by renal biopsy.

   f. Therapy involves the discontinuation of any possible offending medications and supportive care. Although steroid therapy is often used and may hasten the recovery, the data for the utility of steroids in treating AIN are controversial.

   g. Typically patients will have a gradual return of their renal function to baseline.

4. Hepatorenal syndrome (HRS)

   a. HRS describes the syndrome of ARF in the setting of severe hepatic dysfunction.

   b. The pathophysiology involves profound renal vasoconstriction with histologically normal kidneys. Current belief is that this intense renal vasoconstriction is a consequence of the depressed effective circulating volume and activation of neuroendocrine mediators (angiotensin, vasopressin, nitric oxide, etc.) with the intense mesenteric vasodilation seen with advanced liver disease.

   c. Two syndromes of HRS have been described:

      (1) Type I. Rapid and profound deterioration in renal function (increase in serum Cr to >2.5 mg/dl or reduction in Cr clearance by 50% or to <20 ml/min over <2 weeks). It is typically seen with end-stage liver disease and has an identifiable precipitant event, for example, large-volume paracentesis, spontaneous bacterial peritonitis, or gastrointestinal bleeding. It is associated with an extremely high mortality (>90% at 3 months).

      (2) Type II. More insidious onset and modest deterioration in renal function without obligatory progression. Prognosis is significantly better than that of type I HRS.

   d. Although diagnostic criteria for HRS are available, the diagnosis is typically one of exclusion. Indices of function suggest prerenal azotemia, but response to volume loading is typically poor. The urine sediment is usually bland.

   e. Therapy is primarily supportive. Renal vasodilator therapy has not been shown to be of benefit. However, recent small studies suggest that mesenteric vasoconstrictors (midorine, octreotide, the vasopressin analogues terlipressin and ornipressin), and the antioxidant NAC may be of benefit in select patients. **Transjugular intrahepatic portosystemic shunt** (TIPS) procedures have also shown benefit in treating patients with HRS who were not candidates for liver transplantation. The role of dialysis is controversial.

  f. Liver transplantation is the definitive treatment. Renal function usually recovers completely following transplantation.

5. Toxins

  a. Aminoglycosides (see Chapter 11)

    (1) Pathophysiology is related to proximal tubular cell toxicity. The urine sediment may contain tubular casts. FENa is typically elevated.

    (2) Drug dosing is a critical factor in disease initiation, and accurate estimation of GFR and close pharmacologic monitoring are crucial. High trough drug levels appear more predictive of deterioration in renal function.

    (3) There is some evidence that once-daily dosing regimens have equivalent therapeutic efficacy with decreased nephrotoxicity when compared to traditional multiple daily dosing regimens.

    (4) Prognosis is usually good, with return of renal function to baseline or near-baseline levels in most patients.

  b. Amphotericin B (see Chapter 11)

    (1) Amphotericin B is associated with a high incidence of nephrotoxicity (approximately 30%).

    (2) Risk factors include male gender, maximum daily dose ($\geq$60 mg/d), duration of therapy, preexisting renal disease, critical illness at the onset of therapy, and concurrent use of cyclosporine.

    (3) Pathophysiology involves injury to multiple tubular segments including the proximal tubule, ascending limb, and collecting system from direct toxicity and intrarenal vasoconstriction. The resulting abnormalities can include a type I (distal) renal tubular acidosis and potassium and magnesium wasting.

    (4) Associated with increased mortality.

    (5) Prevention

      (a) Saline loading is used to minimize tubuloglomerular feedback and intrarenal vasoconstriction.

      (b) Use of less nephrotoxic amphotericin preparations such as **liposomal amphotericin B** or **amphotericin B colloid dispersion.** (see Chapter 11).

c. Heme pigment

(1) Rhabdomyolysis represents the primary cause of heme pigment–associated nephrotoxicity.

(2) Pathophysiology is related to hypovolemia (fluid shift into injured muscle), intrarenal vasoconstriction, direct tubular toxicity, and intratubular cast formation.

(3) Manifestations can include muscle pain and weakness, "doughy" muscles, or evidence of compartment syndrome.

(4) Diagnosis. The FENa is typically low. The pathognomonic finding is cola-colored urine with a heme-positive dipstick result but without red blood cells on microscopic exam of the sediment. The urine sediment may also contain pigmented granular casts. Hyperkalemia, hyperphosphatemia, hyperuricemia, hypocalcemia, and an anion-gap metabolic acidosis are frequently evident.

(5) Treatment is primarily supportive. Calcium repletion during the initial stages of injury should be undertaken with caution because during the recovery phase, hypercalcemia often occurs as calcium is released from recovering tissues.

(6) Prevention

i. Volume repletion

ii. Alkalinization of the urine to a pH greater than 6.0 is advocated to prevent the crystallization of myoglobin with the tubules. There is no clear evidence of superiority to volume repletion alone. Urine alkalinization can be achieved by infusing 5% dextrose (D5W) with 150 mEq/L of sodium bicarbonate.

iii. Mannitol has a potential benefit through an antioxidant effect. As with alkalinization, there is no clear evidence of superiority over volume repletion alone. When mannitol is administered it is often infused as a mixture with 5% dextrose in half-normal saline (D5 1/2NS) to which 40 mEq/L of sodium bicarbonate and 10 g/L of 20% mannitol are added.

VIII. Management of acute renal failure

A. Pharmacologic

1. Prevention

a. Volume repletion. Hypovolemia is a major risk factor for ARF under almost every circumstance. Therefore, volume repletion with a goal of optimizing renal perfusion is crucial in preventing renal failure. Although there is some evidence suggesting a benefit of using sodium bicarbonate in specific instances such as in the prevention of RCN, there is no evidence overwhelmingly supporting one fluid choice over another.

b. Discontinuation of potentially nephrotoxic agents in patients at high risk.

c. Use of nonionic, low-osmolality radiocontrast agents in patients at high risk of RCN.

d. Other than the use of periprocedure **NAC** and **sodium bicarbonate** in patients at high risk for RCN, current evidence does not support the use of pharmacologic agents in the prevention of ARF (including dopamine, fenoldopam, mannitol, and atrial natriuretic peptide).

2. Treatment

a. Whereas numerous agents have been extensively investigated in treating or limiting injury in the setting of ARF, there is no evidence supporting the use of any agent in the treatment of ARF.

(1) Dopamine. Dopamine, when infused at low rates (0.5–2 μg/kg/min), increases renal plasma flow, GFR, and renal sodium excretion. Although some anecdotal evidence exists for the use of dopamine with ARF, all randomized, prospective trials have shown no benefit in terms of disease progression, need for renal replacement, or mortality.

(2) Fenoldopam. Fenoldopam, a selective agonist of the dopamine type I receptor, is the only Food and Drug Administration–approved drug in the United States for the treatment of hypertensive emergencies.

i. When infused at low doses (0.03–0.1 μg/kg/min), fenoldopam has been shown to increase renal plasma flow and reduce the aberrant renal hemodynamics seen with aortic cross-clamping without significantly affecting systemic hemodynamics.

ii. However, there are no prospective, randomized, controlled data supporting the use of this agent in the treatment of ARF.

(3) Diuretics. Although it is known that nonoliguric renal failure is associated with better prognosis than oliguric renal failure, there is no evidence showing that using diuretics to convert oliguric renal failure to a nonoliguric form has any benefit in terms of mortality, disease progression, or need for renal replacement therapy. In fact, a recent retrospective analysis suggested that **high-dose loop diuretics may worsen outcome with ARF.** This study also showed that impaired responsiveness to loop diuretics is a poor prognostic indicator with ARF.

  i. Atrial natriuretic peptide (ANP) increases GFR through its hemodynamic effects and by dilation of the afferent arteriole. The evidence does not support the use of ANP in the treatment of ARF.

  ii. Insulin-like growth factor 1 (IGF-1) has been shown to accelerate renal recovery in experimental models of ischemic ARF. However, the clinical evidence shows no benefit in terms of renal recovery, need for renal replacement, or mortality.

B. Renal replacement therapy (RRT) is often indicated in the management of patients with ARF in the ICU. Controversy exists regarding the timing of dialysis or filtration, but the trend has been toward earlier initiation. Several forms of renal replacement therapy are available.

1. **Acute peritoneal dialysis (PD)** has largely been replaced by continuous venovenous therapy. PD catheter insertion often led to leakage of PD fluid, infection, catheter malfunction, and, rarely, perforation of a viscus.

2. **Hemodialysis (HD)**
   a. Intermittent HD remains a viable and efficient option for hemodynamically stable patients.
   b. Some studies suggest that daily hemodialysis may be associated with a better prognosis.
   c. HD requires the establishment of vascular access in the femoral, internal jugular, or subclavian vein.
   d. Anticoagulation can be avoided in the acute setting by periodically flushing the filter.
   e. Complications of HD include hypotension, arrhythmias, bleeding, and infection of the access.

3. **Continuous renal replacement therapy** is the preferred modality in the unstable patient.
   a. **Access** is the same as for HD.
   b. **Anticoagulation/base replacement** can be with heparin or citrate serving as a regional anticoagulant and with use of prostacyclin.
   c. **Continuous venovenous hemofiltration (CVVH)** is the most commonly used form of continuous renal replacement therapy.
   d. The **ultrafiltration rate** is generally 1.6 to 3.2 L/h with replacement fluid calculated to achieve the desired body balance.
   e. It has been shown that the dose of dialysis can impact mortality, and that an ultrafiltration rate of at least 35 ml/h/kg should be used. High-volume hemofiltration has been proposed as a therapy for sepsis, but there is insufficient data to support its use at this time.

  f. Hemofiltration has also been shown to be effective in preventing RCN.

  g. Complications

    (1) Citrate toxicity can occur when citrate is used, particularly in patients with liver disease. Features of citrate toxicity include normal to high serum calcium, low ionized calcium, a high anion gap, and worsening metabolic acidosis.

    (2) Other complications include infection, bleeding, metabolic alkalosis, and hypophosphatemia, especially with prolonged therapy.

 4. Other modalities include continuous arteriovenous hemofiltration (CAVH) and continuous venovenous hemofiltration with dialysis (CVVHD).

IX. Management of the complications of ARF

 A. Volume overload

  1. An average individual requires a minimum of about 500 ml of fluid each day to carry nonvolatile solute. Fluid intake is offset by urinary, gastrointestinal, wound, and insensible losses. In patients with renal failure, the inability to balance fluid intake by urinary elimination may lead to volume overload.

  2. Most patients in the ICU require the administration of fluid volumes in the form of drugs and nutrition that are far in excess of the volume required to carry solute.

  3. Treatment options for minimizing the risk of or for treating fluid overload include the following:

   a. Induced diuresis. Fluid management often can be facilitated when oliguria responds to diuretic therapy. Forced diuresis may have specific benefits in a limited number of conditions such as rhabdomyolysis and tumor lysis syndrome, but should never be attempted until prerenal azotemia has been excluded.

   b. Minimize exogenous fluid administration

    (1) Use low-flow, constant-flush systems on pressure-monitoring catheters and infusion pumps.

    (2) Concentrate drugs to their solubility or safety limits.

    (3) Avoid any unnecessary fluid administration (e.g., convert medications to enteral formulations whenever practical).

  4. Renal replacement therapy will inevitably be required in the anuric patient or when conservative therapy fails.

 B. Hyponatremia (see also Chapter 7) most often results from excessive antidiuretic hormone (ADH) secretion, but may also develop as a result of defective concentrating mechanisms. The first line of treatment in either of these cases is fluid restriction (<800 ml/d). Treatment with normal saline and a loop diuretic may be necessary.

C. Metabolic acidosis

1. Metabolic acidosis is typically associated with an increased anion gap from the retention of organic acids.
2. Organic acids are normally produced at a rate of 1 mEq/kg/d, but production may be greatly increased in the catabolic critically ill. Serum bicarbonate may decrease at a daily rate of 2 mEq/L or more.
3. Treatment is usually not necessary, and overaggressive correction of acidosis may precipitate acute hypocalcemia.
4. When needed, sodium bicarbonate, 40 to 80 mEq/d, can be used to maintain pH within the normal range.
5. Dialysis may be necessary when the acid load is very high or when volume overload or hypernatremia limits the amount of sodium bicarbonate that can be safely administered.

D. Hyperkalemia

1. **Electrocardiographic (ECG) changes** may be diagnostic (see also Chapter 7). Peaked T waves and a shortened QT interval usually are the earliest changes, followed by prolongation of the PR interval and a decrease in the amplitude of the P wave. As hyperkalemia progresses, depression of the ST segment and widening of the QRS complex follow, eventually producing a sinusoidal waveform.
2. Treatment depends on the degree of hyperkalemia and the severity of ECG changes. The presence of a widened QRS complex is an indication for prompt treatment with intravenous calcium, bicarbonate, glucose, and insulin. Less pronounced changes such as T-wave peaking may be managed with the more slowly acting cation exchange resins.
3. **Specific treatment guidelines**
   a. **Calcium gluconate** (15–30 mg/kg intravenously [IV]) or **calcium chloride** (5–10 mg/kg IV), administered over 2 to 5 minutes, directly antagonizes the effect of potassium on the myocardium.
   b. **Sodium bicarbonate,** 50 to 100 mEq IV, will partly reverse the acidosis and cause a redistribution of potassium into cells. In mechanically ventilated patients, hyperventilation can be used to create a respiratory alkalosis, which will have the same effect.
   c. **Glucose and insulin.** One to two ampules of 50% glucose (dextrose) in water and 10 units of regular insulin IV should be given over a 5-minute period. Redistribution of potassium into the cell occurs within minutes.
   d. Sodium polystyrene sulfonate **(Kayexalate)** is a sodium–potassium ion exchange resin given via the gastrointestinal tract that directly removes potassium from the body. Kayexalate (25–50 g

in 100 ml of a 20% sorbitol solution) may be given orally or as a retention enema. Because of its slow rate of potassium removal, it should not be used as sole therapy for life-threatening hyperkalemia. Excessive use of Kayexalate with sorbitol has been associated with bowel perforation.

   e. Dialysis is indicated for the urgent treatment of life-threatening hyperkalemia. Hemodialysis is far more effective than continuous hemofiltration therapy for acute management of hyperkalemia.

E. Hypermagnesemia (see also Chapter 7) is rarely seen in renal failure, except when supplemental magnesium, such as in some antacids, is administered.

F. Hyperphosphatemia (see also Chapter 7) is common in ARF. Although phosphorus has no toxic effects, in excess it decreases serum calcium concentration. Severe elevations of the phosphate, as seen in tumor lysis syndrome, can be associated with metastatic calcifications. Phosphorus-binding antacids (Amphogel, Alternagel) usually are given to decrease plasma phosphorus levels and maintain calcium levels within a normal range. Calcium-based phosphate binders such as calcium acetate and non–calcium-based binders such as Svelamar can also be used. Overuse of antacids may produce hypophosphatemia.

G. Anemia in patients with ARF has many causes. Erythropoietin (EP) is produced by the kidney and stimulates erythrocyte production within the bone marrow. Absence of EP likely contributes to anemia in ARF. EP therapy is used routinely for patients with chronic renal failure and has been shown to decrease transfusion requirement in the critically ill.

H. Encephalopathy

   1. Altered mental status with renal failure is due to retention of endogenous waste.

   2. Manifestations range from tremor, myoclonus, asterixis, and frank seizures to lethargy, disorientation, and coma.

   3. Uremic encephalopathy usually improves with dialysis.

   4. Many other metabolic derangements and drug effects can contribute to encephalopathy in critically ill patients (see Chapter 29).

I. Decreased drug elimination. A large number of drugs are eliminated by the kidneys, including several neuromuscular blocking agents and potentially toxic drugs such as aminoglycosides and digoxin. The doses of renally excreted drugs must be adjusted when renal function is impaired. It should be remembered that in early ARF, the serum creatinine concentration does not fully reflect the reduction in GFR.

J. Uremic pericarditis occurs for unknown reasons and can be complicated by cardiac tamponade and infective pericarditis. Patients should be examined daily for the presence of a **pericardial friction rub.** Cardiac tamponade should be considered if unexplained cardiovascular decompensation occurs. Pericarditis may be an indication for emergency dialysis.

K. **Bleeding abnormalities** are common in patients with renal failure and are generally attributed to abnormal platelet function. Management of bleeding problems (see also Chapter 10) may include the following:

1. HD temporarily corrects platelet abnormalities, but also may activate complement and platelets and exacerbate a coagulopathy.

2. Desmopressin acetate **(DDAVP),** 0.3 to 0.4 μg/kg IV, subcutaneously, or intranasally, may improve platelet function in uremic patients.

3. Conjugated **estrogen therapy** produces a long-lasting improvement in the bleeding tendency of uremic patients.

L. **Infectious complications** are responsible for the majority of deaths in patients with ARF. Uremia impairs the ability to fight infection and blunts the usual manifestations of infection.

M. **Nutritional support** (see Chapter 9) is an important ancillary measure in critically ill patients with ARF.

1. Management of nutritional support in ARF is complicated by the need for volume restriction and the concern that supplemental protein may result in production of additional nitrogenous wastes.

2. Carbohydrates have a protein-sparing effect. Nutritional supplements, when administered with essential amino acid preparations, can be provided that do not significantly increase serum urea nitrogen concentration.

3. Enteral nutrition is preferred to parenteral nutrition, when possible.

4. Continuous renal replacement therapies permit an increased volume of feedings with less concern about volume overload. Renal replacement therapies also eliminate nutrients, as they do wastes. Glucose is usually infused with the replacement fluid, and amino acid solutions may be increased to compensate for the loss.

SELECTED REFERENCES

Anavekar NS, McMurray JJ, Velazquez EJ, et al. Relation between renal dysfunction and cardiovascular outcomes in myocardial infarction. *N Engl J Med* 2004;351:1285–1295.

Angeli P, Volpin R, Gerunda G, et al. Reversal of type I hepatorenal syndrome with the administration of midodrine and octreotide. *Hepatology* 1999;29:1690–1697.

Block CA, Manning HL. Prevention of acute renal failure in the critically ill. *Am J Respir Crit Care Med* 2002;165:320–324.

Doty JM, Saggi BH, Blocher CR, et al. Effects of increased renal parenchymal pressure on renal function. *J Trauma* 2000;48: 874–877.

Forni LB, Hilton PJ. Continuous hemofiltration in the treatment of acute renal failure. *N Engl J Med* 1997;336:1303–1309.

Go AS, Chertow GM, Fan D, et al. Chronic kidney disease and the risk of death, cardiovascular events and hospitalization. *N Engl J Med* 2004;351:1296–1305.

Kay J, Chow WH, Mao T, et al. Acetylcysteine for prevention of acute deterioration of renal function following elective coronary angiography and intervention. *JAMA* 2003;289:553–558.

Kellum JA, Mehta RL, Angus DC, et al. The First International Consensus Conference of Continuous Renal Replacement Therapy. *Kidney Int* 2002;62:1855–1863.

Marenzi G, Marana I, Lauri G, et al. The prevention of radiocontrast agent-induced nephropathy by hemofiltration. *N Engl J Med* 2003;349:1333–1340.

Mehta RL, McDonald B, Gabbai FB, et al. A randomized trial of continuous versus intermittent dialysis for acute renal failure. *Kidney Int* 2001;60:1154–1163.

Merten GJ, Burgess WP, Gray LV, et al. Prevention of contrast-induced nephropathy with sodium bicarbonate. *JAMA* 2004;291:2328–2334.

Mueller C, Buerkle G, Buettner HJ, et al. Prevention of contrast media-associated nephropathy. *Arch Intern Med* 2002;162:329–336.

Ronco C, Bellomo R, Homel P, et al. Effects of different doses in continuous veno-venous haemofiltration on outcomes of acute renal failure: a prospective randomised trial. *Lancet* 2000;356:26–30.

Stone GW, McCullough PA, Tumlin JA, et al. Fenoldopam mesylate for the prevention of contrast-induced nephropathy. *JAMA* 2003;290:2284–2291.

Thadhani R, Pasqual M, Bonventre JV. Acute renal failure. *N Engl J Med* 1996;334:1448–1460.

Acute Liver Failure

William J. Benedetto and Kenneth L. Haspel

I. **Postoperative complications after liver surgery**
   A. **Hemorrhage**
      1. **Insufficient surgical hemostasis.** Bleeding must be anticipated. Surgical techniques respecting the segmental structure of the liver (i.e., anatomic resection) and the use of argon beam coagulators have decreased intra- and postoperative blood loss. Wedge resections tend to bleed more postoperatively than lobectomies because more of the raw surface remains.
      2. **Postoperative coagulopathy** (see also Chapter 10).
      3. **Management**
         a. Restoration of **normovolemia** with crystalloids, colloids, and packed red blood cells.
         b. Restoration of **normothermia.**
         c. If the hematocrit does not stabilize or hemodynamics do not stabilize despite the aforementioned measures, ongoing bleeding must be suspected that requires **surgical reintervention.** Hepatic **angiography and embolization** are also options.
   B. **Coagulopathy** may occur secondary to massive operative blood losses, hypothermia, hyperfibrinolysis, or a decreased production of clotting factors by the hepatic tissue. Correction of coagulopathy is carried out with transfusion of fresh-frozen plasma, platelets, cryoprecipitate, and so on.
   C. **Fever.** Postoperative pyrexia may reflect resorption of hematoma or necrotic tissue or may be a sign of peritonitis or abscess formation.
   D. **Biliary fistula.** Leaking bile ducts may form bile collections. Suction drains should be left in place or new drains should be inserted by interventional radiology. Usually biliary fistulas close on their own within 3 weeks.
   E. **Hepatic aneurysm.** Anemia, leukocytosis, and abdominal pain may be indicators of a late complication after hepatic trauma, namely the development of a false aneurysm after an injury of the hepatic vasculature. Therapeutic embolization is considered the treatment of choice.
   F. **Intra- or perihepatic abscess.** The risk of abscess formation is increased with concomitant colonic or pancreatic injury, large collections of hematoma or bile, and open drains. Prolonged postoperative pyrexia in combination with leukocytosis and increasing right upper quadrant pain should raise the suspicion of a peri/intrahepatic abscess. Treatment includes drainage by interventional radiology or surgical revision in combination with intravenous antibiotics.

G. **Postoperative liver failure.** In otherwise normal livers (i.e., liver surgery for removal of a metastatic lesion or adenoma), resections of up to 80% of the liver mass are generally well tolerated. Complications may arise in the following circumstances:

1. The remaining liver is too small to maintain full hepatic function.
2. Alterations in hepatic blood flow lead to ischemia.

II. **Postoperative liver dysfunction after nonhepatic surgery**

A. **Etiologies** include

1. Infections (e.g., viral hepatitis, exacerbation of chronic hepatitis, sepsis).
2. Ischemia secondary to hypotension, congestive heart failure, and hepatic artery ligation or injury.
3. Hypoxia.
4. Drug and toxin induced (e.g., alcohol, halothane, acetaminophen).
5. Bile duct obstruction or injury.
6. Pancreatitis.
7. Bilirubin overload secondary to hematomas, blood transfusions, hemolysis, and so on.

B. **Preexisting hepatic disease** makes the liver much more vulnerable to the foregoing stress factors.

C. **Symptoms** are often nonspecific and include right upper quadrant pain, nausea, vomiting, indigestion, pruritus, fatigue, fever, and mental confusion or encephalopathy.

D. **Signs** include jaundice, right upper quadrant tenderness, palmar erythema, spider nevi, splenomegaly, ascites, portosystemic collaterals (e.g., *caput medusae,* hemorrhoids, gastroesophageal varices), coagulopathy, anemia, and gynecomastia.

E. **Management.** See section III.C.

III. **Fulminant hepatic failure**

A. **Fulminant hepatic failure** is characterized by a fast onset of severe impairment of liver function. Patients with chronic liver disease are excluded. It may be subdivided further into **hyperacute** (0–7 days), **acute** (8–28 days), and **subacute** (29 days–12 weeks) failure depending on the time interval between first symptoms and signs of liver failure.

B. **Causes**

1. **Infections**
   a. **Viral** (e.g., hepatitis A, B, C, D, E, yellow fever, cytomegalovirus, Epstein-Barr virus).
   b. **Bacterial** (e.g., liver abscess, *Legionella* sepsis, Q-fever).
2. **Toxins/drugs/chemicals** (e.g., acetaminophen, carbon tetrachloride, designer drugs such as "ecstasy," mushroom toxins such as that of *Amanita phalloides,* halothane, isoniazid, valproic acid).
3. **Ischemia and/or hypoxia** of any cause, but also specifically due to venous congestion of the liver (e.g., right ventricular failure, Budd-Chiari syndrome),

tumors that impair blood flow to the liver, and trauma to the liver and its supplying vessels.

4. **Metabolic** causes (e.g., Reye's syndrome, acute fatty liver of pregnancy, Wilson's disease, heat stroke).

C. **Complications and management**

1. **Cerebral edema** is the leading cause of death in fulminant hepatic failure. Cerebral edema is present in up to 80% of cases of hepatic failure that proceed to stage IV encephalopathy (see Table 25-1). Theories for the development of cerebral edema include impaired cerebral autoregulation and decline of cerebral blood flow, disruption of the blood–brain barrier, and intracellular accumulation of osmotically active molecules. Focal neurologic signs usually do not occur and may indicate intracranial bleeding or early herniation. Management of cerebral edema is discussed in Chapters 13 and 29.

2. **Cardiovascular.** Arteriovenous shunting and vasodilation due to decreased clearance of vasoactive metabolites by the liver produce a high-output state characterized by tachycardia, increased cardiac output, and decreased systemic vascular resistance. An important differential diagnosis in these immunocompromised patients is sepsis. See Chapters 1, 2, 11, and 28 for diagnosis and management. Increased intracranial pressure (ICP) may be present, and attention to maintenance of adequate cerebral perfusion pressure is prudent.

3. **Respiratory**

   a. **Endotracheal intubation** may be required if protective airway reflexes are lost.

   b. **Hypoxemia** may occur in patients with hypoventilation, atelectasis, pleural effusions, pulmonary shunting, and pulmonary edema, and may require intubation and artificial ventilation.

   c. **Hyperventilation** may be necessary as a temporary treatment for increased intracranial pressure (see Chapter 13).

4. **Coagulopathies** can be secondary to decreased production of clotting factors and/or increased thrombolysis. Thrombocytopenia and impaired platelet function are common. Transfusion of coagulation factors in the

Table 25-1. Clinical stages of hepatic encephalopathy

Stage 1. Altered behavior, impairment of sleep, change of handwriting, slurred speech

Stage 2. Drowsiness, disorientation, restlessness, brisk tendon reflexes, increased muscle tone, clonus

Stage 3. Somnolent, but arousable, marked confusion, disturbance of speech, hyperreflexia, miosis

Stage 4. Coma, mydriasis, hypo- or areflexia, unresponsiveness to painful stimuli absence of active bleeding is controversial, but may be indicated prior to invasive procedures or when invasive ICP monitoring devices are in place.

5. **Renal failure** complicates about half of the cases of fulminant hepatic failure and commonly is due to **hepatorenal syndrome (HRS)**. Renal failure and hepatic disease are discussed in detail in section IV.

6. **Electrolyte and acid-base disorders** are varied and include
   a. Respiratory alkalosis.
   b. Metabolic acidosis as an early sign of acetaminophen intoxication or a late sign of lactic acidosis when the liver is no longer able to metabolize lactic acid adequately.
   c. Hypokalemia.
   d. Hyponatremia secondary to reduced free water clearance.
   e. Hypernatremia secondary to dehydration after mannitol therapy.
   f. Hypoglycemia due to impaired glycogen mobilization, gluconeogenesis, and insulin metabolism.

D. **Liver transplantation in fulminant hepatic failure**
   1. **Indications.** Orthotopic liver transplantation may be an option for patients with fulminant hepatic failure. Accurate predictions of whether a patient's liver will be able to recover with medical treatment alone may avoid unnecessary liver transplantation or suggest early transplantation, which may improve outcome. The **King's College criteria for liver transplantation** (Table 25-2) provide a comparatively fast and inexpensive assessment of liver function that can be frequently repeated. **Factor V levels** also have been

Table 25-2.   King's College criteria for liver transplantation in fulminant hepatic failure

Acetaminophen intoxication
   Arterial pH <7.3 irrespective of grade of encephalopathy
   Or a combination of:
      Encephalopathy grade III or IV
      Prothrombin time >35 sec
      Serum creatinine >3.4 mg/dl
Nonacetaminophen patients
   INR >7.7 irrespective of grade of encephalopathy
   Or any three of the following variables
      Age <10 or >40 years
      Etiology is hepatitis C, halothane hepatitis, or idiosyncratic drug reaction
      Duration of jaundice before onset of encephalopathy >7 days
      Prothrombin time >25 sec
      Serum bilirubin >18 mg/dl

used to determine indications for liver transplantation in patients with viral hepatitis. Encephalopathy associated with a factor V level of less than 20% of normal in patients younger than 30 years of age or less than 30% of normal in patients older than 30 years of age is considered an indication for transplantation. Because these assessment protocols are not perfect, it has been advocated that all patients with fulminant hepatic failure be listed for transplantation as soon as the diagnosis is made. The patient is reevaluated when a donor liver becomes available, and the decision to transplant or continue to follow is made at that time.

2. **Contraindications** to transplantation include sepsis, acute respiratory distress syndrome, and cerebral edema that is unresponsive to treatment. **Relative contraindications** include rapidly developing hemodynamic instability requiring increasing vasopressor support, psychiatric disturbances (e.g., noncompliance with medications, multiple suicide attempts), and advanced age.

E. Liver support systems

1. Available types include cell-based or non–cell-based systems. Non–cell-based systems, including the molecular adsorbent recycling system (MARS) and the HemoTherapies Liver Dialysis Unit, expose patient plasma or blood to an absorbent medium such as albumin (MARS) or charcoal (Liver Dialysis Unit) to dialyze circulating toxins. Cell-based systems, including the extracorporeal liver assist device (ELAD), the bioartificial extracorporeal liver support (BELS) system, and the HepatAssist Liver Support System, use immortalized human or porcine hepatocytes to metabolize these toxins. The intended use is as a bridge to recovery from an acute insult or to transplant.

2. Experience with these devices remains somewhat limited, though investigation continues. An early meta-analysis of studies demonstrated a benefit for acute-on-chronic liver failure, but did not find a demonstrable effect on acute liver failure.

IV. Liver cirrhosis can be seen as an irreversible final pathway of different chronic liver diseases. Hepatocyte necrosis and destruction of the connective tissue network lead to irregular nodular regeneration of hepatic parenchyma, extensive fibrosis, and distortion of the hepatic vasculature.

A. Etiologies include

1. **Alcoholic** cirrhosis, which accounts for most cases in the Western world.

2. **Viral hepatitis** following chronic hepatitis B, C, and D infection. Twenty percent of chronic hepatitis C infections progress to cirrhosis.

3. **Primary biliary cirrhosis.**

4. **Secondary biliary cirrhosis** as a result of prolonged obstruction of the biliary tract.

5. **Longstanding congestive heart failure.**

6. **Metabolic diseases** (e.g., hemochromatosis, Wilson's disease, glycogen storage diseases, and α-1-anti-trypsin deficiency).

7. **Drug-related toxicities** (e.g., methotrexate, isoniazid, methyldopa).

8. **Parasitic infections** (e.g., *Echinococcus* infection, schistosomiasis).

B. **Portal hypertension and bleeding from gastro-esophageal varices.** Although there are other causes (e.g., Budd-Chiari syndrome, portal vein thrombosis), cirrhosis is the most common underlying disease leading to portal hypertension. Cirrhosis creates portosystemic collaterals that may form varices with a risk of bleeding.

1. **Patients with esophageal bleeding** present with hematemesis, melena, and hematochezia. The diagnosis must be confirmed by esophagogastroscopy because bleeding frequently occurs from duodenal or gastric ulcers or the Mallory-Weiss syndrome.

2. **Endoscopic sclerotherapy and variceal ligation** are commonly used to manage esophageal varices and esophageal bleeding. The procedures are highly successful and can immediately follow diagnostic esophagogastroscopy.

3. **Portal vein pressures** may be measured by catheterization of the portal vein (percutaneous transhepatic) or indirectly by transjugular or transfemoral catheterization of the hepatic veins.

4. **Nonselective β-adrenergic blockers** like **propranolol** administered prophylactically reduce the risk of bleeding, although mortality is unaffected. Propranolol reduces portal pressure by constriction of the splanchnic vasculature and to a smaller degree by cardiac output reduction.

5. **Vasopressin** reduces blood flow and pressure in the portal system including its collaterals. Vasopressin should be administered through a central line because infiltration may cause tissue necrosis. The infusion dose is 0.1 to 0.4 units/min. Note that this dose is as much as 10 times higher than the "replacement" dose of vasopressin suggested as therapy of septic shock (Chapter 28). Side effects include myocardial ischemia, gastrointestinal ischemia, acute renal failure, and hyponatremia. Concomitant infusion of **nitroglycerin** may reduce the side effects of vasopressin.

6. **Somatostatin** is a naturally produced peptide hormone that acts as a vasoconstrictor in supraphysiologic doses. Fewer side effects are reported with somatostatin than with vasopressin.

7. **Octreotide** is a synthetic analogue of somatostatin that has a much longer half-life. The dose is 25 to 50 μg/h.

8. **Balloon tamponade** is only recommended if medical or sclerotherapy/variceal ligation is unsuccessful. Different tubes are available. The

Sengstaken-Blakemore tube is a triple-lumen tube with a gastric balloon, an esophageal balloon, and a gastric tube. The **Minnesota tube** has an additional port for esophageal aspiration and a larger gastric balloon. The **Linton-Nachlas** tube has only a gastric balloon. When tubes with a double balloon are used, the gastric balloon is inflated first and placed on gentle traction. If the bleeding does not stop, the esophageal balloon is also inflated. Major complications include esophageal rupture and aspiration. Aspiration risks can be reduced by endotracheal intubation prior to insertion of the esophageal tube.

9. **Emergency surgical shunt operations** and **surgical ligations** are only used as a last resort. **Transjugular intrahepatic portosystemic shunt (TIPS)** procedures use a percutaneously placed expandable metal stent to form a direct portocaval channel within the liver. All these procedures are associated with high complication rates, and are usually reserved for patients who have recurrent bleeding despite repeated sclerotherapies.

C. **Hepatic encephalopathy** appears to be caused by multiple factors. Hepatic clearance of cerebrotoxic substances such as ammonia, mercaptans, and short-chain fatty acids is reduced. In addition, experimental evidence suggests that the damaged liver is no longer able to produce certain substances that are crucial for normal brain function. The isolation of benzodiazepine-like compounds from brains of patients with hepatic encephalopathy and partial antagonism of hepatic encephalopathy by flumazenil suggest that the gamma-aminobutyrate (GABA)-minergic system may be altered.

1. **Diagnosis of hepatic encephalopathy** is made clinically. Ammonia levels do not correlate with the severity of the encephalopathy. In contrast to fulminant hepatic failure, increased intracranial pressure is only rarely associated with chronic hepatic encephalopathy.

2. **Management** includes the elimination of any precipitating factors (such as gastrointestinal bleeding) if possible. A nasogastric tube should be inserted to document and evacuate any upper gastrointestinal bleeding (if present) and permit administration of lactulose.

3. **Lactulose** acidifies the bowel contents and increases diffusion of ammonia into bowel lumen where it can be eliminated. The initial dose is 20 ml/h orally or by nasogastric tube until diarrhea occurs. The dose is then adjusted to produce three to four soft stools per day. Lactulose also can be administered as an enema (300 ml of 50% lactulose in 700 ml of water three times daily). Side effects include hypokalemia, dehydration, and hypernatremia. Alternatively, **neomycin,** 1 g orally or by nasogastric tube, four times daily, may be helpful.

D. **Ascites** is produced in cirrhosis by the combination of portal hypertension, hypoalbuminemia, and fluid retention. Greater than 500 ml of ascites can usually be detected clinically by a distended abdomen, bulging flanks, everted umbilicus, shifting abdominal dullness, and an abdominal fluid wave. The diagnosis can be confirmed by ultrasonography. Other causes of ascites should be excluded by a diagnostic paracentesis. Ascites can be classified as transudative or exudative.

1. **Transudative ascites** is caused by movement of fluid across the hepatic sinusoids and the intestinal capillaries and is due to increased hydrostatic pressure from portal hypertension. In transudative ascites due to portal hypertension, the total protein content tends to be less than 2.5 g/dl and the difference between the albumin concentrations of the serum and ascites is frequently greater than 1 g/dl. **Other causes** of transudative ascites include congestive heart failure, inferior vena cava occlusion, Budd-Chiari syndrome, and Meigs' syndrome.

2. **Exudative ascites** develops secondary to exudation of the fluid from the peritoneum. Portal hypertension is absent. In exudative ascites (with normal portal pressure), the protein content usually exceeds 2.5 to 3 g/dl and the difference between the albumin concentrations of the serum and ascites is often less than 1 g/dl. **Other causes** of exudative ascites include neoplasms (e.g., peritoneal carcinomatosis), peritoneal infections (e.g., tuberculosis, pyogenic peritonitis), chylous ascites, pancreatitis, and nephrogenic ascites.

3. On **diagnostic paracentesis,** the ascites should be sent for cell count, Gram's stain, bacterial culture, amylase level, lactate dehydrogenase, carcinoembryonic antigen, and triglycerides.

4. **Mainstays of therapy for ascites** in cirrhosis are a salt-restricted diet, containing as little as 11 mmol of sodium per day to induce a negative sodium balance and limit ascitic fluid accumulation. Diuretics are added if necessary. Because one cause for the fluid retention in cirrhosis is secondary hyperaldosteronism, **spironolactone** is the diuretic of first choice. Other diuretics may be added cautiously if needed. Overly aggressive diuresis may result in azotemia and hypotension secondary to hypovolemia. The effectiveness of the treatment is monitored by daily weighing. Daily weight loss should not exceed 0.5 to 1 kg. Patients refractory to medical therapy may require additional paracenteses. Plasma and urinary electrolytes should be monitored regularly, especially during diuretic treatment.

E. **Splenomegaly** may produce thrombocytopenia or pancytopenia, but rarely requires treatment.

F. **Spontaneous bacterial peritonitis (SBP)** is an infection of ascitic fluid without a primary intraabdominal focus (see also Chapter 28).

1. **Signs and symptoms** may range from subtle to severe abdominal pain with rebound tenderness, fever, chills, nausea, and vomiting. Because symptoms may be absent, **diagnostic paracentesis** for culture and cell count is recommended in the assessment of patients with ascites. Gastrointestinal hemorrhage, which is often associated with bacteremia, puts the cirrhotic patient at risk of developing SBP. The most important sources of contamination of the ascites are the gastrointestinal tract, urinary tract, pneumonias, and endoscopic procedures. Greater than 90% of the cases of SBP are caused by a single organism. Enteric gram-negative bacteria are most frequently isolated (70%), followed by gram-positive cocci (*Streptococcus pneumoniae, Enterococcus, Staphylococcus*) in about 20% of the cases and anaerobes in approximately 5%. **Polymicrobial infections in SBP are rare** and should trigger a search for bowel perforation.

2. **Treatment.** Because the mortality of untreated SBP is high, antibiotic therapy should be initiated immediately after samples of the ascites are taken. Empiric antibiotics that are active against gram-negative, gram-positive, and anaerobic bacteria should be administered initially and then modified based on cultures. Potential regimens include the following:

   a. A β-lactam such as **ampicillin** plus **aminoglycoside.**

   b. A third-generation nonpseudomonal cephalosporin such as **ceftriaxone** or **cefotaxime.**

   c. A β-lactam/β-lactamase inhibitor such as **timentin.**

   d. **Vancomycin** should be added to each of the foregoing regimens if methicillin-resistant *Staphylococcus aureus* (MRSA) is suspected.

3. **Prophylaxis.** Patients with cirrhosis who are admitted with gastrointestinal bleeding may be prophylactically treated with cefotaxime. To prevent recurrence of SBP, prophylactic treatment with a fluoroquinolone or trimethoprim-sulfamethoxazole may be considered, especially for liver transplant candidates.

G. **Hepatopulmonary syndrome.** Pathologic **dilation of intrapulmonary vessels** in cirrhosis increases right-to-left shunting of blood flow through the lungs. The diagnosis can be made with contrast-enhanced echocardiography or radiolabeled macroaggregated albumin. The degree of hypoxemia is variable, and is inconsistently improved by administration of supplemental oxygen. Partial or complete improvement of hypoxemia after liver transplantation has been reported.

H. **Hepatorenal syndrome (HRS)** is characterized by worsening renal function, sodium retention, and oliguria without an identifiable cause in a patient with cirrhosis and ascites. Renal failure is thought to be caused by

Table 25-3. Child-Pugh classification

	Classification Points		
	1	2	3
Encephalopathy	None	Grades 1 and 2	Grades 3 and 4
Ascites	Absent	Slight–moderate	Tense
Bilirubin (mg/dl)	<2.0	2–3	>3.0
Bilirubin (mg/dl) if primary biliary cirrhosis	<4	4–10	>10
Albumin (g/dl)	>3.5	2.8–3.5	<2.8
PT (seconds above control)	1–4	4–6	>6

Points from each of the five categories are summed to yield a total score: class A, 5–6 points; class B, 7–9 points; class C, 10–15 points. The mortality of cirrhotic patients rises dramatically with increasing Child scores. The 1-year mortality rate is 0%–10% for Child's A, 20%–30% for Child's B, and 50%–60% for Child's C. PT, prothrombin time.

inappropriate renal **vasoconstriction,** which reduces renal blood flow and glomerular filtration rate. Significant morphologic abnormalities are absent. Clinical signs usually include oliguria, azotemia, hyperkalemia, and hyponatremia. Other causes of renal failure, such as prerenal azotemia, acute tubular necrosis, and glomerulonephritis, must be excluded (Chapter 24). In HRS, the urinary sediment is unremarkable, and significant sodium retention is present. The urinary sodium is often less than 5 mmol/L, which is less than that observed in prerenal azotemia, and is unresponsive to volume expansion. Treatment of HRS syndrome is often unsuccessful and the mortality rate is high. Treatments with TIPS and arteriolar vasoconstrictors have been attempted, but have met with limited success. Liver transplant remains the only definitive therapy.

  I. Grading of liver disease. Originally designed to assess the surgical risk in patients undergoing surgery, Pugh's modification of Child's classification (Table 25-3) is also used to assess the course of patients with cirrhosis.

V. Drug-induced liver disease

  A. The liver is the central organ for the metabolism of most drugs. Drug excretion through the kidneys and the bile is made possible by transformation to more hydrophilic compounds (biotransformation). In most cases, hepatotoxicity is not caused by the originally administered drug, but by its metabolites.

  B. Hepatotoxicity has been classified into direct hepatotoxic reactions and idiosyncratic reactions.

    1. Direct hepatotoxins damage the liver in a dose-dependent fashion and characteristically produce hepatocyte necrosis in a particular region of the liver lobule.

2. **Idiosyncratic reactions** account for the majority of cases, are unpredictable, and occur even when the drugs are administered in the normal therapeutic range. The histology shows diffuse liver injury consisting of necrosis and/or cholestasis, and usually is associated with a significant inflammatory reaction. Rash, febrile reaction, eosinophilia, or a serum sickness syndrome may be present. In some instances, autoantibodies to cytochrome P-450 and other microsomal enzyme groups can be demonstrated.

3. This classification is blurred, however, because of considerable interindividual variation in susceptibility to direct hepatotoxins. Some idiosyncratic reactions seem to occur when a combination of host factors and/or environmental factors is present. Variables like enzyme polymorphism, interactions among drugs, age, and obesity influence the extent of both direct and idiosyncratic hepatotoxic reactions.

C. **Diagnosis** is based on a history of exposure to a certain drug (reactions usually occur within 90 days after first administration), but is especially difficult in the intensive care unit (ICU) setting, where patients are exposed to multiple drugs. Clinical and laboratory data are used to support the diagnosis. Other causes of liver dysfunction must be excluded.

D. **The differential diagnosis** of drug-induced liver disease includes viral hepatitis, worsening of chronic liver disease, biliary obstruction (e.g., tumor, gall stones, injury), postoperative liver dysfunction, sepsis, congestive heart failure, and pancreatitis.

E. Some drugs are associated with characteristic histologic lesions, whereas others may vary or show considerable overlap in their histologic presentation. Results of liver biopsies often are inconclusive. Table 25-4 lists some examples of drugs associated with liver disease. Virtually any drug, however, may injure the liver.

VI. **Total parenteral nutrition (TPN) and liver disease**

A. **Steatosis ("fatty liver").** Parenteral feeding may be associated with complications that affect the liver. Serum hepatic aminotransferases and bilirubin concentrations may increase progressively with increasing duration of TPN. The histopathologic correlate in adults usually is a fatty liver (i.e., macro- and microvesicular steatosis). It is usually asymptomatic and benign in character. Overfeeding (see Chapter 9) appears to be the most important factor contributing to the steatosis.

B. **Cholestasis.** Cholecystokinin (CCK), a hormone derived from the intestine, is released after stimulation by food. Total parenteral nutrition creates a fasting-like state for the gut and decreases CCK release. This diminishes gallbladder emptying and promotes biliary sludge formation. Acalculous and calculous forms of cholecystitis may be distinguished by ultrasonography.

Table 25-4. Classification of drug-induced hepatic disease

Type of Lesion	Examples	Comments
Acute viral hepatitis-like reaction	Diclofenac, halothane, isoflurane, isoniazid, methyldopa, phenytoin	Mortality rate much higher than that of viral hepatitis; histologic pattern of bridging necrosis in severe cases
Zonal necrosis	Acetaminophen, carbon tetrachloride	Dose dependent; negligible inflammatory response; lesions predominantly restricted to one lobular zone
Steatohepatitis, alcoholic hepatitis-like reaction	Amiodarone, perhexiline, nifedipine, valproic acid	
Steatohepatitis, microvesicular	Aspirin, tetracycline, zidovudine	
Cholestasis	Angiotensin-converting-enzyme inhibitors, carbamazepine, chlorpromazine, cimetidine, cotrimoxazole, dextropropoxyphene, erythromycin, estrogens, flucloxacillin, haloperidol, sulfonamides, tricyclic antidepressants	Histologically, inflammatory, noninflammatory, and forms with bile duct destruction can be recognized
Granulomatous hepatitis	Allopurinol, diltiazem, quinidine, phenytoin, procainamide, sulfonamides	Histiocytes and eosinophiles in the granulomas reflect a hypersensitivity reaction
Veno-occlusive disease	Chemotherapeutic drugs	Lesions are dose dependent
Chronic hepatitis	Amiodarone, aspirin, diclofenac, isoniazid, methyldopa, phenytoin, nitrofurantoin, trazodone	Occurs with continued exposure to a drug; in most cases, hepatitis resolves after discontinuation of the drug
Adenomas, hepatocellular carcinomas	Estrogens, anabolic hormones	

SELECTED REFERENCES
Caraceni P, Van Thiel DH. Acute liver failure. *Lancet* 1995;345:163–169.

Christenson E, Schlichting P, Fauerholdt L, et al. Prognostic value of Child-Turcotte criteria in medically treated cirrhosis. *Hepatology* 1984;4:430–435.

Kjaergard L, Lise L, Liu J, et al. Artificial and bioartificial support systems for acute and acute-on-chronic liver failure: a systematic review. *JAMA* 2003;289:217–222.

Lee WM. Drug-induced hepatotoxicity. *N Engl J Med* 2003;349:474–485.

McCormick PA. Improving prognosis in hepatorenal syndrome. *Gut* 2000;47:166–167.

Menon KVN, Kamath PS. Managing the complications of cirrhosis. *Mayo Clin Proc* 2000;75:501–509.

O'Grady JG, Alexander GJ, Hayllar KM, et al. Early indicators of prognosis in fulminant hepatic failure. *Gastroenterology* 1989;97:439–445.

Patzer JF. Advances in bioartificial liver assist devices. *Ann N Y Acad Sci* 2001;944:320–333.

Shellman R, Fulkerson W, DeLong E, et al. Prognosis of patients with cirrhosis and chronic liver disease admitted to the medical intensive care unit. *Crit Care Med* 1988;16:671–678.

Sherlock S, Dooley J. *Diseases of the liver and biliary system*, 10th ed. Oxford: Blackwell Science, 1997.

Gastrointestinal Disease

Patricia R. Bachiller and Jean Kwo

I. Patients may be admitted to the intensive care unit (ICU) because of **gastrointestinal (GI) diseases,** such as acute pancreatitis, or after GI surgery. In critically ill patients, the GI tract may be compromised by severe multiple organ system disease and may also result in dysfunction of other systems. GI pathology in the critically ill may pose a diagnostic and therapeutic challenge because the classic presentations seen in the otherwise healthy patient are less likely.

II. **GI bleeding**

   A. **Initial assessment and stabilization**

      1. Symptoms of **acute GI bleeding** include hematemesis, melena, hematochezia, and shock.

      2. **Initial assessment and stabilization** must be simultaneous and follow the principles of resuscitation. Patients at high risk for aspiration (e.g., with hematemesis and impaired level of consciousness) require intubation for airway protection. Large-bore intravenous (IV) access (at least two 16-gauge peripheral IVs) is needed for fluid replacement to ensure adequate perfusion.

         a. Investigate the patient's **history** for use of aspirin, nonsteroidal antiinflammatory drugs (NSAIDs), alcohol, or cigarettes. Other significant history includes prior GI bleeding, renal failure, coronary artery disease, peripheral vascular disease, and prior surgery. The **physical exam** must include vital signs, orthostatic heart rate (HR), and blood pressure (BP) measurements and a rapid search for signs of underlying GI or other major comorbid illness (e.g., stigmata of liver disease or heart murmurs).

         b. **Initial assessment** includes preparing for possible massive volume resuscitation and deciding on appropriate levels of invasive monitoring (e.g., arterial catheter, urinary catheter, central venous pressure monitor, cardiac output measurement). Blood should be cross-matched and transfused if needed. Hematocrit and coagulation studies are followed serially. Patients with the following markers have the highest mortality: age older than 60 years, HR greater than 100 beats per minute (bpm), systolic BP less than 100 mm Hg, major comorbidity, stigmata of ongoing or recent bleeding on endoscopy, bleeding due to upper GI malignancy, and secondary bleeding (i.e., in an already-hospitalized patient).

B. Diagnosis and localization

  1. The ligament of Treitz defines the boundary between **upper and lower GI hemorrhage.** Hematemesis (regurgitation of blood) indicates an upper GI source. Melena (dark blood per rectum) occurs when more than 50 to 100 ml of blood has remained in the GI tract long enough for bacterial degradation to occur and thus suggests an upper GI source. Hematochezia (red blood per rectum) is due to lower GI bleeding in 85% to 90% of cases. A nasogastric (NG) tube should be placed and gastric aspiration performed; coffee-ground material or blood confirms an upper GI source. A nonbloody NG aspirate is nonspecific and may be found in about 20% of patients with upper GI bleeding and half of patients with duodenal bleeding.

  2. **Localization of the source of GI bleeding**

     a. Upper GI bleeding

     (1) **Esophagogastroduodenoscopy (EGD)** is diagnostic in 90% to 95% of cases and allows for immediate therapy. It should be performed emergently for massive bleeding. Major complications of EGD occur in 0.5% of patients and include perforation, bleeding, aspiration, and more rarely death.

     (2) Two separate EGDs are recommended prior to proceeding with other diagnostic modalities, such as **angiography.**

        i. Successful angiographic detection requires ongoing bleeding of 0.5 to 1 ml/min (about 3 units of blood per day) and is useful from the distal esophagus to the colon.

        ii. Angiography may direct endoscopic or surgical treatment or it may be therapeutic via embolization or selective intraarterial vasopressin infusion.

        iii. Complications associated with angiography are rare and include contrast-induced nephrotoxicity and distal embolization of vessel wall plaque.

     b. Lower GI bleeding

     (1) **Colonoscopy** for lower GI bleeding is diagnostic in 72% to 86% of cases and is usually undertaken after a colonic purge, and thus requires up to 24 hours for patient preparation. EGD is often performed first to rule out an upper GI source. If bleeding is massive and precludes colonoscopy or if colonoscopy is nondiagnostic, the patient may require radionuclide imaging or angiography.

     (2) **Radionuclide imaging** may identify a general area of bleeding in preparation for therapy via endoscopy, angiography, or surgery. Technetium-99m sulfur colloid can detect 0.05 to 0.1 ml/min of bleeding but is only useful with constant bleeding because it is cleared by

the reticuloendothelial system within 10 minutes. Technetium-99m–labeled red blood cells (RBCs) detect 0.1 ml/min of bleeding and remain in the bloodstream for 24 hours, thus allowing multiple imaging sessions and making possible the detection of intermittent bleeding.

(3) **Angiography** is an important modality for obscure GI bleeding not localized by two EGDs or by colonoscopy. Its yield in lower GI bleeding is 40% to 92%.

(4) **Newer promising techniques** for detecting a bleeding source include helical computed tomography (CT) after intraarterial contrast injection, and magnetic resonance imaging (MRI) with intravascular contrast injection.

C. **Common causes of GI bleeding**
  1. **Upper GI bleeding**
    a. From 30% to 40% of patients with portal hypertension develop **variceal bleeding,** which may originate in the esophagus, stomach, or duodenum (see Chapter 25).

    (1) The **mortality** for one episode of variceal bleeding ranges from 10% to 70%, depending on liver disease severity, and the risk of rebleeding is 70% within 6 months.

    (2) **Complications** associated with acute variceal bleeding include aspiration of gastric contents, hepatic encephalopathy (due to increased protein and ammonia in the gut), infection, and renal failure.

    (3) Initial **management** of an acute bleed is as described previously (section **II.A.2**). Treatment with nonspecific **β-blockers** (propranolol or nadolol) and/or **nitrates** lowers the portal venous pressure gradient. Varices rarely bleed with a gradient of less than 12 mm Hg. These therapies have demonstrated a survival benefit in treated outpatients.

    (4) **Early endoscopy** is crucial as 30% to 50% of patients with known varices bleed from other upper GI sources. Endoscopic variceal band ligation and sclerotherapy control bleeding in 80% to 90% of cases. Band ligation is increasingly used because there is a 10% to 20% complication rate associated with sclerotherapy.

    (5) **Octreotide** (50-μg bolus plus 5-day infusion at 50 μg/h) or the combination of **vasopressin** (0.4 U/min) and **nitroglycerin** is recommended as a medical adjunct to endoscopy. Octreotide is a long-acting analogue of **somatostatin.** Octreotide and vasopressin are splanchnic vasoconstrictors that reduce portal pressure. Vasopressin has a 20% to 30% rate of systemic side effects such as

myocardial and cerebral ischemia. Its safety
is improved by administration with nitroglycerin. Once a patient with variceal bleeding is
hemodynamically stable, β-blockers and nitrates can be started.

(6) **Balloon tamponade** controls esophageal or
gastric variceal bleeding in 60% to 90% of
cases when endoscopy and medical therapy
fail (see Chapter 25). However, this is a temporary measure because most patients rebleed
on balloon deflation. Because of the risk of
pressure necrosis, deflation must occur within
24 to 48 hours. Esophageal rupture occurs
in 3% of the patients. Other major complications include aspiration, tracheal rupture,
tracheoesophageal fistula, and esophageal ulcerations.

(7) **Transjugular intrahepatic portosystemic shunting (TIPS)** controls refractory
variceal bleeding in up to 90% of cases by
reducing the portal pressure gradient to
less than 15 mm Hg. Using a transjugular
approach and radiographic guidance, a stent
is placed in the liver to connect a branch of the
portal vein with a hepatic vein. TIPS may be
complicated by shunt occlusion, accelerated
liver failure, and the development of hepatic
encephalopathy.

b. **Mallory-Weiss tears** are mucosal lacerations
within 2 cm of the gastroesophageal (GE) junction
that are likely due to increases in pressure occurring during vomiting. Most of these lesions stop
bleeding spontaneously and have a less than 10%
chance of rebleeding. However, actively bleeding
Mallory-Weiss tears are best addressed endoscopically. Addition of IV **vasopressin** can be effective
in refractory cases.

c. **Peptic ulcers,** found in the stomach or duodenum, cause 50% of upper GI bleeding with a mortality of 6% to 7%. A discussion of peptic ulcer
disease follows in section **VI.B.**

(1) **EGD** is the initial diagnostic and therapeutic
choice. The **endoscopic appearance** of an
ulcer has prognostic significance. Ulcers with
a spurting artery or a visible vessel have a
high rebleeding risk (50%–100%). Ulcers with
adherent clot or a red or black spot are at moderate risk, whereas ulcers with a clean base
are at low risk (<5%) for rebleeding.

(2) **Treatment** starts with prompt resuscitation.
From 75% to 80% of peptic ulcer bleeding resolves spontaneously. **Endoscopic therapy,**
with electrocautery, thermal coagulation,
and/or epinephrine injection, reduces the risk
of rebleeding to less than 10%. **Angiographic**

embolization is successful in stopping bleeding in 80% to 88% of peptic ulcers. Approximately 10% of patients require **surgery** to control the hemorrhage.

(3) Acid suppression with **histamine-2 (H₂) antagonists** and **proton-pump inhibitors (PPIs)** aids in ulcer healing and reduces rebleeding rates. PPIs show more consistent acid suppression than H₂ blockers.

(4) **Eradication of *Helicobacter pylori* (*H. pylori*) infection** decreases the rate of future rebleeding more than antisecretory therapy alone, although there is little role for *H. pylori* eradication in the acute setting.

d. **Stress ulceration,** also called stress-related erosive syndrome, erosive gastritis, or hemorrhagic gastritis, leads to upper GI bleeding in 1% to 7% of ICU patients.

(1) **Stress ulcers** are mucosal erosions typically found in the gastric fundus and body. Their pathogenesis is thought to involve mucosal hypoperfusion and increased gastric acidity occurring in critically ill patients.

(2) **EGD** is the modality of choice for initial evaluation and treatment. Angiography with selective embolization (often of the left gastric artery) achieves hemostasis in about 67% of cases. Surgery is reserved for severe refractory hemorrhage.

e. **Aortoenteric fistulas** are connections between the GI tract, most commonly the distal duodenum, and either the native aorta (primary) or an aortic vascular graft (secondary). Secondary fistulas are more common, occurring in 0.6% to 1.5% of patients after aortic reconstructive surgery. Patients often present with an initial "herald" bleed soon followed by massive hemorrhage.

(1) **Endoscopy, CT, and angiography** can be used to localize the fistula prior to surgery. A hemodynamically unstable patient requires fluid resuscitation and emergent exploratory laparotomy. Even with rapid intervention, mortality is approximately 60%.

f. **Dieulafoy's lesion** is an abnormally large artery protruding through the mucosa, most often into the gastric lumen (fundus or body). Bleeding can be massive and recurs in 15% of cases despite endoscopic therapy. Typically, surgical resection is performed once the patient is stabilized.

2. **Lower GI bleeding** (below the ligament of Treitz) accounts for 24% of GI bleeding and has a mortality of 2% to 4%.

a. **Mesenteric ischemia,** involving either the small bowel or the colon, can present with lower GI bleeding (see section **VIII.B**).

b. **Small-bowel bleeding** is suspected after two negative EGDs and a negative colonoscopy.

(1) **Angiodysplasia** is the most common cause of GI hemorrhage between the ligament of Treitz and the ileocecal valve. Other causes include tumors, inflammatory bowel disease, Meckel's diverticulum, NSAID-induced ulcers, and Dieulafoy's lesions.

(2) **Diagnosis** is difficult but may be made in about 50% to 70% of cases by push enteroscopy (which examines the jejunum) or wireless video capsule endoscopy. If the bleeding is brisk, radionuclide scans or angiography may be useful.

(3) **Treatment** of sources of bleeding within the small intestine is directed to the underlying disease.

c. Twenty percent of **colonic bleeding** is due to diverticula. Other common causes are hemorrhoids, ischemic colitis, and angiodysplasia.

(1) **Diverticular bleeding** is usually self-limited but can recur in 14% to 53% of patients. Colonoscopy or angiography can locate the site of bleeding and offer therapy. Endoscopic therapy may reduce the rebleeding rate from 50% to zero. Operative resection is indicated when bleeding and hemodynamic instability persist.

(2) **Colonic angiodysplasias** account for 20% to 30% of acute lower GI bleeding and are more frequent in patients older than the age of 60 years. Most lesions are found in the ascending colon, and most patients have multiple lesions. Colonoscopy or angiography is very successful for diagnosis and treatment, and surgery is reserved for failures of these modalities.

(3) **Colorectal neoplasms** can present with acute lower GI bleeding, though chronic or occult blood loss is more common. Colonoscopy may yield the diagnosis, whereas treatment involves surgical resection, chemotherapy, or radiation. Occult bleeding or iron-deficiency anemia in an elderly patient warrants a search for neoplasm.

(4) **Hemorrhoids** make up 2% to 9% of cases of severe acute hematochezia. Treatment is with sitz baths and fiber supplementation. Surgery is reserved for refractory cases.

(5) **Inflammatory bowel disease** (Crohn's disease or ulcerative colitis) may lead to bloody diarrhea or hematochezia. Colonoscopy usually reveals a diffuse mucosal inflammation. Medical therapy involves hydration, bowel rest, and steroids, and is best directed

by a gastroenterologist. Recurrent bleeding, which is not infrequent, may require surgery.

III. The GI tract as a source of infection

A. The acute abdomen may present insidiously in the critically ill patient. ICU patients are difficult to assess because the classic signs of an acute abdomen, tenderness and guarding, may not be apparent. Nonspecific findings such as fever, positive blood cultures, and hemodynamic instability may suggest intraabdominal infection but are not diagnostic. Consequently, one must maintain a high index of suspicion for occult abdominal infections. Some of the more frequent entities in ICU patients are acalculous cholecystitis, mesenteric ischemia, and any perforation or leakage. For discussion of specific infectious processes, see Chapter 28.

1. **Diagnostic evaluation**
    a. A good **history and physical exam** may provide clues, and serial abdominal exams may be invaluable. Directed laboratory testing (bilirubin, lactic acid, etc.) may be helpful. **Plain films** of the abdomen can support but not exclude a diagnosis of obstruction or perforation.
    b. **Ultrasonography** (US) evaluates the hepatobiliary system well. **Computed tomography** (CT) can localize and characterize abdominal masses (e.g., abscesses) and organs and also sensitively detects free intraperitoneal air. Both US and CT may guide percutaneous drainage of intraabdominal collections.
    c. **Laparoscopy** or **laparotomy** is an option for patients in whom intraabdominal pathology is strongly suspected but US and CT are negative or contraindicated. Unless there is relatively clear evidence of intraabdominal pathology requiring surgery, the high mortality of laparotomy in critically ill patients may outweigh the possible benefit of the operation.

B. Translocation of intestinal bacteria across the gut wall normally occurs constantly; intraluminal bacteria move through and between mucosal cells and migrate to the mesenteric lymph nodes. In critically ill patients, these bacteria may spread hematogenously and potentially lead to infection or sepsis. Patients whose GI mucosa is disrupted or more permeable (due to perforation, ischemia/hypoperfusion/shock, thermal injury, systemic infection from another source, or malnourishment) may have higher counts of translocating bacteria. In addition, bacteria may more easily reach the mesenteric lymph nodes and the bloodstream and cause systemic illness in patients with impaired immunity. Bacterial overgrowth or changes in the balance of gut flora caused by antibiotics, increased gastric pH, impaired gut motility, or total parenteral nutrition (TPN) may also increase bacterial translocation.

Although no single one of these factors will cause gut bacteria to systemically infect the host, many ICU patients manifest multiple risk factors.

C. **Aspiration** of gastrointestinal contents may lead to pneumonitis or pneumonia. Bacterial overgrowth and impaired intestinal or gastric motility increase the risk of clinically significant aspiration.

1. **Selective gut decontamination** refers to the use of enteral antibiotics to lower intraluminal bacterial counts and thereby bacterial translocation and aspiration. This technique has been shown to reduce the rate of nosocomial pneumonia in critically ill patients but has not been shown to affect mortality. Because of concerns about fostering resistant bacteria, selective gut decontamination is used only in certain situations, such as cirrhotics with GI bleeding or spontaneous bacterial peritonitis, patients with severe pancreatitis, and recipients of liver, intestine, or bone marrow transplants.

D. **Multiple organ dysfunction syndrome (MODS)** in the setting of sepsis, major trauma, head injury, or shock may be partly due to the response of the digestive tract to these insults. Intraluminal endotoxin translocates into the lymph and blood along with bacteria in patients with systemic infections or hemorrhagic shock. In response to such systemic insults, the GI tract releases cytokines that may have a role in acute lung injury as well as in increasing gut permeability (also see Chapter 11).

1. **Enteral nutrition** reduces septic morbidity in patients after major trauma, burns, and surgery. Immune-enhancing enteral nutrients, such as glutamine, arginine, and ω-3-fatty acids, may also reduce septic complications. Bulk-forming fibers, other nutrients such as immunoglobulin A (IgA), fish oil, and prostaglandin E analogues, and probiotics like *Lactobacillus* may be important adjuncts.

IV. **Impaired motility of the GI tract**

A. The term **paralytic ileus** refers to an alteration in GI motility that leads to failure of contents to pass. Ileus can affect the entire GI tract or a localized segment. For example, Ogilvie's syndrome is an isolated colonic ileus (acute colonic pseudo-obstruction).

1. The **pathophysiology** of ileus is thought to involve loss of synchronization of GI epithelial cells leading to chaotic activity without organized peristalsis. Bowel inflammation or dilation may exacerbate the lack of motility by increasing production of nitric oxide, which relaxes smooth muscle.

2. Ileus may be related to a number of **predisposing factors,** listed in Table 26-1. After an uncomplicated abdominal operation, small-bowel motility generally returns within 24 hours. Gastric motility follows within 48 hours and colonic motility returns in 3 to 5 days.

Table 26-1. Causes of ileus

Postoperative
  Especially following operations in the peritoneal cavity
Sepsis
Trauma
Sympathetic hyperactivity
Ascites
Electrolyte derangements
  Hypokalemia
  Hyponatremia
  Hypomagnesemia
  Hypermagnesemia
Drugs
  Catecholamines
  Calcium-channel blockers
  Narcotics
  Anticholinergics
  Phenothiazines
  β-blockers
Gastrointestinal ischemia
Retroperitoneal or intraperitoneal hemorrhage, infection, or
  inflammation
Bowel wall edema
  May occur secondary to massive fluid resuscitation

3. **Diagnosis** is clinical and radiologic. Abdominal radiographs typically show distension of the affected part of the GI tract with intraluminal air throughout. Patients may present with nausea/vomiting, abdominal distension, constipation, diarrhea, intolerance of enteral feeding, and diffuse abdominal discomfort. Rarely, radiographic contrast studies are needed to exclude mechanical obstruction.

4. **Complications** of ileus depend on which portion of the GI tract is involved. A severe ileus can lead to increased intraabdominal pressure, with characteristics of a compartment syndrome (see section **IX**). Gut paresis can lead to bacterial overgrowth, and reflux of bowel contents into the stomach can predispose to aspiration. Fluid sequestration due to intestinal wall inflammation increases bowel wall edema and pressure, compromising the gut's microcirculation. Colonic dilation can lead to ischemia, necrosis, and perforation. Patients with a cecal size greater than 12 cm are at higher risk for perforation, though perforations have been reported with smaller cecal diameters. Patients with chronic dilation may tolerate much larger diameters.

5. **Treatment** begins with **supportive care,** which consists of fluid and electrolyte repletion, and nasogastric drainage. Potential causes of ileus should be reviewed and corrected. If tolerated, fiber-containing

enteral diets or minimal enteral nutrition can promote GI motility. Medications such as metoclopramide, erythromycin, and neostigmine are of limited value. Other potentially helpful measures are mobilization of the patient, placement of a rectal tube, and rectal examination performed every 6 hours. Conservative treatment succeeds in 33% to 100% of cases in about 3 days.

   a. Neostigmine (2–2.5 mg IV given over 3 minutes) can successfully treat Olgivie's syndrome in about 80% of cases. Close monitoring for bradycardia is required.

   6. If conservative measures fail or if perforation appears imminent, **colonoscopic or operative decompression** is indicated.

B. GI hypermotility is seen in some cases of diarrhea secondary to inflammation or infection. Diarrhea is discussed in section **VIII.C.**

V. The esophagus

A. Esophageal perforation is most often iatrogenic, resulting from therapeutic endoscopy (e.g., sclerotherapy, dilation, stenting), NG tube placement, balloon tamponade of varices, endotracheal tube (ETT) placement, or transesophageal echocardiography. Other causes include Boerhaave's syndrome, trauma, pressure necrosis (from foreign bodies or pills), infections, and caustic ingestions. Perforation can occur in the cervical, thoracic, or abdominal esophagus, leading to cervical abscess, mediastinitis/pleuritis, and peritonitis, respectively.

   1. Diagnosis is based mainly on clinical and radiologic features. Patients may have pain, fever, emphysematous crepitus in the neck, mediastinal emphysema, and pleural effusions, often with high amylase content. Contrast studies and CT scans are used to confirm and localize esophageal perforations.

   2. Treatment should be urgent surgery (drainage, drainage and primary repair, or drainage with esophageal diversion or esophagectomy) in patients with sepsis or shock or with large, noncontained perforations because mortality increases when operation occurs after 24 hours. Nonoperative therapy is appropriate in patients with contained perforations, few symptoms, and no preexisting esophageal disease, and consists of broad-spectrum antibiotics (see Chapter 11), acid suppression with a PPI, percutaneous drainage of cervical or pleural collections, and parenteral nutrition.

B. Boerhaave's syndrome is the name for spontaneous esophageal perforation, which may have no obvious precipitant or may be related to retching/vomiting, blunt trauma, weight lifting, or childbirth. Predisposing factors include reflux esophagitis, esophageal infections, peptic ulcer disease, and alcoholism/heavy drinking. Common symptoms/signs are pain, vomiting, dyspnea, and shock. Radiographs often reveal pneumomediastinum and a left pleural effusion because most tears occur in the left distal esophagus. Diagnosis is often difficult and therefore delayed. Broad-spectrum antibiotics, TPN, and acid suppression are adjuncts to operative therapy.

C. **Ingestions** harmful to the esophagus include foreign bodies and caustic substances.

1. Ingested **foreign bodies,** most commonly food boluses, can present with dysphagia, odynophagia, chest pain, or airway obstruction. Blunt objects less than 2 cm in size traverse the GI tract uneventfully, whereas objects greater than 6 cm will obstruct within the duodenum, if not in the esophagus. Most objects that do not pass spontaneously may be removed endoscopically; this should be done relatively early due to the risk of perforation from pressure-induced necrosis of the esophageal wall.

2. **Acids** (pH <2) and **alkalis** (pH >12) cause severe burns when ingested. Acids are usually liquid and often spare the esophagus, passing into the stomach. Alkalis, such as drain cleaners, dishwasher detergents, and certain denture and household cleaners, tend to be solids and thus remain in the esophagus.

   a. **Caustic burns** are classified similarly to skin burns. Grade 2b burns (friable, bleeding, blistered, deeply or circumferentially ulcerated esophagus with damage extending through the mucosa, submucosa, and muscularis propria) and grade 3 burns (extensive necrosis that is completely transmural) develop esophageal strictures as late sequelae. Patients with grade 3b injuries have a 65% mortality.

   b. **Initial management** consists of basic **resuscitation.** The airway should be evaluated by direct laryngoscopy followed by preemptive intubation or tracheostomy if any edema is seen, depending on the severity of the injury. Fluid requirements may be high due to inflammation of the mediastinal tissues. Radiographs of chest and abdomen should be obtained to evaluate for evidence of perforation. There is no role for gastric lavage, induced emesis, milk, water, or activated charcoal.

   c. **Endoscopy** should be performed early unless a grade 3 burn is observed in the hypopharynx. Endoscopy is controversial between 24 hours and 3 days after the injury because mucosal sloughing, inflammation, and formation of granulation tissue are beginning and the wounded area is very soft. Between 5 and 15 days postinjury, endoscopy is contraindicated because collagen deposition may not yet have started. Spontaneous esophageal perforation should be suspected during the first 2 weeks if the patient's clinical condition deteriorates.

d. Patients with grade 1 and grade 2a injuries (i.e., no deep or circumferential ulcerations) may start oral intake immediately after endoscopy and are often discharged from the hospital within days. Patients with more severe injuries require ICU admission and nutritional support.

e. Patients should receive acid suppression therapy. Steroid therapy (**methylprednisolone** 40–60 mg/d) may reduce the rate of stricture formation in patients with severe burns. Patients on steroids should also receive prophylactic antibiotics.

VI. The stomach

A. **Stress ulceration** is mentioned in section **II.C.1.** and discussed fully in Chapter 12.

B. **Peptic ulcer disease** (PUD) refers to gastric and duodenal ulcers. Risk factors include *H. pylori* infection and NSAID/aspirin use. *H. pylori* eradication and addition of a **PPI** or **misoprostol** (a synthetic prostaglandin) to NSAID therapy can decrease the risk of an ulcer complication.

1. The **diagnosis** of active *H. pylori* infection is most reliably made with the urea breath test or the stool antigen test. Both may be used for retesting (after 4–8 weeks) to confirm eradication. In patients undergoing endoscopy, biopsies can be used for urease testing or histology to diagnose *H. pylori* infection. However, the false-negative rate rises in patients with active or recent bleeding and in patients on PPIs or antibiotics.

2. **Treatment** of *H. pylori* is indicated in most patients based on its association with peptic ulcers, gastric carcinoma, and gastric lymphoma. Recommended first-line treatments are the triple therapies found in Table 26-2. The success rates of these regimens are greater than 80%.

3. **Complications** of PUD include upper GI bleeding, perforation, and, less commonly, obstruction. Therapy for bleeding ulcers is discussed in section **II.C.1.c.** Perforation and obstruction require surgery; urgency and modality (laparoscopic or open) are determined by the patient's clinical status.

VII. The pancreas and biliary tract

A. **Acute pancreatitis**

1. The most common **etiologies** of acute pancreatitis are gallstones and alcohol use. Other causes include post-endoscopic retrograde cholangiopancreatography (ERCP), hypertriglyceridemia, hypercalcemia, ischemia, various viruses, medications (such as azathioprine, didanosine, furosemide, hydrochlorothiazide, estrogens, sulfonamides, tetracyclines, and valproic acid), and idiopathic (10% of cases).

Table 26-2. First-line regimens for eradication of *Helicobacter pylori* infection

Choose one of the following:	AND	Choose two of the following:
PPI (omeprazole 20 mg bid, lansoprazole 30 mg bid, pantoprazole 40 mg bid, rabeprazole 20 mg qd, or esomeprazole 20 mg bid)		Clarithromycin 500 mg bid or tid (regimens are somewhat more effective when clarithromycin is included)
Ranitidine-bismuth-citrate 400 mg bid		Metronidazole 500 mg bid
		Amoxicillin 1 g bid

Or use the following regimen:

A bismuth salt bid to qid (such as bismuth subsalicylate 525 mg or bismuth subcitrate 240 mg) with or without a PPI	AND	Metronidazole 500 mg tid and tetracycline 500 mg qid
		OR
		Furazolidone 100 mg qid and amoxicillin 500 mg tid

bid, twice a day; tid, three times a day; qd, daily; PPI, proton-pump inhibitor.

2. The **pathogenesis** of acute pancreatitis is not fully understood, but early in the disease, pancreatic enzymes, such as trypsin, are prematurely activated. Trypsin activates other enzymes, leading to autodigestion and pancreatic necrosis as well as activation of complement and the coagulation cascade. Other mediators of inflammation and vasodilation are also released. Local and systemic consequences may include peripancreatic necrosis, fat necrosis, capillary leak leading to third spacing of intravascular fluid, shock, respiratory failure/acute respiratory distress syndrome (ARDS), and renal failure.
3. The **diagnosis** is made clinically and with laboratory tests. Patients usually present with severe, constant, poorly localized epigastric and/or back pain as well as nausea/vomiting. The **differential diagnosis** includes acute cholecystitis, hepatitis, cholangitis, perforated ulcer, inferior myocardial infarction, bowel obstruction, ischemic bowel, ruptured ectopic pregnancy, leaking abdominal aortic aneurysm (AAA), and sickle cell crisis.
   a. Simultaneous determination of **amylase and lipase** has a 90% to 95% sensitivity and specificity for making the diagnosis of acute pancreatitis. The serum lipase level is more specific because lipase, for the most part, originates from the pancreas.
   b. **Dynamic CT scanning** with oral and IV contrast is useful in diagnosing acute pancreatitis, determining its severity, and delineating areas of

Table 26-3. Ranson's criteria for determining the severity of pancreatitis

At admission or diagnosis
  Age >55 years
  White blood cell count >16,000/mm^3
  Blood glucose >200 mg/dl
  Serum lactate dehydrogenase (LDH) >350 U/L
  Serum glutamic oxaloacetic transaminase (SGOT) >250 U/dl
During initial 48 hours
  Hematocrit decrease of >10%
  Blood urea nitrogen (BUN) increase of >5 mg/dl
  Serum calcium <8 mg/dl
  Arterial partial pressure of oxygen (PaO$_2$) <60 mm Hg
  Base deficit >4 mEq/L
  Estimated fluid sequestration >6 L

pancreatic necrosis. If the diagnosis is not in doubt, CT scanning is most helpful when performed 1 to 3 days after admission rather than immediately on presentation.

4. **Prognosis**

   a. In most cases of acute pancreatitis, the clinical course is mild and easily treated with fluid replacement, analgesia, and bowel rest. About 10% to 25% of patients develop severe pancreatitis and require intensive care. The overall mortality of pancreatitis is 5% to 10%.

   b. Tools for assessing prognosis include the CT severity index, the Acute Physiology and Chronic Health Evaluation (APACHE) II system, the Glasgow criteria, and **Ranson's criteria** (Table 26-3). Ranson's first five criteria assess the severity of the acute inflammatory process, whereas the criteria measured at 48 hours determine the systemic effects of circulating enzymes and toxins. Mortality is less than 1% in patients with two or fewer, 16% in patients with three or four, and greater than 40% in patients with five or more of Ranson's criteria. Failure of more than one organ system within 3 days of presentation also predicts a high mortality risk.

5. **Clinical course and treatment**

   a. The **initial phase** of acute pancreatitis usually lasts about 1 week and is characterized by a sterile systemic inflammatory response that can lead to **multiple organ system dysfunction.** Commonly involved systems include pulmonary, renal, cardiovascular, central nervous, and coagulation. Within the first 2 days, 60% of patients experience arterial hypoxemia and acute lung injury; 20% of patients develop ARDS. Renal failure afflicts 20% of patients.

(1) **Initial treatment** of acute pancreatitis is largely supportive. Aggressive **fluid resuscitation,** supplemental oxygen, mechanical ventilation, inotropic support, parenteral analgesia, and treatment of specific complications may be needed to reduce the risk of early death. Invasive monitoring beyond an arterial and a urinary catheter may be required. Central venous or pulmonary artery pressures as well as cardiac output can be essential for guiding management, especially in the setting of hypotension and fluid resuscitation with ongoing renal or respiratory failure.

(2) **Nasogastric drainage** is indicated if acute pancreatitis is associated with ileus. **Nutritional support** is crucial. If tolerated, enteral feeding is preferable (see section **III.D.1** and Chapter 9) and may be delivered via a nasojejunal tube. Otherwise, TPN or a combination of both types of nutrition should be used.

(3) Early **ERCP** reduces complications in patients with evidence of a bile duct stone and may be considered in patients with gallstone pancreatitis.

(4) Early treatment with **prophylactic antibiotics** active against enteric organisms is aimed toward preventing infection of pancreatic necrosis. Suggested regimens include 1 to 2 weeks of cefuroxime, imipenem plus cilastatin, or ofloxacin plus metronidazole because of good penetration into pancreatic tissue. The decision regarding the use of prophylactic antibiotics must balance the risks to the patient of inducing resistant bacteria, possibly promoting fungal infection, and antibiotic side effects with the risks of sepsis and infection of pancreatic necrosis.

(5) **Selective gut decontamination** of gram-negative bacteria using oral and rectal antibiotics may reduce morbidity in patients with severe acute pancreatitis.

(6) **Future therapies** for the systemic response to acute pancreatitis may include **lexipafant,** a platelet-activating factor antagonist that may reduce mortality in severe acute pancreatitis.

b. The **second phase** of severe acute pancreatitis is characterized by local pancreatic and intraabdominal complications in addition to multiple organ system failure. The most common of these is pancreatic necrosis. Other complications include fistulas between the pancreatic duct and other structures, pancreatic ascites (distinguished by high amylase content), acute fluid collections, pseudocysts, and pancreatic abscesses.

(1) Pancreatic necrosis occurs in 10% to 20% of patients and has a mortality of 15% to 20%.

   i. The **extent** of pancreatic necrosis should be monitored by periodic CT scans because greater than 50% necrosis in conjunction with clinical deterioration may require surgical necrosectomy. Patients with sterile pancreatic necrosis should be managed conservatively given the high mortality rate (up to 43%) of necrosectomy. Patients with pancreatic necrosis who do not improve clinically should undergo CT-guided fine-needle aspiration of necrotic tissue for Gram stain and culture to detect infection.

   ii. Infected necrosis, with a mortality risk of 20% to 50%, develops after 2 to 3 weeks in 30% to 35% of patients with pancreatic necrosis. Infected pancreatic necrosis should be surgically debrided and treated with broad-spectrum antibiotics with good pancreatic tissue penetration, such as imipenems or fluoroquinolones. The role of antibiotic prophylaxis is controversial (see section **VII.A.5.a.**).

c. Long-term complications

  (1) Rarely, **hemorrhage** may occur due to vessel erosion in the retroperitoneum or peritoneum during acute pancreatitis. More commonly, hemorrhage is associated with a pseudoaneurysm or with erosion into a vessel by a pseudocyst.

  (2) Pseudocysts are encapsulated fluid collections that form 4 to 6 weeks after an episode of acute pancreatitis.

    i. Complications associated with pseudocysts include hemorrhage due to erosion of adjacent vessels, compression of intraabdominal structures, sudden ascites due to rupture, and infection.

    ii. Radiology-guided drainage is indicated for symptomatic pseudocysts as well as those that are greater than 6 cm in size and fail to shrink after 6 weeks.

  (3) Pseudoaneurysms occur most commonly in the splenic artery and have a 75% bleeding rate. These may rupture into a pseudocyst, leading to bleeding from the pancreatic duct (hemosuccus pancreaticus). Pseudoaneurysmal hemorrhage leads to near-certain mortality without quick, aggressive intervention, typically via angiography.

(4) **Splenic venous thrombosis** occurs due to chronic peripancreatic inflammation. Splenic-portal venous obstruction can cause portal hypertension and lead to acute variceal bleeding, and is usually treated with splenectomy. Rarely, thrombosis of the mesenteric vessels, leading to visceral ischemia, also can occur.

B. **Acute cholecystitis** is discussed in Chapter 28. About 20% of patients with acute cholecystitis undergo emergency cholecystectomy due to peritonitis, perforation, or other complications. Patients who have other underlying conditions that make surgery a high risk may be treated with ultrasound-guided percutaneous cholecystostomy.

C. **Acute acalculous cholecystitis** (AAC)

Critically ill patients with trauma, sepsis, burns, and acute renal failure are at risk of developing AAC. Other risk factors include TPN, surgery, atherosclerosis and other vascular disease, and immunosuppression. The mortality rate ranges from 10% to 50%.

1. The **pathogenesis** of AAC is multifactorial and appears related to chemical and ischemic injury to the gallbladder. Risk factors in critically ill patients include stagnant bile due to gallbladder paresis, hypotensive episodes, and/or vascular disease. Pathology specimens reveal an occluded and impaired gallbladder microcirculation, possibly due to inflammation or inappropriate activation of coagulation.

2. **Diagnosis** requires a high index of suspicion because fever may be the only symptom. Other symptoms/signs can include sepsis, right upper quadrant or epigastric pain, nausea/vomiting, and new intolerance of enteral feeding. Laboratory findings may be limited to leukocytosis. Ultrasound and CT are used to confirm the diagnosis.

   a. **Ultrasound** can be performed at the bedside. Findings include gallbladder wall thickness greater than 3.5 mm, gallbladder distension greater than 5 cm, sludge or gas in the gallbladder, pericholecystic fluid, mucosal sloughing, and intramural gas or edema.

   b. **CT** is equal or superior to ultrasound in the diagnosis of AAC. It may also aid in the differential diagnosis by identifying other intraabdominal processes.

3. **Treatment** involves cholecystectomy if the patient can tolerate surgery or ultrasound-guided percutaneous cholecystostomy for drainage. Percutaneous cholecystostomy is successful in 63% to 94% of cases and may be left in place for 6 to 8 weeks. Antibiotic therapy should be directed toward organisms cultured from the gallbladder aspirate, positive in 50% of cases.

D. Cholangitis is an infection of the biliary tract and gall-bladder (see Chapter 28). Patients may present with Charcot's triad of fever, right upper quadrant pain, and jaundice, often aggravated by hypotension and altered mental status. **Treatment** is with antibiotics. Patients who do not respond to antibiotics have nearly 100% mortality without either surgical decompression or ERCP.

VIII. The intestines

A. **Obstruction** results in symptoms and complications similar to those described for ileus in section **IV.A.** Supine and upright abdominal radiographs or abdominal CT confirm the diagnosis.

1. **Small-bowel obstruction** (SBO) is most often due to adhesions. Other causes include hernias, foreign bodies, and tumors.

   a. Patients with partial SBO often respond to conservative therapy, which consists of fluid and electrolyte repletion and nasogastric drainage. Complete SBO should be managed surgically due to high risk for bowel ischemia, necrosis, and perforation.

2. **Large-bowel obstruction** (LBO) is most commonly due to malignancy and thus can develop slowly. Other causes include sigmoid or cecal volvulus, diverticular strictures, and fecal impaction.

   a. **Treatment** is as for SBO (section **VIII.A.1.a**). Sigmoid volvulus may respond to decompression via contrast enema or colonoscopy.

B. **Intestinal ischemia** may be acute or chronic and may affect the small or large intestine. Acute ischemia is more common in patients with risk factors for embolic or thrombotic phenomena (e.g., patients with atherosclerotic disease, dysrhythmias, congestive heart failure, and hypercoagulable states). Chronic mesenteric (affecting the small bowel) or colonic ischemia is typically due to atherosclerotic disease and presents with postprandial pain or chronic colitis.

1. **Acute mesenteric ischemia**

   a. This entity typically presents with severe abdominal pain out of proportion to physical exam findings. Other signs include sudden intolerance of enteral feeding, fever, fecal occult blood, abdominal distension, and altered mental status.

   b. **Leukocytosis** and **metabolic acidemia** are common early laboratory abnormalities, whereas elevated **lactate** and amylase levels are late findings.

   c. **Abdominal radiographs** and **CT** can exclude other pathology. **Angiography** is diagnostic and may be therapeutic. Duplex ultrasound can be used to assess superior mesenteric artery (SMA) flow.

   d. The goal of **general treatment measures** is to reverse ischemia and avoid progression to infarction and necrosis, which can lead to sepsis, myocardial depression, and death. These measures consist of aggressive volume resuscitation, correction of hypotension, nasogastric drainage, avoidance of vasoconstrictive medications, use of broad-spectrum antibiotics, and use of supplemental oxygen. Anticoagulation may be indicated.

   (1) Patients with peritoneal signs or radiographic evidence of necrosis or perforation should undergo immediate **laparotomy** for resection of clearly necrotic areas. Areas of questionable viability are left in place until a reexploration 12 to 24 hours later.

   e. SMA emboli cause 50% of acute mesenteric ischemia and lead to vasoconstriction of surrounding unobstructed arteries. Treatment is with intraarterial **papaverine** infusion (30–60 mg/h) via the angiography catheter. Angiography is repeated every 24 hours (for up to 5 days) to look for a response. If patients with SMA emboli require laparotomy, embolectomy is performed prior to evaluating bowel viability.

   f. SMA thrombi generally occur acutely in patients with chronic mesenteric ischemia due to atherosclerosis. Presence of acute SMA thrombi is treated with intraarterial **papaverine** as well as urgent surgical **revascularization** (thrombectomy or bypass). Intravascular stents are a newer but unproven option.

   g. Nonocclusive mesenteric ischemia results from mesenteric arterial vasospasm and accounts for 20% to 30% of episodes of acute mesenteric ischemia. Mesenteric vasoconstriction is precipitated by hypoperfusion and can persist after the hypoperfusion has resolved. Thus, nonocclusive mesenteric ischemia can manifest hours to days later. Treatment is with intraarterial **papaverine** infusion with daily repeat angiography to confirm response to therapy. Laparotomy is reserved for patients with peritoneal signs.

   h. About 5% to 10% of cases of acute mesenteric ischemia are due to **mesenteric venous thrombosis,** which is best diagnosed by CT. Treatment is with **anticoagulation** (heparin followed by warfarin). Laparotomy is indicated only in cases of suspected gut infarction.

2. Colon ischemia (also called **ischemic colitis**) is most commonly due to thrombosis of an atherosclerotic vessel. Other causes include vasculitis, hypercoagulable states, vasospasm, hypoperfusion, or ligation of the inferior mesenteric artery (IMA) during aortic surgery. IMA ligation injures mainly the left colon, whereas low-flow states predominantly affect watershed areas such as the right colon, splenic flexure, and retrosigmoid junction.

    a. The **diagnosis** of ischemic colitis is suspected in patients with sudden onset of mild left lower quadrant crampy pain, often associated with mild lower GI bleeding, diarrhea, abdominal distension, and nausea/vomiting. Other signs and symptoms include fever, leukocytosis, and mild abdominal tenderness to palpation. The diagnosis is confirmed by colonoscopy or barium enema.

    b. Most cases resolve within days to weeks with **supportive care:** fluid resuscitation, broad-spectrum antibiotics, and colonic decompression with a rectal tube. Indications for surgery include peritonitis, colonic perforation, and clinical deterioration despite adequate medical therapy.

C. Diarrhea occurs when fluid absorption from the GI tract does not match fluid intake into the gut lumen.

    1. Under normal conditions, 9 to 10 L of fluid enters the bowel each day from oral intake and intestinal secretions. The majority of this is absorbed in the small bowel, leaving the remaining 1 to 1.5 L to be absorbed in the proximal half of the colon, with about 100 ml lost daily in stool.

    2. Water is absorbed secondary to osmotic flow as well as active and passive transport of sodium. Changes in GI motility and epithelial mucosal integrity can drastically affect fluid absorption.

    3. Common **etiologies** of diarrhea in the critically ill patient include infections, enteral nutrition, and medications. Ischemic colitis is a concern in **postoperative vascular** patients. Less common causes include fecal impaction, Ogilvie's syndrome, inflammatory bowel disease exacerbation, intestinal fistula, pancreatic insufficiency, sepsis, and hypoalbuminemia.

        a. Infectious diarrhea in the ICU setting is caused most commonly by *Clostridium (C.) difficile* overgrowth in patients treated with antibiotics (see Chapter 28).

            (1) Clinical presentation varies from asymptomatic to fulminant colitis to toxic megacolon.

            (2) Because the sensitivity of the toxin assay for *C. difficile* is greater than 90%, testing one to two stool samples is adequate for diagnosis. Colonoscopy is another option for diagnosis. Treatment is with oral **metronidazole;** surgery is rarely required. Diarrhea in critically ill patients is rarely due to other bacterial and viral infections. Stool cultures and ova and parasite examinations are of low yield after the first 2 days of hospitalization.

        b. Medications implicated in diarrhea are listed in Table 26-4.

        c. Enteral nutrition as a cause of diarrhea is a diagnosis of exclusion. Osmotic diarrhea is

Table 26-4. Medications associated with diarrhea

Antibiotics (particularly erythromycin, ampicillin, clindamycin, tetracycline, cephalosporins)
Magnesium-containing antacids, magnesium or phosphorus supplements
Proton-pump inhibitors, cimetidine
Metoclopramide
Colchicine
Digitalis, theophylline, levothyroxine
Nonsteroidal antiinflammatory drugs
Misoprostol
β-blockers
Cholinergic agents
Chemotherapeutic agents
Immunosuppressants (tacrolimus, cyclosporine, azathioprine)
Antiretroviral medications
Additives such as sorbitol or lactose

secondary to malabsorption of nutrients and usually stops with fasting. Overall nutritional deprivation, manifested as hypoalbuminemia, also plays a significant role in causing malabsorption.

(1) An **osmolar gap** of greater than 70 mOsm suggests an osmotic diarrhea. The osmolar gap is the difference between the measured stool osmolarity and the predicted osmolarity, which is $2 \times ([Na^+] + [K^+])$, based on serum electrolyte measurements.

(2) Treatment of enteral nutrition–related diarrhea involves slowing the rate of feeding, diluting the tube feeds, or temporarily stopping enteral nutrition. Enteral nutrition should be lactose-free. In some patients, peptide-based diets, fiber-rich diets, or elemental diets with reduced fat and residue may be helpful.

d. Fecal impaction can paradoxically lead to diarrhea as a result of decreased fecal tone, mucus secretion, and impaired anorectal sensation.

Table 26-5. Palliative agents used to treat diarrhea

Diphenoxylate with atropine (Lomotil)	A constipating meperidine congener; it is extensively metabolized to the active metabolite difenoxine
Loperamide (Imodium)	Inhibits peristalsis and slows intestinal activity.
Bismuth subsalicylate (Pepto-Bismol)	Has antisecretory, antimicrobial, and antiinflammatory effects
Deodorized or camphorated opium tincture	Antimotility agent

Table 26-6. Causes of constipation

Medications
Narcotics
Anticholinergics
Aluminum hydroxide antacids
Calcium-channel blockers
Iron, barium
Serotonin type 3 (5-HT$_3$) receptor antagonists

Endocrine
Hypothyroidism
Hypercalcemia
Panhypopituitarism
Pheochromocytoma
Glucagonoma
Diabetes
Pregnancy

Neurologic
Cerebral vascular accident
Parkinson's disease
Alzheimer's disease
Spinal cord disease/autonomic neuropathy
Hirschsprung's disease

Systemic
Scleroderma
Amyloidosis
Uremia

Functional
Immobilization
Low-fiber diet
Low fluid intake

---

  e. An **altered enterohepatic circulation,** leading to increased bile acid in the colon, can induce
  net fluid secretion. This is seen in diseases of the
  ileum, fatty acid malabsorption, and altered bowel
  flora.
  4. Management of diarrhea consists of replacement
  of lost fluids and electrolytes and treatment of the
  underlying cause.
  5. Once an infectious etiology is excluded, diarrhea
  can be treated symptomatically with several agents
  (Table 26-5).
  D. Constipation. Many disease states and medications
  can produce constipation. A careful review of the history
  and medications should be undertaken (Table 26-6).
  Treatment is aimed at correcting the underlying disease
  (Table 26-7). Fiber supplementation and various laxatives can be administered once the etiology is identified.
IX. Abdominal compartment syndrome
  A. Abdominal compartment syndrome occurs
  when increased intraabdominal pressure leads to

Table 26-7. **Agents for treating constipation**

Bulk producing	Methylcellulose Psyllium Polycarbophyl	Holds water in stool; most physiologic
Irritant/stimulant	Bisacodyl Senna Cascara Phenolphthalein Casanthranol Castor oil	Direct action on the intestinal mucosa, stimulates motility and secretion
Lubricant	Mineral oil	Retards colonic absorption of fecal water and softens stool
Surfactants	Docusate	Detergent activity, softens stool
Saline based	Magnesium sulfate Magnesium hydroxide Magnesium citrate Sodium phosphate Sodium biphosphate enema	Attracts and retains water in intestinal lumen
Hyperosmolar	Lactulose Glycerin suppository Sorbitol	Osmotically active molecules draw water into the colon

cardiovascular, pulmonary, and renal dysfunction as well as reduced perfusion to intraabdominal organs and to the brain (see Chapter 33).

B. Etiologies include intraabdominal hemorrhage, surgical packing of the abdomen, major abdominal surgery, major burns, massive fluid resuscitation with resultant bowel edema, rapidly accumulating ascites, and ileus or bowel obstruction.

C. Treatment is initially supportive with maintenance of intravascular volume, inotropic support, and mechanical ventilation. Urgent decompressive laparotomy is indicated if there is evidence of organ dysfunction.

SELECTED REFERENCES

Bounds BC, Friedman LS. Lower gastrointestinal bleeding. *Gastroenterol Clin North Am* 2003;32:1107–1125.

Burns BJ, Brandt LJ. Intestinal ischemia. *Gastroenterol Clin North Am* 2003;32:1127–1143.

Huggins RM, Scates AC, Latour JK. Intravenous proton-pump inhibitors versus H$_2$-antagonists for treatment of GI bleeding. *Ann Phamacother* 2003;37:433–437.

Kupfer Y, Cappell MS, Tessler S. Acute gastrointestinal bleeding in the intensive care unit. *Gastroenterol Clin North Am* 2000;29:275–307.

Law NM, Freeman ML. Emergency complications of acute and chronic pancreatitis. *Gastroenterol Clin North Am* 2003;32:1169–1194.

Madl C, Druml W. Systemic consequences of ileus. *Best Pract Res Clin Gastroenterol* 2003;17:445–456.

Proctor DD. Critical issues in digestive diseases. *Clin Chest Med* 2003;24:623–632.

Ranson JH, Rifkind KM, Roses DF, et al. Prognostic signs and the role of operative management in acute pancreatitis. *Surg Gynecol Obstet* 1974;139:69–81.

Villatoro E, Larvin M, Bassi C. Antibiotic therapy for prophylaxis against infection of pancreatic necrosis in acute pancreatitis. In: *Cochrane database of systematic reviews, No. 2,* 2005. Accession number 00075320-100000000-01976.

Endocrine Disorders

Theresa S. Chang, Robert A. Peterfreund, and
Stephanie L. Lee

Endocrine disorders are common comorbid conditions complicating the management of critically ill patients in the intensive care unit (ICU). Early recognition of these conditions facilitates ICU management and the recovery of patients.

I. Diabetes mellitus

Diabetes mellitus (DM) is commonly encountered in the ICU either as the admitting condition or, more commonly, as a comorbid condition complicating critical illness. Recent studies show that **tight glucose control reduces mortality in patients with ICU stays of greater than 5 days.** The greatest reduction of mortality in such cases is secondary to a decline in multiple-organ failure with a proven septic focus. In addition, a reduction in complications including bacteremia, acute renal failure, transfusion requirements, and critical illness polyneuropathy is observed.

A. Physiology.
DM is a chronic systemic disease caused by the lack of insulin action, ultimately resulting in hyperglycemia. Elevated glucose levels normally stimulate the secretion of insulin from pancreatic β-cells. Catecholamines inhibit insulin secretion. Insulin facilitates glucose and potassium transport across cell membranes, enhances glycogen synthesis in the liver, and, in muscle, inhibits lipolysis and increases glucose utilization (glycolysis).

1. **Type 1 DM.** Autoimmune destruction of pancreatic β-cells causes absolute insulin deficiency in type 1 DM. Typically, patients are diagnosed with type 1 DM as a child or an adolescent, but as many as one-third of patients are diagnosed after the age of 20 years. Patients are susceptible to **diabetic ketoacidosis (DKA),** but not obesity. Therapy is with human insulin. **Insulin is absolutely required even during fasting to prevent DKA.**

2. **Type 2 DM** results from a combination of peripheral resistance to insulin and relative insulin deficiency. Patients are classically older, obese, and ketosis resistant. They are often asymptomatic; thus as many as one-third of individuals with the disease are undiagnosed. Type 2 DM is frequently part of a metabolic syndrome known as "syndrome X," "insulin resistance syndrome," or "metabolic syndrome," which is characterized by the clustering of risk factors for coronary heart disease including

hyperinsulinemia (or impaired glucose tolerance), central obesity, hypertension, and atherosclerosis. **Hyperinsulinemia** results in increased free fatty acids and a higher production of hepatic glucose. Resistance to insulin-stimulated glucose uptake causes hyperglycemia. Outpatient management is typically with diet changes, exercise, oral hypoglycemics, insulin sensitizers, or insulin. ICU management is typically with insulin. Practitioners must consider the pharmacologic properties of oral hypoglycemics to appropriately transition patients from oral agents to insulin therapy (Table 27-1).

3. **Other causes** of insulin insufficiency include cystic fibrosis, chronic pancreatitis, hemochromatosis, adverse effects of pentamidine, and pancreatic resection. Glucagonoma, pheochromocytoma, acromegaly, hyperthyroidism, and glucocorticoid excess increase insulin resistance, which may result in hyperglycemia.

B. **Diagnosis.** An outpatient diagnosis of diabetes mellitus requires two independent measurements fulfilling at least one of the following criteria:

1. Casual plasma glucose greater than 200 mg/dl with symptoms of diabetes (polyuria, polydipsia).
2. A fasting plasma glucose level of 126 mg/dl or greater.
3. Plasma glucose of 200 mg/dl or greater 2 hours after an oral glucose load.

Formal criteria for making a new diagnosis of DM in ICU patients are not established. Hyperglycemia in the ICU (casual plasma glucose levels ≥140 mg/dl) necessitates treatment. An elevated hemoglobin A1c level (>6%), which estimates glucose control over the previous 2 to 3 months, is consistent with, but not diagnostic for, DM.

C. **Acute complications**

1. **DKA** occurs almost exclusively in type 1 diabetics. Ketoacidosis results from absolute insulin deficiency or insulin resistance seen during stress (e.g., infection, surgery, myocardial infarction, or trauma). Ultimately, the triad of **hyperglycemia, ketosis,** and **acidosis** is seen. **Insulin** must be administered to correct the metabolic abnormalities. Criteria for the diagnosis of DKA are shown in Table 27-2.

a. Consequences of DKA

i. **Circulatory depression.** Acidosis and metabolic derangements depress myocardial contractility and peripheral vascular tone. Preexisting coronary artery disease (CAD), cardiomyopathy, or peripheral vascular disease (PVD) can contribute to hemodynamic instability. Hyperglycemia (and concurrent hyperosmolarity) produces an osmotic diuresis leading to profound hypovolemia.

ii. **Electrolyte and metabolic abnormalities** include **hyperglycemia** (although glucose is

Table 27-1. Oral agents used in type 2 diabetes mellitus

Agent	Mechanism of Action	Major Side Effects	Time to Onset (hours)	Duration of Action (hrs)
Glyburide, Glimepiride, Glipizide, Repaglinide, Nateglinide Tolbutamide Chlorpropamide	Increase insulin secretion	Hypoglycemia	1 ≤0.25 1 1	10–24, 6–12 3–4 6–12 24–48
Pramlintide	Synergistic with insulin to reduce post prandial hypoglycemia	Hypoglycemia, nausea, gastroparesis	<0.3	3–4
Exentide	Increased insulin secretion and inhibits glucagon secretion	Hypoglycemia when used with sulfonylurea but not metformin	≤0.5	8–12
Rosiglitazone, Pioglitazone	Decrease insulin resistance	Peripheral edema, anemia, potential hepatotoxicity	1	24
Metformin (Glucophage) Glucophage XR	Decreases hepatic glucose output	Lactic acidosis, diarrhea	Days Days	8–12 24
Acarbose, Miglitol	Decrease gastrointestinal glucose absorption	Malabsorption, diarrhea	Immediate	<0.3

**Table 27-2. Criteria for the diagnosis
of diabetic ketoacidosis (DKA) and
hyperosmolar nonketotic coma (HONK)**

Laboratory Parameter	DKA	HONK	Mixed
Serum glucose (mg/dl)	>300	>600	>600
Serum bicarbonate (mEq/L)	<15	≥15	<15
Serum osmolarity (mOsm/L)	≤320	>320	>320
pH	<7.3	≥7.3	
Urinary ketones	>3+	+	+
Serum ketones	+	+	+

+Ketones may be present.

usually <500 mg/dl), intracellular **dehydration, hyperkalemia,** and **hyponatremia.**
Serum potassium concentration is normal or elevated because acidosis drives potassium out of cells even though total body potassium content is actually depressed (3–10 mEq/kg body weight). Measured sodium concentrations are artificially lowered approximately 1.6 mEq/L for every 100 mg/dl that the glucose is elevated. Hypophosphatemia and hypomagnesemia commonly result from urinary losses.

2. **Hyperosmolar nonketotic coma (HONK),** also called "hyperglycemic hyperosmolar syndrome," is a clinical syndrome seen in type 2 DM with physiologic decompensation leading to **hyperglycemia, hyperosmolarity,** and **dehydration** (up to 10- to 12-L deficit). Severe ketosis is not seen, but a mild ketosis and acidemia may occur as a result of starvation or poor perfusion (Table 27-2). The precipitating factors for HONK are similar to those of DKA (Table 27-3). The classic presentation of patients with HONK includes fatigue, blurred vision, polydipsia, polyuria, leg cramps, and weight loss. The laboratory findings in HONK are related to dehydration and hypovolemia. These derangements include abnormal serum electrolytes and elevation in hemoglobin, hematocrit, protein, calcium, amylase, lactate dehydrogenase, transaminases, and creatine phosphokinase levels.

D. **Chronic complications**

1. **Atherosclerosis.** Diabetes mellitus is a strong risk factor for vascular disease, which tends to occur more extensively and at an earlier age than in the general population. Microvascular disease (retinopathy and nephropathy) and macrovascular disease (CAD, PVD, and cerebrovascular disease) have an increased prevalence among diabetics. In the United States, DM is the most common cause of blindness, renal

Table 27-3. Precipitating factors for hyperosmolar nonketotic coma (HONK)

Inciting Events	Pharmacologic Agents
Infection (pneumonia, urinary tract infection, sepsis)	Amphetamines
	Niacin
Noncompliance with insulin regimen or oral hypoglycemic agents	β-Blockers
	Pentamidine
First presentation of diabetes mellitus	β-Agonists
	Protease inhibitors
Dehydration	Diuretics
	Salicylates
Impaired renal function	Glucocorticoids
	Sympathomimetics

failure leading to dialysis, and vascular insufficiency necessitating amputation.

2. **Neuropathy.** Peripheral sensory neuropathies can cause pain and numbness. Central ventilatory responses to hypoxia can be diminished and sensitivity to central nervous system (CNS) depressants can be increased. Autonomic neuropathy is common with postural hypotension, gastroparesis, and bladder atony. A feature of diabetic autonomic neuropathy is symptomatically silent cardiac ischemia. Diabetics have an increased risk of sudden cardiac death caused by autonomic cardiac dysfunction.

3. **Infection** and **poor wound healing** are major complications.

E. **Treatment of hyperglycemia.** Insulin resistance and hyperglycemia are frequent in critically ill patients, even those who do not carry a diagnosis of DM. Recent evidence suggests that a close control of the blood sugar (BS) level of medical/surgical ICU patients is associated with improved outcomes.

1. General principles of management of hyperglycemia in the ICU are as follows:

a. **Blood glucose monitoring**

i. During intravenous (IV) insulin infusion: Check every 2 hours (1 hour or less following insulin dose adjustment).

ii. With regular insulin subcutaneously (SQ): Check 4 hours post administration.

iii. NPH insulin SQ: Check 6 to 8 hours post administration.

b. **Medical management.** Unreliable absorption of SQ or intramuscular (IM) insulin occurs in the setting of tissue edema, hypothermia, hemodynamic instability, and vasopressor therapy. A **continuous IV infusion of regular insulin** in such circumstances is the best choice. The pharmacologic profiles (Tables 27-1 and 27-4) of previously

Table 27-4. Insulin preparations (subcutaneous administration) for therapy of diabetes mellitus

Preparation	Time to Onset (h)	Time of Peak (h)	Duration of Action (h)
Lispro (Humalog)	≤0.25	1	3.5–4.5
Novolog insulin (Aspart)	≤0.25	1	3.5–4.5
Regular	0.5–1	1–5	5–8
Semilente	0.5–3	2–10	12–16
NPH	1–4	4–12	24–28
Lente	1–3	6–15	22–28
Protamine zinc	1–6	14–24	≥36
Ultralente	2–8	10–30	≥36
Glargine (Lantus)	2–4	Peakless	18–24+

Note: When regular insulin is administered IV, the onset of action is immediate and the duration of action is ~1 hour.

administered oral hypoglycemic agents and other insulin preparations must be considered when transitioning patients to IV insulin. Consider the time to **onset, peak,** and **duration of action** of the drugs. All oral agents should be discontinued in a critical care setting because of the risk for drug interactions and drug-specific side effects (Table 27-1). Metformin in particular must be stopped in all critically ill patients because of the risk of lactic acidosis in low-perfusion states and reduced renal function. Patients can be transitioned back to oral medications after leaving the ICU.

c. **Signs and symptoms of hypoglycemia** include evidence of elevated sympathetic outflow (tachycardia, tremulousness, palpitations, diaphoresis) along with headache, seizures, or a depressed level of consciousness ranging from confusion to coma. These may be masked by other features of the critically ill patient's condition. Patients with chronically tight blood sugar control often lose the sympathetic response to hypoglycemia, a condition known as hypoglycemic unawareness.

d. **Guidelines for the continuous infusion of IV insulin** are shown in Table 27-5.

2. **Management of DKA**

a. **Fluids:** Repletion of intravascular volume restores tissue perfusion, improves glomerular filtration, and helps to reverse insulin resistance. Give normal saline (NS) initially to stabilize hemodynamics and urine production, and then switch to one-half NS infusion. Give 5% dextrose in NS when plasma glucose decreases to below 250 mg/dl to prevent hypoglycemia while maintaining insulin infusion.

Table 27-5. Intravenous insulin standard orders in the surgical intensive care unit at the Massachusetts General Hospital

ALL PATIENTS RECEIVING INTRAVENOUS INSULIN MUST HAVE A SOURCE OF DEXTROSE[a]

Goal blood sugar (BS) concentration: 110–140 mg/dl

Monitoring standard
BS every 2 h during "stable-dose" insulin infusion
BS every 1 h during "changing-dose" insulin infusion

Administer bolus to patient with regular insulin prior to starting infusion:
BS: 141–190 $\Rightarrow$ 1 unit
191–240 $\Rightarrow$ 2 units
241–290 $\Rightarrow$ 3 units
291–340 $\Rightarrow$ 4 units
>340 discuss with MD

Infuse 0–15 units of regular insulin in normal saline per hour

Titration of insulin
Start infusion at 0.5–1.5 units/h; when increasing the dose, bolus with the amount of the increase; e.g., to increase rate by 2 units, first bolus the patient with 2 units; in brittle patients, consider increasing or decreasing by 0.5 unit

Hypoglycemia prevention and management
1. For BS = 90, stop insulin infusion, and recheck BS every 30 min × 2
2. For BS = 70, stop insulin infusion, and administer $1/2$ amp of 50% dextrose (D50); recheck BS every 30 min × 2; then, every hour × 2
3. For BS = 50, stop insulin infusion, and administer 1 amp of D50; recheck BS every 20 min × 3; then every 30 min × 2; then every hour × 1

Patients with type 1 diabetes mellitus have a lower insulin requirement than those with type 2 diabetes mellitus. In addition, type 1 diabetics should have insulin delivered without interruption. The guidelines assume that the patient is not in diabetic ketoacidosis. BS = blood sugar.
[a]The administration of exogenous glucose can be waived by the attending physician on an "ad-hoc" basis.

    b. Insulin administration is crucial in DKA because endogenous insulin is absent. First administer a bolus with regular insulin (0.1 U/kg IV or 10 U IV) and then start a continuous infusion of 0.5 to 1.0 U/h. Monitor BS levels every hour after adjusting the insulin infusions. Measure electrolytes every 2 hours.

    c. Electrolytes. Potassium and phosphate are essential for insulin action and should be replaced carefully. Some of the potassium may be given as potassium phosphate and/or potassium acetate to avoid excess chloride levels. Potassium levels require close monitoring and treatment because they will drop with hydration and correction of acidemia. Verify normal kidney function and urine output before treatment:

  i. Serum potassium less than 3 mEq/L: Give K^+, 40 mEq/h.

  ii. Serum potassium less than 4 mEq/L: Give K^+, 30 mEq/h.

  iii. Serum potassium less than 5 mEq/L: Give K^+, 20 mEq/h.

  iv. Serum potassium greater than 5 mEq/L: No replacement necessary.

  d. **Bicarbonate.** Consider for only severe acidosis (i.e., pH <7.0), hemodynamic instability, or in cases of cardiac rhythm disturbances. Following the administration of bicarbonate, arterial pH levels should be monitored every 2 hours.

3. **Management of HONK**

  a. **Fluids.** Fluid administration is crucial. To determine fluid administration rates, first consider the patient's volume status, total body water deficit (see also Chapter 7), serum osmolarity, age, and renal and cardiac function. If the initial serum osmolarity is less than 320 mOsm/kg, give 2 to 3 L of NS. If the patient is hypotensive and not able to tolerate aggressive fluid administration, colloids or vasopressors may be used. Invasive hemodynamic monitoring may help to guide therapy. Give 5% dextrose in the IV fluid once the plasma glucose falls to less than 250 mg/dl.

  b. **Insulin.** Administer a bolus with regular insulin and begin a low-dose continuous IV insulin infusion. If no decrease of glucose levels occurs over the first 2 to 4 hours, increase the insulin infusion rate every hour until a response occurs (see also the guidelines in Table 27-5). HONK patients with DM type 2 are highly insulin resistant and require high doses of insulin.

  c. **Potassium chloride** is usually administered as part of a fluid regimen (see section **I.E.2.c**).

  d. **Bicarbonate** is not given unless lactic acidosis causes the pH to drop to less than 7.0.

  e. **Heparin.** Thromboses/embolic events are common complications of HONK, and prophylaxis should be administered. If thrombosis occurs, a full dose of **heparin** or low-molecular-weight heparin anticoagulation is indicated.

II. Thyroid disease

Like most other endocrine disorders, thyroid disease is usually not the reason for admission into the intensive care unit, but changes in thyroid function do commonly occur in ICU patients.

  A. **Physiology:** Thyroid hormones alter the speed of cellular biochemical reactions, total body oxygen consumption, and heat production. Thyrotropin-releasing hormone (TRH) from the hypothalamus stimulates the secretion of **thyroid-stimulating hormone (TSH)** from the anterior pituitary. TSH controls iodine uptake by the thyroid gland and iodine incorporation into tyrosine residues of thyroglobulin (organification). The hormones **L-thyroxine (T4)** and **triiodothyronine (T3)** are formed and stored in the thyroid gland. A low basal level of thyroid hormone secretion is enhanced by TSH and inhibited by thyroid hormone. Circulating thyroid hormone also exerts negative feedback on the hypothalamus and pituitary to control TRH and TSH release. Both forms of thyroid hormone are extensively (>99%) bound to plasma proteins. Only the free (unbound) thyroid hormone is biologically active. Peripheral tissues convert T4 to T3, which is 50 to 100 times more potent than T4 but has a shorter half-life.

B. **Evaluation/labs:** A careful history and physical examination are essential and should correlate with thyroid function tests. The most useful initial thyroid function test (TFT) in the ambulatory population is the **serum TSH.** However, confounding factors that may depress TSH levels include starvation, glucocorticoids, dopamine, infection and inflammation, and fever. Amiodarone and iodinated radiocontrast agents can also affect thyroid physiology. TSH in critical illness may not accurately reflect thyroid function; free T4 and T3 levels help to establish the diagnosis. The profile of tests results from different thyroid conditions is outlined in Table 27-6. *Note that normal values for thyroid function tests vary among institutions. Local normal values must be used for reference and diagnosis.*

C. **Hyperthyroidism**

   1. Causes:

      a. Graves' disease.

      b. Toxic multinodular goiter.

      c. Subacute thyroiditis (acute phase).

Table 27-6. Laboratory tests of thyroid function

Condition	Total T4	Free T4	T3	FTI[a]	THBR[b]	TSH
Hyperthyroidism	↑	↑	↑[c]	↑	↑	↓
Hypothyroidism 1°	↓	↓	↓[d]	↓	↓	↑
Hypothyroidism 2°	↓	↓	↓[d]	↓	↓	↓/inappropriately Nl
Euthyroid sick						
Mild	Nl to low	Nl	↓	Nl to low	Nl	Nl to low
Severe	↓	Nl to low	↓	↓	Nl[e]	↓
Pregnancy	↑	Nl	↑	Nl to high	↓	Nl[f]

T4, thyroxine; THBR, thyroid hormone binding ratio (similar to T3 uptake); TSH, thyroid stimulating hormone; ↑, increased; ↓, decreased; Nl, normal

[a] Free Tyroxine Index, $T_4 \times THBR$

[b] also T_3RU, T_3U

[c] 5% of patients have only elevated T_3, not T_4

[d] T3 may be maintained in near normal range until severe hypothyrodism

[e] If plasma protein normal.

[f] 13% have transiently low TSH and normal free T_4 at the end of the first trimester.

Table 27-7. Clinical features of thyroid disease

Symptoms	Signs
Hyperthyroidism/thyrotoxicosis	
Nervousness	Motor hyperkinesis
Fatigue	Tachycardia or atrial fibrillation
Weakness	Systolic hypertension
Increased perspiration	Warm, moist skin
Irregular menses	Tremor
Palpitations	Proximal muscle weakness
Increased appetite	Eyelid retraction
Weight loss despite increased appetite	Lid lag, stare
	Elevated liver function tests
Frequent bowel movements/ diarrhea	Decreased cholesterol
	Exophthalmos (Graves' disease only)
Hypothyroidism	
Fatigue	Slow movement
Sleepiness	Slow speech
Depression	Hoarseness
Cold intolerance	Bradycardia
Weight gain	Dry, sallow skin
Constipation	Periorbital edema
Irregular menses with menorrhagia	Nonpitting edema (myxedema)
	Delayed relaxation of deep tendon reflexes
Paresthesias	Enlarged tongue
Carpal tunnel syndrome	Hypertension (especially diastolic)
	Low-voltage electrocardiogram
	Elevated cholesterol
	Elevated creatine phosphokinase
	Enlarged cardiac silhouette on radiography

  d. Toxic adenoma.
  e. Iatrogenic overdosing of thyroid hormone.
  2. Clinical features of hyperthyroidism:
    a. Hyperthyroidism is a hypermetabolic state. Table 27-7 gives a comprehensive list of classic signs and symptoms.
    b. Thyroid storm. In the ICU, decompensated hyperthyroidism, otherwise known as thyroid storm, is life threatening.
      i. Symptoms. Thyroid storm is a state of thyrotoxicosis with physiologic decompensation. It presents with fever out of proportion for infection, dehydration (from fever, vomiting, diaphoresis, or diarrhea), atrial tachydysrhythmias, hypotension often resistant to pharmacotherapy, and alterations in mental status that range from confusion and agitation to psychosis, stupor, and coma. If it is unrecognized, progression to cardiovascular collapse and death occurs in 40% to 50% of

patients. There are no significant differences in thyroid function studies between those with thyroid storm and those with severe hyperthyroidism. Thyroid storm may mimic malignant hyperthermia, neuroleptic malignant syndrome, sepsis, hemorrhage, or drug/transfusion reactions.

ii. **Precipitating factors.** Most patients have a history of partially treated hyperthyroidism or have had symptoms some time before the presentation. Surgical stress can precipitate thyroid storm manifesting 6 to 18 hours postoperatively. Thyroid storm most commonly occurs following infection. Other predisposing factors include myocardial infarction, stroke, parturition, radioiodine therapy, iodinated contrast materials, DKA, and withdrawal or discontinuation of antithyroid medications.

iii. **Pathogenesis.** The mechanisms producing thyroid storm are unclear. Proposed causes include the effects of acidosis or medical illness on thyroid-hormone binding to carrier proteins allowing elevations in free, bioactive, T4 levels.

3. **Treatment**
   a. Chronic thyroid hormone excess is treated with specific antithyroid drugs (**propylthiouracil [PTU]**, **methimazole**). Thyroid hormone levels may not begin to normalize for 2 to 6 weeks. The most serious side effects of antithyroid agents are hepatitis and agranulocytosis. Ablation of the gland can be accomplished with surgery or radioactive iodine therapy.
   b. **Thyroid storm.** The first line of treatment for thyroid storm is cardiovascular resuscitation with volume. Administer dextrose 5% (D5) NS or NS until blood pressure and urine output stabilize, and then switch to D5 half NS. β-Blockers are then used to control tachycardia. Suggestions for additional medical management are listed in Table 27-8.

4. **Special considerations**
   a. **Sympathetic stimulation** can complicate the management of the thyrotoxic patient. If anesthesia is required, thyrotoxic patients may benefit from the sympathectomy produced by regional techniques, particularly neuraxial blockade.
   b. **Hypotension.** Thyroid hormone excess leads to systemic vasodilation and hypotension. Treatment is with direct-acting vasoconstrictors. Fluid resuscitation is important in the patient rendered volume depleted by excessive perspiration and diarrhea.
   c. **Heart failure** Thyrotoxicosis may precipitate heart failure in patients (particularly the

Table 27-8. Treatment of decompensated hyperthyroidism (thyroid storm)

Therapy for controlling thyroid hormones synthesis and release
Thionamides (propylthiouracil, methimazole)
Iodinated medications (iopanoic acid, stable potassium iodide, Lugol's solution)—Graves' disease only
Lithium carbonate

Therapy for blocking conversion of thyroxine to triiodothyronine
Propylthiouracil
Iopanoic acid
Propranolol
Corticosteroids

Therapy for enhancing clearance of thyroid hormones
Gastrointestinal clearance
   Cholestyramine
Blood clearance
   Hemoperfusion
   Plasmapheresis

Therapy for blocking the effects of thyroid hormones
Beta-blockers to control heart rate
Corticosteroids

Supportive measures
Antipyretics (acetaminophen)
Cooling
Meperidine (blocks shivering induced by cooling)
Correction of dehydration
Nutrition
Oxygen
Treatment of congestive heart failure

Therapy for the precipitating illness

---

elderly) with underlying heart disease (ischemia or valvular lesions) who are unable to tolerate tachycardia and thyroid hormone–induced increases in contractility. Such patients may benefit from β-adrenergic blockade. In patients without heart disease, alterations in ventricular contractility with diastolic dysfunction are attributed to sustained elevations in heart rate, as are commonly seen in long-standing thyrotoxicosis. Cardiac function will not normalize until after the treatment of thyrotoxicosis. Patients also can suffer from volume overload with "high-output" failure in the setting of high filling pressures and decreased diastolic filling time. These patients may benefit from diuretics.

d. **Enhanced drug metabolism** is a feature of thyrotoxicosis; one should anticipate high sedative and analgesic requirements. Dose requirements for anticoagulants are decreased because of a reduction in coagulation factor levels.

e. **Myasthenia gravis** may be seen in some Graves' disease patients (30 times increased incidence), so neuromuscular blocking agents should be titrated carefully.

D. Hypothyroidism

1. **Causes:** In adults, Hashimoto's thyroiditis is the most common cause of hypothyroidism. It is associated with other autoimmune processes, including systemic lupus erythematosus (SLE), rheumatoid arthritis, primary adrenal insufficiency, pernicious anemia, type 1 DM, and Sjogren's syndrome. Thyroid ablation (surgery, radioiodine) or radiation therapy can cause hypothyroidism. Iodine deficiency, drug therapy (lithium, amiodarone with thyroiditis), and late-phase subacute thyroiditis also may be causative. Reduced thyroid hormone synthesis can also be congenital. Clinically significant hypothyroidism is unlikely immediately after thyroid surgery because the half-life of T4 is 7 to 10 days. A significant reduction in measured T4 levels is not evident until 3 to 7 days postoperatively.

2. **Clinical features.** Hypothyroidism is a hypometabolic state. Table 27-7 lists symptoms and signs of hypothyroidism.

   a. **Myxedema coma.** Patients with myxedema coma are often seen in the winter when the thermoregulatory stress on the body reaches its peak. Patients typically are older and with known hypothyroidism. Key symptoms include hypothermia and altered mental status. It is associated with hyporesponsiveness to CO_2, congestive heart failure (CHF), and exaggerated signs and symptoms of severe hypothyroidism. Surgery, drugs, trauma, and infection can precipitate this decompensated state. It is a disease characterized by profound hypothyroidism with physiologic decompensation. The term is a misnomer because patients do not always have the features of myxedema nor are they comatose.

   b. **Sick euthyroid state.** This is a condition characterized by central suppression of the thyroid axis. It is also known as nonthyroidal illness syndrome. Lowering tissue energy requirements may be a physiologic adaptation to systemic illness. In such cases, patients have abnormal TFTs in association with various stressors or illnesses. Most patients fit into one of the three following categories: (a) low T3, (b) low T3 and low T4, and (c) low T3, low T4, and low TSH (Table 27-9).

3. **Laboratory diagnosis** is usually based on **TSH** measurements. In the ICU, high-dose glucocorticoid therapy, high-dose dopamine infusions, or severe nonthyroidal illness will blunt the TSH elevation

Table 27-9. Characteristics of euthyroid sick syndrome

Category	Frequency in Hospitalized Patients (%)	Cause	Other Thyroid Function Tests	Prognosis
Low T3	70	$\downarrow$ Extrathyroid conversion of T4 to T3, $\uparrow_r$ t$_3$ production	Within normal limits; possible increased T4	Decrease of T3 proportional to severity of illness
Low T3, T4	50	$\downarrow$ TH production, thyroxine-binding globulin deficiency, TH-binding inhibitors, altered TH metabolism	Within normal limits	Deficit proportional to illness severity

T3, triiodothyronine; T4, thyroxine; TH, thyroid hormone; TSH, thyroid-stimulating hormone; $\downarrow$ = decreased.

Table 27-10. Therapy of myxedema coma

Thyroid hormone	T3 25 micrograms IV every 12 hours T4 load of 300–500 micrograms then 50–75 micrograms/day (up to 2/3–3/4 daily oral dose). If no response switch to T3.
Hypothermia	Gradual rewarming with blankets, increased room temperature (watch for hypotension after vasodilation from warming)
Hypoventilation	Intubation, mechanical ventilation if necessary with warm air; eval w/ ABGs/Xrays
Metabolic disturbances	Hyponatremia: fluid restriction (<1000 ml/day); If Sodium+<120 mEq/L, slow administration of isotonic or hypertonic NaCl
Hypotension	Rule out depressed cardiac function, presence of pericardial effusions, adrenal insufficiency; Echocardiogram can be obtained to assess for effusion vs. hypokinesis. Fluids and vasopressors as necessary knowing the potential for fluid overload, CHF or arrythmias
Glucocorticoid administration	Hydrocortisone 100 mg IV every 6–8 hours × one-two days until symptomatic improvement and adequate HPA axis evaluation.

IV, intravenous; T3, triiodothyronine; T4, thyroxine.

in the hypothyroid patient. Therefore, the degree of TSH elevation may not directly reflect the magnitude of thyroid hormone deficiency. Additional TFTs (free T4, total T4, T3 resin uptake or thyroid-hormone binding ratio, free thyroxine index, total T3) will help to identify the condition. The diagnosis of Hashimoto's autoimmune thyroiditis is confirmed with measurement of antithyroperoxidase antibodies. Myxedema coma patients have an elevated TSH with low levels of free T4 and T3.

4. **Treatment.** Chronic treatment is with exogenous oral supplementation thyroid hormone. Thyroxine requires 7 to 10 days to have an effect. Oral T3 begins to have an effect in 6 hours. Cautious IV thyroid hormone loading will hasten recovery and is indicated for myxedema coma (see Table 27-10). The agent of choice is **T3.** The adult loading dose is 25 to 50 μg; this should be reduced to 10 to 20 μg in cases of known or suspected cardiac disease. The typical T3 requirement is approximately 65 μg /d, administered in divided doses every 4 to 6 hours based on clinical responses. For patients on oral T4 replacement requiring long-term IV thyroid hormone, the convention is to administer T4 daily, starting with 50% of the usual oral dose. TSH levels should be checked after 7 days and the T4 dose adjusted to keep the TSH levels in the normal range. Patients with hypothyroidism are treated with thyroid

hormone replacement. Should myxedema coma arise, further supportive measures are necessary.

a. In patients with nonthyroidal illness, no evidence exists supporting T3 or T4 administration.

b. Hypothermia. Patients with myxedema coma have significant peripheral vasoconstriction. Gradual rewarming is indicated. If rewarming is too rapid, vasodilation may cause hypotension, an increase in oxygen consumption, and eventual cardiovascular collapse. Ultimately, normal body temperature is achieved with the administration of thyroid hormone and passive warming (blankets).

c. Hypoventilation. Patients with myxedema coma often hypoventilate, leading to hypercapnia and hypoxia, ultimately causing a change in mental status secondary to the CO_2 narcosis. Most patients have slow progressive improvement in their mental status within 48 to 72 hours after initiation of thyroid hormone therapy.

d. Hyponatremia and **hypoglycemia.** In most cases of myxedema coma, the hyponatremia from reduced free water renal excretion is usually not severe enough to necessitate aggressive sodium replacement. With thyroid hormone replacement and mild fluid restriction, hyponatremia usually resolves. Severe hyponatremia may cause seizures or mental status changes.

e. Hypotension. Cardiac symptoms typically resolve months after the initiation of thyroid replacement.

f. Glucocorticoid administration. Even if hypoadrenalism is not suspected, the administration of glucocorticoids is advocated because of the potential for panhypopituitarism or autoimmune Addison's disease to coexist with autoimmune hypothyroidism.

g. Potential airway problems include an enlarged tongue, relaxed oropharyngeal tissues, and poor gastric emptying.

III. Calcium metabolism and parathyroid disease

    A. Physiology (see also Chapter 7). Calcium metabolism is governed by the interaction of two hormones, **parathyroid hormone (PTH)** and **vitamin D.** PTH stimulates osteoclastic activity in bone, causing the release of calcium into the extracellular fluid. In the kidney, PTH causes the hydroxylation of vitamin D into its active form and increases **calcium reabsorption** and **phosphorus excretion** at the distal tubule. Vitamin D works primarily to increase calcium absorption in the small intestine. Calcium is crucial for coagulation, muscle contraction, neurotransmission, hormone secretion, and hormone action. Plasma calcium is ionized (60%) or complexed (40%) with protein (mainly albumin) or organic ions. Ionized calcium is the biologically active entity. Acidosis increases and alkalosis decreases ionized calcium because of alterations in albumin binding. Hypoalbuminemia decreases the total serum calcium concentration by approximately 0.8 mg/dl for each gram per deciliter of albumin below the normal value of 4.0 g/dl. Although ionized calcium levels are technically easy to measure, improper sample handling can lead to nonreproducible measurements.

B. Hypercalcemia (see also Chapter 7)

1. **Causes.** This condition occurs when calcium intake from the intestine or bone exceeds renal clearance. Malignant hypercalcemia is caused by the release of a PTH-like molecule (PTH-related protein) from tumors (lung, breast, gut, urinary tract), cytokine-mediated or direct bone destruction resulting in resorption of calcium from the skeleton, or excess production of 1-α-vitamin D hydroxylase, which activates vitamin D. Hyperparathyroidism usually is caused by a parathyroid adenoma. It is characterized by hypercalcemia, hypophosphatemia, and elevated PTH levels. Four-gland parathyroid hyperplasia is found in about 10% of hyperparathyroidism cases. Parathyroid hyperplasia can be associated with medullary thyroid carcinoma and pheochromocytoma in multiple endocrine neoplasia type II as well as secondary hyperparathyroidism of chronic renal failure. Parathyroid cancer is a rare cause of hyperparathyroidism and hypercalcemia.

2. **Clinical features.** Symptoms of hypercalcemia are variable and may depend on the patient's age, comorbid conditions, the duration of the hypercalcemia, and the rapidity of progression (Table 27-11) Hypercalcemia is considered an emergency when the total calcium level is greater than 15 mg/dl.

3. **Medical management** (Table 27-12; also see Chapter 7). Initial management focuses on promoting

Table 27-11.   Hypercalcemia: signs and symptoms

Gastrointestinal	**Osteopenia/osteoporosis**
• Nausea/vomiting	**Weakness/atrophy/fatigability**
• Anorexia	**Central nervous system**
• Constipation	• Seizures
• Pancreatitis	• Disorientation/psychosis
• Peptic ulcers	• Memory loss
Hemodynamic	• Sedation/lethargy/coma
• Dehydration	**Renal**
• Hypertension	• Polyuria
• Electrocardiogram/	• Nephrolithiasis
conduction changes	• Oliguric failure (late)
• Digitalis sensitivity	
• Dysrhythmias	
• Catechol resistance	

Table 27-12. Medical management of symptomatic and/or severe hypercalcemia

Mode of Action	Measure/Substance	Indication	Side Effects/Complications
Intravenous hydration	Isotonic saline administration at 200–300 ml/h (4–6 L/d)	Universal	Volume expansion, hypokalemia, hypomagnesemia
Loop diuretic	Furosemide 20–40 mg, up to 500 mg/d or continuous infusion of 10 mg/h	Universal	Hypokalemia, hypomagnesemia
Bisphosphonates	Pamidronate 60–90 mg IV every 2–4 weeks	Universal if unresponsive to saline diuresis	Fast administration: renal insufficiency, occasional feverish reactions
Calcitonin	200–500 IU/d SQ	Universal (adjuvant)	Nausea, vomiting, escape phenomenon
Steroids	Prednisone 40–100 mg/d	Vitamin D intoxication, sarcoidosis	Iatrogenic Cushing's syndrome
Hemodialysis	Ca-free dialysate	Hypercalcemic crisis and renal insufficiency	Dialysis related
Diet low in calcium and vitamin D	<100 mg Ca/d	Universal	None

IV, intravenous; SQ, subcutaneous.

renal calcium excretion. Treatment of moderate hypercalcemia (calcium >1–2.5 mg/dL above the upper limit of normal) depends on the presence of symptoms, but acute severe hypercalcemia (calcium >2.5 mg/dL above the upper limit of normal) warrants treatment regardless of symptoms. The initial treatment is aggressive intravenous hydration with isotonic saline because most patients are severely volume depleted. Normal saline administered at a rapid rate (2–4 L/h) helps to reverse intravascular volume contraction and promote calciuria. Loop diuretics inhibit reabsorption of calcium at the loop of Henle. Thiazide diuretics should be avoided because they increase calcium absorption at the distal tubule. Renal failure patients intolerant of large-volume resuscitation should be dialyzed with a low-calcium dialysate. **Calcitonin** acts within 24 to 48 hours to lower serum calcium concentrations and is more effective when used in combination with steroids. Bisphosphonates (e.g., **pamidronate**) act by binding to hydroxyapatite in bone and inhibit osteoclastic activity for 2 to 4 weeks. Maximal decrease in calcium concentration occurs between 4 and 7 days and lasts about 2 weeks.

4. **Surgical management.** If the hypercalcemia is secondary to the presence of a parathyroid adenoma or carcinoma, the abnormal gland must be removed. If circulating PTH levels fall by more than 50% 10 minutes after the removal of the adenoma, successful resection has occurred. PTH hyperplasia is surgically treated by removing all abnormal glands with auto transplant of half of one gland into the forearm. Alternatively, a subtotal parathyroidectomy (removal of three and one-half glands) is undertaken.

5. **Critical care considerations**
   a. Hypercalcemia has an unpredictable effect on **neuromuscular blockade.** Hence, neuromuscular blocking agents should be carefully titrated.
   b. Careful **positioning** of the patient in the ICU is required because hypercalcemic patients may have significant osteoporosis.
   c. **After parathyroidectomy,** patients may have transient or permanent hypocalcemia requiring calcium and vitamin D supplementation. The onset of hypocalcemia usually is within a few hours of surgery, but may not occur until a few days postoperatively.
   d. **Volume resuscitation.** Hypercalcemia causes polyuria and volume depletion. Volume status should be corrected with NS.

C. **Hypocalcemia** (see also Chapter 7)
   1. **Causes** (Table 27-13). Total serum calcium levels are decreased in up to 70% to 90% of ICU patients. From 15% to 50% of patients meet criteria for true hypocalcemia. Acute hypocalcemia has been correlated with

Table 27-13. Causes of hypocalcemia

Hypoparathyroidism	**Critical illness**
• Primary	• Alkalosis
• Surgical	• Burns
• Autoimmune	• Toxic shock
• Hypomagnesemia	• Pancreatitis
• Resistance	• Fat embolism
(pseudohypoparathyroidism)	**Anticonvulsant therapy**
• Hemosiderosis	**Hypoalbuminemia**
• Amyloidosis	**Osteoblastic metastases**
Hyperphosphatemia	**Loop diuretics**
• Rhabdomyolysis	**Contrast media containing**
• Phosphate therapy	**EDTA**
• Renal failure	**Intestinal malabsorption**
• Chemotherapy/tumor lysis	**Massive transfusion** (citrate
Vitamin D deficiency	intoxication with chelation
• Liver failure	of calcium)
• Renal failure	
• Lack of sun exposure	
• Dietary deficiency	

EDTA, ethylenediaminetetraacetic acid.

many critical care illnesses including sepsis, pancreatitis, and major trauma. Previous parathyroidectomy (including subtotal removal or removal of three and one-half glands) and a history of previous neck dissection are also risk factors. Hypocalcemia can follow large fluid resuscitations (including transfusions or plasmapheresis) or dialysis with citrate solutions. Like citrate, phosphate also binds calcium; use of a sodium phosphate (phosphosoda) bowel preparation has been associated with hypocalcemia.

2. **Clinical features.** Although the diagnosis of hypocalcemia is made at an albumin-corrected total calcium concentration of 8.5 mg/dl, symptomatic hypocalcemia is unusual until the total serum calcium levels falls below 7.5 mg/dl, especially if the decline is slow. Acute hypocalcemia (e.g. after neck surgery and removal of, or damage to, the parathyroid glands) produces neuromuscular irritability with carpal-pedal spasm and circumoral and acral paresthesias. Severe hypocalcemia results in laryngospasm with stridor, tetany, apnea, and focal or grand mal seizures unresponsive to conventional therapy. Bedside demonstration of facial nerve irritability to percussion (Chvostek's sign) or carpal spasm with tourniquet ischemia for 3 minutes (Trousseau's sign) indicates the need for expeditious calcium supplementation. However, 10% to 15% of normocalcemic patients will have a positive Chvostek's sign. Calcium is a cofactor in the coagulation cascade, and clotting function can be

compromised. Patients may have hypotension with relative insensitivity to beta-adrenergic agonists and a prolonged QT interval on electrocardiogram, which can lead to 2:1 heart block.

3. **Treatment.** Clinically stable ICU patients who are able to take oral medications should receive calcium carbonate or calcium citrate and vitamin D. Patients require 1.5 to 3 g/d of elemental calcium (3,750–7,500 mg of calcium carbonate) in divided doses with food. In acute symptomatic moderate hypocalcemia treated with oral calcium, **calcitriol** (0.25–3 µg/d in divided doses, orally) is given to allow gastrointestinal (GI) absorption. For chronic replacement, oral vitamin D, 50,000 IU one to three times weekly, is given. Therapeutic goals are an albumin-corrected serum calcium concentration near 8 mg/dl and a low urinary calcium level. Phosphorus and magnesium levels should also be evaluated and corrected because hypomagnesemia reduces PTH secretion and function. In emergent situations, 100 to 200 mg of calcium chloride or calcium gluconate can be administered IV through a central vein over 10 minutes by slow IV push. One milliliter of calcium chloride or calcium gluconate is equivalent to 27 and 9 mg of elemental calcium, respectively. Calcium chloride is the preferred preparation for IV therapy because it elevates calcium concentrations for longer time periods and is more concentrated. Therapy can be continued by calcium infusion at a rate of 15 mg/kg over 6 to 8 hours. Parenteral therapy must be monitored by serum calcium measurements every 3 to 4 hours. Elevated phosphorus levels are treated with oral phosphate binders, whereas low magnesium levels (<1 mg/dl) that suppress PTH secretion are treated with parenteral magnesium sulfate.

IV. **Adrenal cortical disease**
   A. **Physiology.** The adrenal gland consists of an outer cortex, which secretes steroid hormones, and an inner medulla, which secretes catecholamines. Together, these hormones maintain homeostasis during states of **physiologic stress,** including surgery, fasting, trauma, or shock. The adrenal cortex produces three classes of steroid hormones: glucocorticoids, mineralocorticoids, and androgens.
      1. **Glucocorticoids. Cortisol** is the principal hormone of this class. **Adrenocorticotropic hormone (ACTH)** from the anterior pituitary stimulates the release of cortisol in a diurnal pattern and in response to stress. **Approximately 30 mg of cortisol is produced daily under basal conditions.** Cortisol has multiple effects on carbohydrate, protein, and fatty acid metabolism. It decreases cellular uptake of glucose and promotes gluconeogenesis and hepatic glycogen synthesis. It is crucial for the conversion of norepinephrine to epinephrine in the

adrenal medulla; it is required for the production of angiotensin II and adequate vascular tone. Cortisol acts as an antiinflammatory agent by stabilizing microsomes and promoting capillary stability. It is metabolized by the liver and also filtered and excreted unchanged by the kidney.

2. **Mineralocorticoids. Aldosterone** is an important regulator of extracellular fluid volume and potassium homeostasis. The **renin–angiotensin** system and, to a lesser extent, potassium concentrations regulate aldosterone secretion. Aldosterone principally acts on the renal tubule to stimulate the absorption of Na and transport it to the extracellular fluid. The resulting excess of anions in the tubule causes a passive transfer of potassium and hydrogen ions into the tubule with excretion in the urine.

3. **Androgens.** Abnormal secretion of these sex hormones may indicate abnormalities in biosynthesis of multiple steroids, including cortisol. The most common cause of increased adrenal androgen secretion is congenital adrenal hyperplasia, resulting in hirsutism and menstrual irregularities in women. Adrenal cortical carcinoma is a rare cause of excess adrenal androgen production.

B. **Adrenal cortical hyperfunction**
   1. **Hypercortisolism** (Cushing's syndrome)
      a. **Causes.** Adrenal cortical hyperfunction is usually secondary to the presence of ACTH-induced adrenal hyperplasia. By definition, patients have Cushing's disease when excess secretion of ACTH from a pituitary tumor drives overproduction of adrenal cortical steroids. Hyperadrenalism from any other cause (e.g., ectopic production of ACTH by tumors, adrenal adenoma, or bilateral adrenal hyperplasia, steroid therapy) is defined as Cushing's syndrome. Cushing's syndrome is commonly iatrogenic, resulting from the therapeutic administration of glucocorticoids.

      b. **Clinical features.** Patients can present with truncal obesity, round facies, hypertension, hypernatremia, excess intravascular volume, hyperglycemia, hypokalemia, or red abdominal striae, poor wound healing, muscle wasting and weakness, osteoporosis, hypercoagulability, mental status changes, emotional lability, pancreatitis, peptic ulceration, glaucoma, and infection. The clinical picture is not always obvious, and suspicion should arise when a patient presents with recent weight gain, impaired glucose tolerance, and high blood pressure. Therefore, those who fit the criteria for metabolic syndrome should be screened for Cushing's syndrome, especially if they are resistant to conventional treatment.

      c. **Diagnosis.** Cushing's syndrome is an uncommon cause of ICU admission. First-line screening tests include the 24-hour urinary free cortisol test, the low-dose dexamethasone suppression test, and the late-night salivary cortisol test. The 24-hour urinary cortisol gives an index of the free (unbound) cortisol that circulates in the blood, and is not affected by factors influencing corticosteroid-binding globulin levels. This test can be repeated up to three times if the index of suspicion for the diagnosis is high enough. However, these tests are generally not interpretable in the ICU because of the physiologic stress responses to critical illness.

   d. Management is based on the surgical resection of the pituitary adenoma, adrenal tumor, or ectopic ACTH-secreting tumor. If transphenoidal surgery is not successful, pituitary irradiation or bilateral adrenalectomy can be attempted. While awaiting surgery, supportive management is crucial. Hypertension may be difficult to treat, and hence the use of a combination of antihypertensive agents in high doses might be required. Excess intravascular volume can be reduced with diuretics; potassium must be replaced. Serum glucose must be monitored frequently. Osteoporosis necessitates careful positioning of the patient. Glucocorticoid replacement is then initiated and then continued for 6 to 36 months after surgery. **Ketoconazole** or **metyrapone** inhibition of cortisol production with cortisol replacement therapy is indicated if surgery is unsuccessful or contraindicated.

2. **Hyperaldosteronism**
   a. Causes. The etiology of hyperaldosteronism in the ICU patient might be from adrenal hyperplasia, adenoma, or carcinoma or from the extra adrenal stimulation of aldosterone with decreased renal perfusion or a renin-secreting tumor.
   b. Clinical features. The manifestation of hyperaldosteronism from any cause includes mild to moderate diastolic hypertension, headache, muscle weakness, polyuria, polydipsia, and electrolyte abnormalities such as hypokalemia, hypernatremia, and metabolic alkalosis.
   c. Laboratory evaluation. Primary hyperaldosteronism is identified by the combination of hypokalemia, decreased plasma renin activity, and high urinary and plasma aldosterone levels in hypertensive patients after sodium replacement. Secondary hyperaldosteronism occurs with increased renin secretion and secondary aldosterone production.
   d. Treatment. Surgical excision of the adrenal aldosteronoma resolves symptoms, but blood pressure may not normalize immediately. Patients are treated supportively with spironolactone and calcium-channel blockers before surgery.

C. Adrenal cortical hypofunction

1. **Causes:** Adrenal insufficiency results from an inadequate basal or stress level of plasma cortisol. The diagnosis is critical because if it is unrecognized, the disorder may be fatal. Preexisting conditions, medications that inhibit steroid synthesis (e.g., etomidate and ketoconazole), and the effects of critical illness can suppress the normal corticosteroid response. Tumors, infection (i.e., fungus, tuberculosis, human immunodeficiency virus, cytomegalovirus), or adrenal hemorrhage may directly damage the adrenal glands. Idiopathic autoimmune atrophy, surgical removal, and radiation therapy can also produce adrenal cortical hypofunction.

2. **Clinical features.** Symptoms may be nonspecific and include weakness, fatigue, anorexia, nausea, vomiting, abdominal pain, myalgias/arthralgias, postural syncope, headaches, memory impairment, cyclical fevers and depression. On physical examination, patients may have hypotension, tachycardia, fever, decreased body hair, vitiligo, and features of hypopituitarism (amenorrhea, cold intolerance). Patients may present with hyperpigmentation (secondary to excess ACTH production), hyponatremia, or hyperkalemia.

3. **Laboratory evaluation.** It has been difficult to define the appropriate glucocorticoid response in a critically ill patient. Several treatment threshold levels have been proposed. Table 27-14 gives one suggested decision tree. Hypoadrenalism is likely if random cortisol levels are less than 15 μg/dl in the ICU setting. Functional hypoadrenalism is unlikely if random cortisol levels exceed 34 μg/dl. A **corticotropin stimulation test** (cosyntropin test) is performed to evaluate possible adrenal insufficiency if a random cortisol is between 15 and 34 μg/dl.

4. **Treatment**

   a. **Acute adrenal insufficiency.** Critically ill patients with hypoadrenalism receive IV **hydrocortisone, 50 mg every 6 hours.** Hypovolemia and hypoglycemia commonly occur.

Table 27-14. Laboratory diagnosis of adrenal insufficiency in critically ill patients

First: randomly timed serum cortisol		
<15 μg/dl	15–34 μg/dl	>34 μg/dl
Hypoadrenalism likely, consider steroid replacement	Perform cosyntropin test	Hypoadrenalism unlikely

Second: cosyntropin test	
Increase of <9 μg/dl	Increase of >9 μg/dl
Hypoadrenalism likely, consider steroid replacement	Hypoadrenalism unlikely

b. Chronic adrenal insufficiency. Glucocorticoid supplementation is also necessary in patients at risk for adrenal suppression during times of stress (including surgery and critical illness). Hydrocortisone, 150 mg/d or greater, is given to patients during the critical phase of the illness. Taper steroid supplementation when the patient stabilizes. Steroid dose equivalents are shown in Table 27-15.

c. Adrenal insufficiency in septic shock (see also Chapter 28). Glucocorticoid therapy improves hemodynamics in patients with septic shock, reduces vasopressor requirements, and may reduce mortality. Treatment should be initiated even before test results return. Glucocorticoid supplementation can be stopped if testing demonstrates appropriate adrenal responses.

5. Critical care considerations

a. Sedative, anesthetic, and vasoactive drugs must be titrated carefully because patients with adrenal hypofunction are exquisitely sensitive to drug-induced myocardial depression.

b. After adrenalectomy, steroid replacement should begin immediately postoperatively. Following **unilateral adrenalectomy,** glucocorticoid supplementation is necessary until the remaining adrenal cortex resumes normal glucocorticoid output, typically after several months. Endogenous mineralocorticoid secretion is usually adequate. Both glucocorticoid and mineralocorticoid replacement are permanently required with bilateral adrenalectomy.

V. Adrenal medullary disease

A. Physiology. Preganglionic fibers of the sympathetic nervous system end in the adrenal medulla and stimulate catecholamine release—norepinephrine (20%) and epinephrine (80%). Catecholamines cause chronotropic and inotropic stimulation of the heart, vasomotor changes, enhanced hepatic glycogenolysis, and inhibition of insulin release. Metanephrine and vanillylmandelic acid (VMA) generated by the liver and kidney are the primary biotransformation products of catecholamines.

B. Pheochromocytoma

1. Physiology. Pheochromocytoma is a rare tumor of the adrenal medulla. It can occur in a variety of other locations, most often within sympathetic ganglia (paraganglionoma). It is a catecholamine-producing tumor, typically solitary, but 10% are bilateral and 10% are metastatic in the adult. ~25% of pheochromocytomas are familial and occur as part of multiple endocrine neoplasia syndrome types II and III; they can also be associated with Von Recklinghausen's disease and mutation of succinate dehydrogeneous subunits B and D. Most tumors secrete both

Table 27-15. Glucocorticoid and mineralocorticoid hormone equivalents

Steroid	Relative Potency		Equivalent Dose (mg)	Duration (h)
	Glucocorticoid	Mineralocorticoid		
Short Acting				
Cortisol	1.0	1.0	20	8–12
Cortisone	0.8	0.8	25	8–12
Aldosterone	0.3	3,000	—	8–12
Intermediate acting				
Prednisone	4.0	0.8	5	12–36
Prednisolone	4.0	0.8	5	12–36
Methylprednisolone	5.0	0.5	4	12–36
Fludrocortisone	10.0	125	—	12–36
Long acting				
Dexamethasone	25–40	0	0.75	>24

epinephrine and norepinephrine, and their release is independent of neurogenic control.

2. **Presentation.** Signs and symptoms result from excess catecholamine release. The classic triad includes palpitations, headache, and diaphoresis in an episodically hypertensive patient, but 10% of patients are not hypertensive. Pheochromocytoma is a rare cause of chronic hypertension. Other signs and symptoms include pallor, anxiety, tremor, hyperglycemia, hypovolemia-induced orthostatic hypotension, polycythemia, and weight loss. Patients with pheochromocytoma are usually dehydrated and hemoconcentrated due to increased insensible losses and vasoconstriction. Chronic exposure to high catecholamine concentrations may ultimately produce a cardiomyopathy. Of note, physical examination (especially of the abdomen) with manipulation of a tumor may cause the release of catecholamines and precipitate a crisis. Ablative surgery is the definitive treatment, but only after pharmacologic and volume stabilization of the patient. Endogenous catecholamine levels return to normal within a few days after successful removal of the tumor.

3. **Management** in ICU and perioperative considerations

   a. **Hypertensive crisis** presents with very high blood pressures, severe headache, visual disturbances, stroke, myocardial ischemia, or CHF. Crises can be precipitated by postural changes, exertion, food or beverage intake, emotional stress, urination, and the use of certain drugs (histamines, ACTH, metoclopramide, tricyclic antidepressants, anesthetic agents). Immediate antihypertensive therapy is critical in such circumstances (see Chapter 8). It is important that β-adrenergic blockade not be implemented before adequate α-blockade has been achieved, to avoid unopposed α-adrenergic activity.

   b. **Shock and hypotension.** A paroxysm of hypertension sometimes precedes severe hypotension. Shock is the presenting problem identified in less than 2% of pheochromocytoma patients. Patients may present with abdominal pain, intense mydriasis, weakness, diaphoresis, and cyanosis. Findings include pulmonary edema, hyperglycemia, and leukocytosis. The mechanisms for such manifestations are not understood.

   c. Rarely, patients with pheochromocytoma present with multiorgan failure known as **pheochromocytoma multisystem crisis.** This occurs when hypertension and/or hypotension are accompanied by multiorgan failure, a temperature great than 40°C, and encephalopathy. This condition can be confused with septicemia, delaying appropriate treatment. If patients suddenly deteriorate despite rigorous medical treatment (including fluid and inotropic agents), emergency tumor removal should be performed.

VI. Pituitary disease

A. Anterior pituitary

1. **Physiology.** The anterior pituitary gland secretes a variety of hormones that regulate the activity of the thyroid and adrenal glands, the ovaries and testes, growth, and lactation. **Growth hormone** (GH) and **prolactin** (PRL) act directly on target tissues, whereas ACTH, TSH, follicle-stimulating hormone (FSH), and luteinizing hormone (LH) act by stimulating other endocrine glands. Control over anterior pituitary hormone production is achieved with stimulation or inhibition by specific hypothalamic factors and feedback inhibition by peripheral hormones. Pituitary tumors are usually benign adenomas characterized by their hormone secretion profile (i.e., nonsecreting, prolactinoma, or GH-, ACTH-, TSH-, and gonadotropin-secreting adenomas). A variety of conditions may lead to pituitary insufficiency.

2. **Hyperfunction**

   a. Hyperfunctioning adenomas are usually benign pituitary tumors that cause no special ICU problems. The hyperthyroidism of a TSH-secreting adenoma and the hyperadrenalism (Cushing's disease) of the ACTH-secreting adenoma are treated as described in previous sections.

   b. **Acromegaly.** This is a growth disorder with skeletal and soft-tissue growth and deformations as well as cardiac, respiratory, neuromuscular, endocrine, and metabolic complications. This condition is caused by excess GH secretion from pituitary or extrapituitary tumors.

      i. **Airway concerns.** Excess GH secretion in the adult lead to prognathism, widening of the maxilla with tooth separation, jaw malocclusion, and overbite. Soft-tissue overgrowth occurs in the lips, tongue, epiglottis, and vocal cords, with subglottic narrowing of the trachea. Difficulties with airway management and endotracheal intubation should be anticipated.

      ii. **Special considerations.** Cardiovascular disease is the most important cause of mortality in acromegaly. Patients are predisposed to CHF, dysrhythmias, and CAD. Cardiac function generally improves after treatment reduces growth hormone levels. Glucose intolerance is commonly encountered; thus, serum glucose levels should be carefully monitored. Peripheral neuropathies and colon carcinoma are associated with acromegaly. Some patients suffer from skeletal muscle weakness or thickening of the upper respiratory tract, which can contribute to respiratory insufficiency. Monoarticular or polyarticular involvement leads to crepitus, stiffness, tenderness, and hypomobility.

3. **Hyposecretion. Panhypopituitarism**
   a. **Causes of pituitary failure.** Postpartum hemorrhagic shock can cause vasospasm and subsequent pituitary necrosis and hypofunction, known as **Sheehan's syndrome.** Other causes include trauma, radiation therapy, pituitary apoplexy, lymphocytic hypophysitis, infiltrative disease (e.g., sarcoidosis or histiocytosis), and tumors (e.g., metastatic carcinoma, macro pituitary adenomas, or craniopharyngiomas). Surgical removal of the pituitary is performed for tumor resection. Pituitary carcinoma is a rare cause of isolated or complete pituitary insufficiency.
   b. **Special considerations**
      i. Glucocorticoid therapy is essential for patients with a history of **adrenal insufficiency.**
      ii. No special treatment or supplementation is necessary for mild to moderate **hypothyroidism.** Management of severe hypothyroidism was discussed previously.
      iii. The onset of pituitary insufficiency after pituitary surgery or apoplexy is delayed. Adrenal insufficiency develops over 4 to 14 days after destruction or removal of the pituitary gland. Glucocorticoid, but not mineralocorticoid, replacement is required. Because of the long half-life of thyroid hormone (7–10 days), symptomatic hypothyroidism does not occur until 2 to 3 weeks following pituitary surgery or apoplexy.

B. **Posterior pituitary**
   1. **Physiology.** The main functions of **oxytocin** are to regulate uterine contractions in labor and milk ejection in lactation. **Antidiuretic hormone (ADH, vasopressin)** regulates plasma osmolarity and extracellular fluid volume by facilitating renal tubular resorption of water and increasing urinary osmolarity. Antidiuretic hormone secretion is enhanced by several commonly encountered stimuli, including decreases in intravascular volume, pain from trauma or surgery, nausea, and positive airway pressure.
   2. **Diabetes insipidus**
      a. **Causes.** Insufficient ADH secretion by the posterior pituitary gland is known as central diabetes insipidus (DI). **Central DI** can be caused by intracranial trauma, hypophysectomy, metastatic disease to the pituitary gland or hypothalamus, and infiltrative diseases such as histiocytosis and sarcoidosis. **Nephrogenic DI** describes

the failure of the renal tubules to respond to ADH. Causes of nephrogenic DI include hypokalemia, hypercalcemia, sickle cell anemia, chronic myeloma, obstructive uropathy, chronic renal insufficiency, lithium therapy, and a rare X-linked hereditary disorder. DI also occurs in the third trimester of pregnancy due to placental vasopressinase.

b. **Diagnosis.** Clinical evidence for DI is a dilute, hypo-osmolar urine production of greater than 400 ml/h in the setting of pituitary surgery or head trauma. Suspected DI is diagnosed by examining simultaneous serum and urine osmolality values. **Serum osmolality is high** (310–320 mOsm/kg) and **urine is inappropriately diluted,** with a specific gravity of less than 1.001 and urine osmolality of less than 200 mOsm/kg. Serum Na levels are elevated.

c. **Central DI.** Clinical features include polydipsia and polyuria. Central DI can be treated with the synthetic vasopressin analogue **desmopressin (DDAVP),** 1 to 2 μg (0.25–0.5 ml) SQ or IV every 6 to 24 hours, as needed. Side effects of DDAVP include hyponatremia and coronary artery vasospasm.

d. **Nephrogenic DI.** The polyuria of nephrogenic DI is associated with an inappropriately hypotonic urine, normal or high levels of plasma vasopressin, and failure of exogenous vasopressin to reduce urinary volume. Patients are limited to a low-sodium diet, and adequate hydration must be assured. Inhibition of prostaglandin synthesis (with ibuprofen, indomethacin, or aspirin) or mild salt depletion with a thiazide diuretic may reduce urine volume.

e. **Management of central DI** includes careful monitoring of urine output and specific gravity, serum sodium levels, plasma volume, and plasma osmolality. The **total body water deficit** in liters (see also Chapter 7) can be estimated as

$$[0.6 \times \text{Body weight (kg)}] \times ([\text{Na}] - 140)/140$$

Initial therapy includes volume expansion and blood pressure support with IV isotonic fluids. Once plasma osmolality falls below 290 mOsm/kg, hypotonic fluids (half-normal saline) are usually used. Mild DI (daily urinary volumes of 2–6 L) does not require treatment in patients with an adequate thirst mechanism who are able to drink fluids freely.

3. **Syndrome of inappropriate ADH secretion SIADH**

a. **Causes.** SIADH is persistent secretion of ADH with hyponatremia in the absence of an osmotic stimulus. SIADH can be caused by carcinoma (bronchogenic, duodenal, pancreatic, ureteral, prostatic, or bladder), other malignancies (lymphoma, leukemia, thymomas, and mesothelioma), CNS disorders (trauma, infections, tumors), pulmonary disorders (tuberculosis, pneumonia, positive-pressure ventilation), drugs (nicotine, narcotics, chlorpropamide, vincristine, vinblastine, cyclophosphamide), hypothyroidism, Addison's disease, and porphyria.

   b. Diagnosis. Patients may complain of a mild headache, anorexia, confusion, or GI disturbances. Suspected SIADH is diagnosed by examining simultaneous serum and urine sodium and osmolality values. SIADH is associated with a high urine osmolality (higher than the serum value), a urinary sodium concentration greater than 20 mEq/L, and a serum sodium concentration less than 130 mEq/L. If serum sodium levels fall below 110 mEq/L, cerebral edema and seizures may result.

   c. Management of mild or chronic SIADH. In some cases, SIADH can be cured by eliminating the tumor, drug, or disease. In other cases, SIADH is self-limited and resolves spontaneously within 2 to 3 weeks. Chronic asymptomatic SIADH with plasma sodium greater than 125 mEq/L has virtually no mortality and does not need treatment. Fluid restriction (800–1,000 ml daily) is the primary treatment for mild to moderate hyponatremia in SIADH.

   d. Management of severe SIADH with profound hyponatremia (sodium <110 mEq/L) or symptomatic hyponatremia (sodium <120 mEq/L) generally requires treatment with isotonic or hypertonic saline. Severely symptomatic patients should be managed in the ICU, where fluid intake, urine output, and serum electrolytes may be monitored frequently. The treatment goal is slow serum sodium correction, no faster than 0.5 mEq/L/h, with a maximum increase of 8 mEq/L/24 h. The therapeutic target is serum sodium 125 mEq/L or serum osmolality approximately 250 mEq/L. The **sodium deficit** can be calculated as

$$\text{Target Na (mEq)} = (135 - \text{Serum Na}) \times 0.5$$
$$\times \text{Weight (kg)}$$

   i. In volume-contracted states, administer isotonic saline alone. If isotonic saline alone does not raise the serum sodium, consider furosemide-induced diuresis to produce a hypotonic urine. If the hyponatremia is especially severe or associated with coma, seizures, or new neurologic symptoms, infuse hypertonic saline (3% saline, 513 mEq/L sodium chloride) for several hours, no faster than 100 ml/h (1 ml/kg/h). Treatment should be evaluated with serum sodium and urine output every hour.

ii. In SIADH associated with volume expansion, administration of **hypertonic saline** is ineffective because the excess sodium is excreted in urine. Hypertonic saline should be given with furosemide to produce a hypotonic urine. Infused at 0.05 ml/kg/min, 3% saline increases the serum sodium by approximately 2 mEq/L per hour. Hypertonic saline is potentially dangerous in volume-expanded, salt-retaining states such as CHF.

VII. Carcinoid

A. Carcinoid tumors
arise from the embryonic foregut (bronchus, stomach, pancreas), midgut (mid-duodenum to mid-transverse colon), or hindgut (descending colon and rectum). They are usually derived from serotonin-producing enterochromaffin cells, but their clinical and biological characteristics differ depending on the site of origin. The most common location of carcinoid tumors is the appendix, followed by the ileum and the rectum. Carcinoid tumors frequently metastasize to the liver. The biochemical hallmark of carcinoid tumors is the overproduction of **serotonin,** the serotonin precursor 5-hydroxytryptophan, or both, along with an increased excretion of the degradation product 5-hydroxyindoleacetic acid (5HIAA) measured in the urine. In addition to serotonin, mediators secreted by carcinoid tumors include bradykinin, histamine, prostaglandins, and kallikrein. Stimuli for the release of mediators include catecholamines, histamine, and tumor manipulation.

B. Carcinoid syndrome.
Clinical features of the carcinoid syndrome depend on the tumor's location and extent of liver metastasis. The syndrome includes episodic flushing, bronchoconstriction, gastrointestinal hypermotility, and mild hyperglycemia. Cardiac manifestations include supraventricular tachycardias and valve cusp distortions. The possibility of left-sided cardiac lesions should not be overlooked. Peripheral vasodilation can produce profound hypotension. Of patients with carcinoids located in the small bowel and the proximal colon, 40% to 50% will have the symptom complex. Symptoms are less frequent with bronchial carcinoids, rare in appendicial carcinoids, and not seen with rectal carcinoid tumors. Compounds released by the tumor are typically metabolized during their first pass through the liver, and symptoms usually are seen only in cases of extensive hepatic metastases or with a tumor located outside the portal system.

C. Management considerations

1. Management of the symptomatic carcinoid patient can be difficult. A carcinoid crisis may be refractory to conventional therapeutic measures such a fluid resuscitation and direct-acting vasopressors (e.g., phenylephrine). Treatment should then be initiated with the somatostatin analogue **octreotide** (50–100 μg IV). This prevents the release of serotonin and its precursors and may block the peripheral actions of serotonin, kinins, and other mediators. Infusions of dilute octreotide (10 μg/ml, rate titrated to blood pressure) can be used for maintenance therapy. Depending on the secretion profile of the particular tumor, other agents that can potentially be used in the management of a carcinoid crisis include H_1 and H_2 histamine antagonists, the kallikrein inhibitor aprotinin, and serotonin antagonists. Newly developed somatostatin analogues with differing specificities for the various somatostatin receptors have been used with improved therapeutic effectiveness in the medical management of carcinoid tumors. Until these are widely available, an alternative treatment is interferon-α, which has been partially effective in controlling hormone secretion, with minimal effects on tumor growth.

2. **Paroxysmal bronchoconstriction** always occurs concurrently with a flushing episode and is associated with release of mediators from the tumor. In addition to the usual treatment of bronchoconstriction, octreotide can be given to decrease mediator release. Note that catecholamines can enhance tumor mediator release, worsening a carcinoid crisis.

3. **Endocardial disease.** Plaquelike thickening on the endocardium of the cardiac valve leaflets, atria, and ventricles occurs in 20% of patients with carcinoid, and usually is associated with high levels of serotonin. Thickening of the endocardium commonly results in pulmonic stenosis and tricuspid insufficiency, which can produce right ventricular failure.

SELECTED REFERENCES

Annane D, Sebille V, Charpentier C, et al. Effect of treatment with low doses of hydrocortisone and fludrocortisone on mortality in patients with septic shock. *JAMA* 2002;288:862–871.

Ariyan CE, Sosa JA. Assessment and management of patients with abnormal calcium. *Crit Care Med* 2004;32:S146–S154.

Axelrod L. Perioperative management of patients treated with glucocorticoids. *Endocrinol Metab Clin North Am* 2003;32:367–383.

Ben-Shlomo A, Melmed S. Acromegaly. *Endocrinol Metab Clin North Am* 2001;30:565–583.

Body JJ, Bouillon R. Emergencies of calcium homeostasis. *Rev Endocr Metab Disord* 2003;4:167–175.

Boord JB, Graber AL, Christman JW, et al. Practical management of diabetes in critically ill patients. *Am J Respir Crit Care Med* 2001;164:1763–1767.

Brouwers FM, Lenders JW, Eisenhofer G, et al. Pheochromocytoma as an endocrine emergency. *Rev Endocr Metab Disord* 2003;4:121–128.

Burman KD, Wartofsky L. Thyroid function in the intensive care unit setting. *Crit Care Clin* 2001;17:43–57.

Cooper MS, Stewart PM. Corticosteroid insufficiency in acutely ill patients. *N Engl J Med* 2003;348:727–734.

Elliott WJ. Hypertensive emergencies. *Crit Care Clin* 2001;17:435–451.

Goldberg PA, Inzucchi SE. Critical issues in endocrinology. *Clin Chest Med* 2003;24:583–606.

Kulke MH. Neuroendocrine tumours: clinical presentation and management of localized disease. *Cancer Treat Rev* 2003;29:363–370.

Kulke MH, Mayer RJ. Carcinoid tumors. *N Engl J Med* 1999;340:858–868.

Lamberts SW, Bruining HA, de Jong FH. Corticosteroid therapy in severe illness. *N Engl J Med* 1997;337:1285–1292.

Lind L, Carlstedt F, Rastad J, et al. Hypocalcemia and parathyroid hormone secretion in critically ill patients. *Crit Care Med* 2000;28:93–99.

Magee MF, Bhatt BA. Management of decompensated diabetes. Diabetic ketoacidosis and hyperglycemic hyperosmolar syndrome. *Crit Care Clin* 2001;17:75–106.

Nishimura M, Uzu T, Fujii T, et al. Cardiovascular complications in patients with primary aldosteronism. *Am J Kidney Dis* 1999;33:261–266.

Ringel MD. Management of hypothyroidism and hyperthyroidism in the intensive care unit. *Crit Care Clin* 2001;17:59–74.

Robertson GL. Antidiuretic hormone. Normal and disordered function. *Endocrinol Metab Clin North Am* 2001;30:671–694.

Vance ML. Hypopituitarism. *N Engl J Med* 1994;330:1651–1662.

Van den Berge G, Wouters P, Weekers F, et al. Intensive insulin therapy in the critically ill patients. *N Engl J Med* 2001;345:1359–1367.

Vaughan ED Jr. Diseases of the adrenal gland. *Med Clin North Am* 2004;88:443–466.

Wilson PW, Grundy SM. The metabolic syndrome: practical guide to origins and treatment: part I. *Circulation* 2003;108:1422–1424.

Wilson PW, Grundy SM. The metabolic syndrome: a practical guide to origins and treatment: part II. *Circulation* 2003;108:1537–1540.

Wong LL, Verbalis JG. Systemic diseases associated with disorders of water homeostasis. *Endocrinol Metab Clin North Am* 2002;31:121–140.

Ziegler R. Hypercalcemic crisis. *J Am Soc Nephrol* 2001;12(Suppl 17):S3–S9.

Zivin JR, Gooley T, Zager RA, et al. Hypocalcemia: a pervasive metabolic abnormality in the critically ill. *Am J Kidney Dis* 2001;37:689–698.

28

Specific Infections

Judith Hellman and Roland Brusseau

This chapter provides an overview of specific infections encountered in critically ill patients and emphasizes their clinical presentation, microbiology, and diagnostic and therapeutic approaches. The reader is referred to Chapter 11 for a review of antimicrobial agents, sepsis, and infectious disease issues in immunocompromised patients. Unless otherwise indicated, the potential antibiotic regimens presented are for the initial empiric treatment of infection. Subsequent therapy should be appropriately tailored to culture data as they become available. Because of the complexity of infectious complications in critically ill patients, management sometimes requires the consultation of infectious disease specialists.

I. Thoracic infections

A. Community-acquired pneumonia (CAP) is an infection of the lower respiratory tract that is acquired outside of the hospital. Although the overall mortality of CAP is low, the mortality in ICU patients with CAP is quite high. Risk factors for poor outcome include advanced age, coexisting chronic diseases (such as heart disease, pulmonary disease, diabetes), immunosuppression, and neoplastic disease. Clinical findings on admission also predict outcome. Increased respiratory rate, hypotension, fever, altered mental status, high or low white blood cell count, hypoxemia, and multilobar or extrapulmonary involvement are associated with higher mortality.

1. **Microbiology.** The most frequent pathogen is *Streptococcus pneumoniae.* CAP is also caused by *H. influenzae* and other gram-negative bacteria such as *Klebsiella pneumoniae* and *Pseudomonas aeruginosa* (particularly in patients with underlying lung disease), gram-positive bacteria such as *S. aureus,* atypical pathogens such as *Legionella pneumophila, Mycoplasma pneumoniae,* and *Chlamydia pneumoniae,* and viruses. *Moraxella catarrhalis* may cause CAP in patients with chronic obstructive pulmonary disease and chronic bronchitis. Immunocompromised patients can develop pneumonia due to the standard pathogens as well as opportunistic organisms.

2. **Diagnosis.** Findings on chest radiography may be variable depending on the pathogen and the underlying condition of the host. Infiltrates may be unilobar or multilobar, and may not be apparent on initial chest radiographs of severely hypovolemic

patients. Whenever possible, the causative microorganism should be identified. Analysis of the sputum by Gram's stain should reveal more than 25 neutrophils and fewer than 10 epithelial cells per low-power field. The causative organism may be suggested by the abundance and morphology of the bacteria on a well-collected sample. In some cases, it may be necessary to perform a bronchoscopy to obtain adequate sputum samples. Sputum cultures may be helpful in identifying the organism and defining the antimicrobial sensitivity. Blood cultures may also be helpful in defining the organism. If pneumonia is accompanied by a significant pleural effusion, the pleural fluid should be analyzed for Gram's stain and culture, pH, lactate dehydrogenase, glucose, and protein concentration. Serologic tests may be useful for identifying infection due to atypical pathogens. *Legionella pneumophila* antigen may be detected in the sputum or urine.

3. **Treatment.** Initial management of CAP is generally empiric, guided by patient condition and the results of Gram's-stained sputum specimens, if available. Outcome is improved with early administration of antibiotics. Clinical presentation does not reliably predict the pathogens involved, and frequently the causative microorganism is not identified. The potential for antibiotic resistance should influence the choice of antibiotics (e.g., *Streptococcus pneumoniae* may be penicillin resistant). Antibiotics for early broad empiric therapy should cover typical as well as atypical microorganisms. Therapy should be adjusted based on results of cultures and serologic tests. Potential empiric regimens for severely ill patients in the ICU include the following:

   a. A third- or fourth-generation cephalosporin such as cefotaxime, ceftriaxone, or cefipime plus an intravenous (IV) macrolide such as azithromycin.

   b. A third- or fourth-generation cephalosporin plus a fluoroquinolone such as levofloxacin.

   c. A β-lactam/β-lactamase inhibitor such as ampicillin/sulbactam plus IV macrolide or fluoroquinolone.

   d. If *Pseudomonas* is a possibility, a β-lactam/β-lactamase inhibitor such as piperacillin/tazobactam or a carbapenem such as imipenem or meropenem plus IV macrolide or fluoroquinolone.

B. **Nosocomial pneumonia** is common in surgical and trauma patients and is associated with the highest mortality of all nosocomial infections. **Ventilator-associated pneumonia (VAP)** is a subset of nosocomial pneumonia that occurs more than 48 hours after intubation. Nosocomial pneumonia has been estimated to occur in approximately 10% to 70% of mechanically ventilated patients. The mortality of patients with nosocomial pneumonia varies among different studies and is estimated to be in the range of 20% to 50%. Bacteria enter the lungs through various routes, including aspiration of oropharyngeal secretions or esophageal/gastric contents, inhalation of airborne droplets, hematogenous spread from other sites, and direct inoculation from colonized hospital personnel or contaminated equipment or devices.

1. **Microbiology.** The microorganisms causing nosocomial pneumonia differ substantially from those causing community-acquired pneumonia. Infections are often polymicrobial. Enteric gram-negative bacteria (such as *E. coli, Klebsiella* spp, *Proteus* spp and *Enterobacter* spp) and *S. aureus* most frequently cause nosocomial pneumonia. Other bacteria include nonenteric gram-negatives such as *Pseudomonas aeruginosa* and *H. influenzae,* anaerobes and gram-positives such as *Enterococcus* spp, and *Streptococcus pneumoniae.* Antibiotic-resistant bacteria are very common.

2. **Diagnosis** of nosocomial pneumonia in intensive care unit (ICU) patients can be difficult. Signs such as fever, leukocytosis, purulent secretions, and even the presence of infiltrates on chest radiographs are nonspecific and may not indicate actual pulmonary infection. There is considerable variability in the approach to diagnostic evaluation. Controversy persists over whether sputum samples should be collected using invasive methods and whether quantitative bacterial cultures (which must be obtained via invasive means) are necessary. With all sampling techniques, the sensitivity of sputum cultures decreases with even short courses of antibiotics prior to sample collection.

   a. **Nonquantitative cultures** are often performed on sputum samples (obtained by noninvasive and invasive means). Most agree that cultures of expectorated sputum and samples from blind endotracheal suctioning are unreliable for definitive diagnosis of pneumonia or for defining with certainty the etiologic microorganism. It is likely, however, that the pathogen will be among the bacteria cultured, and sensitivity data may help to define the antimicrobial resistance patterns.

   b. **Invasive collection** using protected-brush bronchoscopy and/or bronchoalveolar lavage (BAL) provides lower respiratory tract samples for **quantitative cultures.** Quantitative cultures may be more reliable for diagnosis of infection and identification of the specific pathogen(s). Pneumonia is diagnosed for protected-brush bronchoscopy concentrations of greater than 10^3 colony-forming units/ml and BAL concentrations of greater than 10^4 or 10^5 colony-forming units/ml. These samples may also be more useful in defining the specific pathogen. Unfortunately, these techniques can be limited by the invasiveness of the procedures, the lack of standardization for obtaining such samples, and the potential failure to diagnose pneumonia in the early stages when bacterial counts may be lower.

3. **Prophylaxis** of **VAP** is of paramount importance in decreasing morbidity and mortality in the ICU, and is discussed in Chapter 12.

4. **Treatment.** Often antibiotics must be initiated empirically until culture data are available. The clinical setting, including severity of illness, underlying and coexisting diseases, duration of hospitalization, and the local flora of the hospital influence the choice of antibiotics.

   a. **Uncomplicated mild to moderate disease** (i.e., without respiratory failure, hemodynamic instability, or signs of injury to other organs) occurring early during hospitalization (<5 days) is often treated with a single antibiotic such as a third- or fourth-generation cephalosporin, a carbapenem, or a fluoroquinolone in patients who are allergic to penicillins. Numerous studies suggest that **monotherapy** is safe and effective when used properly and may decrease the likelihood of infection due to antibiotic-resistant microorganisms. If anaerobes are a possibility, a β-lactam/β-lactamase inhibitor combination such as ampicillin/sulbactam or ticarcillin/clavulanate can be used as monotherapy. Alternatively, clindamycin or metronidazole may be used in combination with a β-lactam or fluoroquinolone for adequate anaerobic coverage.

   b. **Severe hospital-acquired pneumonia** (i.e., respiratory failure, hemodynamic instability, extrapulmonary organ damage) is treated with **combination therapy.** Combination therapy should also be considered when **mild to moderate pneumonia** occurs later in the hospitalization, occurs in patients with significant comorbidities, or occurs in patients with recent antibiotic exposure. These situations increase the likelihood that pneumonia is caused by *Pseudomonas aeruginosa,* other multiresistant enteric gram-negatives such as *Enterobacter* spp, *Klebsiella* spp, and/or methicillin-resistant *S. aureus* (MRSA). Generally, combination therapy includes any empiric monotherapy agent mentioned previously plus a fluoroquinolone or an aminoglycoside. Linezolid or vancomycin should be added if there is a possibility of MRSA pneumonia.

C. **Lung abscess** results from destruction of the pulmonary parenchyma leading to large, fluid-filled cavities. The most frequent predisposing factor for lung abscess is **aspiration pneumonia,** followed by periodontal disease and gingivitis. Bronchiectasis, pulmonary infarction, septic embolization, and bacteremia also predispose to lung abscess.

1. **Microbiology.** Bacteria causing aspiration pneumonia and subsequent abscess formation differ depending on whether aspiration occurs as an outpatient or as an inpatient. Hospital-acquired aspiration pneumonia is caused by anaerobes, gram-positive bacteria such as *S. aureus,* and gram-negative bacteria such as *Pseudomonas aeruginosa* and *Klebsiella pneumoniae.* Abscesses resulting from hematogenous spread of infection are usually peripheral and multifocal and are most commonly caused by *S. aureus.* Anaerobes and gram-negative bacteria also cause abscesses in this setting. *Mycobacterium tuberculosis, Nocardia,* amebas, and fungi are less frequent causes of lung abscess.

2. **Diagnosis** of lung abscess may be made based on chest radiograph or chest computed tomography (CT). Cultures of expectorated sputum are unreliable. Samples should be collected using protected-brush bronchoscopy or BAL.

3. **Treatment.** Prolonged (2–4 months) antibiotic therapy is the primary treatment for lung abscess. Antibiotic choices will depend on culture isolates. Postural drainage is an important aspect of the management, and bronchoscopy can be helpful in facilitating drainage or removing foreign bodies. Occasionally, a lung abscess is treated with surgical resection; however, this is not a first-line therapy. Complications of lung abscess include empyema, bronchopleural fistula formation, and bronchiectasis.

D. **Empyema** usually originates from intrapulmonary infection such as lung abscess or pneumonia, but also can be introduced from extrapulmonary sites as in trauma or thoracic surgery.

1. **Microbiology.** The most common bacterial cause of empyema is *S. aureus.* Enteric and nonenteric gram-negative bacteria, gram-positive bacteria, anaerobic bacteria, fungi, and *Mycobacterium tuberculosis* also can cause empyema.

2. **Diagnosis** requires direct analysis of pleural fluid for pH, total protein, red blood cell (RBC), and leukocyte (white blood cell [WBC]) count and differential, Gram's-stained and bacterial cultures (anaerobic and aerobic) and possibly fungal smear and culture. Smears and cultures for acid-fast bacilli should be performed if *Mycobacterium tuberculosis* is suspected.

3. **Treatment.** Empyema is treated with a combination of antibiotics and drainage via a thoracoscopy tube. Occasionally, open drainage or decortication of the empyema sac may be required.

E. Mediastinitis can result from spontaneous perforation of the esophagus, leakage from an esophageal anastomosis, trauma, cardiothoracic surgery, head and neck infections, and dental procedures.

1. Microbiology. Mediastinitis following cardiothoracic surgery that does not involve the esophagus is generally monomicrobial and is most often due to gram-positive bacteria, although gram-negative bacteria and fungi also cause mediastinitis. Mediastinitis arising from infections in the head and neck or disruption of the esophagus is usually polymicrobial and is caused by mixed anaerobic bacteria (*Peptococcus* spp, *Peptostreptococcus* spp, *Fusobacterium* spp, and *Bacteroides* spp), gram-positive bacteria, enteric and nonenteric gram-negative bacteria, and fungi (*Candida albicans, Candida glabrata*).

2. Diagnosis. Chest pain may be a presenting symptom. Other manifestations include fever and other systemic signs, crepitus and edema of the head and neck, and sepsis. Widening of the mediastinum, pleural effusion, and subcutaneous or mediastinal emphysema may be evident on chest radiograph and chest CT.

3. Treatment must be initiated rapidly, in most cases with a combination of antibiotics and surgical intervention, including drainage, debridement, and removal or repair of the source of infection. In some situations, contained rupture or small perforations of the esophagus can be treated medically. Broad empiric antibiotic coverage should be employed initially. Antibiotics should then be adjusted based on results of intraoperative cultures. Coverage for head and neck sources (including esophageal disruption) should include anaerobes, gram-positive aerobes, gram-negative aerobes, and facultative anaerobes. Combination therapy with penicillin G or clindamycin plus agents against gram-negatives (such as a third-generation cephalosporin or a fluoroquinolone) is effective. Metronidazole will also provide adequate anaerobic coverage. Broadly active β-lactams such as ticarcillin/clavulanate or carbapenems such as imipenem/cilastatin or meropenem also offer reasonable early coverage. Empiric coverage for postsurgical mediastinitis should include an antistaphylococcal agent such as nafcillin or vancomycin (for MRSA or for patients who are allergic to penicillin).

F. Zoonotic pneumonias (including the severe acute respiratory syndrome [**SARS**]) are pneumonias whose etiologic agents have nonhuman reservoirs. These pneumonias are rare, and presumptive diagnoses are generally made by contact history.

1. Microbiology. Bacteria responsible for zoonotic pneumonias include *Chlamydia psittaci,* which causes psittacosis (from contact with parrots and their relatives), *Coxiella burnetii,* which causes Q-fever (from sheep and parturient cats), and *Francisella tularensis,* which causes tularemia (from rabbit, deer, or deerfly bites). **Viral** causes of zoonotic pneumonias include the SARS-associated coronavirus (SARS-CoV), the purported etiologic agent of **SARS.** The prognosis for zoonotic infection is generally good with the exceptions of Q-fever, which can be complicated by subacute bacterial endocarditis, and SARS, which is often fatal.

2. **Diagnosis.** Because zoonotic agents are difficult (and often dangerous) to grow, diagnosis is often made through serologic testing. SARS may be diagnosed by either viral isolation or SARS-specific serologic testing. Additional serologic tests should be performed to exclude influenza A as well as *Legionella* spp and *Francisella tularensis,* which can mimic the influenza-like presentation of SARS.

3. **Treatment**
    a. **Bacterial zoonotic infections.** Extended therapy (2–5 weeks) with either doxycycline or a fluoroquinolone is recommended for zoonotic bacterial infections.
    b. **SARS.** Options are limited and treatment is generally supportive. Antiviral therapies are limited because there are no recommended antiviral agents with reliable anti–SARS-CoV activity. Ribavirin and oseltamivir have been used with limited success. Some studies suggest that corticosteroids and interferons may be beneficial.

G. **Bioterror agents** represent a group of bacterial and viral pathogens that can cause severe pneumonias and other potentially life-threatening syndromes in large populations. Known or suspected agents that cause acute pneumonias in this category include **inhalational anthrax, tularemia pneumonia,** and **pneumonic plague.**

1. Prognosis for disease caused by these agents is generally related to the size of the inhaled inoculum, host comorbidities, and the rapidity of initiating antimicrobial therapy.

2. **Microbiology.** Inhalational anthrax results from inhalation of the spores of *Bacillus anthracis,* a naturally occurring gram-positive bacillus. Tularemia pneumonia is caused by *Francisella tularensis,* which finds its natural home in rabbit and deer species. Pneumonic plague is caused by *Yersinia pestis,* which has the potential for person-to-person spread.

3. **Diagnosis.** Inhalational anthrax is typically biphasic in its presentation, with an initial and resolving influenza-like prodrome followed by bacteremia and rapid deterioration. Definitive diagnosis is made by culturing *Bacillus anthracis* from blood, pleural fluid, or cerebrospinal fluid (CSF). Tularemia pneumonia is confirmed by serology of respiratory

fluid or blood and will appear as gram-negative rods on staining. Pneumonic plague caused by *Yersinia pestis* may appear similar to tularemia pneumonia clinically, but is distinguishable by both serology and the presence of bipolar-staining gram-negative bacilli in *Yersinia pestis*–affected sputum.

4. **Treatment.** *B. anthracis* is highly susceptible to the majority of antibiotics, and penicillins have traditionally been the mainstay of therapy. *Francisella tularensis* and *Yersinia pestis* have both traditionally been treated with streptomycin. However, given concern for potential antibiotic resistance in modified or manipulated agents and the potential that there has been exposure to one or more agent, empiric therapy with doxycycline or a fluoroquinolone should be considered while awaiting results of cultures and other diagnostic tests.

II. **Intraabdominal infections** usually arise from sources within the gastrointestinal (GI) tract. Infection can also result from contiguous spread from the urogenital/reproductive tract or hematogenous or lymphatic spread, and can be introduced from the outside (as occurs with trauma or surgery). Infections are often polymicrobial and include enteric gram-negative rods (*E. coli, Klebsiella* spp, *Enterobacter* spp, and *Proteus* spp), *Pseudomonas aeruginosa,* aerobic gram-positive cocci (*Enterococcus* spp and *Streptococcus* spp), and gram-positive and gram-negative anaerobes (*Clostridium* spp, *Bacteroides* spp, *Fusobacterium* spp, and *Peptostreptococcus* spp). Management of intraabdominal infection depends on the cause and the site(s).

A. **Microflora of abdomen and pelvis**

1. **GI tract.** Normally, concentrations of bacteria increase progressively from the stomach through the small bowel and colon. Bacteria in the stomach and proximal small bowel include *Streptococcus* spp and *Lactobacillus* spp as well as anaerobes such as *Peptostreptococcus* spp but generally not *Bacteroides* spp. The concentrations of enteric gram-negative rods such as *E. coli* and anaerobic gram-negatives such as *Bacteroides* spp increase progressively in the distal small bowel and colon. Colonic bacteria include enteric gram-negative rods, gram-positive bacteria such as *Enterococcus* and *Lactobacillus,* and anaerobes such as *Bacteroides* spp, *Clostridium* spp, and *Peptostreptococcus* spp. Many factors alter either the quantity or the quality of the GI microflora, resulting in increases in the concentration as well as a shift in the spectrum of bacteria to include antibiotic-resistant bacteria, including nonenteric strains such as *Pseudomonas aeruginosa.* Such factors include the following:

a. pH (antacids, histamine-2 blockers).

b. Antibiotics.

c. GI dysmotility.

  d. Small-bowel obstruction, ileus, regional enteritis.
  e. Bowel resection or intestinal bypass procedures.
  f. Hospitalization or residence in a chronic nursing facility prior to developing infection.
 2. Genital tract microflora include gram-positive aerobic bacteria such as *Streptococcus* spp, *Lactobacillus* spp, and *Staphylococcus* spp as well as anaerobic bacteria such as *Peptostreptococcus* spp, *Clostridium* spp, and *Bacteroides* spp.
B. Peritonitis. Peritoneal infections can occur spontaneously, can result from perforation of an abdominal viscus, or can be introduced from the outside (as with trauma or the presence of foreign bodies such as peritoneal dialysis catheters).
 1. Spontaneous bacterial peritonitis (SBP) occurs in susceptible individuals, including those with ascites from chronic liver disease or congestive heart failure, and is believed to result from hematogenous or lymphatic spread or translocation of bacteria across the bowel wall. Symptoms/signs of SBP include fever, abdominal pain, GI dysmotility, worsening liver function/hepatic encephalopathy, and renal failure. However, patients with SBP may be asymptomatic or have only minor symptoms.
  a. Microorganisms. Generally SBP is caused by a single organism. Enteric gram-negatives followed by nonenterococcal streptococci are most common. SBP is sometimes caused by enterococci. Anaerobes rarely cause SBP. The presence of anaerobic bacteria or mixed flora suggests the possibility of secondary peritonitis.
  b. Diagnosis. A diagnostic paracentesis should be performed prior to the administration of antibiotics if SBP is suspected. Ascites fluid should, at minimum, be sent for cell counts and Gram's stain and culture. A polymorphonuclear leukocyte (PMN) count of greater than 250 is highly suggestive of SBP. If the ascites fluid is hemorrhagic, the PMN count should be adjusted based on the RBC count. Cultures of ascites fluid are often negative despite a cell count that is consistent with SBP. Use of blood culture bottles (anaerobic and aerobic) to culture ascites fluid may increase the likelihood of detecting the bacteria. Blood cultures should also be obtained.
  c. Treatment. Empiric antibiotic therapy should be initiated prior to obtaining the results of cultures if the ascites fluid PMN counts are greater than 250 cells/mm^3 (adjusted for RBC counts). Antibiotics should be modified appropriately when culture and sensitivity data become available. Potential empiric regimens include the following:
   i. Cefotaxime is the primary regimen for SBP. High doses (2 g IV every 4 hours) are used for life-threatening SBP.

      ii. A β-lactam/β-lactamase inhibitor combination, such as ampicillin/sulbactam, piperacillin/taxobactam, or ticarcillin/clavulanate.

      iii. Ceftriaxone.

      iv. Ertapenem.

      v. If resistant enteric gram-negatives are a possibility, imipenem or meropenem, or a fluoroquinolone should be considered

2. Secondary peritonitis usually results from perforation or necrosis of a solid viscus or suppurative infections of the biliary and female reproductive tracts.

  a. Diagnosis is often made with assistance of plain abdominal radiograph films and scans (e.g., CT, magnetic resonance [MR] imaging, ultrasonography). Exploratory laparotomy may be necessary to diagnose and treat the source of peritonitis.

  b. Treatment requires identification and control of the source of infection. Treatment usually involves a combination of surgery or placement of drainage catheters and broad-spectrum antibiotics that are active against gram-negative and gram-positive bacteria and anaerobes. Knowledge of local resistance patterns should influence the ultimate choice of empiric antibiotics.

    i. Peritonitis that occurs very early in the hospitalization and **without recent antibiotic therapy** in patients who are not in chronic care facilities is unlikely to result from antibiotic-resistant bacteria. Potential regimens include the following:

      (a) A β-lactam/β-lactamase inhibitor such as ampicillin/sulbactam.

      (b) A third-generation cephalosporin (ceftriaxone, cefotaxime) plus an anti-anaerobe (clindamycin or metronidazole).

      (c) A carbapenem.

      (d) Fluoroquinolone plus an anti-anaerobe (clindamycin, metronidazole).

      (e) The traditional "triple-antibiotic" regimen of ampicillin, gentamicin, and metronidazole.

      (f) Ampicillin, levofloxacin, metronidazole.

    ii. Peritonitis that develops during hospitalization or residence in a chronic nursing facility or in the context of recent therapy with antibacterial agents may be caused by antibiotic-resistant microorganisms.

      (a) Monotherapy with a carbapenem (imipenem/cilastatin or meropenem).

      (b) A third- or fourth-generation cephalosporin (ceftazidime or cefepime if *Pseudomonas* spp are suspected) plus an anti-anaerobe. Consider adding a fluoro-quinolone if infection with *Pseudomonas* spp or *Enterobacter* spp is suspected. If ceftazidime is used, an additional agent with gram-positive coverage should be added.

(c) An anti-anaerobe with coverage of aerobic gram-positives (clindamycin) and a fluoro-quinolone may be useful in patients who are allergic to β-lactams or if infection with *Pseudomonas* spp is suspected.

(d) Vancomycin or linezolid should be added to each of the aforementioned regimens if infection with MRSA is a possibility.

C. **Intraabdominal abscess** may result from persistence of bacteria after secondary peritonitis or hematogenous spread of extraabdominal infection. Abscesses can cause fever, peritonitis, sepsis, and multiple-organ dysfunction syndrome.

1. **Microorganisms** commonly cultured from abscesses include *Bacteroides* spp (especially *Bacteroides fragilis*), gram-negative and gram-positive bacteria such as *Enterococcus* spp, and *S. aureus.*

2. **Diagnosis.** Computed tomography is useful for diagnosing and localizing abscesses. Ultrasonography can be done at the bedside, and can be particularly useful in diagnosis of right upper quadrant, renal, and pelvic abscesses. Indium-labeled WBC and gallium scans are occasionally useful in localizing abscesses but have low specificity and must be followed up with more definitive tests. Rarely, exploratory laparotomy must be performed for diagnosis.

3. **Treatment** of intraabdominal abscess includes drainage and antibiotics. The method of drainage (percutaneous under CT or ultrasound guidance versus operative) depends on a variety of factors including the abscess location, whether the abscess is associated with perforation or gangrene, and the presence of loculations that make drainage with a single catheter unlikely. Often culture data are available to guide antibiotic selection. For initial empiric coverage, it is reasonable use one of the combinations suggested previously for treating secondary peritonitis in hospitalized patients. Ceftazidime or cefepime may be favored over ceftriaxone because they have better activity against *Pseudomonas aeruginosa.*

D. **Infections of the hepatobiliary system**

1. **Acute cholecystitis** results from biliary tract obstruction or instrumentation of the biliary tract and involves the gall bladder (GB) and cystic duct.

a. **Complications** include GB perforation with subsequent peritonitis, empyema of the GB from cystic duct obstruction, emphysematous cholecystitis, and empyema of the GB, which can cause gram-negative sepsis.

b. Microbiology. Bacteria include enteric gram-negative bacteria such as *E. coli, Klebsiella* spp, *Proteus* spp, and *Enterobacter* spp, gram-positive bacteria such as *Enterococcus* spp, and anaerobes such as *Clostridium* spp and *Bacteroides* spp. Emphysematous cholecystitis is caused by *Clostridium* spp and gram-negative bacteria.

c. Diagnosis. Abdominal ultrasonography may reveal gallstones, thickening of the GB wall, a dilated gallbladder, or a pericholecystic fluid collection.

d. Treatment includes antibiotics and surgery. The timing of surgery depends on a number of factors. Surgery is often performed on an urgent basis when the more severe complications of acute cholecystitis as just described occur. Surgery may be delayed for stabilization of the patient or for preparation of the patient with serious medical conditions. Cholecystitis can be treated with the antibiotic regimens previously described for secondary peritonitis.

2. Cholangitis is usually caused by partial or complete common bile duct (CBD) obstruction.

a. Diagnosis. The classic presentation is jaundice, fevers, chills, and biliary colic. Blood cultures are often positive.

b. Treatment differs depending on whether there is partial or complete CBD obstruction. **Nonsuppurative cholangitis,** which results from partial CBD obstruction, will often respond to antibiotic therapy. **Suppurative cholangitis,** which is due to complete CBD obstruction causing pus under pressure, bacteremia, and septic shock, must be treated as early as possible with a combination of antibiotics and surgical or endoscopic decompression. Cholangitis can be treated with the antibiotic regimens described previously for secondary peritonitis.

3. Liver abscess. Abscesses can be solitary or multiple. Manifestations range from fever with leukocytosis and right upper quadrant pain to sepsis. Liver abscesses can result from local or hematogenous spread of infection. The most common local source is the biliary system.

a. Microbiology. The organisms depend on the source.

   i. Biliary tract: gram-negative bacteria and *Enterococcus* spp.

   ii. Peritoneal infections: gram-positive and gram-negative bacteria and anaerobes.

   iii. Hematogenous spread: generally a single organism such as *S. aureus* or *Streptococcus* spp. Candidal abscesses also occur.

b. Diagnosis is generally made by CT scan or ultrasonography.

    c. Treatment includes drainage and antibiotics. The initial antibiotic choice depends on the origin of the infection. Abscess arising from the biliary tract or peritoneum should be treated with antibiotics directed against the organisms involved in the initial infection. Abscess resulting from hematogenous spread should be treated with agents active against gram-positive bacteria.

E. Splenic abscess is rare, but has high mortality if left untreated. It usually results from hematogenous spread, but can result from splenic trauma or contiguous spread. The diagnosis of splenic abscess should prompt a search for **bacterial endocarditis** as the source.

    1. Microbiology. The most common organisms isolated on culture are *Streptococcus* spp followed by *S. aureus. Salmonella* spp and, rarely, anaerobic bacteria also cause splenic abscess.

    2. The **diagnosis** is suggested by left upper quadrant pain, fever, leukocytosis, and a left-sided pleural effusion.

    3. Treatment. Splenic abscess is usually treated with splenectomy and antibiotics.

F. Pseudomembranous or ***Clostridium difficile (C. difficile)* colitis** occurs as a complication of antibiotic therapy and is caused by overgrowth of *C. difficile,* an anaerobic, gram-positive, spore-forming bacillus that produces toxins that damage the bowel wall. The carrier rate is 3% in the general population and 20% in patients treated with antibiotics. Although clindamycin, cephalosporins, and ampicillin are the most frequent offenders, almost all antibiotics have been implicated, including vancomycin and metronidazole. Antibiotics alter the normal flora, providing an environment for the conversion of *C. difficile* spores to vegetative forms leading to rapid replication and toxin production. Epidemic outbreaks can occur because of environmental contamination, transmission by health care workers, and oral–fecal spread. **Manifestations** include watery and/or bloody diarrhea, abdominal cramps, toxic megacolon, perforation of the bowel, and peritonitis. Leukocytosis can be marked, sometimes in excess of 50,000 cells/μl.

    1. Diagnosis. Stool examination may reveal leukocytes, red blood cells, and *C. difficile* toxin. Stool cultures for *C. difficile* are not helpful. Sigmoidoscopy with visualization of "pseudomembranes" can be helpful in making the diagnosis.

    2. Treatment. *C. difficile* colitis is treated with metronidazole (preferably enteral if able) or enteral vancomycin and, if possible, with discontinuation of causative antibiotic(s). IV vancomycin is not effective. Unless contraindicated, therapy should begin with metronidazole to decrease the selection pressure for vancomycin-resistant gram-positive bacteria. Treatment with intravenous metronidazole is used when patients are unable receive treatment via the enteral route. Generally, treatment is continued for 10 to 14 days, although some practitioners favor continuing treatment until antibacterial agents are discontinued. Suggested enteral doses are as follows:

a. Metronidazole 250 mg orally every 6 hours or 500 mg every 8 hours.

b. Vancomycin 125 to 500 mg orally every 6 hours.

III. **Wound infections.** Multiple factors influence the development and severity of wound infections. The incidence of postoperative wound infection due to antibiotic-resistant bacteria increases with the length of hospitalization prior to surgery. Prophylactic measures are effective in preventing wound infections.

A. **Classification of surgical wounds**

1. **Clean.** No entry into internal organs that harbor bacteria.

2. **Clean-contaminated.** Organs are entered in elective surgery without spillage of contents.

3. **Contaminated.** Spillage of organ contents occurs without formation of pus.

4. **Dirty.** Spillage of contents occurs with pus formation.

B. **Microbiology.** Microorganisms reflect the site of origin and are altered by recent treatment with antibiotics, prolonged preoperative hospitalization, and coexisting diseases. **Clean surgical wound infections** are most often caused by *S. aureus,* coagulase-negative *Staphylococcus,* and *Streptococcus* spp. Severe wound infections that occur in the first 48 hours after surgery may be caused by *Clostridium* or group A streptococcus (*Streptococcus pyogenes*). Infections of **contaminated wounds** will reflect the origin of contamination (respiratory, GI, or genitourinary [GU] tract).

C. **Clinical presentation and diagnosis.** Wound infections vary in severity from superficial infections of the skin and subcutaneous tissues to deep and severe infections involving the underlying fascia and/or muscles. Superficial wound infections are most frequently manifested by erythema, warmth, and swelling. Fever is variably present.

D. **Prevention.** Detection and treatment of infection at other sites, limiting the duration of hospitalization before surgery, proper surgical technique, and proper preoperative scrubbing of the patient and the surgical team are important measures. Whereas recommendations vary for clean procedures that do not involve placement of foreign material, **prophylactic antibiotics** are routinely administered for clean procedures involving placement of foreign material and for all procedures that enter, or are complicated by spillage from, internal organs. Prophylactic antibiotics should be given within the 30 minutes prior to incision, and for clean or clean-contaminated operations should be discontinued within 24 hours of surgery to minimize the risk of colonization with antibiotic-resistant organisms. Longer courses of antibiotics are generally given for contaminated or dirty wounds. Choices of prophylactic antibiotics are guided by site and type of surgery, duration of hospitalization prior to surgery, and recent use of antibiotics. Many institutions have established specific guidelines for prophylactic antibiotics.

E. **Treatment**

1. **Mild superficial wound infections** may be treated with removal of sutures or staples and opening of the wound to drain fluid collections.

2. **Severe wound infections** are usually treated with a combination of parenteral antibiotics and surgical debridement. Cultures of fluid or tissue collected in a sterile fashion should be used to guide antimicrobial therapy. Initial empiric antibiotic coverage will be dictated by the setting. First-generation cephalosporins offer reasonable coverage for uncomplicated postoperative wound infections. Clindamycin is an alternative in patients allergic to β-lactams. Vancomycin, linezolid, or daptomycin should be reserved for cases where there is a reasonable possibility that the infection is caused by MRSA. Gram-negative coverage should be considered for infections originating in the GI, GU, and respiratory tracts.

F. **Necrotizing soft tissue infections. Necrotizing fasciitis** and **myonecrosis** (clostridial and nonclostridial) are life-threatening deep infections that involve the fascia and subcutaneous tissue (necrotizing fasciitis) and muscle (myonecrosis). These infections have the propensity to spread rapidly and cause severe systemic toxicity early in the course of infection. The mortality due to necrotizing soft tissue infections is high, particularly if there are delays in surgical or medical intervention.

1. **Microbiology**

a. **Necrotizing fasciitis.** *Streptococcus* spp are most commonly isolated from wound cultures. Polymicrobial infections with anaerobes, enteric gram-negatives, and *Streptococcus* spp also occur.

b. **Myonecrosis.** Clostridial myonecrosis (gas gangrene) is a severe, fulminant skeletal muscle infection caused by *Clostridium* spp. Exotoxins released by bacteria are important in the pathogenesis of clostridial myonecrosis. Nonclostridial myonecrosis is generally polymicrobial due to *Streptococcus* spp, enteric gram-negative rods (*E. coli, Klebsiella pneumoniae, Enterobacter* spp, etc.), and anaerobic bacteria.

2. **Diagnosis.** Early features include pain out of proportion to the local external findings and systemic

toxicity. Crepitus may be present due to gas in soft tissues.

3. **Treatment**

a. **Debridement.** Immediate recognition and prompt surgical exploration and debridement are critical. Frequent surveillance of the wound is essential, and repeated surgical debridement is often necessary.

b. **Antibiotics** are chosen based on the presentation and the likely source of infection. Gram's stain of intraoperative wound samples can guide initial therapy. Empiric therapy should be broad and include coverage of *Streptococcus* spp and *Staphylococcus* spp, enteric gram-negative bacteria, and anaerobes. Because clindamycin is a bacterial protein synthesis inhibitor, some practitioners add clindamycin to regimens for treatment of suspected exotoxin-producing necrotizing soft-tissue infections to attempt to reduce exotoxin production.

c. The role of **hyperbaric oxygen** for necrotizing soft tissue infections caused by anaerobic bacteria is not clear.

IV. **Urinary tract infections.** The range of severity of urinary tract infections (UTIs) varies from urethritis and cystitis, which are often treated in the outpatient setting, to pyelonephritis and renal or perinephric abscess, which can produce septic shock. Urinary tract infections are the most common nosocomial infection, and cause up to 30% of gram-negative bacteremias in hospitalized patients. Fungal urinary tract infections are discussed in section **VIII.**

A. **Predisposing factors.** Indwelling urinary catheters, neurologic or structural abnormalities of the urinary tract. and nephrolithiasis. **Prophylaxis** of UTIs in the ICU is discussed in Chapter 12.

B. **Microbiology.** Bacteria usually enter the urinary tract via the urethra and spread to more proximal segments. Thus the same microorganisms tend to cause both upper and lower urinary tract infections. Occasionally, hematogenous seeding (especially with *S. aureus*) or spread from contiguous peritoneal infection can result in upper urinary tract infections (especially perinephric and renal abscesses). The most common organisms cultured from the urine are gram-negative rods, including *E. coli, Klebsiella* spp, *Proteus* spp, and sometimes *Enterobacter* spp. *Serratia* spp and *Pseudomonas* spp are additional causes of catheter-related infections. Gram-positive organisms, including *Staphylococcus saprophyticus, Enterococcus* spp, and *S. aureus,* are sometimes involved. Urethritis can also be caused by *Chlamydia trachomatis, Neisseria gonorrhoeae, Trichomonas, Candida* spp, and herpes simplex virus (HSV).

C. **Diagnosis.** Analysis of the urinary sediment for leukocytes in conjunction with urine cultures can be useful in distinguishing colonization from true infection. The urinary sediment is also helpful in determining whether the infection is in the upper or the lower urinary tract. White blood cell casts suggest that infection involves the kidneys or tubules. Urine cultures are essential for guiding antimicrobial therapy.

D. **Specific urinary tract infections**

1. **Cystitis** is infection of the bladder characterized by dysuria and frequency, cloudy or bloody urine, and localized tenderness of the urethra and suprapubic regions. More severe symptoms such as high fever, nausea, and vomiting suggest renal involvement.

2. **Acute pyelonephritis** is a pyogenic infection of the renal parenchyma and pelvis. It is characterized by costophrenic angle tenderness, high fevers, shaking chills, nausea, vomiting, and diarrhea. Laboratory analysis reveals leukocytosis, pyuria with leukocyte casts, and occasional hematuria. Bacteria are often visible on Gram's stain of unspun urine. Evaluation of the urinary tract should be considered because a significant proportion of pyelonephritis is associated with structural abnormalities. Treatment includes antibiotics and removal or correction of the source. Complications include papillary necrosis, impaired urine-concentrating ability, urinary obstruction, and sepsis.

3. **Renal and perinephric abscesses** are uncommon and usually are due to ascending infection from the bladder and ureters. Major risk factors include nephrolithiasis, structural urinary tract abnormalities, urologic trauma or surgery, and diabetes mellitus. Most common isolates are *E. coli, Klebsiella* spp, and *Proteus* spp. *Candida* spp may also cause renal and perinephric abscesses. Renal and perinephric abscesses may present nonspecifically with fever, leukocytosis, and pain (flank, groin, abdomen). Urine cultures may be negative, particularly if the patient has already received antibiotics. Diagnosis can be made by abdominal ultrasound or CT scan. Treatment is drainage and antibiotics.

4. **Prostatitis** is an infrequent infection in the ICU that can occur as a result of bladder catheterization. Symptoms and signs include fevers, chills, dysuria, and an enlarged, tender, and boggy prostate. Treatment includes antibiotics and, if possible, removal of the urinary catheter.

E. **Treatment of urinary tract infections.** Prior to receiving culture results, empiric broad therapy should be initiated that cover likely organisms. Fluoroquinolones or third- or fourth-generation cephalosporins are often used. Ceftazidime or cefepime may be selected if infection with *Pseudomonas* spp is likely. If *Enterococcus* spp is suspected, broader coverage may be obtained with ampicillin plus an aminoglycoside. Rarely, imipenem/cilastatin is used for infections that are caused by antibiotic-resistant bacteria.

V. Intravascular catheter-related infections can be localized to the site of insertion (site infections) or can be disseminated (catheter-related bloodstream infections). Catheters in the central circulation (central venous and pulmonary artery) are responsible for most catheter-related infections. **Risk factors** for catheter-related bloodstream infections (BSI) include total parenteral nutrition **(TPN),** which increases the risk of fungal infections, and prolonged catheterization. **Fever** is the most common presenting feature, and localized signs of infection at the insertion site are often absent. Site infections or unexplained fever should prompt assessment for line infection.

A. Microbiology. The most common pathogens are coagulase-negative *Staphylococcus* followed by *S. aureus*. A variety of gram-negative and other gram-positive bacteria also cause catheter-related infections. *Candida* spp account for close to 10% of catheter-related BSI.

B. Prevention of catheter-related infections is discussed in detail in Chapter 12.

    1. Strict sterile technique during placement and care of catheters is the most important factor in preventing catheter-related infections.

    2. Skin antisepsis. Two percent chlorhexidine has been shown to be superior to 10% povidone-iodine or 70% ethanol in preventing catheter-related BSI.

    3. Antibiotic-impregnated catheters have been shown to reduce the rates of catheter-related BSI.

C. Management

    1. Catheter removal. Institutional practices for management of suspected catheter-related infections vary. Some institutions/intensive care units favor replacement of catheters at a fresh site if catheter-related infection is a possibility. Others routinely change catheters over a guidewire and perform quantitative cultures. When the line has been changed over a guidewire, if blood or quantitative tip cultures are positive, the rewired catheter is removed and a new line is placed at a fresh site. A strong suspicion that the catheter is the source of fever or septic complications should prompt a change in site and, at a minimum, blood cultures.

    2. Antibiotics. The choice of antibiotics is dictated by the clinical situation and culture data. Empiric therapy often is started with vancomycin if there are systemic signs of infection or if preliminary blood culture results indicate gram-positive bacteremia. Often an additional agent is added to cover gram-negatives or for synergistic coverage of *Enterococcus* spp. Further therapy should be tailored to the specific organism identified. For uncomplicated catheter-related bacteremia, antibiotics are generally continued for

7 to 14 days (14 days if *S. aureus* is isolated from the blood). Fungal infections are treated for a longer time, particularly in immunocompromised hosts.

VI. Infective endocarditis (IE). Infective endocarditis is caused by microbial invasion of the endocardium. IE most commonly involves the cardiac valves, but can also occur in the septal or mural myocardium. IE can involve native valves **(native valve endocarditis [NVE])** and prosthetic valves **(prosthetic valve endocarditis [PVE]).** PVE that occurs within 2 months of valve replacement (early PVE) results from colonization of the valve by microbes at the time of surgery and most commonly is caused by *Staphylococcus* spp. Late PVE is similar to NVE. Microorganisms gain entry into the bloodstream via direct inoculation during procedures (GI, GU, and dental procedures, bronchoscopy, endotracheal intubation) or from a focus of existing infection such as pneumonia or dental abscess. **Acute IE** is characterized by abrupt onset and rapid progression. **Subacute IE** is characterized by insidious onset and slower progression.

A. Predisposing factors include abnormalities of the heart (such as those due to rheumatic heart disease and degenerative valvular lesions) and IV drug abuse. Endocarditis can occur in previously normal hearts. Intravascular devices such as central venous catheters, pacemaker wires, hemodialysis shunts, and prosthetic valves increase the chance of developing IE.

B. Microbiology. IE is most commonly caused by bacteria, but can be caused by fungi, viruses, and rickettsiae.

   1. Gram-positive bacteria. *Streptococcus* spp are the most common pathogens, particularly the viridans group (such as *sanguis, mutans,* and *intermedius*). *Enterococcus* spp also cause endocarditis, particularly in elderly patients who have undergone GU procedures and in IV-drug abusers. *Staphylococcus* spp, particularly *S. aureus,* often cause IE. *S. aureus* endocarditis is often severe and is more commonly complicated by myocardial and valve ring abscesses, emboli, and metastatic lesions (such as lung, CNS, and splenic abscess). Identification of *Streptococcus bovis* as the causative organism should prompt a workup for a GI source such as colon cancer.

   2. Gram-negative bacteria infrequently cause infective endocarditis. IV-drug abusers and patients with prosthetic valves are more susceptible. IE due to gram-negative bacteria is often severe and has an abrupt onset and high mortality. A characteristic NVE of abnormal valves is caused by a group of bacteria collectively called HACEK group bacteria (*Haemophilus* spp, *Actinobaccillus actinomycetemcomitans, Cardiobacterium hominis, Eikenella corrodens,* and *Kingella* spp) and is characterized by a subacute course, large vegetations, and frequent embolic events.

C. Diagnosis

1. **Physical examination** may reveal a heart murmur, petechiae, nail-bed splinter hemorrhages, retinal hemorrhages (Roth's spots), red or purple nodules on digital pads (Osler's nodes), and flat red lesions on the palms or soles (Janeway lesions).

2. **Blood cultures** are moderately sensitive for IE. Several (three or more) sets of blood cultures should be obtained within the first 24 hours if IE is suspected. Rarely, blood cultures are negative, particularly when IE is due to intracellular organisms such as rickettsiae, anaerobic bacteria, the HACEK group of bacteria, and fungi. Special media may be necessary to isolate the responsible microorganism.

3. **Echocardiography** is an important tool for diagnosing and managing IE. Transthoracic echocardiography (TTE) is far less sensitive than transesophageal echocardiography (TEE) for detecting vegetations, particularly in patients receiving mechanical ventilation. Echocardiography can be used to follow the progression of vegetations and to identify and follow complications such as valvular insufficiency, valve ring or myocardial abscesses, pericardial effusions, and heart failure.

D. Treatment

1. **Antibiotics.** Prolonged courses of bactericidal antibiotics are used to treat IE. For acute bacterial endocarditis, it may be necessary to begin antibiotics prior to definitive diagnosis. However, blood cultures should be obtained prior to the first dose of antibiotics.

   a. **Empiric therapy.** Sometimes treatment of subacute NVE is delayed until results of blood cultures are available.

      i. **Indications for empiric therapy**
         (a) Critically ill and strong suspicion of endocarditis.
         (b) Likely to have endocarditis and is to undergo cardiac surgery.
         (c) Positive blood cultures.
         (d) When the diagnosis seems certain (e.g., vegetations documented by echocardiography in the setting of fever and other clinical parameters consistent with IE).
         (e) Suspected of having PVE.

      ii. **Empiric initial therapy for acute NVE** should include agents that are active against *Streptococcus* spp, *Enterococcus* spp, and *Staphylococcus* spp. Potential regimens include the following:
         (a) Ampicillin or penicillin plus nafcillin plus aminoglycoside (gentamicin).

           (b) Vancomycin plus aminoglycoside (gentamicin). Enterococcal infection should be treated with a combination of ampicillin or vancomycin plus an aminoglycoside because ampicillin and vancomycin are only bacteriostatic for *Enterococcus* spp.

      iii. Empiric initial therapy for early or late PVE

           (a) Vancomycin plus aminoglycoside (gentamicin) plus rifampin.

  b. Subsequent antibiotic therapy should be based on blood culture data. Determinations of minimum inhibitory and bactericidal concentrations (MIC and MBC, respectively) are extremely important in deciding the optimal regimen. Blood cultures should be obtained during therapy to verify clearance of bacteremia. Failure to clear bacteremia may indicate abscess.

  2. Surgery. Valve replacement or valvulectomy (tricuspid) may be necessary. Indications for surgery vary depending on the valve, and include severe and refractory heart failure, valve obstruction, fungal endocarditis, prosthetic valve instability, and failure to clear bacteremia with appropriate antibiotic therapy. Surgery also may be indicated for recurrent IE, extension to the myocardium or paravalvular region, two or more embolic events, or periprosthetic leaks.

E. Complications of infective endocarditis

  1. Cardiac

    a. Valvular insufficiency and heart failure. Heart failure is the most common cause of death in patients with IE.

    b. Myocardial and paravalvular abscess.

    c. Heart block may result from extension of a paravalvular abscess.

    d. Obstruction. Rarely, large vegetations may cause obstruction, particularly when IE is caused by fungi.

    e. Purulent pericarditis occurs most commonly with IE due to *Staphylococcus* spp.

  2. Extracardiac

    a. Immune complex disease can damage distant organs such as the kidneys.

    b. Embolic events can lead to ischemia and infarction. Abscesses may occur at sites of embolization. Left-sided endocarditis predisposes to emboli to the kidneys, brain, spleen, and heart, whereas right-sided endocarditis predisposes to pulmonary emboli.

    c. Mycotic aneurysms result from local infection of the blood vessel with dilation of the vessel. Mycotic aneurysms in the CNS can present with catastrophic subarachnoid or intracerebral hemorrhage. Mycotic aneurysms can also occur outside of the CNS.

        d. Neurologic complications. Toxic encephalopathy, meningitis, cerebritis, brain abscess, stroke (infarction or hemorrhage), subarachnoid or intracerebral hemorrhage.

        e. Renal failure

        f. Sepsis

VII. Miscellaneous infections

    A. Sinusitis. Facial trauma and the presence of nasotracheal and/or nasogastric tubes predispose ICU patients to sinusitis.

        1. Microbiology. Sinusitis is usually caused by gram-negative bacteria, *S. aureus,* and anaerobes.

        2. Diagnosis can be difficult. Many experts recommend CT scans of the face and sinuses. Needle aspiration of the sinuses may provide helpful bacteriologic data, particularly in patients who have been hospitalized for prolonged periods and may be infected with antibiotic-resistant organisms.

        3. Treatment is often initiated based on the clinical constellation of fever of unclear etiology, presence of nasal tubes or history of head and neck trauma, and purulent nasal discharge. Treatment includes removal of nasal tubes to allow drainage of the obstructed sinus outflow tract, nasal humidification and decongestants, and antibiotics that target likely pathogens. Surgical drainage is rarely indicated.

    B. Central nervous system infections:

        1. Meningitis. Generally, infection is limited to the subarachnoid space and cerebral ventricles and does not involve the brain parenchyma, but occasionally meningitis is complicated by brain abscess. Bacterial meningitis may result from hematogenous seeding, direct invasion from trauma or surgery, or extension of infection from a contiguous structure such as rupture of a brain or epidural abscess into the subarachnoid space.

        a. Microbiology. Many organisms cause meningitis. Community-acquired pathogens include *Streptococcus pneumoniae, H. influenzae, Neisseria meningitidis,* and *Listeria monocytogenes.* Meningitis caused by enteric and nonenteric gram-negative bacteria and *S. aureus* may result from trauma, neurosurgery, or bacteremia. *S. aureus* meningitis may originate from infections at other sites such as pneumonia, sinusitis, and endocarditis. Meningitis associated with CSF shunts are most often caused by *Staphylococcus epidermidis.*

        b. Diagnosis. Collection of CSF for analysis of glucose, protein, cell count and differential, Gram's stain, and bacterial culture is essential. Other specialized tests of CSF, including test for cryptococcal antigen, the Venereal Disease Research Laboratory slide test, bacterial antigen tests, and fungal smear and culture, may be indicated depending on other patient factors such as immunocompromise. In patients suspected of having cerebral edema, a CT scan of the brain should be performed prior to the lumbar puncture. Blood cultures should be obtained prior to starting antibiotics.

c. **Treatment.** The choice of antibiotics will be determined by the clinical situation and the ability of various antibiotics to penetrate the CNS. Because host defenses are impaired in the CNS, bacterial meningitis must be treated with bactericidal antibiotics. Emergence of penicillin-resistant community-acquired pathogens has resulted in a shift in treatment to third-generation non-antipseudomonal cephalosporins such as ceftriaxone, which penetrates the CNS well. Vancomycin is often added if there is concern about resistance to β-lactam antibiotics. *Listeria monocytogenes* meningitis should be treated with penicillin G or ampicillin, or trimethoprim/sulfamethoxazole in penicillin-allergic patients, possibly in conjunction with an aminoglycoside. Meningitis caused by gram-negative bacteria is frequently treated with a third-generation cephalosporin. If *Psuedomonas aeruginosa* or other resistant gram-negative bacteria are suspected, ceftazidime, cefepime, or meropenem should be considered. Additional coverage should be added to ceftazidime if gram-positive infection is a possibility, and vancomycin should be considered if MRSA is a possibility. *S. aureus* meningitis is usually treated with nafcillin or vancomycin in penicillin-allergic patients or if MRSA is the pathogen.

2. **Paradural abscesses include epidural and subdural abscesses.** Epidural abscesses most frequently occur in the vertebral column, whereas subdural abscesses usually occur in the cranium. Paradural abscesses result from trauma, neurosurgery, invasion of the paradural space (such as with epidural catheter placement), local spread from contiguous structures (such as the paranasal sinuses or paravertebral region), and hematogenous spread from distant sites. Paradural abscess can rapidly progress and can cause considerable irreversible damage to underlying neural structures. Thus, rapid diagnosis and institution of therapy is essential. Drainage of the abscess is crucial for microbiologic diagnosis as well as for treatment.

a. **Microbiology.** Bacteria causing subdural abscesses reflect the source of infection. Infections may be caused by *Streptococcus pneumoniae, Staphylococcus* spp, *H. influenzae,* enteric gram-negatives, and anaerobes. *S. aureus* is the most common cause of epidural abscess. Enteric gram-negatives also cause epidural abscesses, particularly in patients with urinary tract infections or following vertebral surgery.

b. **Diagnosis.** Severe localized spinal pain is the most common presenting symptom of epidural abscess. Computed tomography scans are helpful in diagnosing and localizing subdural abscesses. Magnetic resonance imaging is the diagnostic test of choice for epidural abscesses. Computed tomography and myelography also can be helpful.

c. **Treatment** includes antibiotics and drainage. Initial antibiotic therapy should be based on likely pathogens for the situation and then modified based on results of cultures. *S. aureus* should be treated with nafcillin. Vancomycin or linezolid may be substituted in penicillin-allergic patients or if MRSA is the pathogen. Third- or fourth-generation cephalosporins (antipseudomonal if *Pseudomonas aeruginosa* is the pathogen) are often used for gram-negative infections.

VIII. **Fungal infections.** Fungi act as opportunistic or, less commonly, as virulent pathogens and cause a variety of different syndromes ranging from superficial mucocutaneous infection to systemic infection with visceral organ involvement.

A. *Candida*

1. *Candida* **spp** are the most common cause of opportunistic fungal infections in surgical and medical ICUs. The incidence of nosocomial candidal infections has increased dramatically, and *Candida* species are now among the most common organisms isolated from blood cultures.

2. **Risk factors** include treatment with broad-spectrum antibiotics, presence of indwelling devices (urinary, peritoneal, and intravascular), immunocompromise (HIV infection, transplantation, hematologic malignancy, chemotherapy, neutropenia, and burns) and total parenteral nutrition.

3. **Clinical manifestations**

a. **Candiduria** may be due to infection or may reflect colonization of an indwelling urinary catheter. Candiduria should raise concerns about possible fungal balls, pyelonephritis, or candidemia.

b. **Mucocutaneous infections** include oropharyngeal candidiasis, esophagitis, GI candidiasis, vulvovaginitis, and intertrigo.

c. **Candidemia** is characterized by positive blood cultures, and can be associated with dissemination to visceral organs. The mortality is very high, especially with *Candida glabrata*. Patients with positive blood cultures should be evaluated closely for indwelling vascular line and/or deep organ infection. Quantitative cultures of catheter tips can be performed.

d. Disseminated or invasive candidiasis. Deep organ infections can result from hematogenous spread, by direct extension from contiguous sites, or by local inoculation. Diagnosis can be difficult because blood cultures are frequently negative. Positive superficial cultures (e.g., urine, sputum, and wounds) may represent colonization or contamination, and diagnostic serologic tests are not available. A high level of suspicion must be maintained in patients with the risk factors described previously. Definitive criteria for disseminated infection include positive cultures from the infected tissue or peritoneal fluid, actual invasion (histologically) of burn wounds, and endophthalmitis. Suggestive criteria include two positive blood cultures at least 24 hours apart, with one positive culture drawn at least 24 hours after the removal of vascular cannulae and, in the right population, three or more colonized sites.

   i. Hepatosplenic candidiasis is most common in patients with hematologic malignancy. The diagnosis is suggested by right upper quadrant pain, persistent fevers, elevated alkaline phosphatase, and multiple "bull's eye" lesions on abdominal ultrasonography or CT scan, although the liver may also appear homogeneous in these studies. Diagnosis can be confirmed by histologic analysis of a liver biopsy.

   ii. Candidal peritonitis results from perforation of the intestines or stomach or infection of a peritoneal dialysis catheter.

   iii. Cardiac candidiasis includes myocarditis, pericarditis, and endocarditis. Valvular vegetations can be quite large, and major embolic events are common and devastating.

   iv. Renal candidiasis arises from ascending infection from the bladder resulting in fungus balls and papillary necrosis, or from hematogenous spread resulting in pyelonephritis and abscess formation.

   v. Ocular candidiasis can cause blindness.

   vi. Other sites of disseminated candidiasis include the central nervous system and the musculoskeletal system.

4. **Treatment of candidal infections.** There have been few controlled trials to define the best therapeutic modalities. Antifungal therapy should be tailored to available culture data with particular attention to the presence of fluconazole-resistant organisms.

   a. Candiduria can be treated with amphotericin or nystatin bladder irrigation or oral fluconazole. The choice should be guided by the organism identified (*Candida glabrata* is often resistant to fluconazole) as well as the likelihood of renal involvement. Because urinary catheters often have thick fungal sediments attached, replacement of indwelling urinary catheters is also recommended.

   b. **Mucocutaneous candidiasis** is initially treated with a topical agent such as nystatin, mycostatin, clotrimazole, or ketoconazole. Systemic therapy with oral fluconazole may be indicated when patients do not respond to topical therapy.

   c. **Candidemia** is treated with systemic antifungal therapy. Venous and arterial catheters should be replaced at new sites and catheter tips should be cultured. Tunneled central venous lines are often left in place unless there is failure to clear the fungemia with antibiotics. The decision to treat with fluconazole, amphotericin, or caspofungin is based on the patient's overall clinical status and the fungal isolate. *Candida glabrata* and *Candida krusei* are often resistant to fluconazole. Amphotericin and caspofungin are both options for the treatment of severe infection. In unstable patients, amphotericin or caspofungin is generally favored over fluconazole.

   d. **Disseminated candidiasis** requires a combination of systemic antifungal therapy, drainage or debridement of infected areas, removal of intravascular catheters, and sometimes removal of infected valves and other foreign bodies. Although there is general consensus that *Candida* spp grown from the peritoneal cavity (i.e., not just peritoneal drains) should be treated, opinions differ with respect to whether amphotericin, caspofungin, or fluconazole should be used, and whether the toxic agent 5-fluorocytosine should be added for synergy. The same is true for hepatosplenic candidiasis. Lack of response to fluconazole is an indication to change the antifungal coverage. Severe endophthalmitis is treated with amphotericin B.

B. **Aspergillus** is a cause of invasive opportunistic infection in immunocompromised ICU patients. Distinguishing colonization from infection can be difficult. Diagnosis of infection is based on serologic data, tissue histology, and cultures. Positive sputum cultures do not necessarily indicate disease and negative cultures do not rule out disease. Thus, it is helpful, although not always clinically feasible, to get pulmonary tissue for analysis.

   1. **Clinical manifestations** range from localized pulmonary disease to disseminated disease.

      a. **Invasive pulmonary disease** occurs in immunocompromised patients, and presents with fever and pulmonary infiltrates. Pathologic analysis reveals infarction and hemorrhage. Pulmonary thrombosis can occur when the organisms invade vessel walls. Diagnosis is made by direct analysis of pulmonary tissue. A significant proportion of patients with locally invasive disease also have disseminated disease.

b. **Dissemination** to a variety of organs occurs due to vascular invasion. Abscesses occur in the CNS, lung, liver, and myocardium. Budd-Chiari syndrome and myocardial infarctions may occur.

c. **Other pulmonary manifestations**

    i. **Aspergillomas** are fungus balls that occur in cavities in the upper lobes of the lungs, especially in bullae and occasionally in old tuberculous cavities. Patients present with cough, hemoptysis (which can be life threatening), fever, and dyspnea.

    ii. **Allergic bronchopulmonary aspergillosis** causes episodic asthmatic symptoms and usually occurs in patients with chronic asthma or cystic fibrosis. Radiographic findings range from segmental infiltrates to transient nonsegmental infiltrates. Eosinophilia is present in the sputum and blood.

2. **Treatment of aspergillosis**

a. **Disseminated disease** and **invasive pulmonary disease** are treated with intravenous amphotericin or voriconazole. In some cases, disseminated disease is treated with a combination of amphotericin and voriconazole. Caspofungin is also approved by the U.S. Food and Drug Administration for treating patients with invasive aspergillosis who have failed to respond to or are intolerant of amphotericin. Surgical resection may be indicated when systemic antifungal therapy has failed.

b. **Localized pulmonary manifestations**

    i. **Aspergilloma.** Surgery is indicated in patients with recurrent hemoptysis. There may also be a role for corticosteroid treatment. Systemic amphotericin B does not improve outcome compared with supportive measures.

    ii. **Allergic bronchopulmonary aspergillosis** is treated with systemic corticosteroids (aerosolized steroids are not of benefit) and sometimes aerosolized antifungals. The benefits of long-term corticosteroid therapy have not been shown.

IX. **Viral infections**

A. **Cytomegalovirus (CMV)** is an important cause of infection in immunocompromised patients. It is the most common cause of infection in solid-organ and bone marrow transplant recipients. Primary infection occurs in seronegative individuals, whereas secondary infection occurs when there is activation of latent infection or reinfection of a seropositive host. Primary infection in immunocompetent hosts is often asymptomatic, although, rarely, severe disease occurs. Diagnosis of CMV infection requires detection of viral components or an increase in antibodies directed to CMV.

1. **Manifestations of CMV in immunocompromised patients**
   a. **Self-limited febrile illness** is common.
   b. **Interstitial pneumonitis.** CMV pneumonitis resulting in respiratory failure requiring mechanical ventilation has high mortality.
   c. **CMV hepatitis** is usually mild, but can be severe, particularly in liver transplant patients.
   d. **GI.** Diarrhea, GI bleeding.
   e. **Retinitis**
2. **Treatment.** CMV infection is very difficult to treat, and infection recurs rapidly after cessation of antiviral agents. **Ganciclovir** and **foscarnet** are both used to treat CMV retinitis in AIDS patients. Ganciclovir is also given for CMV infection in organ transplant recipients. Foscarnet is used in patients with CMV who are intolerant of ganciclovir. Life-threatening CMV infection (such as CMV pneumonitis) may be treated with the combination of ganciclovir and high-dose intravenous CMV immunoglobulin. Administration of hyperimmune globulin to bone marrow transplant recipients with pneumonitis has resulted in improved outcome.

B. **Herpes simplex virus (HSV) I and II.**
1. **Manifestations** of HSV infection include the following:
   a. **Mucocutaneous** and **genital** disease.
   b. **Respiratory tract infection**
      i. Tracheobronchitis.
      ii. HSV pneumonia generally occurring in debilitated or immunocompromised patients.
   c. **Ocular infection** such as blepharitis, conjunctivitis, keratitis, corneal ulceration, and blindness.
   d. **Esophagitis.**
   e. **Encephalitis, meningitis.**
2. **Disseminated HSV** usually occurs in patients who are extremely debilitated or immunocompromised, but occasionally occurs during pregnancy. Manifestations include necrotizing hepatitis, pneumonitis, cutaneous lesions from hematogenous spread, fever, hypotension, disseminated intravascular coagulation, and CNS involvement.
3. **Diagnosis.** Wright's Giemsa's stain (Tzanck smear) or Papanicolaou's stain of material scraped from lesions can be helpful, but are insensitive and do not distinguish between HSV and varicella-zoster virus (VZV) infection. Viral culture, histologic examination of tissue or skin biopsy, and DNA or protein staining of viral antigens are other diagnostic tests. Brain

biopsy may be necessary for diagnosis of HSV encephalitis.

4. **Treatment**

   a. **Severe HSV infections,** including CNS infections, pneumonitis, and disseminated HSV, are treated with IV **acyclovir. Foscarnet** may be used to treat acyclovir-resistant HSV.

   b. **Mucosal, cutaneous, and genital infections** may be treated with **acyclovir, famciclovir,** or **valacyclovir.** Although normal hosts do not always require treatment, consideration should be given to treating critically ill or debilitated patients even if they do not fit classic criteria for immunocompromise.

   c. **Ocular infection** may be treated with topical agents such as acyclovir, and should be managed in consultation with an ophthalmologist.

C. **Varicella-zoster virus** infection may be encountered in the ICU as a primary infection (chicken pox) or reactivation infection (herpes zoster or shingles), and can cause mild to life-threatening disease.

   1. **Primary VZV** infection in adults may have severe systemic effects and pulmonary involvement that causes respiratory failure. Immunocompromised patients are prone to severe systemic disease with involvement of lungs, kidneys, CNS, and liver.

   2. **Herpes zoster** usually manifests as a dermatomal cutaneous infection from reactivation of VZV that has been dormant in the sensory ganglia. Rarely, reactivated herpes zoster causes CNS disease such as encephalitis and cerebral vasculitis.

   3. **Treatment.** IV acyclovir is used for serious VZV infection (pneumonia, encephalitis) in immunocompromised or immunocompetent hosts.

SELECTED REFERENCES

Bowton DL. Nosocomial pneumonia in the ICU—year 2000 and beyond. *Chest* 1999;115(3 Suppl):28S–33S.

Cohen J, Powderly WG. *Infectious diseases*, 2nd ed. New York: Elsevier, 2004.

Cunha BA, ed. Infectious disease in critical care medicine. New York: Marcel Dekker, 1998.

Darling RG, Catlett CL, Huebner KD, et al. Threats in bioterrorism. I. CDC category A agents. *Emerg Med Clin North Am* 2002;20: 273–309.

Goodman EL. Practice guidelines for evaluating new fever in critically ill adult patients. *Clin Infect Dis* 2002;35:503–511.

Mylonakis E, Calderwood SB. Infective endocarditis in adults. *N Engl J Med* 2001;345:1318–1330.

Niederman MS. Guidelines for the management of adults with community-acquired pneumonia. Diagnosis, assessment of severity, antimicrobial therapy, and prevention. *Am J Respir Crit Care Med* 2001;163:1730–1754.

O'Grady NP, Alexander M, Dellinger EP, et al. Guidelines for the prevention of intravascular catheter-related infections. Centers for Disease Control and Prevention. *MMWR Recomm Rep* 2002;51(RR-10):1–29.

Ortiz-Ruiz G, Caballero-Lopez J, Friedland IR, et al. A study evaluating the efficacy, safety, and tolerability of ertapenem versus ceftriaxone for the treatment of community-acquired pneumonia in adults. *Clin Infect Dis* 2002;34:1076–1083.

Pappas PG, Rex JH, Sobel JD, et al. Guidelines for treatment of candidiasis. *Clin Infect Dis* 2004;38:161–189.

Stroke, Seizure, and Encephalopathy

Leigh R. Hochberg and Lee H. Schwamm

Nontraumatic acute cerebral dysfunction can be the reason for initial hospital presentation, accompany underlying illness, or complicate medical or perioperative management. The majority of etiologies require specific and urgent intervention, and understanding acute dysfunction of the brain is of paramount importance. Common disorders include ischemic stroke, intracerebral hemorrhage, subdural hemorrhage, subarachnoid hemorrhage, seizures, and encephalopathy (of infectious, inflammatory, hypo/hypertensive, or toxic/metabolic origin). The neurologic examination is critical in distinguishing focal versus generalized processes and can help to identify the likely etiology.

I. **Stroke** is the acute onset of a focal neurologic deficit or disturbance in the level of arousal due to cerebral ischemia, hemorrhage, or venous occlusion. Therapy is aimed at restoring adequate cerebral blood flow and preventing secondary brain injury.
   A. **Acute ischemic stroke** is due to acute vascular occlusion. Symptoms often include sudden onset of visual loss, weakness or numbness on one side of the body, ataxia, unexplained falling, dysarthria, or aphasia. Thrombosis-in-situ may occur in diseased segments of small penetrating vessels (i.e., lacunar stroke) or larger arteries (e.g., atherosclerotic stenosis, arterial dissection), and emboli may be liberated from proximal sites (e.g., heart, aorta, carotid artery) to lodge in otherwise normal major cerebral arteries or their distal branches.
      1. **Lacunar strokes** tend to occur in patients with diabetes and chronic hypertension and may be clinically silent or present as pure motor hemiparesis, pure sensory loss, or a variety of well-defined syndromes (e.g., dysarthria-clumsy hand, ataxic-hemiparesis). Descending compact white matter tracts or brainstem gray matter nuclei are injured, often producing widespread and striking initial deficits. However, the prognosis for recovery with lacunar stroke is better than with large-artery territory stroke. Nevertheless, because the risk of hemorrhagic transformation in these patients is low, many centers favor the use of **intravenous (IV) thrombolysis** in all but the most clinically mild lacunar strokes. Because initial small-vessel clinical syndromes may sometimes be due to large-artery thrombosis affecting end vessels, all patients presenting with acute ischemic symptoms should undergo some form of acute neurovascular

imaging to establish large vessel patency (e.g., computed tomographic angiography [CTA], magnetic resonance angiography [MRA], ultrasound, or conventional contrast angiography). This should not delay IV thrombolysis using recombinant **tissue plasminogen activator (tPA,** alteplase) in appropriate patients.

2. **Large-artery occlusion** is divided into disorders of the anterior (internal carotid artery and branches) and posterior (vertebrobasilar arteries and branches) circulations. These strokes carry a risk of swelling and hemorrhagic transformation. The "ischemic penumbra" refers to a region of brain with inadequate blood supply that still may be salvaged with rapid restoration of normal blood flow. Although the center of an ischemic zone (the core) may be irreversibly injured before the patient obtains medical attention, the surrounding ischemic penumbra may be saved by rapid intervention.

   a. **Middle cerebral artery (MCA) occlusion** is characterized by weakness of the contralateral face and arm with hemianopia and a preference of the eyes and head toward the side of the involved hemisphere ("looking toward the lesion"). Additional findings include aphasia in dominant-hemisphere strokes, hemineglect in nondominant-hemisphere strokes (patient "ignores" the left side of the body, the surroundings, or the presence of the deficit itself), and a variable degree of leg weakness depending upon how much of the middle cerebral artery stem is involved (and thus how much of the underlying white matter or basal ganglia is affected). Involvement restricted to branches of the MCA may produces fragments of this syndrome, often with sparing of leg strength.

   b. **Anterior cerebral artery (ACA) occlusion** is rare, and causes isolated weakness of the lower limb. If both ACAs are affected, a generalized decrease in initiative (abulia) may also occur.

   c. **Border zone** or "watershed" infarction is the result of insufficient blood flow to parts of the brain supplied by the distal territories of more than one of the major cerebral vessels. This develops most commonly in the setting of severe, sustained hypotension (e.g., cardiac arrest) or in the presence of severe atherosclerotic narrowing of one or both carotid arteries. Because the region most commonly affected is the white matter underneath the motor areas (the ACA/MCA border zone), the classic presentation is that of proximal arm/leg weakness with preservation of distal strength, the so-called "person in a barrel."

   d. **Posterior circulation** infarction involves the brainstem, cerebellum, thalamus, and occipital and mesial temporal lobes. As a result, patients can present with bilateral limb weakness or sensory disturbance, cranial nerve deficits (sensory and/or motor), ataxia, nausea and vomiting, visual field deficits, or decreased level of consciousness, including coma. The full-blown syndrome results from occlusion of the basilar artery trunk, with fragments of the syndrome produced by branch occlusions. Edema and mass effect from cerebellar stroke may be life threatening due to the confined space of the posterior fossa, with resulting upward or downward transtentorial herniation (see section on cerebellar hemorrhage).

3. **Conditions mimicking stroke** include seizure, migraine, toxic-metabolic derangement, and amyloid spells. Diffusion-weighted MR imaging helps to distinguish cerebral infarction from stroke mimics by identifying areas of intracellular swelling (i.e., cytotoxic edema) associated with ischemia.

   a. Whereas partial complex **seizures** may mimic stroke, especially if speech is impaired, postictal neurologic deficits (Todd's phenomena) may masquerade as any focal neurologic deficit, including weakness, sensory loss, or aphasia lasting hours to days after a seizure.

   b. The aura associated with a **migraine** headache may include focal neurologic deficits such as weakness, numbness, or aphasia, and may occur in the absence of headache ("typical aura without headache"). Patients with recurrent migraine headaches are at a somewhat increased risk for true ischemic stroke. Patients who present with persistent symptoms similar in quality to their typical migrainous aura or who present with a new focal deficit accompanied by their typical aura should be evaluated for stroke.

   c. **Toxic-metabolic states** such as hypo- or hyperglycemia, hyponatremia, hypoxia, or intoxication may produce focal or global neurologic deficits. Laboratory evaluation including electrolytes should be performed in all cases. Occult infections can also exacerbate deficits from old strokes and masquerade as new or recurrent stroke.

   d. Patients with **amyloid angiopathy** may have transient neurologic dysfunction associated with microscopic hemorrhages that are suggestive of transient ischemic attacks (TIAs). Diagnosis of cerebral amyloid angiopathy may be suggested by MR imaging gradient-echo sequences, which easily identify areas of hemosiderin deposition.

4. **Important etiologies of ischemic stroke** include cardiac and arterial **thromboembolism,** intracranial and extracranial **atherosclerosis,** endocarditis, paradoxical emboli, arterial dissection, vasculitis, and inherited and acquired hypercoagulable disorders. Carotid or vertebral artery **dissection** may occur spontaneously, after trauma, or in connective

tissue disease (e.g., fibromuscular dysplasia). Dissection can be recognized on angiography or axial T1 fat suppression MR imaging. **Vasculitis** may occur in primary central nervous system (CNS) disease or as part of a systemic syndrome such as systemic lupus erythematosus (SLE) or polyarteritis nodosa. **Hypercoagulability** may be due to clotting factor imbalance (protein C, protein S, antithrombin III deficiency) or autoimmunity (antiphospholipid antibodies). Sickle cell disease can also lead to focal cerebral arterial occlusion. Special attention should be given to the possibility of dissection, hypercoagulable states, autoimmune syndromes, and hemoglobinopathies when evaluating stroke in the young.

5. **Acute evaluation** for IV **thrombolysis** should be performed in all patients presenting within 3 hours of symptom onset to an appropriate facility. This includes accurate neurologic assessment, CT or MR imaging to exclude hemorrhage and early ischemic changes, laboratory exclusion of stroke mimics, hemostatic profile (platelets, prothrombin time [PT], activated partial thromboplastin time [aPTT], electrocardiogram [ECG]), and historical/imaging findings consistent with acute ischemia. If available, echoplanar MR with diffusion- and perfusion-weighted imaging or functional CT may provide further insight into vascular anatomy and tissue injury (Fig. 29-1).

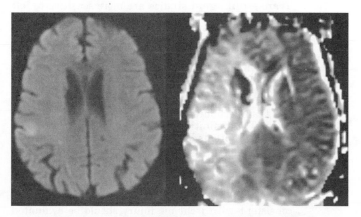

Fig. 29-1. Diffusion-weighted image (DWI) (*left*) and perfusion image (*right*) in a 70-year-old woman with new-onset left hemiparesis and neglect. The small area of hyperintensity seen on DWI identifies an infarction, but is insufficient to explain her clinical syndrome. The perfusion image shows a dramatic deficit in the right middle cerebral artery (MCA) territory, caused by occlusion of a branch of the right MCA. The oligemic, dysfunctional cortex accounts for her weakness and neglect. This "diffusion/perfusion mismatch" represents cortical territory at risk for infarction that may be rescued by appropriate medical and/or interventional neuroradiologic management.

Alternatively, ultrasound may permit rapid and repeatable neurovascular assessment of the carotid bifurcation, cervical vertebral arteries, and intracranial arterial branches. Specialized centers may offer endovascular approaches to reperfusion, including intraarterial (IA) thrombolysis, mechanical thrombectomy, or angioplasty. These approaches may provide benefit beyond the 3-hour window of IV tPA, extending this window up to 6 or more hours in the anterior circulation and perhaps up to 24 hours in the posterior circulation. The only drug approved for use in acute ischemic stroke remains IV tPA, though others are undergoing clinical trials. See http://www.acutestroke.com for the Massachusetts General Hospital Acute Stroke Service protocols, and http://www.strokecenter.org for completed and active clinical trials in cerebrovascular disease.

6. **Subacute evaluation** should identify the cause and help define the risk for recurrent stroke. **Echocardiography** with agitated saline contrast injection should be performed to exclude intracardiac thrombus and to assess left ventricular size and function, left atrial size, mitral and aortic valvular disease, and right-to-left shunt. An adequate assessment for intracardiac shunt, including patent foramen ovale (PFO), must demonstrate full opacification of the right atrium and physiologic evidence of an increase in right atrial pressure sufficient to demonstrate shunting. **Transesophageal** studies are more sensitive to left atrial thrombus and atheromatous disease of the aortic arch. A 24-hour Holter monitor may identify paroxysmal atrial fibrillation. Particularly in young patients, the cause of the stroke should be vigorously pursued, including evaluation for inherited or acquired hypercoagulable syndromes.

7. **Transient ischemic attacks** are traditionally considered to be sudden, focal neurologic deficits that last less than 24 hours and are believed to be of vascular origin. This definition is falling out of favor because ischemic symptoms lasting more than several hours almost always are associated with evidence of infarction on advanced imaging techniques (diffusion-weighted imaging [DWI]), and occasionally symptoms lasting only a few minutes also have imaging that demonstrates infarction. Therefore, even transient symptoms consistent with ischemic injury should be evaluated as potential ischemic stroke. Recent data suggest that 5% of TIAs are followed by a stroke within 48 hours, and 10% of patients with a TIA will have a stroke within 3 months. Urgent evaluation of TIAs is imperative for assessing cerebral arterial patency, identifying risk factors for recurrent ischemia, and initiating treatment(s) that can reduce the risk of subsequent stroke.

8. **Acute treatment.** If the time of onset is clearly established to be less than 3 hours and cranial CT excludes intracranial hemorrhage or well-established stroke, all patients with a significant nonresolving deficit and the clinical diagnosis of ischemic stroke are potential candidates for **IV tPA.** A 0.9-mg/kg (maximum 90 mg) dose is infused over 60 minutes with 10% of the total dose administered as an initial IV bolus over 1 minute. Contraindications to IV tPA are summarized in Table 29-1. Following IV tPA, no aspirin, heparin, or warfarin should be given for 24 hours. Patients with severe strokes (National Institutes of Health Stroke Scale [NIHSS] >20) have a higher rate of hemorrhage after tPA; however, many centers favor treatment of these patients, given their otherwise unfavorable prognosis. Proximal artery occlusions are less likely to recanalize with IV tPA and are more likely to produce severe clinical deficits. Further treatments to improve revascularization are being studied, including the use of transcranial ultrasound during IV tPA therapy and the use of other thrombolytic agents with or without concomitant antiplatelet agents.

   a. **Intraarterial thrombolytic** (tPA, urokinase) administration should be considered in experienced centers for patients with confirmed large-artery occlusion (by CTA, MRA, or angiography) who are past the 3-hour IV tPA window according to locally developed protocols. Doses of up to 1.25 million units of urokinase or up to 22 mg of intraarterial tPA have been used in conjunction with mechanical clot disruption to recanalize proximal arteries and restore function. **Mechanical clot retrieval** devices are also being studied, and one has recently been approved by the Food and Drug Administration.

   b. Continuous intravenous **unfractionated heparin,** although without proven benefit in acute stroke, is sometimes used in patients ineligible for thrombolysis and can be considered in patients with basilar stenosis, internal carotid or extradural vertebral artery dissection, fluctuating deficits, or symptomatic critical carotid stenosis without large MCA infarct. The aPTT should be monitored every 6 hours and the heparin dose adjusted to maintain the aPTT in the range of 1.5 to 2.5 times the baseline. Initial heparin bolus may raise the risk of hemorrhage and is deferred except in fluctuating deficits or acute basilar thrombosis. Whereas chronic anticoagulation reduces the risk of recurrent stroke in patients with atrial fibrillation, in patients with large infarcts, initiation is often deferred for days to weeks to minimize the risk of hemorrhagic transformation. Any patient who experiences a clinical deterioration on heparin must be

Table 29-1. Inclusion and exclusion criteria for administering intravenous tissue plasminogen activator to patients with acute stroke

Inclusion criteria
- A significant neurologic deficit expected to result in long-term disability
- Acute ischemic stroke symptoms with onset or time last known well, clearly defined, less than 3 hours before tPA will be given

Absolute exclusion criteria
- Hemorrhage or well-established acute infarct on CT
- Central nervous system lesion with high likelihood of hemorrhage status post intravenous tPA (e.g., brain tumors, abscess, vascular malformation, aneurysm, contusion)
- Established bacterial endocarditis

Relative contraindications
- Mild or rapidly improving deficits
- Significant trauma within 3 months
- Cardiopulmonary resuscitation with chest compressions within last 10 days
- Stroke within 3 months
- History of intracranial hemorrhage, or symptoms suspicious for subarachnoid hemorrhage
- Major surgery within last 14 days
- Minor surgery within last 10 days, including liver and kidney biopsy, thoracocentesis, lumbar puncture
- Arterial puncture at a noncompressible site within last 14 days
- Pregnant (up to 10 days postpartum) or nursing woman
- Gastrointestinal, urologic, or respiratory hemorrhage within last 21 days
- Known bleeding diathesis (includes renal and hepatic insufficiency)
- Life expectancy <1 year from other causes
- Peritoneal dialysis or hemodialysis
- Partial thromboplastin time >40 seconds; platelet count <100,000
- INR >1.7 (prothrombin time >15 if no INR available) with or without chronic oral anticoagulant use
- Systolic blood pressure >180 mm Hg or diastolic blood pressure >110 mm Hg, despite basic measures to lower it acutely
- Seizure at onset of stroke (this relative contraindication is intended to prevent treatment of patients with a deficit due to postictal Todd's paralysis or with seizure due to some other CNS lesion that precludes recombinant tPA therapy; if rapid diagnosis of vascular occlusion can be made, treatment may be given in some cases)
- Glucose <50 or >400 mg/dl (this relative contraindication is intended to prevent treatment of patients with focal deficits due to hypo- or hyperglycemia; if the deficit persists after correction of the serum glucose, or if rapid diagnosis of vascular occlusion can be made, treatment may be given in some cases)
- Consideration should be given to the increased risk of hemorrhage in patients with severe deficits (NIHSS >20), age >75 years, or early edema with mass effect on CT

From the Massachusetts General Hospital Acute Stroke Services (www. acutestroke.com).
CT, computed tomography; NIHSS, National Institutes of Health Stroke Scale; INR, International Normalized Ratio; tPA, tissue plasminogen activator.

imaged immediately to rule out hemorrhagic transformation.

c. **Antiplatelet therapy** should be considered for patients who do not qualify for thrombolytic therapy. **Aspirin** in doses ranging from 160 to 1,300 mg daily may benefit patients with acute stroke for whom thrombolytics or anticoagulants are not indicated. Other antiplatelet agents such as IV **abciximab** or **eptifibatide** (see Chapter 17) are being studied in acute ischemic stroke. Combination aspirin plus extended-release **dipyridamole** has been shown to be superior to aspirin alone for secondary stroke prophylaxis. **Clopidogrel,** another antiplatelet agent, is useful for reducing the risk of recurrent vascular events in patients with peripheral vascular disease.

d. Urgent **carotid revascularization** may be indicated in cases of stroke in which there is a critical degree of carotid stenosis, a small distal infarction, and a large territory of vulnerable brain. Revascularization of larger strokes may be associated with acute reperfusion injury and should be delayed by weeks to months.

e. In some patients with stenosis of major vessels, **pharmacologically induced hypertension** with **phenylephrine** may improve neurologic function acutely and rescue viable brain tissue, perhaps due to penumbral salvage. Early studies suggest that induced hypertension is safe in patients without cardiac comorbidities, such as angina or congestive heart failure (CHF).

9. **Subacute treatment.** Hypovolemia and hyponatremia should be avoided, and intravascular volume should be maintained with isotonic solutions. **Fever** should be aggressively controlled because even mild hyperthermia worsens outcome. Swelling is maximal at 2 to 5 days after stroke onset, and standard increased intracranial pressure (ICP) management should be initiated (see Chapters 13 and 34). In massive hemispheric or cerebellar infarction, decompressive surgery can be life saving and may improve outcome in survivors.

B. **Primary intracerebral hemorrhage (ICH).** The broad differential diagnosis for intracranial bleeding includes ICH, epidural and subdural hemorrhage (see Chapter 34), subarachnoid hemorrhage (described subsequently), venous sinus thrombosis (also described subsequently), and, rarely, isolated intraventricular hemorrhage. These can often be distinguished initially by noncontrast CT scan, though more advanced imaging (to be discussed) may be required. The most common locations for ICH are basal ganglia, thalamus, cerebral white matter, pons, and cortical lobar surface, but 8% to 10% of incidents occur in cerebellum. **Long-standing hypertension** is the most common cause (75%), although other etiologies are recognized, such as aneurysm, trauma, vascular malformations, amyloid angiopathy, coagulopathies, neoplasms, sympathomimetic drugs, septic emboli, and vasculitis. Metastases, especially adenocarcinoma and melanoma, may present with intracerebral hemorrhage or swelling. ICH as a primary process should be differentiated from hemorrhagic transformation of ischemic infarction, in which a bland ischemic stroke develops petechial bleeding or turns into a space-occupying hematoma.

1. **Clinical syndromes.** ICH often presents with headache, nausea, vomiting, and focal neurologic signs similar to those seen in ischemic strokes. The evolution of symptoms may occur more slowly than in ischemic stroke or may cause an acute, devastating picture. As a rule, patients with ICH present with systolic hypertension. In patients who were normotensive at baseline, this usually resolves over the first week; in chronic hypertensive patients, aggressive, multiple-drug treatment is often required to control blood pressure. In contrast to most cortical hemorrhages, the progression to death from cerebellar hemorrhage may be rapid.

   a. **Supratentorial** ICH presents with symptoms referable to the site of bleeding. With rebleeding or development of vasogenic edema or hydrocephalus, there is often worsening of symptoms with decline in arousal. Transtentorial herniation is the mode of death in massive hemorrhage.

   b. **Midline infratentorial** hemorrhage produces only dysequilibrium on standing, walking, and sometimes sitting. Romberg sign cannot be assessed because balance is already impaired with eyes open. If gait is not tested, this lesion may not be detected until other cerebellar signs emerge secondary to brain swelling. **Lateral cerebellar hemispheric** lesions produce symptoms ipsilateral to the lesion. Patients complain of limb incoordination and demonstrate ataxia with falling toward the side of lesion, dysmetria (overshoot) on finger-nose-finger testing, dysdiadokinesia (inaccuracy on rapid alternating movements), intentional tremor (exaggerated on approaching the target), and nystagmus (worse looking toward lesion). Speech may be dysarthric (slurred) or explosive.

2. **Acute evaluation** of patients with suspected ICH consists of brain imaging; both CT and MR are very sensitive. In addition, toxicology screen, PT, aPTT, and platelets should be checked and signs of occult malignancy excluded. Hemorrhage volume correlates with outcome, and can be estimated easily in cubic centimeters on unenhanced head CT using the "ABC/2" method, where A is the greatest diameter of the hemorrhage on a single slice, B is the hemorrhage diameter perpendicular to A on the same slice, and C is the approximate number of axial CT slices revealing

hemorrhage multiplied by slice thickness in centimeters. Thirty-day mortality for patients with a parenchymal hemorrhage volume of greater than 60 cm^3 on their initial CT and a Glasgow coma scale (GCS) score of 8 or less is 90%, and for those with a volume of less than 30 cm^3 and a GCS score of 9 or greater it is 20%. **Subacute evaluation** should identify the etiology by imaging and history. MR imaging with susceptibility may identify areas of prior occult cortical hemorrhage and suggest a diagnosis of amyloid angiopathy in patients with lobar ICH. Repeat MR in 3 to 6 weeks may also detect lesions (e.g., tumor) masked by acute hemorrhage. Rarely, aneurysmal hemorrhage may result in primarily parenchymal hematoma, mimicking ICH. Conventional contrast angiography or CTA is indicated in any suspicious case. Prognosis is based on clinical presentation and imaging findings. Patients with cerebellar lesions less than 2 cm in diameter or with self-limited cerebellar signs usually do well, those with 3-cm lesions or progressive drowsiness do poorly without intervention, and 20% have lesions greater than 3 cm and a poor prognosis regardless of treatment. Prognosis in patients with cortical ICH is also related to hematoma size. It should be noted, however, that the most common cause of death in large ICH is withdrawal of supportive care, and the prognosis for large ICH with extended rehabilitation is less clear.

3. **Acute treatment** consists largely of supportive care, blood pressure control, reversal of coagulopathy, and ICP monitoring or surgical intervention in selected cases. To correct elevated PT, **vitamin K,** 10 mg infused at 1 mg/min, should be given intravenously, accompanied by rapid transfusion of fresh-frozen plasma (FFP); **protamine** is used for elevated aPTT. Platelets should be provided to patients with platelet counts less than 100,000; patients who have uremic or pharmacologic (e.g., aspirin) platelet dysfunction may benefit from **desmopressin.** Reduction of systolic blood pressure to below 180 mm Hg is important to prevent rebleeding; overly aggressive reduction may precipitate ischemia in patients with concurrent major-vessel stenosis or a history of chronic hypertension. Beta-blockers such as **labetalol** are preferred for blood pressure control, given their additional benefit of being antiarrhythmic; conversely, nitrates may paradoxically increase ICP by dilating the cerebral vasculature. IV calcium-channel blockers such as **nicardipine** may be useful if further reduction in blood pressure is needed. **Neurosurgical consultation** should be obtained early, especially in cerebellar hemorrhage of diameter 2 cm or greater. Resection of lobar or basal ganglia ICH can be life-saving. Surgical methods include open craniotomy and stereotactic drainage. Intraventricular tPA may also improve outcome in patients with intraventricular extension of the ICH.

Recombinant activated **factor VIIa** has recently been reported to improve outcome and reduce hematoma expansion following ICH. **Obstructive or communicating hydrocephalus** may develop, and usually requires external ventricular drainage, although it may not need permanent ventricular shunting. Corticosteroids do not appear to be of benefit in ICH unless there is further deterioration due to vasogenic edema. **Anticonvulsant therapy** is indicated in cases with seizure, where the hematoma extends to the cortex, or when the consequence of a seizure itself would be deleterious (e.g., refractory ICP, coagulopathy, unstable fractures). Detailed **Massachusetts General Hospital guidelines for management of intracerebral hemorrhage** are available at www.acutestroke.com.

4. When **ICH** is suspected **in patients who received thrombolysis for acute stroke,** a head CT should be obtained immediately, along with neurosurgical and hematologic consultation, PT, aPTT, complete blood count (CBC), and D-dimer and fibrinogen concentrations. Treatment of verified symptomatic hematoma includes use of 2 units of fresh-frozen plasma **(FFP)** to replete factors V and VII, 20 units of **cryoprecipitate** to replete fibrinogen, and 6 units of **platelets.** Patients treated with heparin should receive **protamine** IV push, 1 mg per each 100 units of unfractionated heparin given in the preceding 4 hours. If an anticoagulant dose of low-molecular-weight heparin had been used, the maximum dose of protamine (50 mg) should be given. The foregoing laboratory values should be repeated every hour until bleeding is brought under control. If these measures fail to control bleeding, **aminocaproic acid,** 5 g IV over 1 hour, may be given.

C. **Cerebral venous thrombosis (CVT)** most commonly occurs in the sagittal, transverse, or straight sinus (often called venous sinus thrombosis), although the clot may extend into the vein of Galen or the internal jugular vein. Smaller, cortical venous thromboses can also occur, as can cavernous sinus thrombosis. CVT may occur in the setting of infection, tumor, trauma, hypovolemia, coagulation disorders, systemic inflammatory diseases, oral contraceptive use, pregnancy, and the puerperium. Despite a thorough diagnostic evaluation, nearly 25% of cases will be deemed idiopathic.

1. The **clinical syndrome** includes signs of increased intracranial pressure (ICP) such as headache, nausea, and vomiting, often more pronounced after prolonged recumbency. Focal neurologic signs or seizures may be seen in the setting of vasogenic edema or venous infarction. Without recanalization, altered sensorium can progress to coma. If the diagnosis is not considered, it is often overlooked until venous hemorrhage has occurred.

2. **Acute evaluation** relies on an imaging. CT with contrast may demonstrate filling defects in the superior sagittal sinus and torcula ("empty delta" sign) in up to 30% of patients, parenchymal abnormalities suggestive of deranged venous drainage in up to 60% of patients, small ventricles from increased ICP, or contrast enhancement of the falx and tentorium from venous hypertension. CT or MR venography provides enhanced sensitivity. Transfemoral angiography is diagnostic if MR is inconclusive. Lumbar puncture may demonstrate an elevated opening pressure, increased protein and red cells, and mild pleocytosis.

3. **Acute treatment** is effective if initiated early, but prognosis for recovery worsens significantly without treatment. Continuous IV unfractionated **heparin** titrated to aPTT of 60 to 80 should be given and maintained until the patient stabilizes or improves. Heparin should be given even in the presence of hemorrhage. In certain cases of extensive thrombosis or rapid deterioration in patient condition, transvenous thrombolysis with locally injected chemical thrombolytic or mechanical clot disruption should be considered at experienced centers. Measures to control ICP elevation and prophylaxis for seizures must be undertaken, and factors that exacerbate clotting (e.g., dehydration) must be avoided.

D. **Subarachnoid hemorrhage** (SAH) may be traumatic or nontraumatic. Nontraumatic SAH is caused most commonly by the **rupture of a cerebral aneurysm.** The majority of aneurysms arise from the carotid artery circulation, most commonly the ACA and less frequently the posterior communicating artery (PCA) or the MCA. Posterior circulation aneurysms commonly arise from the basilar tip or may also result from intradural vertebral dissections with pseudoaneurysm formation and rupture. Aneurysms may exist on a congenital basis, arise in the setting of atherosclerosis, or more rarely occur due to infection (mycotic) or emboli. Rupture of cerebral aneurysms releases blood into the subarachnoid space and causes up to 30% mortality in the first 24 hours. The primary brain injury may be anything from minimal to lethal, and abrupt loss of consciousness at onset is characteristic. Rebleeding of untreated aneurysms occurs in up to 30% of patients in the first 28 days, with 70% mortality. Hypotension, aspiration pneumonia, neurogenic pulmonary edema, seizures, obstructive hydrocephalus, or ischemia due to vasospasm may produce secondary brain injury. Serial examination and brain imaging can identify symptoms suggestive of most of these complications, but separate techniques are necessary to distinguish vasospasm.

1. **Clinical syndromes.** The "worst headache of my life" complaint should raise suspicion of SAH. Nausea, vomiting, altered sensorium, and focal cranial nerve defects (especially third-nerve palsy) are

Table 29-2. Classification of patients with intracranial aneurysms according to surgical risk (Hunt and Hess classification system)

Grade	Characteristics
I	Asymptomatic or minimal headache and slight nuchal rigidity
II	Moderate to severe headache, nuchal rigidity, no neurologic deficit other than cranial nerve palsy
III	Drowsiness, confusion, mild focal deficit
IV	Stupor, moderate to severe hemiparesis, possibly early decerebrate rigidity, vegetative disturbances
V	Deep coma, decerebrate rigidity, moribund

Table 29-3. Classification of subarachnoid hemorrhage according to risk of vasospasm (Fisher group classification system)

Group	Characteristics of Subarachnoid Hemorrhage on Computed Tomography Scan
1	No detectable subarachnoid blood, or trace diffuse blood
2	Diffuse blood with clot less than 3 × 5 mm (in axial plane) and less than 1 mm in vertical layer
3	Blood clot greater than 3 × 5 mm (in axial plane) or greater than 1 mm invertical layer
4	Intracerebral or intraventricular blood with no detectable subarachnoid or only minimal diffuse subarachnoid blood

The Fisher system does not refer to progressive grades of vasospasm risk, but rather to distinct groups. Only group 3 was associated with a risk of severe symptomatic vasospasm (>95%).

associated with SAH. A warning headache may occur due to a sentinel bleed in which blood may be confined to the aneurysm wall without true SAH. Clinical grading predicts outcome (Table 29-2) and risk of vasospasm (Table 29-3).

2. **Acute evaluation. CT scan** is the best initial test for SAH, and will detect SAH in about 95% of cases. Lumbar puncture should be performed in cases where SAH is suspected and CT is negative. Xanthochromia is a helpful sign of old blood products in the CSF, but it takes at least 4 hours to develop. Angiography should be performed urgently if SAH is suspected. A small proportion of SAH cases will have normal angiography. Follow-up imaging is needed in most cases, and attention should be given to base-of-skull arteriovenous fistulas and aneurysms compressed by hematoma. MR or CTA may also reveal aneurysms and may

help with surgical planning. With improved surgical
and anesthetic techniques, early aneurysm localization with angiography and early definitive aneurysm
repair have greatly improved outcome. Concerns that
angiography itself might lead to aneurysmal rebleeding have proven unwarranted.

3. **Subsequent evaluation.** Transfemoral angiography remains the gold standard for documenting vasospasm; however, it is invasive and carries some risk.
Vasospasm may develop at any time, but is most frequent between days 4 to 14 postrupture. Many centers
perform **serial transcranial Doppler ultrasound**
to detect presymptomatic narrowing of cerebral vessels at the base of the brain. Risk of clinically significant vasospasm can be predicted by grading of blood
collections around the basal arteries on the 24-hour
CT scan (Fisher groups 1–4; see Table 29-3).

4. **Acute treatment** consists of definitive obliteration of
the culprit aneurysm (clipping or endovascular therapy) and prevention of delayed ischemic deficits. Systolic arterial blood pressure should be strictly controlled (<120 mm Hg) until the aneurysm is secured.
Surgery, endovascular therapy, or both are performed
urgently; intervention choice is based on aneurysm location, anatomy, patient comorbidities, surgical and
endovascular risk, and operator experience. A calcium-
channel antagonist, **nimodipine,** 60 mg orally every
4 hours given for 21 days, reduces ischemic symptoms from 33% to 22%. Further therapy is focused
on maximizing cerebral blood flow and oxygen utilization to minimize the clinical sequelae of vasospasm.
This is generally accomplished by creating a hyperdynamic state with induced hypertension, hypervolemia,
and optimal oxygen-carrying capacity. Release of natriuretic factors causes **cerebral salt wasting** and
subsequent volume loss, with resultant serum hypo-
osmolarity and urine hyperosmolarity. The **treatment
for cerebral salt wasting is volume repletion** with
IV saline, either normal saline (0.9%) or **hypertonic
saline** solutions. Volume restriction, which would be
appropriate for syndrome of inappropriate antidiuretic
hormone (ADH) secretion (SIADH), should be avoided
because it leads rapidly to hypovolemia, hypotension,
and decreased blood flow distal to areas of vasospasm.
Oral NaCl tablets and mineralcorticoid administration
(**fludrocortisone,** 0.1 mg orally twice a day) may also
be useful. **Albumin** (250 ml of 5% albumin every 6–
8 hours) is often used in addition to normal saline to
keep central venous pressures at 8 to 12 mm Hg. It
has been the practice for patients with Fisher group 3
hemorrhage or evidence of vasospasm to be given blood
transfusions to maintain a hemoglobin concentration
of at least 9.0 gm/dl; the intention is to support an optimal balance of oxygen-carrying capacity and blood viscosity in areas with compromised cerebral perfusion.

Recent studies in other clinical scenarios have raised some question about the relative benefit of transfusion. Induced hypertension with an α-adrenergic agonist such as **phenylephrine** is safe and effective at reversing ischemic symptoms due to decreased cerebral blood flow in patients with vasospasm. The hypercatecholaminergic state following SAH can trigger the development of a stunned myocardium and acute heart failure; this condition, although usually fully reversible, can result in several days of marked global cardiac hypokinesis. When combined with the need for induced hypertension, this requires in some patients invasive hemodynamic monitoring and inotropic support with agents such as **norepinephrine** or **dobutamine.** In refractory vasospasm or in patients who cannot tolerate induced hypertension, intraarterial vasodilators such as **nicardipine** or **papaverine** or the use of **balloon angioplasty** may alleviate cerebral ischemia. Despite higher initial risk, they have become a mainstay of therapy. Newer, multimodal intracerebral monitors, including brain tissue oxygenation and cerebral microdialysis catheters, may provide early warning signs of vasospasm and help to guide appropriate therapy. Evidence for prophylactic anticonvulsant therapy is limited, but it may be helpful in the first 2 weeks, especially in those patients in whom seizure would be deleterious, such as patients with markedly increased ICP. No benefit from corticosteroids has been demonstrated in patients with SAH.

II. **Seizures** may occur in more than 10% of patients during their ICU stay. Repeated tonic-clonic seizures may be easily recognized and they must be treated early; uncontrolled generalized motor seizures that persist for greater than 60 minutes are associated with significant increases in neuronal injury and mortality. Conversely, nonconvulsive seizures are often undetected; up to 8% of comatose patients *with no outward evidence of seizure* have been found to have ongoing nonconvulsive seizures. Whereas single seizures should prompt a search for etiology and subsequent correction of inciting conditions and/or seizure prophylaxis, **status epilepticus** (continuous seizure lasting longer than 5 minutes, or more than one seizure without restoration of appropriate mental status) is a medical emergency. Table 29-4 summarizes common causes of seizures in the ICU.

A. **Clinical syndrome.** Seizures may be categorized into multiple subtypes. The most relevant in the ICU are generalized tonic-clonic, partial complex, and an unremitting form of either (status epilepticus). In **generalized tonic-clonic seizures,** patients present with stiffening, followed by limb jerking and impaired consciousness, often accompanied by hyperdynamic vital signs. Seizures with subtle motor manifestations may go unrecognized in critically ill patients; careful observation of a patient may reveal subtle but evident rhythmic limb or facial movements indicative of seizure. **Partial complex seizures**

**Table 29-4.   Common etiologies of
seizures in the intensive care unit**

Neurologic pathology
Neurovascular
  Ischemic or hemorrhagic stroke
  Vascular malformation
Tumor
  Primary
  Metastatic
Infection
  Abscess
  Meningitis
  Encephalitis
Inflammatory disease
  Vasculitis
  Acute disseminated encephalomyelitis
Trauma
Primary epilepsy
Inherited central nervous system metabolic disturbance
Complications of critical illness
Hypoxia
Drug/substance toxicity
Drug/substance withdrawals
  Anticonvulsants
  Barbiturates
  Benzodiazepines
  Alcohol
Fever (febrile seizures)
Infection
Metabolic abnormalities
  Hyponatremia
  Hypocalcemia
  Hypophosphatemia
  Hypoglycemia
  Renal/hepatic dysfunction
Surgical manipulation (craniotomy)

Adapted from Varelas PN, Mirski MA. Seizures in the adult intensive care unit.
J Neurosurg Anesthesiol 2001;13:163–175.

produce a decrease in responsiveness without a complete loss of consciousness. They may be accompanied by stereotypic limb movements (e.g., chewing, blinking, swallowing), but not rhythmic limb jerking.

B. Other conditions mimicking seizure include benign entities (myoclonus, fasciculations, tremor, spasticity) and potentially dangerous entities (brainstem ischemia, rigors, metabolic encephalopathy). For example, sudden onset of bilateral arm and leg posturing coupled with impaired eye movements is often seen in acute basilar artery occlusion. When in doubt, neurologic consultation and electroencephalogram (EEG) should be requested.

C. **Acute evaluation** consists in confirming the diagnosis and identifying potential causes. In many cases, EEG is not required due to obvious motor signs. All patients should undergo laboratory screen including CBC, electrolytes, blood urea nitrogen (BUN), creatinine, glucose, Ca, Mg, PO_4, liver function tests (including NH_3), anticonvulsant medications levels, blood and urine toxicology screen, and, when indicated, pregnancy test and arterial blood gases. CT scan and lumbar puncture may be necessary to establish the underlying diagnosis once seizures are controlled. Physical examination should look for signs of occult head trauma, substance abuse, fever, meningismus, and diabetes. Always check for Medical Alert bracelets or wallet information, and try to contact relatives or neighbors to determine prior medical and seizure history. Nonconvulsive status epilepticus can only be diagnosed by EEG. An EEG can also document triphasic waveforms suggestive of metabolic encephalopathy. Long-acting muscle relaxants in the absence of EEG monitoring have **no role** in the initial management of uncontrolled seizures, except in patients who cannot otherwise be adequately ventilated.

D. **Acute treatment** consists in safely aborting seizures as early as possible with the appropriate degree of intervention. Most patients require no intervention and will spontaneously recover after one seizure. Some patients require **benzodiazepines** and **phenytoin** without intubation, whereas some extreme cases may require **pentobarbital** anesthesia. Management by defined protocol is the best method for assuring that patients are treated promptly, and a thorough evaluation must be completed as soon as the patient is stabilized. A standard protocol approach is outlined in Table 29-5.

E. Proper **phenytoin drug maintenance** dosing can be confirmed by sending phenytoin levels 20 min after the loading dose in patients who are still seizing. When treating status epilepticus, aim for uncorrected levels of 20 to 30 μg/ml. Once seizures are controlled, phenytoin maintenance dosing is 300 to 400 mg/d, with a target serum level of 10 to 20 μg/ml. Because phenytoin is largely albumin bound and renally excreted, **correction for hypoalbuminemia** or acute renal failure is necessary once the acute episode is controlled: Phenytoin (corrected) = Phenytoin(measured)/[(0.2 × Albumin) + 0.1] for low albumin, and Phenytoin (corrected) = Phenytoin(measured)/[(0.1 × Albumin) + 0.1] for low albumin and acute renal failure.

III. **Encephalopathy**
A. **Toxic-metabolic** injury to the CNS is a frequent and reversible cause of impaired cognition in the ICU, but always remains a diagnosis of exclusion. Frequent causes include medication effects, perturbations in electrolyte, water, glucose, or urea homeostasis, acute renal or hepatic failure, sleep disturbances, and psychiatric disturbances. Treatment is supportive, with removal of the

Table 29-5.   Protocol for treating status epilepticus

0–2 minutes	Assess basic life support.
	• Start supplemental oxygen; monitor O_2 saturation
	• Initiate seizure precautions (e.g., padding bed rails)
	• Obtain seizure history
	• Look for evidence of head trauma or toxic ingestion/injection
	• Send urine and blood toxicology, electrolytes, blood urea nitrogen, creatinine, glucose, Ca, Mg, osmolarity, anticonvulsant drug levels
	• Consider prophylactic therapy (e.g., phenytoin)
2–5 minutes	**If the initial seizure has not stopped, or has stopped and restarted**
	• Give 2 mg IV **lorazepam,** every 2 minutes, up to 0.1 mg/kg
	-If lorazepam is not immediately available, diazepam 10–20 mg or midazolam 2–5 mg can be substituted
	• Start **phenytoin** 20 mg/kg IV load at ≤50 mg/min
	-Phenytoin IV can cause bradycardia, hypotension, and full-blown cardiovascular collapse, and therefore must be given in a monitored setting
	-In a patient with epilepsy presumed on phenytoin, give 10 mg/kg while awaiting drug levels
	-Fosphenytoin can be substituted for phenytoin at a dose of 20 mg phenytoin equivalents (PE)/kg IV at ≤150 mg PE/min
	• Begin IV normal saline, give **thiamine** 100 mg IV and **dextrose** 25–50 g IV if blood glucose is <60 mg/100 dl
	• Treat fever with acetaminophen and ice packs
	• Consider intubation to maintain airway patency
	• Check arterial blood gas
6–30 minutes	• Monitor electrocardiogram, airway; check blood pressure every 60 seconds
	• Repeat benzodiazepines every 15 minutes for continued motor seizures during phenytoin load
	• Determine presumptive pathophysiologic mechanism
31–50 minutes	• Give **phenobarbital** 10–20 mg/kg IV at ≤70 mg/min
	- Many patients require endotracheal intubation and mechanical ventilation by this point in the protocol
	• Call for urgent continuous EEG monitoring and obtain expert consultation

(Continued)

Table 29-5. *Continued*

>**50** minutes	• Give **pentobarbital** 3–5 mg/kg IV to induce burst suppression (see Fig. 29-2); in most adults, pentobarbital bolus 400 mg over 15 minutes then 100 mg every 15–30 minutes until burst suppression appears is reasonably well tolerated, followed by an infusion at 0.3–9.0 mg/kg/h to maintain burst suppression
	 - Alternative agents include the following:
	   Midazolam drip (may be preferable if blood pressure is unstable) 0.2 mg/kg slow IV push, followed by 0.1–2.0 mg/kg/h to stop electrographic and clinical seizures; or
	   Propofol 2–mg/kg load and 2–10 mg/kg/h to stop clinical and electrographic seizures or maintain burst suppression on EEG
	   Valproate 15–mg/kg IV load may be useful as an adjunctive agent.
	 • For all infusions, decrease the infusion periodically to check the EEG pattern that is being suppressed; if electrocerebral silence ("flatline") occurs, always decrease the dose until bursts are seen again
	 • Prepare an infusion of alpha-agonist (e.g., phenylephrine) for treatment of anticipated hypotension

EEG, electroencephalogram; IV, intravenous.

offending agent when possible. Patients receiving intravenous or epidural opioids who experience sudden or unexplained postoperative changes in mental status should receive **naloxone** to rule out opioid toxicity. Intensive blood sugar control (see Chapter 27) may improve outcome in a wide range of critically ill patients. Hyperammonemia with or without signs of liver abnormality can cause profound encephalopathy and increased ICP, and often responds to oral **lactulose** and reduction of nitrogen (protein) intake. Wernicke's encephalopathy, secondary to thiamine deficiency (usually in alcoholics, and occasionally in persons on severe diet regimens or other rapid reduction in nutrition), presents with ataxia, eye movement paralysis, nystagmus, apathy, or confusion. Treatment includes **thiamine** 100 mg IV, which should be continued daily for at least 5 days.

B. Hypertensive encephalopathy is due to sustained, severe hypertension or relative hypertension with impaired autoregulation. Early, reversible symptoms are likely due to blood–brain barrier disruption and vasogenic edema; with sustained hypertension, cerebral hemorrhage and irreversible injury may occur. Because acute elevations in blood pressure may be seen commonly in many types of brain injury in which antihypertensive therapy could

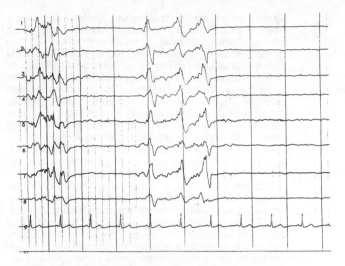

Fig. 29-2. Burst suppression during electroencephalographic monitoring. The bottom line is a tracing from an electrocardiographic lead.

be deleterious (e.g., ischemic stroke, traumatic brain injury), accurate diagnosis is essential. Clinical manifestations range from headache and visual scotoma to confusion, seizures, and coma. The likelihood of recovery depends on the extent of injury prior to treatment. **Head CT** is insensitive and may reveal bilateral posterior-predominant subcortical hypodensity. **MR** imaging reveals T2 and apparent diffusion coefficient hyperintensity with a posterior predilection, which may also involve diffuse subcortical white matter, cortical gray matter, and cerebellum; gradient-echo sequences often reveal microscopic petechial hemorrhages. Management of hypertensive crisis is outlined in Chapter 8. Most patients with hypertensive encephalopathy have underlying chronic hypertension. This shifts upward the range of pressures at which cerebrovascular autoregulation occurs. Thus, a rapid reduction in blood pressure in a chronically hypertensive patient might cause acute global hypoperfusion at a pressure that would be well tolerated in normotensive patients. Cyclosporine and FK-506 are among the chemotherapeutic agents that can produce a **toxic leukoencephalopathy;** reduction in dose or switching agents often results in symptom resolution and gradual reversal of the changes seen on MR imaging.

C. **Infectious/inflammatory**
   1. The most treatable **viral encephalitis** (and second most common after HIV) is due to acute **herpes simplex** infection. Patients present with headaches, fever,

seizure, or cognitive impairments. Early in the course there is a CSF lymphocytosis (5–500 cells/mm^3) with normal glucose and mild increases in protein, followed by hemorrhagic necrosis with bloody CSF. The EEG shows characteristic bursts of periodic high-voltage slow waves, and MR imaging reveals temporal and inferior frontal lobe involvement. CSF polymerase chain reaction (PCR) is extremely sensitive, although false negatives can occur, especially in the setting of very high CSF leukocytosis. Because therapy with **acyclovir** (10 mg/kg every 8 hours) reduces mortality and morbidity, it should be instituted in any suggestive case. Other forms of viral encephalitis, including those due to human herpes viruses 6 and 7, Epstein-Barr virus, cytomegalovirus, and varicella-zoster virus, may respond to specific antiviral treatments. Encephalitis due to arboviruses (arthropod-borne viruses) such as eastern equine, California, and St. Louis encephalitis, do not respond to acyclovir but can present in a similar manner. West Nile encephalitis commonly presents with paraparesis in addition to headache, fever, and encephalopathy. Vasogenic edema, seizures, and increased ICP may occur in all of these disorders, and patients require close monitoring in an ICU setting.

2. **Bacterial meningitis** must be diagnosed and treated rapidly, although in the early hours it may be clinically indistinguishable from viral meningoencephalitis. Acute onset of headache, meningeal signs (neck stiffness, photophobia), fever, and altered sensorium should suggest the diagnosis of acute bacterial meningitis. Etiology, diagnosis, and treatment of meningitis are outlined in Chapter 28.

3. **Acute disseminated encephalomyelitis (ADEM) and acute hemorrhagic leukoencephalitis (AHL).** Often preceded by a routine viral illness or mycoplasma pneumonia, these infections present with cerebral demyelination (ADEM) or hemorrhage (AHL) and **malignant cerebral edema.** Initial presentations have variable localizing signs, but encephalopathy, stupor, and coma ensue rapidly. Early brain MR can reveal characteristic demyelination, edema, and/or widespread petechial hemorrhage, with markedly increased CSF protein concentration. High-dose IV **methylprednisolone** and supportive care should be provided. ADEM has a better prognosis than AHL.

4. **Other infectious agents and inflammatory conditions.** Granulomatous diseases such as sarcoidosis as well as fungal, mycobacterial, and protein infectious (prion) agents can also affect the central nervous system and lead to encephalopathy. Characteristic imaging or CSF analysis may be helpful, but tissue biopsy is often required to diagnose these more uncommon etiologies.

SELECTED REFERENCES

Bousser MG. Cerebral venous thrombosis: diagnosis and management. *J Neurol* 2000;247:252–258.

Broderick JP, Adams HP Jr, Barsan W, et al. Guidelines for the management of spontaneous intracerebral hemorrhage: a statement for healthcare professionals from a special writing group of the Stroke Council, American Heart Association. *Stroke* 1999;30:905–915.

de Gans J, van de Beek D, and the European Dexamethasone in Adulthood Bacterial Meningitis Study Investigators. Dexamethasone in adults with bacterial meningitis. *N Engl J Med* 2002;347:1549–1556.

Fisher CM, Kistler JP, Davis JM. Relation of cerebral vasospasm to subarachnoid hemorrhage visualized by computed tomographic scanning. *Neurosurgery* 1980;6:1–9.

Johnston, SC, Cross DP, Browner, WS, et al. Short-term prognosis after emergency department of TIA. *JAMA* 2000;284:2901–2906.

Kidwell CS, Alger JR, Saver JL. Beyond mismatch: evolving paradigms in imaging the ischemic penumbra with multimodal magnetic resonance imaging. *Stroke* 2003;34:2729–2735.

Mayberg MR, Batjer HH, Dacey R, et al. Guidelines for the management of aneurysmal subarachnoid hemorrhage. A statement for healthcare professionals from a special writing group of the Stroke Council, American Heart Association. *Circulation* 1994;90:2592–2605.

Rordorf G, Koroshetz WJ, Ezzeddine MA, et al. A pilot study of drug-induced hypertension for treatment of acute stroke. *Neurology* 2001;56:1210–1213.

Shneker BF, Fountain NB. Assessment of acute morbidity and mortality in nonconvulsive status epilepticus. *Neurology* 2003;61:1066–1073.

van Gijn J, Rinkel GJ. Subarachnoid haemorrhage: diagnosis, causes and management. *Brain* 2001;124:249–278.

Varelas PN, Mirski MA. Seizures in the adult intensive care unit. *J Neurosurg Anesthesiol* 2001;13:163–175.

30

Acute Weakness

David Greer and Edward George

I. **Introduction**
   A. **Acute weakness in the intensive care unit (ICU)** can be caused by diseases affecting the central nervous system (CNS), the peripheral nervous system (PNS), or muscle. A **careful history** can often elucidate the underlying cause and cue the correct workup. This should include recent neurologic symptoms, injuries, current medications, alcohol or illicit drug use, travel, potential envenomations or neurotoxin exposures, and accompanying sensory or autonomic symptoms.
   B. Focal or lateralizing signs on examination should suggest a CNS cause, including a cerebrovascular event (ischemic or hemorrhagic), focal abscess or encephalitis, traumatic brain injury, or brainstem process.
   C. Injury to the brainstem may cause symmetric weakness in the extremities, and the key to the examination is a careful cranial nerve examination (pupillary reactions, corneal responses, eye movements). Central pontine myelinolysis also causes symmetric weakness, with prominent eye movement abnormalities. Brainstem processes commonly cause a depressed level of consciousness.
   D. Injury to the cervical spinal cord initially causes a flaccid quadriparesis, areflexia, and a sensory level loss depending on the level and extent of the injury.
   E. As a rule, **myopathic disorders** cause weakness primarily of proximal muscles, with relative sparing of deep tendon reflexes (DTRs) and sensation. **Neuropathic disorders** cause more-distal weakness, loss of sensation, dysautonomia, and depressed DTRs. In the ICU setting, critical illness neuropathy and myopathy often coexist. Diseases of the neuromuscular junction often affect the respiratory muscles early, and involve the cranial musculature (especially eye movements) and proximal (limbgirdle) muscles.
   F. **Laboratory evaluation** should include a complete blood count with eosinophil count, erythrocyte sedimentation rate to aid in the diagnosis of vasculitis and myositis, liver function tests, blood urea nitrogen, creatinine, urinalysis, electrolytes, calcium, magnesium, phosphorus, and creatine phosphokinase (CPK). Patients with respiratory symptoms should have chest radiography, which may reveal, in addition to intrinsic lung disease, a potential cause for weakness (e.g., thymic enlargement with myasthenia gravis, lung mass with paraneoplastic disease, etc.). In certain cases, additional laboratory tests are indicated, such as aldolase, lactate level, and an anti-acetylcholine receptor antibody. A lumbar puncture

should be performed if Guillain-Barré syndrome is considered. Electromyography with nerve conduction studies (EMG/NCS) may be needed to help establish a diagnosis, with nerve and/or muscle biopsy occasionally required.

II. **Central nervous system causes**
   A. **Stroke,** either ischemic or hemorrhagic. The **sudden onset of neurologic symptoms and signs** prompts an immediate evaluation. The level of consciousness may be affected, depending on the size and location of the stroke (e.g., brainstem or ventricular system). The initial steps in the workup, after stabilization of the patient, include neuroimaging. Noncontrast computed tomography (CT) should be performed to exclude an intracranial hemorrhage, and then CT angiography and CT perfusion if needed (see Chapter 29).
   B. **Primary brainstem processes** in addition to ischemic or hemorrhagic stroke can include **central pontine myelinolysis** (Chapter 29). This occurs after rapid correction of a hypo-osmolar state (typically hyponatremia) that has been present for at least 48 hours. Patients have an impaired level of consciousness, ranging from confusion to coma. Paresis involves the upper extremities more than the lower extremities, and sixth-nerve palsies and rigidity are common. Other ocular abnormalities include miotic or mydriatic pupils, conjugate gaze palsies, and ocular bobbing. The purported cause for the abnormal response in the pons is that oligodendrocytes in the pons are located close to the highly vascularized gray matter, causing it to be particularly susceptible to damage from vasogenic edema and leakage of myelinotoxic substances from the vessel. Other areas of brain that are affected include midbrain, basal ganglia, white matter of the folia cerebelli, and the deep layers of the cerebral cortex and adjacent white matter. The diagnosis is made typically by magnetic resonance imaging (MRI). EMG/NCS are normal. There is no specific treatment, and prognosis is poor for extensive lesions.
   C. **Encephalitis or abscess** should be considered in patients with fever, confusion, meningismus, focal neurologic signs, or seizures. Therapy is directed at the causative agent (bacterial, viral, or fungal). Surgical treatment is warranted for large, loculated lesions or those refractory to medical (antibiotic) therapy.

III. **Myopathy**
   A. Acutely, myopathic disorders cause **proximal** greater than distal weakness, with preserved DTRs and sensation. Chronically, patients may develop atrophy and distal weakness as well. Causes include steroid use, alcoholism, immobility, connective tissue disorders (polymyositis, dermatomyositis), infection (trichinosis), toxic (extended paralytic use, neuroleptics, heavy metal/toxin exposure), and metabolic (hyper- or hypokalemia) factors. Electromyographic/nerve conduction studies and muscle biopsy are often indicated to establish a diagnosis.

B. **Critical illness myopathy** occurs in the setting of sepsis, neuromuscular blockade, and corticosteroid use. Neuropathic features include abnormal fiber size, atrophy, angulated fibers, internalized nuclei, rimmed vacuoles, fatty degeneration, fibrosis, and single-fiber necrosis. Variations include **thick-filament myopathy,** seen in patients who have received **corticosteroids** for severe asthma or organ transplantation, with or without concomitant **neuromuscular blocking agents,** and necrotizing myopathy, often distinguished by a markedly elevated serum CPK. No specific therapies for these different myopathies have been found to be helpful, other than removing the causative agents as early as possible. Muscle biopsy should be considered to rule out an inflammatory myopathy. **Critical illness myopathy** may be differentiated from **critical illness polyneuropathy** (CIP) on the basis of clinical presentation because critical illness polyneuropathy demonstrates proximal and distal impairment as well as loss of DTRs. An additional method of differentiation between myopathy and polyneuropathy may be made on the basis of the nature of progression and duration of symptoms. CIP is often self-limiting, and recovery is relatively rapid and complete. However, critical illness myopathy is frequently more severe with regard to symptoms and duration. It can involve a prolonged recovery phase, with patients still experiencing marked physiologic compromise and diminished quality of life as long as 1 year after the initial presentation. EMG/NCS and muscle biopsy may be required for a definitive diagnosis.

C. **Acute rhabdomyolysis** occurs with traumatic crush injuries, drug overdose, toxin exposure, severe metabolic abnormalities, and infections. Patients have swollen, tender muscles, with localized or diffuse weakness. There is breakdown of skeletal muscle, with leakage of its intracellular contents, causing secondary organ damage. **CPK** is highly elevated, and there may be leukocytosis, hyperkalemia, hyperuricemia, hypo- or hypercalcemia, hyperphosphatemia, lactic acidosis, thrombocytopenia, and disseminated intravascular coagulation (DIC). Management should be directed toward hydration with a goal of urine output in excess of 2 ml/kg body weight. To minimize renal compromise associated with myoglobinuria, the urine is alkalinized by the addition of sodium bicarbonate to intravenous fluids, with a target urine pH greater than 6.5 in the setting of serum CPK concentrations greater than 5,000 to 6,000 U/L. Threshold for treatment can be lower in the setting of acidemia, hypovolemia, and/or underlying renal disease. Controlling renal failure (which may require temporary hemodialysis) and correcting metabolic abnormalities and DIC are primary goals of the therapeutic plan.

D. **Neuroleptic malignant syndrome** is a rare disorder that occurs in the setting of neuroleptic use (but also may be seen with atypical neuroleptics, metoclopramide, and selective serotonin-reuptake inhibitors). It presents with severe muscle rigidity, hyperthermia, and autonomic dysfunction. Patients commonly have a leukocytosis and elevated CPK. It is felt to be caused by sudden and profound dopamine blockade, and young, dehydrated male patients are particularly susceptible. Treatment consists in discontinuing the offending agent, providing hydration, using antipyretic measures, and administering bromocriptine (2.5–7.5 mg three times a day), and dantrolene (1–10 mg/kg intravenously or in divided oral doses of 50–600 mg/d).

IV. **Neuropathy** can be axonal or demyelinating. Causes of neuropathy observed in the ICU include **CIP, Guillain-Barré syndrome, metabolic disorders** (diabetes, porphyria, hypophosphatemia, alcoholism), **vitamin B$_{12}$ deficiency, infections** (Lyme disease), **endocrine disorders** (hypothyroidism), and **toxins** (diphtheria, arsenic, thallium, shellfish poisoning).

   A. **Critical illness polyneuropathy (CIP)** typically occurs in older patients who are severely ill, often with sepsis. It is a self-limited process, often with a good recovery if the underlying critical condition(s) can be treated. Additional risk factors include the duration of mechanical ventilation, hyperosmolality, parenteral nutrition, nondepolarizing neuromuscular blocking agents, and severity of illness on admission. The clinical exam is significant for motor and sensory system involvement, with a flaccid tetraparesis and muscle atrophy. Deep tendon reflexes are commonly reduced. EMG/NCS reveal a distal axonal sensorimotor polyneuropathy, with fibrillations and positive sharp waves in the proximal and distal muscles, with relative sparing of the facial muscles. Biopsy reveals predominantly axonal degeneration and denervation atrophy of both proximal and distal muscles. Succinylcholine should not be given to patients with CIP because of the risk of developing hyperkalemic cardiac arrest. Treatment consists of supportive care, treatment of the underlying conditions, and prolonged physical therapy.

   B. **Guillain-Barré syndrome** (GBS; acute inflammatory demyelinating polyneuropathy) is an acute/subacute demyelinating inflammatory neuropathy with a number of variants, including motor-sensory GBS, pure motor GBS, Miller Fisher variant (MFS), bulbar variant, and primary axonal GBS. The incidence is 1 to 2 per 100,000 adults. It is frequently precipitated by an infectious illness, including infection with *Campylobacter jejuni,* cytomegalovirus, and herpes simplex virus, and upper respiratory tract infections. It can also be induced by surgery and immunizations. The process consists in complement activation triggering of myelin destruction in the peripheral nervous system. Axonal involvement is seen in 15% of cases, most typically with *Campylobacter* infection.

      1. **The clinical presentation** is of migratory symmetric weakness, sensory dysesthesias, and hyporeflexia. MFS presents with ataxia, ophthalmoplegia, and hyporeflexia, without appendicular weakness.

2. **Evaluation** includes cerebrospinal fluid (CSF) analysis and EMG/NCS. The CSF reveals elevated protein with normal cell counts (albuminocytologic dissociation), but the protein may be normal in the first week. If a marked pleocytosis (>20 cells) is present, an evaluation for HIV and Lyme disease should be undertaken. Characteristic findings on EMG/NCS include motor nerve conduction block, prolonged distal conduction, and slowing of nerve conduction. An important early finding is prolongation, dispersion, or absence of F waves, indicative of root demyelination. Antibody testing is also performed to distinguish the different variants of GBS.

3. **Management** should place emphasis on supportive care of the complications, particularly **respiratory failure** and **autonomic dysfunction.** Indications for intubation include a vital capacity of less than 15 ml/kg and a maximum negative inspiratory pressure of less than 30 mm Hg as well as the clinical appearance of a tiring patient. Patients with early cranial nerve dysfunction are more susceptible to aspiration and dysautonomia. **Early tracheostomy** should be considered in patients with severe weakness. Extubation attempts should be delayed in patients with ongoing dysautonomia because the stress of weaning can cause dramatic fluctuations in blood pressure as well as cardiac dysrhythmias. Dysautonomia typically consists of rapid, wide fluctuations in blood pressure, but other causes of hypotension in GBS patients include sepsis, pulmonary embolus, venous pooling, and electrolyte disturbances. Patients tend to be hypersensitive to both vasopressor medications as well as intravenous (IV) antihypertensive medications, and hypotension is best treated with fluid boluses and Trendelenburg position. Betablockade should be avoided in patients with bradycardia because their use has been linked to cardiac arrest. Dysrhythmias are generally of minor significance, but sinus bradycardia, sinus arrest, and atrioventricular block can occur; tachydysrhythmias, such as supraventricular tachycardia and ventricular tachycardia, may occur in the setting of tracheal intubation or suctioning. Complete heart block is treated with a temporary pacemaker. Other important features of management include pain control (often responsive to neuropathic pain agents, nonsteroidal antiinflammatory drugs, and narcotics), deep vein thrombosis prophylaxis, and splinting to prevent contractures.

4. **Specific therapies** for GBS include **plasma exchange (PE)** and **IV immunoglobulin (Ig).** Relative contraindications to treatment with PE include sepsis, myocardial infarction within 6 months, marked dysautonomia, and active bleeding. Side effects of PE include vasovagal reactions, hypovolemia, anaphylaxis, hemolysis, hematoma formation, hypocalcemia, thrombocytopenia, hypothermia, and hypokalemia.

Standard therapy consists of five exchanges each of 2 to 4 L over 90 to 120 minutes with 5% albumin repletion, over alternating days. IV Ig does not require placement of a central venous catheter, is less expensive than PE, and does not produce hemodynamic instability. Side effects include aseptic meningitis, anaphylaxis (especially in immunoglobulin A [IgA]-deficient patients), acute renal failure, and thromboembolic events (including ischemic stroke). Some studies have suggested a higher relapse rate with IV Ig compared with PE. The dose of IV Ig is 0.4 g/kg/d for 5 days. Corticosteroids have no benefit in the treatment of GBS.

V. Neuromuscular junction. Transmission of neural impulses can be affected by myasthenic syndromes, botulism, hypermagnesemia, organophosphate poisoning, nerve agents (e.g., sarin), and prolonged effects of paralytic agents.

A. Myasthenia gravis is an autoimmune disease with antibodies directed against the acetylcholine receptor (in approximately 80% of cases), leading to destruction/simplification of the synaptic cleft. Its prevalence is 14 per 100,000 adults. It occurs in individuals of all ages, with a peak in women in the third and fourth decades and in men in the sixth and seventh decades. Typically, symptoms increase in severity within the first 3 years of onset and are punctuated by spontaneous, brief remissions. Common presenting signs include ophthalmoparesis, ptosis, jaw weakness, proximal limb weakness, and progressive respiratory failure. **Myasthenic crisis** presents as a dramatic worsening, particularly of respiratory symptoms, often triggered by a viral infection, surgery, childbirth, or an exacerbating medication. Bulbar function should be assessed early to determine the need for elective intubation. **Cholinergic crisis** can also present with respiratory decompensation, and occurs with overmedication with cholinergic agents. Symptoms include excessive salivation, thick bronchial secretions, muscle fasciculations, abdominal cramping, diarrhea, and miosis (myasthenic patients typically have mydriasis).

B. Diagnosis of myasthenia gravis is by EMG/NCS, antibody testing, and the **edrophonium (Tensilon) test,** which must be performed in an ICU or emergency department setting. Markers of improvement include an increase in sustained upward gaze, ptosis, or dynamometry of a muscle or muscle group in an extremity. The dose is 1 ml of edrophonium in a 10-mg/ml solution. One-tenth of a milliliter (1 mg) is given as a test dose, waiting 30 seconds for excessive muscarinic effects. The remainder is then given over 1 minute. Edrophonium has a rapid onset (30 seconds) and short duration of action (2–20 minutes). The test is considered positive if there is unequivocal improvement in an objectively weak muscle. Atropine, 0.5 mg IV, should be given if abdominal cramps, bronchospasm, vomiting, or bradycardia occurs. If the bradycardia persists and is accompanied by hypotension, an additional 1 mg of atropine should be given. Edrophonium can also be given if the differential between myasthenic and cholinergic crisis is considered, although in a smaller dose (1 mg); patients without myasthenia may be unchanged or worsened by the test.

C. EMG/NCS testing should be performed after discontinuation of anticholinesterase medications for 12 hours. Surface electrodes are used for repetitive stimulation at a rate of 2 to 5 Hz before and after maximal voluntary contraction of the tested muscle. An abnormal result is defined as a 15% or greater reduction in the compound muscle action potential (CMAP) amplitude between the first and fourth responses with supramaximal stimulation.

D. All patients with myasthenia should have a chest CT or MRI performed to detect the presence of a **thymoma** or enlargement of the thymus gland. If a thymoma is detected, it is an absolute indication for removal unless the patient is considered a poor surgical candidate. Patients undergoing thymectomy should undergo preoperative plasma exchange.

E. **Treatment** of myasthenia gravis involves stabilization of the patient, especially from a respiratory standpoint. ICU monitoring should be considered for patients with respiratory symptoms, and bedside pulmonary function tests are notoriously poor indicators for the need for mechanical ventilation; these patients can experience a rapid deterioration. When the vital capacity has fallen to less than 15 ml/kg or is less than 25% of the predicted value, respiratory failure should be considered to be imminent. Specific therapies include **immunomodulation** and **anticholinesterase agents.** Plasma exchange standard therapy is five exchanges each of 2 to 4 L over 90 to 120 minutes with 5% albumin repletion over alternating days. The IV Ig dose is 0.4 g/kg/d for 5 days. **Corticosteroids** are typically initiated during the acute setting, but their benefit is typically delayed by several days, and they are continued for 1 month or more. **Pyridostigmine** may also be used in the acute setting, but its use is tempered by respiratory side effects, such as increasing bronchial secretions.

F. Medications that can worsen myasthenic symptoms include antibiotics (clindamycin, aminoglycosides, tetracycline, gentamycin, bacitracin, trimethoprim-sulfamethoxazole), hormones (corticotropin, thyroid hormone, oral contraceptives), cardiovascular agents (quinidine, propanolol, procainamide, proctolol, lidocaine, verapamil, nifedipine, diltiazem), psychotropic agents (chlorpromazine, promazine, phenelzine, lithium, diazepam), anticonvulsants (phenytoin, trimethadione, carbamazepine), paralytics, and miscellaneous agents (penicillamine, chloroquine).

G. The **differential diagnosis** for myasthenia gravis should include Lambert-Eaton myasthenic syndrome, which may be the initial presentation of an occult malignancy; congenital myasthenic syndromes; Graves disease; botulism; progressive external ophthalmoplegia;

and intracranial mass lesions. The Lambert-Eaton syndrome is paraneoplastic syndrome affecting the presynaptic release of acetylcholine. In contrast to myasthenia gravis, autonomic and sensory symptoms are seen with this disorder, and the EMG reveals an incremental *improvement* with higher-frequency repetitive stimulation.

SELECTED REFERENCES

Berrouschot J, Baumann I, Kalischewski P, et al. Therapy of myasthenic crisis. *Crit Care Med* 1997;25:1228–1235.

De Jonghe B, Sharshar T, Lefaucher JP, et al. Paresis acquired in the intensive care unit: a prospective multicenter study. *JAMA* 2002;288:2859–2867.

Deem S, Lee CM, Curtis JR. Acquired neuromuscular disorders in the intensive care unit. *Am J Respir Crit Care Med* 2003;168:735–739.

Fulgham JR, Wijdicks EFM. Guillain-Barré syndrome. *Crit Care Clin* 1997;13:1–15.

Grand'Maison F. Methods of testing neuromuscular transmission in the intensive care unit. *Can J Neurol Sci* 1998;25:S36–S39.

Greer DM. Intensive care management of neurological emergencies. In: Layon AJ, ed. *A textbook of neurointensive care.* Philadelphia: WB Saunders, 2004;397–436.

Herridge MS, Cheung AM, Tansey CM, et al. One-year outcomes in survivors of the acute respiratory distress syndrome. *N Engl J Med* 2003;348:683–693.

Hund E. Neurological complications of sepsis: critical illness polyneuropathy and myopathy. *J Neurol* 2001;248:929–934.

Lampl C, Yazdi K. Central pontine myelinolysis. *Eur Neurol* 2002; 47:3–10.

Pelonero AL, Levenson JL, Pandurangi AK. Neuroleptic malignant syndrome: a review. *Psychiatr Serv* 1998;49:1163–1172.

Van der Meché FGA, Van Doorn PA, Meulstee J, et al. Diagnostic and classification criteria for the Guillain-Barré syndrome. *Eur Neurol* 2001;45:133–139.

Vassilakopoulos T, Petrof BJ. Ventilator-induced diaphragmatic dysfunction. *Am J Respir Crit Care Med* 2004;169:336–341.

31

Drug Overdose, Poisoning, and Adverse Drug Reactions

Richard M. Pino and John C. Klick

I. Introduction

A. **Drug overdose and poisoning** are frequently cared for in the intensive care unit (ICU). Although an overdose of prescription or nonprescription drugs might poison, that is, injure or kill cells, in this chapter the term "poisoning" will be reserved for compounds not used for therapy and for animal toxins. Drug overdose and poisoning might be iatrogenic (e.g., coagulopathy secondary to warfarin during adjustment), secondary to intentional (e.g., suicide attempt) or unintentional (e.g., a child taking his or her grandparent's digitalis) ingestion of a drug, due to an animal bite (e.g., rattlesnake), the result of inhalation (e.g., carbon monoxide), or a result of substance abuse (e.g., cocaine). A recent survey revealed 1,153 annual deaths from poisonings, of which approximately half were suicides. Of the total number of exposures, 85% were unintentional and 8% were due to therapeutic errors. This chapter presents the most common forms of intoxication.

B. **Initial treatment and stabilization** might include giving cardiopulmonary support, administering an antidote, beginning the elimination of an ingested drug by gastrointestinal decontamination with activated charcoal, and initiating correction of acid-base alterations. The intensivist needs to understand the sequelae of each drug taken in overdose.

C. In view of the large number of drugs and poisonous substances, the physician should be familiar with reference resources in each institution and the telephone number of the area **poison control center.** Hospitals often have readily available texts and on-line drug and toxicology information.

D. Each overdose should be approached in a systematic manner to determine the following:

1. The substance (s) taken.
2. The last dose of the drug and its dosing frequency.
3. The reason for the medication.
4. Other medications usually taken.
5. Coexisting disease.
6. The effects of the overdose, e.g., hypotension, respiratory failure, or life-threatening dysrhythmias.
7. Whether the effects of the drug can be reversed or the drug can be eliminated without further harm to the patient.

II. Overdose and adverse effects of prescription and nonprescription drugs

A. Acetaminophen (APAP) is the most commonly overdosed medication in the world and a leading cause of hepatic failure.

1. Most APAP is metabolized by glucuronization and sulfation to inactive compounds. Less than 10% is converted by a cytochrome P-450 mixed-function oxidase to N-acetyl-p-benzoquinoneimine (NAPQI), which has a half-life of nanoseconds. If NAPQI is not neutralized by conjugation with glutathione, it injures the bilipid layer of the hepatocyte. APAP overdose (7.5 g for adult, 150 mg/kg for children) overwhelms the hepatic glutathione stores, resulting in cell death.

2. **Baseline and daily laboratory tests** include the prothrombin time (PT), alanine leucine aminotransferase (ALT), aspartate serine transferase (AST), and bilirubin.

3. **Treatment** is the enteral administration of N-**acetylcysteine (NAC).** NAC serves as a glutathione substitute, enhances glutathione synthesis, and increases the amount of APAP that is conjugated by sulfation. If the elapsed time after APAP ingestion is 4 hours or less or additional overdosed drugs are suspected, activated charcoal is given and an APAP level is drawn. The serum APAP level is then plotted on a nomogram as a function of time after ingestion. The nomogram has three lines indicating lower limits for possible, probable, and high-risk groups. Individuals who have APAP levels above the possible line are treated with an NAC loading dose of 140 mg/kg orally diluted in a fruit juice or carbonated beverage. Because of its objectionable taste, it is often administered via a gastric lavage or nasotracheal tube. Aggressive antiemetic therapy may be needed when the elapsed time is 8 hours or longer; the initial loading dose is given prior to obtaining an APAP level. Additional doses are 17 mg/kg every 4 hours for 17 doses or until the APAP levels are in the nontoxic range. Doses are repeated when a patient vomits an NAC dose within 1 hour of administration. An IV form of the drug is available. Dosing is 150 mg/kg over 15 minutes, followed by 50 mg/kg infused over 4 hours, then 100 mg/kg over 16 hours. This drug has a high incidence of anaphylactoid reactions (see VIII B).

4. **Severe hepatotoxicity** secondary to the overdose of APAP is indicated by an ALT or AST greater than 1,000 IU/L. This hepatotoxicity may progress to fulminant hepatic failure and eventually lead to liver transplantation or death secondary to sepsis, cerebral edema, hepatorenal syndrome, and metabolic acidosis (72–96 hours). There is complete

resolution of hepatic dysfunction (4–14 days) in survivors.

B. Antipsychotic agents are derived from several classes of compounds in addition to the classic phenothiazines. They are used for the treatment of acute and chronic psychiatric disease, the control of acute agitation, and the treatment of migraine headaches, as antiemetics (e.g., droperidol, promethazine, prochlorperazine), prokinetics (e.g., metoclopramide), and as part of some anesthetic regimens (e.g., droperidol).

1. **Haloperidol,** a butinophenone, is frequently used for the treatment of delirium. These drugs work via dopamine (D_2)-receptor blockade, but also have variable affinity for α_2-adrenergic, M_1-muscarinic, H_1-histamine, and $5HT_{2A}$-serotonin receptors.

2. **Phenothiazines** have antidysrhythmic effects similar to those of quinidine. Metabolism is mostly hepatic. The elimination half-lives of many of these drugs administered orally or intramuscularly are long (10–40 hours) and extended up to 3 weeks in depot preparations.

3. **Toxic manifestations** of antipsychotics include seizures, hypotension, cardiac conduction delays manifested by prolonged QT intervals, ventricular dysrhythmias, especially *torsades de pointes,* extrapyramidal symptoms, and the neuroleptic malignant syndrome. The judicious use of intravenous haloperidol in the ICU is not usually associated with any of these. However, because of its long half-life, prolonged sedation may occur, especially in the elderly, after sequential escalated doses.

4. **Treatment** of antipsychotic overdose is supportive. Gastrointestinal decontamination is employed.

   a. **Seizures** can be treated initially with benzodiazepines, progressing to barbiturate therapy if needed. As for any patient with seizures, other causes (e.g., hypoxemia, cerebral hemorrhage, embolic disease, other drugs, etc.) should be ruled out.

   b. **Hypotension** can be treated with phenylephrine or norepinephrine. Epinephrine in lower doses and dopamine may further decrease blood pressure secondary to unopposed β_2-receptor stimulation. The α effects of dopamine might not be present secondary to the reduction in postsynaptic norepinephrine stores.

   c. **Lidocaine** may be more useful for the treatment of ventricular dysrhythmias than agents that prolong intraventricular conduction.

   d. **Physostigmine** (1–2 mg intravenous [IV] for adults, 0.2 mg/kg for children) with repeated doses as needed every 0.5 to 1.5 hours is used for the treatment of an anticholinergic syndrome.

   e. **Dystonic reactions** can be treated with diphenhydramine (25–50 mg).

5. Neuroleptic malignant syndrome (NMS) is a relatively rare life-threatening reaction to antipsychotics within 24 to 72 hours after administration. It is characterized by an altered mental status (which may initially be attributed to a treatment failure) prior to the development of fever, muscle rigidity, and autonomic dysfunction.

   a. Fever occurs from an imbalance of dopamine in the hypothalamus, which causes a change in the mechanisms for temperature homeostasis, and centrally mediated muscle rigidity. This is in contrast to the accelerated calcium-associated skeletal muscle metabolism in **malignant hyperthermia (MH)** (see section **VII**). The onset of NMS is slower, with less severe symptoms than with MH. The postoperative patient usually has a common reason (e.g., atelectasis, wound infection) for an increase in temperature before MH and NMS are considered. NMS has been seen after the use of prochlorperazine and promethazine as antiemetics and should be considered as a source of fever in an ICU patient receiving haloperidol, metoclopramide, or droperidol. Initial treatment is the discontinuation of the drug in question and cardiopulmonary support followed by cooling.

   b. Dantrolene (initial IV dose of 1–2.5 mg/kg every 6 hours, followed by 100–300 g orally [PO] per day or 1 mg IV/kg every 6 hours for 24–72 hours) is used to control skeletal muscle rigidity and hypermetabolism. At these doses, there is profound muscle weakness, which might necessitate intubation and mechanical ventilation. The mannitol in dantrolene will create a brisk diuresis as treatment for myoglobin-induced renal failure secondary to rhabdomyolysis.

   c. Bromocriptine (2.5 mg thrice daily), a dopamine agonist, is given to offset the action of the antipsychotic on the dopamine receptor.

   d. Amantidine (100–200 mg enterally, twice a day) and **levodopa/carbidopa** (25/250 enterally four times a day) have also been used.

   e. Laboratory studies include creatinine phosphokinase (CPK) levels, urinary myoglobin, and electrolytes.

C. β-blockers inhibit the pathway of G-protein → cyclic adenosine monophosphate (cAMP) production → myocyte protein kinase → calcium release → excitation–contraction coupling. The more lipid-soluble β-blockers (e.g., propranolol, metoprolol, and labetalol) also have a membrane-stabilizing function. These agents are used to decrease myocardial contractility, the automaticity of pacemaker cells, and the conduction velocity through the atrioventricular node. β-blockers are divided into β_1 and β_2 classes based on actions at *therapeutic* doses. With therapeutic doses in susceptible patients or with increased drug levels of a β-selective agent, both β_1 and β_2 effects can be present [e.g., bronchospasm (β_2 blockade) induced with esmolol (β_1)].

1. **Lipophilic β-blockers** are metabolized by the liver with their bioavailability increased in hepatic disease or by inhibitors of hepatic enzymes such as cimetidine and erythromycin. Nonlipophilic β-blockers are eliminated by the kidney. Renal insufficiency or the use of drugs affecting renal perfusion, for example, nonsteroidal antiinflammatory drugs (NSAIDs), increases blood levels. Most patients with β-blocker toxicity have symptoms within 4 hours and resolution within 72 hours. The toxic effects of sotolol may not be noticed for several days after ingestion because of its long half-life.

2. **Hypotension** secondary to decreased myocardial contractility can occur even in the absence of a severe bradycardia. **Bradydysrhythmias** (sinus, junctional rhythm, atrioventricular [AV] block, and idioventricular rhythm), widening of the QRS complex, widening of the QT interval, and asystole have been associated with β-blocker toxicity, especially for the lipophilic agents. Lipophilic β-blocker overdose has been associated with **central nervous system (CNS)** symptoms ranging from a decreased level of consciousness to seizures and coma.

3. **Electrocardiography** is essential in the diagnosis of β-blocker toxicity. Digitalis and calcium-channel blocker toxicity (see later discussion) should be considered because these drugs are often given with β-blockers to control heart rates. As for any patient with neurologic symptoms, electrolytes and serum glucose should be checked. Computed tomography of the head is useful to eliminate the possibility of an intracranial process (e.g., neoplasm, hematoma, aneurysm) as a basis for these symptoms.

4. **The initial treatment** of β-blocker toxicity is cardiopulmonary support, gastrointestinal decontamination with activated charcoal, and correction of hypoglycemia, with electrolytes as needed.

   a. **Glucagon** is the pharmacologic agent of choice because the myocardial receptor for glucagon is not affect by β-antagonists. The increase in cAMP via stimulation of adenylate cyclase by glucagon increases myocardial contractility and heart rate, thereby overcoming the effects of the β-blockade. The initial dose of glucagon is 50 to 150 μg/kg (up to a total dose of 10 mg if needed) followed by an infusion of 0.07 mg/kg.

   b. The use of **phosphodiesterase inhibitors** for β-blocker overdose treatment has been reported. Although it would seem logical that the administration of β-agonists would readily reverse bradycardia and hypotension, in reality the response is extremely variable even at more than five times the usual maximum dose.

    c. Epinephrine is the β-agonist of choice. Atropine and pacing are not usually effective except for sotolol.

    d. Sotolol-induced dysrhythmias can be treated with overdrive pacing in addition to lidocaine and magnesium.

D. Calcium-channel antagonists comprise one of the largest leading classes of antihypertensives and antidysrhythmics. The antihypertensive effect is through inhibiting the influx of extracellular calcium through slow voltage-gated slow membrane channels in vascular smooth muscle. This is the sole action of the dihydropyridine family (nifedipine, amlodipine, and felodipine). Myocardial depression may also occur in some compromised individuals and in overdose secondary to the effects on atrial and ventricular myocytes.

    1. Calcium-channel antagonists are highly protein bound, with variable bioavailability and half-lives. Metabolism is hepatic. Verapamil and diltiazem are converted to active metabolites. They are also potent inhibitors of microsomal metabolizing enzymes and may increase the concentration of drugs that are metabolized by this pathway, for example, phenytoin and theophylline. Conversely, the elimination of calcium-channel antagonists is decreased by inhibitors of these hepatic enzymes, for example, cimetidine.

    2. Bradycardia, conduction defects (e.g., asystole, idioventricular rhythms, bundle-branch blocks), and **hypotension** are the hallmarks of verapamil and diltiazem toxicity. Overdose of the dihydropyridines results in hypotension with reflex tachycardia. A common finding with excess of calcium-channel blocker is an **ileus** in a patient who had been tolerating enteral nutrition. Other symptoms are related to hypotension (e.g., stroke, lethargy, coma).

    3. Treatment initially consists of cardiovascular support. **Calcium chloride** (1 g) or **calcium gluconate** (3 g) is repeated as needed until the blood pressure rises, the heart rate increases, or there is no effect after four to five administrations. As with β-blockade overdose, **glucagon** administration (see section **I.C.4.a**) might be effective.

    a. Cardiac pacing and vasopressor inotropes (norepinephrine, dopamine) should be considered if the heart rate and/or blood pressure do not respond to the former treatments.

    b. Nonabsorbed drug should be removed via gastrointestinal decontamination with activated charcoal. This might require several doses because many of the calcium-channel antagonists are usually taken in extended-release forms.

E. Digitalis preparations (digoxin, digitoxin) are widely used for the treatment of cardiomyopathies and for ventricular rate control in atrial fibrillation and atrial flutter. Because of a narrow therapeutic window, renal dysfunction, and changes in bioavailability secondary to drug interactions, mild digitalis toxicity is relatively uncommon. Through the inhibition of the Na^+/K^+-ATPase pump by digitalis, cardiac myocytes gain intracellular Ca^{2+}, a positive inotrope especially in the failing heart. Digitalis has a chronotropic effects by several mechanisms. An increase in central nervous system vagal tone decreases the rate of sinoatrial (SA) node depolarization and prolongs the refractory period of the bundle of His. With the exception of the SA node, the increase of Na^+ increases phase 4 depolarization and increases excitability as well as delayed afterpotentials.

1. **Digoxin,** the most commonly administered form of the drug, is eliminated by renal clearance after an enterohepatic circulation. **Digitoxin** is cleared by hepatic metabolism. The therapeutic index of digitalis is narrow, and plasma levels can be affected by several factors. The addition of quinidine, amiodarone, and verapamil to a therapeutic regimen will significantly increase established digitalis levels. Increased levels may also be seen in patients given antibiotics by an alteration of the gastrointestinal flora that leads to a decreased metabolism. Hypokalemia, hypocalcemia, and hypomagnesemia will increase the sensitivity of the myocardium to digitalis.

2. **Initial symptoms** of digitalis toxicity are **gastrointestinal:** anorexia, nausea, and vomiting. Toxicity may not be readily diagnosed because these symptoms may stem from a variety of causes other than digitalis. **Dysrhythmias,** especially in patients with compromised hearts, are more common indicators of toxicity when other reasons have been excluded. Digitalis toxicity may be manifested by almost any rhythm or conduction disturbance. The most common are premature ventricular contractions (PVCs), first-degree AV block, and atrial fibrillation. A characteristic ST depression is seen on the electrocardiogram (ECG). Serum digitalis levels may be influenced by a variety of factors and are secondary in the diagnosis of expected toxicity.

3. **Treatment** of digitalis toxicity can be difficult. **Atropine and/or cardiac pacing** are effective for treating bradydysrhythmias. The administration of **magnesium, lidocaine, or phenytoin** will often treat ectopy. With a significant overdose, the inhibition of the Na^+/K^+-ATPase will result in significant hyperkalemia, which may be refractive to most treatments. This will eventually result in a loss of total body potassium that must be repleted when the overdose is treated. The most effective method of digitalis overdose treatment is the removal of free digitalis by Fab fragments **of antidigitalis immunoglobulin G (IgG) (Digibind).** This enhances the clearance of digitalis from the circulation by renal elimination.

The removal of digitalis at tissue sites is also accelerated. The dose of Digibind is calculated from a formula based on the body load of digitalis. This calculation requires a digoxin level that may not be available. It is simpler to administer Digibind (40 mg/vial) until the dysrhythmias are effectively treated or until the maximum dose of 800 mg (20 vials) is reached. Digoxin levels, although elevated, will reflect both the drug bound to the Fab fragments and the unbound drug.

F. **Lithium** is used for the treatment of manic-depressive disorder. Lithium toxicity may be the result of a suicide attempt, increased levels during chronic treatment, or increased levels after the new administration of a thiazide diuretic or placement on a low-sodium diet. The exact mechanism of lithium's action is unknown, but it may increase hippocampal serotonin release, enhance norepinephrine reuptake, and/or inhibit adenylate cyclase. Gastrointestinal absorption is rapid, the element is distributed in whole-body water, and there is renal elimination with significant reabsorption. The half-life of lithium is 30 hours.

1. **Serious toxicity** is present at serum lithium levels of 2.5 to 3.5 mEq/L, with life-threatening complications at levels greater than 3.5 mEq/L. A change in renal function that permits increased resorption of lithium in the proximal convoluted tubule (e.g., hypovolemia, hyponatremia, NSAIDs) will increase serum lithium levels. Nephrogenic diabetes insipidus is the most common toxicity seen. Dysrhythmias and circulatory collapse have been reported.

2. **Treatment** is gastrointestinal decontamination if an intentional overdose is suspected. Half-normal saline (0.45%) should initially be given to restore euvolemia because the patient usually has a high serum osmolality. The administration of a thiazide diuretic or amiloride may help to control the polyuria. Hemodialysis is required for a life-threatening lithium overdose.

G. **Salicylates. Acetylsalicylic acid (ASA, aspirin)** is the most commonly used salicylate and has traditionally been the agent of salicylate overdose. With the advent of child-proof containers, the restriction of child aspirin to 81 mg/tablet and 36 tablets per container, the awareness of **Reye's syndrome,** and the availability of nonsalicylate analgesics, the incidence of salicylate overdose secondary to ASA has markedly diminished. **Methylsalicylate** is found in topical formulations used to treat musculoskeletal pain and in oil of wintergreen. Chronic use on excoriated skin may result in salicylism. **Bismuth subsalicylate** is found in antidiarrheal preparations.

1. **ASA is absorbed** in ionized form in the stomach and in enteric form in the distal small intestine.

Hydrolysis of ASA to salicylic acid with elimination by renal filtration and excretion is the major metabolic pathway. There are several secondary metabolic pathways for salicylic acid. In severe overdose, these pathways become overwhelmed and the elimination half-life of salicylic acid is prolonged to up to 30 hours. A toxic salicylate concentration is greater than 30 mg/dl. Initially, hyperventilation, via direct CNS stimulation by the drug, produces a respiratory alkalosis. Bicarbonate is renally excreted and hypokalemia ensues in a compensatory fashion. An anion-gap metabolic acidosis occurs secondary to the uncoupling of oxidative phosphorylation and inhibition of the tricarboxylic acid cycle in the liver. Patients may be agitated and have tinnitus. Hyperglycemia or hypoglycemia may be present. Often, hypernatremia with dehydration exists that is related to a large insensible loss with hyperventilation. Uncommon events are pulmonary edema, coma, hyperpyrexia, and gastrointestinal bleeding.

2. **Laboratory tests** include plasma salicylate levels until the peak level is obtained, electrolytes, blood urea nitrogen (BUN), creatinine, glucose, liver function tests, and arterial blood gas tensions and pH as needed.

3. **Initial treatment** is gastrointestinal decontamination with activated charcoal, cardiovascular and respiratory support, replacement of electrolytes, glucose, and fluids, and alkalinization of the urine to "ion trap" salicylic acid and prevent reabsorption by the proximal convoluted tubules. Hemodialysis should be considered when there is renal dysfunction or when salicylate levels are greater than 80 mg/dl.

H. Theophylline is a central respiratory stimulant, a smooth muscle relaxant (decreased peripheral vascular resistance, bronchodilation, relaxation of the gastroesophageal sphincter), a positive chronotrope and inotrope, and a diuretic. An increase in cAMP-mediated actions via the inhibition of the breakdown of adenylate cyclase by phosphodiesterase is the "classic" mechanism of theophylline. It is now thought that this does not occur at therapeutic levels, and theophylline's actions may be through an increase in catecholamines, competitive antagonism of adenosine, and a direct action on intracellular transport.

1. **Metabolism** is by hepatic cytochrome P-450 to 3-methylxanthine (active) and an inactive hydroxylated compound. Although few drugs enhance the elimination of theophylline (barbiturates, phenytoin, carbamazepine, cigarette smoking), plasma theophylline concentrations may be increased by many commonly used drugs that are inhibitors of the cytochrome P-450 system (including macrolides,

fluoroquinolones, and cimetidine), primary hepatic disease, and a reduction of hepatic blood flow during congestive heart failure.

2. **Toxicity** is dependent on the duration of intoxication. Overdose is often the result of a drug calculation or administration error.

   a. **Symptoms** include nausea, vomiting, diarrhea, hypotension, cardiac dysrhythmias (usually sinus tachycardia, but a supraventricular tachycardia, ventricular tachycardia, or ventricular fibrillation may occur), agitation/anxiety, seizures, and muscle tremors. A relative hypokalemia with normal total body potassium stores may be present.

   b. **Acute toxicity** produces minor symptoms at 20 to 40 μg/ml, moderate symptoms at 40 to 80 μg/ml, severe symptoms at 70 to 80 μg/ml, and death at 100 μg/ml or greater. Increasing age, comorbid disease, and decreasing age in children increase the severity of a chronic intoxication for a given plasma level. It is more difficult to predict the effects of acute-on-chronic intoxication.

3. **Initial treatment** is cardiopulmonary support as needed. Theophylline levels and serum electrolytes should be obtained on a periodic basis, especially for acute intoxications. A relative hypokalemia may exacerbate theophylline-induced tachydysrhythmias.

   a. Supraventricular tachycardias may be treated with **adenosine,** an antagonist of theophylline. Hypotension, tachycardia, and hypokalemia may be reversed with **propranolol** unless the patient has a history of bronchospastic disease. **Lidocaine** has been show to be effective for ventricular dysrhythmias. **Benzodiazepines** have been effective for the treatment of seizures.

   b. Theophylline will readily diffuse from the circulation and adsorb to **activated charcoal** in the lumen of the gastrointestinal tract. One gram of activated charcoal per kilogram should be administered every 4 hours with aggressive antiemetic therapy to prevent theophylline-induced vomiting. Repeated administration of activated charcoal to remove theophylline has been associated with an ileus. Sustained-release preparations may form bezoars that might be difficult to remove.

   c. **Charcoal hemoperfusion** has been the gold standard for removal of theophylline. With the advent of more efficient membranes, **hemodialysis** is now considered equivalent to hemoperfusion. Hemodialysis should be considered for patients who cannot tolerate repeated doses of activated charcoal or who have levels greater than 60 μg/ml after activated charcoal, or for initial serum theophylline concentrations greater than 80 μg/ml.

I. **Tricyclic antidepressant (TCA)** toxicity is the most common cause of prescription-related drug deaths and usually occur within 24 hours of ingestion. The onset of toxic symptoms occurs within hours. In general, TCAs decrease the neuronal reuptake of epinephrine and norepinephrine by inhibiting fast sodium channels and blocking cholinergic, histamine, and gamma-aminobutyric acid (GABA) channels. **Trazodone** does not block the reuptake of norepinephrine, but does block adrenergic receptors. **Amoxapine** blocks dopamine receptors.

1. TCAs are quickly absorbed from the gastrointestinal tract and are rapidly distributed to tissue sites. Elimination is by hepatic hydroxylation and demethylation. The enzymes responsible for hydroxylation are saturated at high concentrations of substrate, resulting in a prolonged elimination. TCAs have half-lives of 8 to 30 hours in therapeutic concentrations, which may be prolonged to 81 hours in an overdose.

2. **Initial signs of TCA toxicity** are anticholinergic: tachycardia, hyperthermia, ileus, mydriasis, urinary retention, dry mucous membranes and skin, and altered mental status.

   a. **Manifestations of serious TCA toxicity** are dysrhythmias, hypotension, respiratory depression, pulmonary edema, self-limited seizures, and coma. Life-threatening toxicity is present with serum concentrations of greater than 1 μg/ml, with fatality at greater than 3 μg/ml.

   b. **The ECG** in an overdose usually demonstrates a sinus tachycardia with a first-degree AV block, nonspecific intraventricular conduction delay (secondary to an inhibition of phase 0 depolarization), and rightward axis. An atrial electrocardiogram with an esophageal lead might be useful for distinguishing this pattern from ventricular tachycardia, which is also common with TCA overdose.

   c. **Hypotension** is caused by decreased myocardial contractility (due to blockade of the fast sodium channels), depletion of norepinephrine reserves in neurons, and vasodilation (due to alpha blockade). The usual cause of death is refractive hypotension.

   d. **Treatment** consists of initial gastrointestinal decontamination with activated charcoal and cardiopulmonary support as needed. Refractive hypotension should be treated by repletion of intravascular volume and administration of norepinephrine. Administration of sodium bicarbonate also effectively treats TCA cardiotoxicity, either through the alkalinization of the blood (to pH 7.5) or through supplementing Na^+, but not by drug trapping, because there is minimal renal elimination.

III. Alcohols

A. Ethanol (EtOH) is the most extensively used nonprescription drug. It is also present in a variety of cough and cold preparations, mouthwashes, and perfumes.

1. **Ethanol is absorbed** from all levels of the gastrointestinal tract, but primarily in the stomach and small intestine, with blood levels achieved within 60 minutes of ingestion. It is initially metabolized to acetaldehyde by alcohol dehydrogenase in the liver. A cytochrome P-450–dependent pathway is used for less than 10% of metabolism, but is increased in chronic drinkers. Acetaldehyde is metabolized to acetate via acetaldehyde dehydrogenase. Ethanol elimination may be as low as 12 mg%/h in nondrinkers to 50 mg%/h in chronic alcoholics. The blood alcohol level will reflect the peak amount of ethanol ingested.

2. **The effects of ethanol intoxication** depend on whether there is chronic or acute use and the amount ingested. The standard values for blood alcohol levels are only valid for the nondependent person.

   a. **Acute intoxication** in the "nonalcoholic" may be manifested by euphoria to total circulatory and respiratory collapse. A frequent cause of morbidity is hypoxemia secondary to **aspiration** of gastric contents after loss of airway reflexes. **Dehydration** may be present from an ethanol-induced depression of antidiuretic hormone. A "holiday heart" syndrome of **atrial fibrillation** or **flutter** associated with ethanol use in nonalcoholics that corrects with cessation of use is well known.

   b. **Chronic intoxication** is a spectrum of comorbid conditions. Many patients have no symptoms other than an increased tolerance for ethanol. Malnutrition, peptic ulcer disease, bone marrow suppression, and immunosuppression may be subtle. Pulmonary complications secondary to concomitant tobacco and ethanol use are common. More severe forms of chronic ethanol intoxication include cardiomyopathy, dysrhythmias, Wernicke's encephalopathy, Korsakoff's psychosis, cerebella ataxia, ketoacidosis, hepatic cirrhosis, and gastrointestinal hemorrhage.

3. **Treatment** of the EtOH-intoxicated patient in the ICU is initially focused on the reason for admission (e.g., subdural hematoma, aspiration, musculoskeletal trauma, co-ingestion) in addition to cardiopulmonary support.

   a. **Other causes for altered mental status** (e.g., sepsis, encephalopathy, hypoglycemia, or head trauma) should be ruled out. The emergence of focal neurologic signs should prompt a detailed workup (e.g., the beginning of an acute subdural hematoma might not be evident on an admission computed tomography but be evident several hours later).

b. **Fluid losses** secondary to alcohol-induced diuresis, decreased oral intake, and vomiting need to be repleted. Cardiovascular support will depend on the level of intravascular volume depletion and degree of cardiomyopathy.

c. **Attention to pulmonary function** and secretion clearance is important in view of the high probability of pulmonary dysfunction secondary to smoking. Although antibiotic coverage for aspiration of community-acquired flora is usually not needed, empiric administration of a broad-spectrum antibiotic (e.g., ampicillin/sulbactam) may be prudent in the initial stages of treatment if malnutrition or immunosuppression is suspected.

d. **Vitamin therapy** with thiamine and folate and repletion of electrolytes should be initiated. Alcoholic ketoacidosis requires volume resuscitation and glucose administration in a manner similar to resuscitation for diabetic ketoacidosis.

e. **The altered coagulation profile** of patients with cirrhosis, including the thrombocytopenia of splenomegaly, does not require treatment unless there is a clinical indication. Bleeding esophageal varices may require endoscopic or surgical intervention.

4. **EtOH withdrawal** is often seen following elective surgery or an emergent admission. Symptoms include anxiety, tremors, irritability, hypertension, and hallucinations that generally peak approximately 24 hours after cessation of EtOH but may appear within 10 hours. These symptoms might easily be attributed to a mild postoperative effect of drugs or disorientation in a "pleasantly confused" elderly patient.

a. **Denial** and underestimation of one's EtOH daily consumption is commonplace. Clearly, some elderly patients who have had "one glass of wine a night" for years will exhibit signs of withdrawal. A tactful and nonjudgmental approach often elicits a more accurate history in such situations.

b. **Tonic-clonic seizures** may occur within 48 hours after a decrease in EtOH use.

c. **Delirium tremens (DTs)** is a life-threatening syndrome marked by autonomic instability (hypertension, tachycardia, hyperpyrexia, tremors, and diaphoresis) that may be present 3 to 5 days following the cessation of EtOH.

5. **Benzodiazepines,** through their binding the GABA receptors, are cross-tolerant with EtOH. All benzodiazepines have been used with success. Intravenous or EtOH **diazepam** or **lorazepam** can be administered on a dosage schedule that is appropriate for the patient's age, size, and physical condition. The long activity of diazepam secondary to its active

metabolite nordiazepam should be considered in subsequent dosing schedules.

  a. For the treatment of seizures and severe DTs, the intravenous route is used with escalating doses.

  b. Tracheal intubation and mechanical ventilation may be required if respiratory depression occurs due to the needed high doses of benzodiazepines.

  c. Immediately following a seizure, an arterial blood gas measurement will usually exhibit metabolic acidosis with a pH sometimes lower than 7.0. Measurement is not indicated in this setting because the acidosis will spontaneously correct after the seizure.

 6. Haloperidol is useful for the psychotic reactions accompanied by ethanol withdrawal. It can be given intravenously beginning at 1 mg, with doubling of the dose after each intervention. Because of the long half-life, prolonged sedation, but without respiratory depression, may occur after sequential administrations. The QT segment on the ECG should be checked for prolongation during haloperidol treatment (see Chapter 19).

B. Methanol (MtOH) (wood alcohol) is a commonly used solvent. It is often ingested after synthesis in home distilleries (i.e., "moonshine") or by alcoholics seeking any form of alcohol. Peak levels are reached within 90 minutes of ingestion. The fatal dose may be as little as 60 ml. The majority of the MtOH is initially converted by alcohol dehydrogenase to formaldehyde, followed by oxidation by several enzymes to formic acid.

 1. Signs and symptoms include blurred vision/ blindness, gastrointestinal reactions (nausea, vomiting, severe abdominal pain, diarrhea), a severe anion-gap metabolic acidosis, and respiratory depression.

 2. Treatment of MtOH poisoning, in addition to cardiopulmonary support, is the administration of **intravenous EtOH** to achieve a blood level of 100 mg%. Start with a loading dose of 0.6 g/kg followed by 66 to154 mg/kg depending on the past ethanol use pattern of the patient. The EtOH will compete with MtOH for metabolism by alcohol dehydrogenase and reduce the production of formaldehyde. **Hemodialysis** is initiated to remove nonmetabolized MtOH. **Fomepizole,** an inhibitor of alcohol dehydrogenase that is used for the treatment of ethylene glycol toxicity (see later discussion), is also efficacious in treating MtOH ingestion.

C. Ethylene glycol, commonly used as antifreeze and also found in other solvents, is usually lethal after an ingestion of 100 ml if not treated swiftly. Like EtOH and MtOH, ethylene glycol is initially metabolized by alcohol dehydrogenase. Subsequent metabolic products are lactic acid, aldehydes, glycolate, and oxalic acid.

 1. Intoxication is marked by a severe anion-gap metabolic acidosis, a large osmolal gap (increased osmolality not accounted for by glucose, sodium, or BUN), and tissue damage secondary to the deposition of oxalate crystals. Hypocalcemia results from the chelation of calcium by the oxalate. Patients may be admitted in coma and have seizures, neuromuscular dysfunction secondary to hypocalcemia (myoclonic activity, loss of deep tendon reflexes, tetany), acute renal failure, and congestive heart failure and pulmonary edema (both related to deposition of oxalate).

2. **Treatment** of ethylene glycol toxicity includes cardiopulmonary support, treatment of the metabolic acidosis, intravenous EtOH administration as for MtOH poisoning (see prior discussion), and hemodialysis. **Fomepizole** (Antizol) is a competitive inhibitor of alcohol dehydrogenase that treats ethylene glycol poisoning and prevents renal injury by limiting the formation of toxic metabolites. The initial dose is 15 mg/kg, followed by 10 mg/kg every 12 hours for four doses, and then 15 mg/kg every 12 hours (all given as infusions over 30 minutes) until the ethylene glycol levels are less than 20 mg/dl.

IV. **Substance abuse**

A. **Amphetamine and cocaine intoxications** can be the primary reason for admission, or comorbidities of trauma. **Amphetamines** are indirect sympathomimetics that increase postsynaptic catecholamines by inhibiting the presynaptic uptake and storage of catecholamines as well as their destruction by oxidase. **Cocaine** works in a similar fashion, and also binds to the dopamine-reuptake transporter. Both have been associated with seizures, intracerebral hemorrhage, ischemic strokes, hypertension, tachycardia, myocardial ischemia and infarctions, dysrhythmias, hyperpyrexia, rhabdomyolysis, acute renal failure, disseminated intravascular coagulation, and pulmonary edema. Pulmonary edema may occur several days after drug use, and initially appears as acute respiratory distress with hypoxemia followed by a noncardiogenic pulmonary edema. Treatment is supportive care for the organ systems involved and aggressive control of hyperpyrexia, if present. Unopposed β-blockade should be avoided because it worsens outcome. Hyperadrenergic symptoms can be treated with benzodiazepine administration.

B. **Barbiturates** are used to treat seizure disorders, induce general anesthesia, and produce conscious sedation in children. They are a source of substance abuse and have been implicated in suicides. Co-ingestion of other substances must be considered. These highly lipid-soluble drugs are absorbed rapidly from the gastrointestinal tract and rapidly distributed to the brain. Barbiturates are oxidized by enzymes in the smooth endoplasmic reticulum of hepatocytes and are cleared to a variable extent by the kidney. Induction of the oxidative enzymes may increase elimination of compounds metabolized by the same pathways and also produce tolerance to barbiturates.

1. **Severe acute barbiturate overdose** is manifested by coma, hypoventilation, hypothermia, and hypotension (secondary to cardiovascular depression).

2. **Treatment** includes cardiopulmonary support and the removal of barbiturate by alkaline diuresis and gastrointestinal decontamination with activated charcoal. Neurologic status is assessed with frequent physical examinations, computed tomography to determine the presence of focal lesions, and lumbar puncture to rule out meningitis. An **isoelectric electroencephalogram** may indicate suppression of neuronal activity by the barbiturate rather than brain death.

C. **Benzodiazepines** have sedative, anxiolytic, anticonvulsant, and hypnotic actions and high abuse potential. They enhance the binding of GABA to its receptor and potentiate neuronal inhibition through hyperpolarization of the plasma membrane.

1. Oral formulations are easily absorbed from the gastrointestinal tract and appear in the systemic circulation within 30 minutes. The metabolism of all benzodiazepines is by hepatic cytochrome P-450 with transformation to secondary products and conjugation to inactive compounds that are cleared by the kidney. The metabolic products (desalkylflurazepam, desmethyldiazepam) of some benzodiazepines retain the affinity for the GABA receptor and have half-lives greatly exceeding those of their parent compounds. As for other drugs that use the cytochrome P-450 pathway, their metabolism can be increased by increased age, hepatic disease, and inducers (e.g., EtOH, barbiturates) or decreased by inhibitors (e.g., cimetidine, erythromycin).

2. **The toxicity** of benzodiazepines taken in overdose is minimal due to a high therapeutic index. Patients will exhibit CNS depression marked by drowsiness, stupor, or ataxia. Coma, respiratory depression, and death are rare. If co-ingested with EtOH, barbiturates, TCAs, or antipsychotics, however, the safety margin of benzodiazepines is markedly diminished. Profound CNS depression, cardiovascular instability, and respiratory failure may be present.

3. **Diazepam** is frequently used for sedation in concert with opiates to facilitate mechanical ventilation (see Chapter 5). Toxicity due to elevated diazepam and desmethyldiazepam levels may be seen if the initial dose is not decreased after a few days, especially for elderly patients. Profound sedation may confound the physical examination to the point of requiring an invasive and expensive neurologic investigation (e.g., lumbar puncture, computed tomography).

4. **Treatment** is supportive after gastrointestinal decontamination with activated charcoal. **Flumazenil**

is a benzodiazepine antagonist that will reverse the effects of an overdose. The dose is 0.5 to 5 mg IV. Because the half-life is almost 1 hour, redosing after 1 to 2 hours is required to prevent resedation. Seizures from co-ingested drugs (e.g., TCAs, EtOH) may occur when flumazenil use reverses the therapeutic effects of the benzodiazepine.

D. Opioid overdose in the ICU is often iatrogenic. Manifestations include somnolence, decreased respiratory drive with hypercarbia, and, rarely, apnea. Symptoms are treated by temporarily stopping or reducing the source of the opiate, administering naloxone in 40-μg increments to reverse the respiratory depression without compromising pain control, and providing ventilatory support as needed.

1. Patients admitted to the ICU after illicit use of opioids may have had respiratory depression reversed by naloxone or nalmefene in the emergency department, need further monitoring for respiratory depression and continued treatment with naloxone, have a requirement for mechanical ventilation, or need treatment for an overdose of co-ingested substances.

2. **Heroin** may cause the rapid onset of noncardiogenic pulmonary edema, similar to neurogenic pulmonary edema. This can occur several days after heroin use and is often initially diagnosed as acute respiratory distress syndrome (ARDS). Resolution follows ventilatory support with positive end-expiratory pressure and appropriate diuresis.

3. **Withdrawal** of therapeutic or abused opiates is often associated with an abrupt increase in sympathetic output. Agitation, severe hypertension, tachycardia, and pulmonary edema may result. α-2-adrenergic blockade with **clonidine** (0.1–0.3 mg/d, by mouth or by a weekly patch) will relieve some of the symptoms. Benzodiazepines can be used treat anxiety and concomitant ethanol withdrawal. **Early consultation** with specialists in substance abuse facilitates continuity of treatment.

E. Designer drugs are "recreational" drugs that are produced through small modifications of the chemical structure of a variety of compounds. Because of these structural changes, the drugs may fall outside current classifications of illicit compounds. The designer drugs used in a community and their precise effects vary, but are usually well known to law enforcement agencies and emergency room personnel. Treatment is usually supportive.

V. Poisonings

A. Carbon monoxide (CO) is a common cause of poisoning because CO is undetectable and ubiquitous whenever there is incomplete oxidation of propane, natural gas, kerosene, and gasoline. It is a frequent prehospital cause of death following smoke inhalation (see Chapter 35). An unappreciated source is through the metabolism of methylene chloride that is inhaled or absorbed from commercial paint products. CO binds to any heme protein and cuproprotein with an affinity greater than that of oxygen.

1. Mild symptoms include headache and nausea. The signs and symptoms of more serious exposures may reflect tissue hypoxia and reperfusion injury: ataxia, dyspnea, myocardial ischemic, dysrhythmias, hypotension, lactic acidosis, seizures, and coma. The diagnosis is made on clinical suspicion and the level of arterial or venous carboxyhemoglobin (COHg) measured spectrophotometrically with a co-oximeter. Because oxyhemoglobin and COHg absorb light at the same wavelength, pulse oximetry cannot be used as an indicator of CO poisoning. The delayed onset of a wide range of neuropsychiatric symptoms (Parkinsonism, dementia, personality changes, psychosis, incontinence) may occur 3 to 240 days after exposure to CO, with a 1-year recovery of 50% to 75%. Advanced age may be one risk factor. There are no predictive laboratory or clinical tests for this syndrome.

2. **Treatment** of CO poisoning is 100% O_2 to compete with CO bound to hemoglobin. The half-life of CO is 2 to 7 hours. This is reduced to an average of 90 minutes with 100% O_2 via face mask, 60 minutes by endotracheal administration, and 23 minutes with hyperbaric O_2 (HBO) at 2.8 to 3 atmospheres absolute (2,128–2,280 mm Hg) (see also Chapter 35).

B. **Cyanide**-containing compounds are widely used in industry and found in many synthetic compounds, insecticides, and cleaning solutions.

1. **Cyanide** can be released from many burning plastics during structure fires (see Chapter 34).

2. **Amygdalin,** a supposed herbal antineoplastic remedy from apricot pits, and similar plant compounds will release cyanide when degraded in the gastrointestinal tract.

3. **Sodium nitroprusside** (SNP) is metabolized to nitric oxide and cyanide. In the liver, the cyanide reacts with thiosulfates via the enzyme rhodanase to form thiocyanates, which are cleared by the kidney. Both cyanide and thiocyanates bind to the ferric iron of mitochondrial cytochrome oxidase, uncouple oxidative phosphorylation, and cause histotoxic hypoxia. Cyanide toxicity may occur when SNP is used at high doses, over periods usually longer than 3 to 4 days, in patients with renal insufficiency (decreased elimination of thiocyanate), and in hepatic insufficiency (increased cyanide levels secondary to decreased thiocyanate formation).

4. **Symptoms** of mild cyanide toxicity, as seen with SNP use, include lethargy, confusion, agitation,

increasing tachycardia, tachyphylaxis, and a lactic acidosis. In the appropriate clinical scenario, lactate levels have been considered one of the best markers for cyanide toxicity because cyanide levels are usually not readily available. The difference between the arterial and mixed venous oxygen saturation pressure increases to greater than 70% because tissues cannot utilize oxygen. Severe poisoning produces coma, seizures, cardiac collapse, and respiratory failure.

5. **Treatment** of SNP-induced toxicity is supportive after discontinuation of the drug. Gastrointestinal decontamination with activated charcoal is used for ingested cyanide compounds. **Sodium nitrite** (300 mg IV over >5 minutes in a volume of 100 ml of 5% dextrose) can be administered. Rapid administration of sodium nitrite will cause hypotension. The nitrite reacts with hemoglobin to form methemoglobin. The cyanide complexed to cytochrome oxidase will then form methemoglobin-cyanide, thereby restoring active enzyme. In severe toxicity, inhaled **amyl nitrite** has been used as quick source of nitrite. Subsequent treatment with **sodium thiosulfate** (12.5 g) leads to the formation of thiocyanate that can be removed by the kidney. If needed, additional half doses of sodium nitrite and sodium thiosulfate can be given.

VI. Envenomations

A. The incidence of bites from venomous snakes in the United States is estimated to be between 7,000 and 8,000 per year, with a mortality of fewer than 10 patients per year. Bites due to *Elapidae* (coral snakes) and *Crotalidae* (pit vipers) are the most common in the southwestern regions of the United States. The Crotalidae are in virtually every state and every climate. Coral snake bites are relatively rare.

B. **Crotilad venom** nonenzymatically damages microvascular endothelial cells, producing transudation of intravascular fluid.

1. Symptoms occur within 12 hours of the envenomation.

a. With severe bites, **hypovolemic shock** secondary to intravascular depletion, hemoconcentration, and hypoproteinemia is produced. An enzymatic degradation of the subendothelial tissues worsens shock via the extravasation of erythrocytes.

b. An enzyme-mediated **disseminated intravascular coagulopathy (DIC)-like process** occurs by primary fibrinogenolysis. Unlike true DIC, some hemostasis is maintained because thrombin formation is maintained, the D-dimer is not positive because the venom does not activate factor XIII to cross-link fibrin, and the administration of procoagulant blood products will not be useful because this is not a consumptive coagulation process. Thrombocytopenia is due to a loss of platelets at the disrupted envenomation site.

c. **Destruction of muscle** by digestive enzymes or from a compartment syndrome at the site of the bite is possible with the sequelae of acute renal failure secondary to myoglobinuria. With the exception of the bite of the Mojave rattlesnake, neuromuscular blockade is not produced.

2. **Treatment** includes fluid resuscitation and cardiopulmonary support.

a. **Compartment pressures** in the region of the bite should be monitored and fasciotomies and debridements performed if indicated.

b. **Crotilad antivenin** is administered according to the suppliers' recommendations. Because the polyvalent antivenin is a serum of equine origin, skin testing should be performed to determine whether the patient has an immune reaction to horse antigens. If the test is positive and the antivenin is required, the patient should be pretreated with diphenhydramine and a histamine-2 (H_2) blocker. One should be prepared to treat an anaphylactoid reaction (see section **VIII**) to the antivenin. Serum sickness may develop.

c. **Laboratory tests** every 4 hours include a complete blood count with platelets, prothrombin time, partial thromboplastin time, fibrinogen, and fibrin split products. Because the antivenin contains horse proteins, blood samples for typing and cross-matching should be obtained prior to its administration.

C. **Coral snake venom** contains polypeptides that bind to the postsynaptic receptors of the neuromuscular junction. The result is a competitive, nondepolarizing **neuromuscular blockade** characterized by a slow onset (>10 hours), precipitous manifestation, and prolonged duration (up to 2 months). There is little local tissue damage.

1. Patients are observed for at least 24 to 48 hours. The bite area should be vigorously scrubbed with soap to remove residual venom on the skin that can enter the circulation through breaks in the integument.

2. An infusion of **coral snake antivenin** should be administered according to the guidelines of the manufacturer. Because the antivenin is in serum of equine origin, skin testing should be performed as described previously to determine whether the patient has an immune reaction to horse antigens. A new alternative is an ovine Crotalidae polyvalent immune Fab. Initial control of the coagulopathy may be difficult, and a delayed onset of hematotoxicity may occur with this drug.

3. Patients who develop neuromuscular blockade should be treated with mechanical ventilation and supportive care until resolution.

VII. MH is an inherited hypermetabolic state caused by the inability of skeletal muscle sarcoplasmic reticulum to reuptake calcium after exposure to volatile anesthetics or succinylcholine. The precise pathophysiologic mechanism of MH is not known. It usually occurs immediately after induction of anesthesia, especially if succinylcholine is administered, or at some time during the anesthetic. MH can also occur several hours into the postoperative period.

    A. Signs of MH reflect its hypermetabolic state: severe hypercarbia that is difficult to correct with increased ventilation, metabolic acidosis, tachycardia, and a temperature increase of 1°C to 2°C every 5 minutes. Initially, signs of MH may be considered mild and mistaken for atelectasis or infection. The true extent of hypercarbia and metabolic acidosis is best measured in a sample of central venous blood, which may reveal a partial dioxide pressure of 90 mm Hg in contrast to an arterial partial carbon dioxide pressure of 60 mm Hg. Hyperkalemia, hypertension, hypercalcemia, a CPK increasing to 20,000 units or greater within the first 12 to 24 hours, and myoglobinuria are also seen. Dysrhythmias stem from the hypercarbia and the combined metabolic and respiratory acidosis. Disseminated intravascular coagulation may occur due to the release of tissue thromboplastin from damaged muscle tissue.

    B. Initial treatment of MH hinges on the administration of **dantrolene** to inhibit the release of calcium from the sarcoplasmic reticulum and decrease the intracellular calcium concentration. The initial dose is 2.5 mg/kg with doses repeated until the hypercarbia, heart rate, temperature, and acidosis resolve. A total initial dose greater than the recommended maximum of 10 mg/kg is sometimes required. A dose of 1 mg/kg IV or orally can be repeated every 6 hours for 48 to 72 hours to prevent the recrudescence of MH.

        1. Metabolic acidosis requires treatment with sodium bicarbonate if respiratory compensation is inadequate.

        2. Persistent dysrhythmias are controlled with procainamide.

        3. Hyperthermia can be treated with external cold packs and gastric and rectal lavage with cold saline.

        4. Myoglobinuria is initially treated with the mannitol that is admixed with the dantrolene [each ampoule of dantrolene (20 mg) contains 3 mg of mannitol].

        5. Hypokalemia and hypocalcemia are common after treatment of the crisis.

    C. Therapy for MH is often begun prior to the knowledge of CPK and blood gas measurements. **In the face of a normal value** or an incomplete clinical picture, the use of dantrolene should be discontinued because it can produce muscle weakness so severe that mechanical ventilation will be required.

VIII. Anaphylaxis and anaphylactoid reactions

A. **Anaphylaxis** is a life-threatening immunologic response to an antigenic stimulus usually within a few minutes after exposure.

1. **Common drugs** known to cause anaphylaxis in susceptible individuals are the thiobarbiturates, penicillins, cephalosporins, protamine in patients receiving NPH insulin, and intravenous contrast dye for radiology procedures. Many patients have a known anaphylaxis to bee stings and foods such as shellfish, peanuts, soybeans, and eggs. Simplistically, following an initial sensitization, some individuals synthesize high titers of immunoglobulin E (IgE). On reexposure, the antigen binds to specific IgEs on the surfaces of mast cells and basophils, initiating activation of the cells. A rapid, massive release of mediators of the immune response (e.g., histamine, prostaglandins, leukotrienes, kinins) subsequently occurs.

2. **Signs and symptoms.** The "classic" cutaneous manifestations of urticaria and flushing may not be evident prior to life-threatening symptoms of respiratory distress, hypotension, hypovolemia, pulmonary hypertension, and dysrhythmias.

3. **Treatment** for a severe reaction includes endotracheal intubation before airway edema becomes severe, rapid infusion of crystalloid to replete the lost intravascular volume (liters will be needed), and the parenteral administration of epinephrine (begin with 300–500 μg IV).

a. **Epinephrine** will increase blood pressure through effects on vascular tone (α_1) and augmentation of cardiac output (β_1), will inhibit the release of mediators (β_2), and is a potent bronchodilator (β_2). Bronchodilation can be maintained with an infusion of epinephrine titrated to effect (>1–2 μg/min) with the caveat that lower doses (0.5–1 μg/min) may cause vasodilatation through β_2 activity on vascular smooth muscle.

b. **Secondary treatment** includes the blockade of H_1 and H_2 receptors with **diphenhydramine** (0.5–1.0 mg/kg, IV) and the administration of **corticosteroids** (1–2 g of methylprednisolone) to further inhibit the immune response.

c. **Subsequent management** includes immunologic testing as needed and the standard intensive care management of resolving respiratory and cardiovascular sequelae of the anaphylaxis and resuscitation. The choice of invasive monitors will depend on the comorbidity and severity of the reaction in a given patient.

B. **Anaphylactoid reactions,** in contrast to anaphylaxis, do not involve presensitized IgE. Anaphylactoid reactions may involve the IgG- or complement-mediated release of immunologic mediators or be the result of an idiosyncratic interaction of the drug with mast cells or basophils.

1. Many drugs that may cause anaphylaxis in some individuals will cause an anaphylactoid reaction in others (thiobarbiturates, protamine).

2. **Mild anaphylactoid reactions** caused by drug-induced histamine release produce transient hypotension, flushing, and urticaria. Such reactions are frequently noted with atracurium (but not *cis*-atracurium), *d*-tubocurarine, morphine, and vancomycin. These are easily treated with crystalloid administration, low doses of ephedrine, and time.

3. **Severe anaphylactoid reactions** are clinically indistinguishable from anaphylaxis and are treated in the same manner.

IX. **Nerve agent toxicity.** The treatment of injury secondary to nerve agents employed as chemical weapons is a daunting task due to multiple logistical, psychological, and medical issues. Tabun, sarin, and soman are colorless and odorless fluorinated cyanide-containing volatile organophosphates (GX agents). VX agents are sulfur-containing organophosphates that are more persistent liquids. These compounds bind covalently to the enzymatic site of acetylcholinesterase (AChE). This bond becomes stronger with time (called "aging"). Soman ages AChE within minutes of contact. Exposure to these agents results in a rapid accumulation of acetylcholine at nicotinic and muscarinic receptors within *seconds*. Only synthesis of AChE corrects the depletion. Activation of neuromuscular nicotinic receptors result in a depolarizing blockade with progression to a complete blockade and respiratory arrest. In the CNS, confusion, convulsions, and coma will occur. Muscarinic stimulation leads to bradycardia with likely asystole, bronchorrhea, bronchoconstriction, excessive salivation, urination, lacrimation, and diarrhea.

A. **Protection of health care providers** is a prerequisite to patient care. Protective gear that will specifically isolate the wearer from exposure to the chemical agent must be utilized prior to entering environment where further exposure is possible or treating someone who has not been adequately decontaminated by established protocols.

B. **Initial treatment** is the administration muscarinic agonists, pralidoxime chloride (2-PAM), and anticonvulsants.

1. **Muscarinic blockers**

a. **Atropine.** The dose of atropine for controlling toxic symptoms is 10 to 20 mg during the first 3 hours after exposure. The starting dose is 2 mg IV for adults and 0.02 mg/kg IV for children. To fully antagonize the muscarinic activity, the patient is basically put into an anticholinergic overdose that may require up to 50 mg/24 hours to achieve.

b. **Scopolamine** (0.25 mg IV initially, then intra-muscularly [IM] every 4–6 hours) may limit the anticholinergic effect.

2. **Benzodiapines** are freely used for sedation and for their anticonvulsive properties.

3. **2-PAM** (1–2 g IM; children 15–25 mg/kg IM) and obidoxime (used in some countries) are reactivators of AchE by competing with the generation of the co-valent bond between the toxin and the active site of the enzyme.

C. **Definitive hospital care.** Most individuals who are exposed to high concentrations of chemical agents will die before treatment. Patients who reach definitive care are those who have been minimally exposed to chemi-cal agents or who have received an initial antidote and supportive care.

1. **Medical treatment** will continue as described pre-viously. Analgesia, sedation, and supportive care for multisystem organ involvement are required.

2. **Evaluation of concurrent trauma** is essential. Patients may be triaged to an intensive care unit be-fore a standard trauma workup has been performed.

3. **Symptoms of other injuries** may be absent or diffi-cult to assess. For example, a recovering patient may have abdominal pain from a perforated viscus that is masked by pain secondary to 2-PAM or the effects of the AChE inhibitor. Depth of sedation may be dif-ficult to ascertain with atropine-induced miosis.

4. **Logistics** of medical supply are important. In the scenario of a mass casualty requiring mechanical ventilation, there may be insufficient equipment such as ventilators and bronchoscopes. Critical care will be provided outside of the intensive care unit. Similarly, intensivists will necessarily provide emer-gency medical care as needed.

SELECTED REFERENCES

Ben Abraham R, Rudick V, Weinbroum AA. Practical guidelines for acute care of victims of bioterrorism: conventional injuries and concomitant nerve agent intoxication. *Anesthesiology* 2002;97:989–1004.

Brent J, McMartin K, Phillips S, et al. Fomipazole for the treatment of ethylene glycol poisoning. *N Engl J Med* 1999;340:832–838.

Brent J, McMartin K, Phillips S, et al. Fomipazole for the treatment of methanol poisoning. *N Engl J Med* 2001;344:424–429.

Ernst A, Zibrak JD. Carbon monoxide poisoning. *N Engl J Med* 1998; 339:1603–1608.

Gold BS, Dart RC, Barish RA. Bites of venomous snakes. *N Engl J Med* 2002;347:347–356.

Haddad LM, Shannon MW, Winchester JF, eds. *Clinical management of poisoning and drug overdose*, 3rd ed. Philadelphia: WB Saunders, 1998.

Kenar L, Karayilanoglu AT. Prehospital management and medical intervention after a chemical attack. *Emerg Med J* 2004;21:84–88.

Mowry JB, Furbee RB, Chyka PA. Poisoning. In: Chernow B, ed. *The pharmacologic approach to the critically ill patient*, 3rd ed. Baltimore: Williams & Wilkins, 1994: 975–1008.

Watson WA, Litovitz TL, Rodgers GI, et al. 2002 annual report of the American Association of Poison Control Centers Toxic Exposure Surveillance System. *Am J Emerg Med* 2003;21:353–421.

Woolf AD, Chrisanthus K. On-site availability of selected antidotes: results of a survey of Massachusetts hospitals. *Am J Emerg Med* 1997;15:62–66.

Wright RO, Wang RY. Poison antidotes: guidelines for rational use in the emergency department. *Emerg Med Rep* 1995;16:201–212.

Dermatologic Considerations

Bonnie T. Mackool

I. Purpura

A. The descriptive term **purpura,** defined as nonblanching erythema, encompasses many of the most serious cutaneous disorders encountered in the intensive care unit (ICU) setting. Purpura results from either dysfunction of the blood vessel or hematologic disturbances. **Palpable purpura** represents vasculitis, excepting perhaps a traumatized lesion into which an individual has bled, in which case there is not a primary inflammatory process around the vessels causing the palpable purpura. Vascular tumors are also purpuric.

B. **Vasculitis** implies damage to blood vessels by an inflammatory infiltrate, which may be caused by a primary vasculitic process such as **Wegener's granulomatosis, polyarteritis nodosa,** and **allergic angioitis and granulomatosis (Churg-Strauss syndrome).** In the **infectious vasculitis** entities, an infectious organism may lodge itself in the smallest vessels causing an inflammatory response damaging vessels, as in **meningococcemia, gonococcemia, yeast, deep fungal infections,** and **endocarditis.**

1. **Systemic inflammatory vasculitis**

   a. Skin findings occur in nearly one-half of patients with **Wegener's granulomatosis,** a necrotizing granulomatous vasculitis classically involving the upper airways, lungs, and kidneys. Skin lesions are the initial presentation in only 13% of patients. Palpable purpura of the lower extremities is the most common cutaneous presentation. Ulcers, papules, and nodules may occur. Oral ulcerations occur frequently and may be the initial presentation. Laryngeal, pulmonary, neurologic, and ocular diseases often are present. The latter symptoms include conjunctivitis and scleritis. **Skin or tissue biopsy** shows necrotizing vasculitis, although skin biopsy alone may show only a leukocytoclastic vasculitis. An antineutrophil cytoplasmic antibody (c-ANCA) test is often positive. Cutaneous Wegener's granulomatosis without systemic involvement can occur.

   b. In **polyarteritis nodosa (PAN),** a livedo or netlike pattern of purpura is often present with papules, nodules, or ulcers in a linear distribution. Palpable purpura of the lower extremities is another presentation. PAN represents a necrotizing vasculitis of the small and medium muscular arteries; it can involve the renal, hepatic, and coronary arteries. PAN may be associated with hepatitis B surface antigen as well as a positive p-ANCA. Purely cutaneous cases have been reported.

c. **Allergic angioitis and granulomatosis** occurs in patients with a history of asthma and eosinophilia. Cutaneous lesions are present in two-thirds of cases. Skin findings consist of palpable purpura on the extremities. Tender subcutaneous nodules on the extremities and scalp may occur. Multiple organs can be involved. In more than 60% of patients, peripheral neuropathy occurs presenting as mononeuritis multiplex. Skin biopsy shows a leukocytoclastic vasculitis and/or granulomas and/or eosinophils.

2. **Infectious vasculitis**

a. **Endocarditis** can produce characteristic purpuric macules or papules on the palms (**Janeway lesions,** and, when more prominent, **Osler's nodes**), **petechiae** (often scant in number), and **splinter hemorrhages** on the nails (a more reliable sign when present on multiple fingers and the proximal nail bed). **Purpuric pustules** or, in sepsis, large areas of purpura and necrosis may occur. Blood cultures confirm infection. Necrotizing vasculitis may be present on skin biopsy. Red blood cells may be present in the urine.

b. Both **meningococcemia and gonococcemia** are characterized by small pustules on a purpuric base. In the latter, the lesions are scant in number and are located over joints. Petechiae may be numerous or scant in meningococcemia and may be the only cutaneous feature. These lesions may range in size and number and have no characteristic distribution. Prompt treatment for meningococcemia is crucial.

c. **Rocky Mountain spotted fever** (RMSF) initially presents with small, lightly erythematous macules or papules on the wrist and on the palms. The papules then spread up the arms centrally on the trunk and concomitantly become purpuric. The lack of purpura with the initial lesions often causes the physician to overlook the possibility of the diagnosis of RMSF. The average incubation period is 4 to 8 days, with a range of 1 to 14 days. Petechiae may be the only cutaneous sign of RMSF. Prior to or accompanying the rash of RMSF, patients appear abruptly ill with fevers, headaches, diffuse myalgias and arthralgias. Patients often experience abdominal pain, which can mimic an acute abdomen. If abdominal pain occurs before the rash, exploratory abdominal surgery can ensue. The fatality rate is high. Any suspicion necessitates prompt antibiotic therapy [e.g., doxycycline (except in pregnancy or for children), chloramphenicol (for children)]. Laboratory tests, which should not delay treatment, include serologic testing and direct immunofluorescent staining of the antigen in skin biopsies (not offered at many centers). Serodiagnosis is optimal at 14 to 21 days after the onset of illness, and therefore is not useful at the time when disease should be treated. Patients who are treated within 48 hours of symptom onset may not develop convalescent antibodies and may appear seronegative upon testing. Hyponatremia and thrombocytopenia may be present at the time of illness.

3. **Hypersensitivity vasculitis.** Apart from palpable purpura as a sign of vasculitis, petechiae combined with larger areas of purpura can represent the hypersensitivity vasculitis known as **Henoch-Schönlein purpura (HSP)** in patients of age less than 21 years. In adults 21 years old and older, it is simply called **hypersensitivity vasculitis.** It is characterized by petechiae on the lower legs with larger purpuric papules or plaques. Lesions can extend from the lower legs to the upper thighs on to the buttocks. Skin lesions often are preceded or accompanied by arthralgia, abdominal pain, diarrhea, hematochezia, renal failure, and elevated liver function tests. Monitoring of hepatic and renal function is imperative. If cutaneous lesions are absent, the initial abdominal pain may precipitate exploratory abdominal surgery for an acute abdomen. Attacks are often recurrent. Skin biopsy shows a leukocytoclastic vasculitis, and if performed within 12 to 24 hours of lesion onset may demonstrate staining of perivascular immunoglobulin A (IgA)-containing immune complexes. Eosinophilia and anemia may be present. The antigen is often a drug or an infection. In addition to supportive treatment and elimination of the offending organism, prednisone sometimes in combination with cytotoxic immunosuppressive agents such as cytoxan can be used in severe cases.

C. **Depositional disorders.** These disorders represent damage to the blood vessels, with resultant extravasation of blood and purpura.

1. In depositional disorders like **systemic amyloidosis,** material is deposited within the vessel causing the vessel to be fragile. A sign that is highly suggestive of amyloidosis is the development of purpura in response to pinching a thin-skinned area such as the eyelid. Macroglossia and smooth erythematous or purpuric papules can occur.

2. In **cryoglobulinemia,** cryoglobulin deposition within the wall of the blood vessel renders the blood vessel susceptible to trauma. Purpuric lesions in cryoglobulinemia occur most distally in cooler areas (fingers, toes, hands, feet, and ears). Diagnosis is typically made by demonstrating circulating cryoglobulins. Skin biopsy of a purpuric lesion may help to confirm the diagnosis.

3. **Cholesterol emboli** characteristically manifest on the distal skin, mainly hands and feet. A livedo or netlike pattern of purpura is characteristic; cyanosis and digital gangrene and ulceration may occur. Diagnosis is typically clinical. Superficial skin biopsy is usually of low yield. If biopsy is necessary, a deeper wedge excision is of higher yield in demonstrating cholesterol clefts. Renal failure can ensue days to even months later. Early onset of renal failure indicates a poor prognosis.

D. **Purpura due to hematologic disorders.** In addition to inherent blood vessel deficiencies, hematologic disorders can also cause purpura.

1. **Disseminated intravascular coagulation (DIC).** Large, stellate-shaped purpuric macules appear in an asymmetric fashion on the body. Lesions can appear at any location and can be several centimeters in diameter. Petechiae may also be present.

2. **Protein C and protein S deficiency.** Patients with abnormal or deficient protein C or protein S may present with large areas of purpura, which may subsequently undergo necrosis. Patients with one of these deficiencies are most at risk for cutaneous infarction when Warfarin or heparin therapy is initiated or when doses are loaded. In Warfarin necrosis, fatty areas such as the breast and the calves are most prone.

3. **Heparin-related thrombosis.** Distal purpura and even necrosis can result from heparin-induced antibodies.

E. **Purpura with pain and induration. Calciphylaxis** is a poorly understood disorder that occurs most frequently in patients with renal failure and secondary hyperparathyroidism. It occurs more often in women and possibly in patients with type 1 diabetes mellitus. Massive amounts of calcium precipitate with phosphate and are deposited in the skin. It appears that deficient or dysfunctional protein C or S plays a role in precipitating the depositional process. The calcium/phosphate product may be normal at time of symptom onset with pain and induration. Purpura ensues as vessels become more damaged, and ulceration follows. Calciphylaxis is frequently fatal. Partial or total parathyroidectomy appears to decrease or halt progression in some cases. Debridement of ulcers or affected areas and intravenous (IV) antibiotics may be necessary. Warfarin or heparin loading should be avoided, if possible, in patients at risk. If anticoagulation is required, low-molecular-weight heparin should be substituted whenever possible. Treatment with biphosphonates may possibly attenuate disease progression. In all cases, phosphate and calcium levels must be monitored and balanced. Hyperbaric oxygen treatment has been reported to be of benefit in some cases. Early diagnosis is critical. **Skin biopsy** is imperative for the diagnosis.

II. Erythema

A. **Erythema** is caused by dilation of the dermal blood vessels. Epidermal change is signified by scale. Patients with widespread erythema covering literally almost the entire surface of their body are described as **erythrodermic**.

B. **Diagnosis.** The **differential diagnosis of erythroderma** is broad and includes drug eruption, previously existing skin disorders (e.g., psoriasis, atopic dermatitis, pityriasis rubra pilaris, contact dermatitis), erythema multiforme major, cutaneous T-cell lymphoma, scabies crustosa (previously called Norwegian scabies), toxic shock syndrome, graft-versus-host disease, and *Staphylococcal* scalded-skin syndrome. A skin biopsy should be performed of a characteristic area to determine the cause of the erythroderma. Morphologic and other clues are often lost with disease progression.

1. Any medication may cause a **drug eruption.** Sulfonamides, penicillins and anticonvulsants are common culprits. An exanthematous eruption may progress to erythroderma. Hypersensitivity syndrome may accompany a severe cutaneous eruption and is characterized by fever, malaise, and internal organ involvement. Reactions often occur within 1 week of starting the drug, but onset may occur later. Pruritus may be mild to severe or absent.

2. **Psoriasis.** Psoriasis is characterized by symmetrically distributed plaques with coarse, silvery scale. It may involve the scalp and intergluteal cleft. Nail changes with yellowish discoloration of the nail plate, pitting, and onycholysis (lifting up of the nail plate from the nail bed) are common features. Pustular psoriasis has small, white pustules, which may coalesce into lakes. Patients are often febrile, have an elevated white blood cell (WBC) count, appear very ill, and often complain of joint pain.

3. **Erythema multiforme** is characterized by erythematous macules or papules with a variety of hues of erythema, eventually creating target lesions that have three hues of erythema. Erythema multiforme minor has a limited distribution of target lesions. Erythema multiforme major is characterized by mucosal membrane erythema and erosiveness and large areas of cutaneous involvement.

   a. **Stevens-Johnson syndrome (SJS)** refers to large areas of involvement with target lesions and mucosal membrane involvement, which may include ocular involvement in the form of conjunctivitis.

   b. **Toxic epidermal necrolysis (TEN)** is the most feared form of erythema multiforme major, involving death of the epidermis with subsequent necrosis and sloughing. TEN is often characterized by flaccid bullae that, when compressed, extend beyond the visible boundaries of the bullae creating the so-called positive Nikolsky sign. An acute form of graft-versus-host disease as well as linear IgA bullous dermatosis may resemble TEN. Linear IgA bullous dermatosis has been reported with medications, notably vancomycin.

  c. **Potential causes of erythema multiforme** apart from medications are infections with herpes simplex virus and *Mycoplasma pneumoniae*. Skin biopsy will help confirm the diagnosis of erythema multiforme. Any erosive mucosa area should be cultured for herpes simplex virus, and a chest radiograph should be performed to look for pneumonia. For a very quick diagnosis, rolling dead elevated skin around a swab and submitting this to pathology is another method of diagnosing toxic epidermal necrolysis.

  d. **Treatment of** erythema multiforme is palliative. If a patient has begun to slough the skin, which suggests evolving toxic epidermal necrolysis, steroids are not advised because of the risk of infection. Immediate transfer to a burn unit is advised for patients suspected of having TEN. Observation for signs of pulmonary compromise, including pneumonia, is important because all visceral mucosa, including pulmonary and gastrointestinal mucosa, may shed. Although intravenous immunoglobulin (IVIG) has been used in the treatment of TEN, studies with IVIG show varying results. Thus, at our institution, the use of IVIG in TEN is considered experimental.

3. **Atopic dermatitis** generally is characterized by a light-intensity, diffuse erythema with scale. Areas may be impetiginized with a characteristic yellow crusting appearance.

4. **Pityriasis rubra pilaris (PRP)** is characterized by orange discoloration, prominent hair follicles, and islands of sparing particularly in the periumbilical area. Palms and soles often pass through a brief period of orange or yellow discoloration. PRP is often misdiagnosed as psoriasis. Skin biopsy may help to avoid misdiagnosis of PRP as psoriasis.

5. **Cutaneous T-cell lymphoma** is characterized by papules, plaques, and nodules. Erythrodermic patients with cutaneous T-cell lymphoma by definition have an advanced stage of this disease. The intensity of erythema often is deep compared to that of atopic dermatitis, which is characterized by a light-intensity erythema.

6. **Staphylococcal scalded-skin syndrome (SSSS)** is characterized by painful erythema that may be localized or generalized, with or without flaccid bullae. Bullae may lead to erosions. Erythema begins in periorificial and intertriginous areas and then becomes generalized. Because the disease is toxin mediated, the bullae do not contain *Staphylococcus* organisms unless

it is the site of inoculum. Children and individuals with renal failure are at increased risk because of their inability to eliminate the toxin.

7. **Toxic shock syndrome (TSS)** is another toxin-mediated illness that can cause generalized erythema from *Staphylococcus aureus* or from group A *Streptococcus*. Manifestations, including fever, hypotension, weakness, diarrhea, dyspnea, and seizures, which can be abrupt in onset. The rash has a variety of presentations including widespread erythema or a scarlet fever–like eruption with small, rough papules. Mucosal membrane involvement is common, including a strawberry tongue and other oral findings, and ocular involvement. The rash is often more prominent around the infected site. A diffuse scarlatina-like eruption occurs in only 10% of cases of *Streptococcus* TSS. Desquamation of the skin is most prominent on the palms and soles and occurs 1 to 2 weeks after generalized erythema.

C. **Laboratory data.** Patients with erythroderma are often hypokalemic, hypoalbuminemic, and dehydrated with a corresponding azotemia. Hypersensitivity syndromes can cause elevated WBC counts. Eosinophilia may or may not be present in drug hypersensitivity. Patients with pustular psoriasis may have WBC counts in the range of 20,000 cells/μl. Erythrocyte sedimentation rates are often elevated in all forms of erythroderma. Pustules in pustular psoriasis are usually negative on culture. *S. aureus* is sometimes cultured because patients can be colonized from prior hospitalizations or from contact with other people. Patients with *Staphylococcus* TSS rarely have positive blood cultures, whereas approximately 60% of patients with *Streptococcus*-associated TSS have positive blood cultures.

D. **Treatment.** The patient who is erythrodermic is generally very cold, shivering, and highly uncomfortable. Initial treatment is arranged to alleviate these symptoms.

1. **Fluid replacement** and close monitoring of electrolytes are crucial.

2. **Suspected medications** in the case of drug hypersensitivity should be stopped, and all potentially cross-reacting medications avoided (i.e., for phenytoin hypersensitivity, phenobarbital and carbamazepine should be avoided).

3. **Topical steroids** with occlusion are used for noninfectious, inflammatory processes (e.g., psoriasis, atopic dermatitis). They are vasoconstrictive, which decreases heat and fluid loss. In pustular psoriasis, it is suggested that topical steroids be used without occlusion. Plastic wraps or occlusive suits are applied over a medium-potency topical steroid such as fluocinolone acetonide 0.025% twice daily. The areas are occluded for 2 hours twice a day. As with systemic steroids, topical steroids can cause hypokalemia, increased blood glucose levels in predisposed patients, and adrenal

insufficiency, especially when applied over large areas and/or under occlusion. In addition, the erythroderma by itself predisposes to hypokalemia. The maximum duration of topical steroid therapy should not exceed 2 to 3 weeks, and should be shorter for face and skin folds. Occlusion should be discontinued after approximately 3 to 5 days.

4. **Treatment** in addition to or after the short-term use of topical steroids is directed at the underlying cause of the erythroderma.

   a. For a drug eruption, a period of 2 to 3 weeks generally leads to improvement, and care is supportive.

   b. In psoriatic patients, systemic therapy with immunosuppressive biologic agents, systemic retinoids, or phototherapy for a severe flare are options. If phototherapy is anticipated, additional lubrication and topical steroid treatments are administered to decrease scale and allow for the penetration of light therapy. Systemic steroids are *not* a treatment for psoriasis.

   c. Pityriasis rubra pilaris is treated with retinoids often in combination with phototherapy (PUVA or narrow band UVB) or methotrexate.

   d. Intravenous antibiotics are administered to patients with SSSS and TSS.

   e. Treatment for cutaneous T cell lymphoma is based on the clinical stage of disease, and includes psoralens plus ultraviolet A light (PUVA), UVB and narrowband UVB (perhaps in early stages), topical nitrogen mustard, bexarotene gel (used for <15% of body surface area), electron beam, extracorporeal photochemotherapy, chemotherapy, and alpha-interferon.

   f. Treatment for graft-versus-host disease includes systemic steroids, PUVA, topical steroids, extracorporeal photopheresis, and various combinations of immunosuppression.

   g. **Scabies crustosa** is treated overnight with an antiscabetic agent such as permethrin cream (Elimite), which is rinsed off 8 hours after application. The drug is reapplied approximately 7 days later to treat remaining eggs. However, weeks of subsequent treatment are generally required in scabies crustosa. Sheets should be cleaned before and after treatment. Clothing worn prior to treatment should only be worn again after being washed or after 3 days have elapsed since wear. Oral ivermectin is often administered in cases of scabies crustosa because even weeks of topical treatment may still result in failure to completely eradicate the parasite.

III. **Generalized erythema without erythroderma**

   A. Generalized erythema may present as a **drug eruption** or **another hypersensitivity reaction to an antigen such as a virus or parasite.** A decreased inflammatory response imposed by steroids may allow a parasite to proliferate, and a hypersensitivity response will then worsen. Thus, pruritus or erythema that is worsened with systemic steroid administration should prompt a search for a parasite such as an intestinal parasite.

B. **Viral infections** that may cause generalized erythema include **parvovirus** B19 (associated with erythema infectiousum or fifth disease), **measles (rubeola), and German measles (rubella).**

1. In **rubeola,** small, bright-red oral lesions (Koplik's spots) occur on the buccal mucosa. Koplik's spots may precede the rash and become less distinct with rash progression. Coryza is prominent. Erythematous macules and papules begin in the posterior auricular areas and in the forehead and extend inferiorly over the face, neck trunk, and extremities.

2. The rash of **rubella** begins on the face and progresses rapidly to the neck, arms, trunk, and legs. Erythematous macules and papules are discrete and become coalescent on the trunk. The rash changes rapidly over a few hours, tending to fade as it spreads. Lymphadenopathy may be prominent, particularly the suboccipital and postauricular nodes. Petechiae on the soft palate may be seen during the prodrome.

3. **Acute human immunodeficiency virus (HIV) conversion** may also cause a generalized macular or papular erythematous eruption.

C. **Scarlet fever** caused by group A *Streptococcus* (and occasionally *S. aureus*) is characterized by light-intensity erythema, often consisting of fine papules. The papules give the skin a "sandpaper-like" feel, which can generalize and be accentuated in skin folds (Pastia's lines). Scarlet fever is treated with penicillin V. Macrolides or cephalosporins are used in penicillin-allergic patients.

IV. **Vesicular and pustular disorders**

A. **Herpes simplex virus (HSV) infections** are commonly seen in critically ill patients (Chapter 28). HSV infections are characterized by vesicles and/or pustules that may be hemorrhagic and are grouped on the nose, lips, or other areas. Traumatic procedures to these areas, such as endotracheal intubation and nasogastric tube placement, tend to predispose individuals to outbreaks of herpes simplex. Genital herpes lesions when cleansed or traumatized, especially in patients that have any type of urinary or bowel incontinence or diarrhea, can spread from inoculation of herpes simplex to irritated areas. Monomorphic erosions, papules, vesicles, or pustules and pain in any erythematous or scaly area should raise the possibility of herpes simplex.

1. Uncomplicated episodes of HSV in adults can be treated as follows:

a. Initial episodes: **acyclovir** (200 mg) orally, five times daily or (400 mg) orally three times daily for 7 to 10 days, or **famciclovir** (250 mg) orally twice daily for 5 to 10 days, or **valacyclovir** (for initial genital infections) 1 g orally twice daily for 5 to 10 days. Valacyclovir dosing in oral cold sores is 2 g twice daily for 1 day. Doses of acyclovir, famciclovir, and valacyclovir must be decreased in renal insufficiency.

    b. Recurrent episodes: **acyclovir** (400 mg) orally three times daily or 800 mg orally twice daily for 5 days, or **famciclovir** (125 mg) orally twice daily for 5 days, or **valacyclovir** for recurrent genital herpes (500 mg) orally twice daily for 5 days. Doses of acyclovir, famciclovir, and valacyclovir must be decreased in renal insufficiency.

    2. In immunocompromised adults, HSV can be treated with IV **acyclovir** (5 mg/kg; the dose must be decreased in renal insufficiency) every 8 hours for 3 to 10 days. With improvement, drug administration can be switched to the oral route

B. Herpes zoster is characterized by grouped vesicles or pustules in a dermatomal distribution. In immunosuppressed patients, lesions of herpes zoster may be atypically papular or nodular. Herpes zoster frequently begins with pain, absence of skin findings, and localized erythema, initially without any vesiculation. In these cases, erythema may be misdiagnosed as cellulitis. Similarly, preeruptive zoster, depending on its location of pain, can be misdiagnosed as nephrolithiasis, angina, or an acute abdomen. Herpes zoster in the perianal area can cause diarrhea and temporary bowel incontinence. At the time that erythema presents it is useful to perform a complete skin exam to look for isolated vesicles outside of the dermatome. A small number of isolated vesicles occur outside of involved dermatomes.

    1. Herpes zoster can be treated in adults with **acyclovir** (800 mg) orally five times daily for 7 to 10 days, **famciclovir** (500 mg) orally three times daily for 7 days, or **valacyclovir** 1,000 mg orally three times daily for 7 days. Doses of all three agents must be decreased in renal insufficiency.

    2. In immunocompromised adults, varicella zoster can be treated with **acyclovir** (10 mg/kg) every 8 hours (the dose must be decreased in renal insufficiency).

C. Varicella-zoster infection is characterized by fever, malaise, and light-intensity erythematous plaques with a central vesicle. Lesions can be scant or numerous. Small erosive lesions can occur on the buccal mucosa or on the tongue. Lesions of varicella zoster may become impetiginized, especially in children with atopic dermatitis. When this occurs, isolated bullae with yellow crust occupy the sites of previous vesicles. **Treatment** in children 2 years of age or older is acyclovir 20 mg/kg per dose orally four times daily for 5 days. In adults and in children greater than 40 kg, the oral acyclovir dose is 800 mg four times daily for 5 days. Dose must be decreased in renal insufficiency.

D. **Vesicular and pustular drug eruptions.** Any drug can cause a vesicular or pustular drug reaction. Vesicles can become pustular, or pustules may occur as the primary lesion. Initial vesiculation should also raise the possibility of evolving bullous erythema multiforme or toxic epidermal necrolysis.

E. **Pustular reaction (early).** Pustules may represent infectious etiologies such as cutaneous candidiasis, *S. aureus*, or other staphylococcal infections. On the feet, superficial fungal infections may manifest as either vesicles or pustules.

F. **Sweet's syndrome (acute febrile neutrophilic dermatosis) and pyoderma gangrenosum (PG).** Lesions frequently start as the pustule on an erythematous base and enlarge into nodules that can be several centimeters in diameter. Patients often exhibit high WBC counts and fevers during eruptive periods. The surface is described as having a hint of vesiculation, but the lesions do not produce fluid. Lesions are often painful. It is estimated that 20% of patients with Sweet's syndrome have an associated malignancy; approximately 85% of these patients have a hematologic malignancy, most commonly acute myeloid leukemia. Although ulcerative colitis frequently occurs in patients with PG, only 0.6% to 5% of patients with ulcerative colitis have PG. PG may also be associated with leukemia, paraproteinemia, myeloma, and other disease. Both neutrophilic disorders are histopathologically characterized by a neutrophilic infiltrate in the dermis and epidermis.

1. **Avoid debridement.** Sweet's syndrome and pyoderma gangrenosum are commonly misdiagnosed as bacterial infections and subsequently debrided. It is important to consider these diagnoses and avoid debridement until a biopsy is performed to avoid accelerating disease progression. It is well known that in PG, trauma elicits pathergy that is a manifestation of disease activity, most commonly exhibited as progressive ulceration.

2. **Treatment** for Sweet's syndrome and PG is with high-dose systemic steroids usually beginning with IV methylprednisolone, which is later replaced by oral prednisone at a dose of approximately 60 mg daily. **Intralesional steroid injections** of the expanding rim is another often-used treatment option, given alone in mild cases or in combination with systemic steroids in more severe cases. Cyclosporine, azathioprine, dapsone, and mycophenolate have been used in the treatment of PG. The application of cromolyn, a mast cell inhibitor, is complementary therapy. Potassium iodide has been reported to be effective in Sweet's syndrome. Additional treatments reported to have been used in Sweet's syndrome include topical steroids in mild cases, colchicine, indomethacin, clofazamine, cyclosporine, and dapsone.

V. Ulcerative processes

A. **Skin breakdown on the heels and sacrum as well as the posterior scalp and scapular area** can occur in the ICU setting, where patients are immobile for long periods of time. Patients with **vascular disease** are more susceptible to ulceration from pressure and trauma. **Herpes simplex** is common in perianal and hip areas, and ulcer edges should be examined for a scalloped shape characteristic of previously coalescent vesicles. A Tzanck preparation or viral culture should be performed as needed. Ulcers should be cultured for bacteria and yeast, if such are suspected. Treatment of pressure ulcers involves frequent side-to-side turning and placement of padding under pressure areas such as the heels. Wet-to-dry dressings are preferable if pressure ulcers are infected, and occlusive dressings should be avoided in these areas except to prevent infection from fecal incontinence. Systemic antibiotics may be necessary.

B. **Cancers** that metastasize to the skin may cause ulceration. Frequently the surface of the ulcer is nodular or undulating. Metastatic carcinomas can cause deep induration around the ulcer.

C. **Infectious causes** of ulcerative processes include the initially nodular entities of **ecthyma gangrenosum and ecthyma. Meleney's ulcer** is an insidious process in which synergistic staphylococcal and streptococcal infections result in an aggressive ulcerative process that only responds to debridement and IV antibiotics.

D. **Warfarin-induced necrosis** is characterized by ulceration in fatty areas such as the breasts, abdomen, calves, and buttocks. Purpura often borders theses areas, and the initial lesion often is a purpuric plaque. Warfarin-induced necrosis can occur in patients that are deficient in protein C or its cofactor protein S.

E. **Calciphylaxis** is discussed under purpura (see section **I.E**).

F. **Lesions of pyoderma gangrenosum and Sweet's syndrome may ulcerate** (see section **IV. D.2**).

VI. Bullae may begin as vesicles and become enlarged.

A. **Bullous hypersensitivity reactions** can result from any drug. A skin biopsy is necessary to distinguish them from **bullous pemphigoid, bullous erythema multiforme,** and **toxic epidermal necrolysis.**

B. Bullae also can be caused by local ischemia (e.g., in DIC or in cholesterol emboli). In these cases, bullae are generally preceded by purpura.

C. **Contact dermatitis** can present with bullae on an erythematous and scaly base, often in a geometric pattern. Bullae may also result from peripheral edema, which commonly occurs on the lower extremities.

D. **Toxic epidermal necrolysis and pemphigus vulgaris** are characterized by short-lived flaccid bullae. The skin sloughs very easily, and both diseases demonstrate diffuse mucosal ulceration. All mucosa should be examined, including ocular, oral, anal, and genital mucosa. Pemphigus vulgaris has characteristic histopathology and immunofluorescent staining. **Paraneoplastic pemphigus,** most frequently associated with lymphoproliferative disease, tends to be refractory to treatment and demonstrates ocular and prominent oral involvement.

E. Intact bullae, often tense, are seen in **bullous impetigo, bullous lupus erythematosus, bullous pemphigoid,** and **bullous diabeticorum.** When compressed, the bullae do not expand, thereby exhibiting a **negative Nikolsky sign.** Bullous lupus erythematosus and bullous pemphigoid have specific findings on histo–pathology and direct immunofluorescent staining. The lesions of bullous diabeticorum are nonspecific. In bullous impetigo, the bullous fluid grows *S. aureus* or *Streptococcus* spp.

F. *Vibrio (V.)* infections of the skin are characterized by purpuric plaques and hemorrhagic bullae. Pustules and lymphangitic erythema can occur. Lesions can progress to ulcers and necrotizing fasciitis. Although *V. vulnificus* characteristically involves skin infections, other *Vibrio* strains, including *V. cholerae,* may cause similar lesions. Infection can occur through ingestion of infected raw seafood, handling infected fish or shellfish, or skin penetration of organisms on the shells of infected shellfish (i.e., oysters, clams). Patients with hemochromatosis and liver disease are most at risk. Septicemia from *V. vulnificus* has a mortality rate of approximately 50%. The diagnosis of *V. vulnificus* can be confirmed by stool culture and that of *V. cholerae* by Gram's stain, dark-field microscopy, or culture of stool. *V. vulnificus* can be cultured from blood and skin. Treatment options for *V. vulnificus* infections in adults include tetracycline combined with cefotaxime or levofloxacin as alternate therapy. Necrotic lesions should be debrided.

G. **Treatment guidelines.** The area should be cleaned with sterile saline and then dried. A moist covering with a dressing such as Xeroform is optional. Lesions susceptible to breakage can be drained by piercing the edge of the lesion once or twice with a sterile needle. However, in inflammatory processes, it is advisable that the bullae remain intact to provide a protective covering of the dermis. The underlying process such as **bullous pemphigoid, pemphigus vulgaris,** or **bullous lupus erythematosus** frequently requires systemic immunosuppressive therapy. Bullous pemphigoid in mild to moderate cases can be treated with potent topical steroids. Pemphigus vulgaris and moderate to severe cases of bullous pemphigoid initially require systemic steroids along with an agent such as azathioprine or mycophenolate. Methotrexate, cyclosporine, dapsone, and intravenous immunoglobulin have also been used to treat bullous pemphigoid and pemphigus vulgaris.

SELECTED REFERENCES

Abramson JS, Givner LB. Rocky Mountain spotted fever. *Pediatr Infect Dis J* 1999;18(6):539–540.

Champion RH, Burton JL, Burns DA, et al., eds. *Rook / Wilkinson / Ebling Textbook of dermatology*, 6th ed. London: Blackwell Science, 1998.

Chaudhary K, Wall BM, Rasberry RO. Livedo reticularis: an underutilized diagnostic clue in cholesterol embolization syndrome. *Am J Med Sci* 2001;321(5):348–351.

Cohen PR, Kurzrock R. Sweet's syndrome revisited: a review of disease concepts. *Int J Dermatol* 2003;42:761–778.

Fitzpatrick TB, Johnson RA, Wolff R, et al. *Color atlas and synopsis of clinical dermatology*, 4th ed. New York: McGraw-Hill, 2001.

Freedberg IM, Eisen AZ, Wolff K, et al., eds. *Fitzpatrick's Dermatology in general medicine*, 6th ed. New York: McGraw-Hill, 2003.

Jolles S. A review of high-dose intravenous immunoglobulin (hdIVIg) in the treatment of the autoimmune blistering disorders. *Clin Exp Dermatol* 2001;26(2):127–131.

Langford CA, Sneller MC. Update on the diagnosis and treatment of Wegener's granulomatosis. *Adv Intern Med* 2001;46:177–206.

Mehta RL, Scott G, Sloand JA, et al. Skin necrosis associated with acquired protein C deficiency in patients with renal failure and calciphylaxis. *Am J Med* 1990;88:252–257.

Piette WW, Stone MS: A cutaneous sign of IgA-associated small dermal vessel leukocytoclasis vasculitis in adults (Henoch-Schönlein Purpura). *Arch Dermatol* 1989;125(1):53–56.

Roujeau JC, Kelly JP, Naldi L, et al. Medication use and the risk of Stevens-Johnson syndrome or toxic epidermal necrolysis. *N Engl J Med* 1995;333:1600–1607.

Stevens DL, Tanner MH, Winship J, et al. Reappearance of scarlet fever toxin A among streptococci in the Rocky Mountain West: severe group A streptococcal infections associated with a toxic shock-like syndrome. *N Engl J Med* 1989;321:1–7.

Tacket CO, Brenner F, Blake PA. Clinical features and an epidemiologic study of vibrio vulnificus infections. *J Infect Dis* 1984;149:558–561.

Critical Care of the Trauma Patient

Adrian A. Maung and Robert L. Sheridan

I. **Introduction.** In the United States, traumatic injury is the leading cause of death among individuals between the ages of 1 and 44 years. It kills more Americans between the ages of 1 and 34 years than all other causes combined. Injury accounts for approximately one out of six hospital admissions, with almost 20% of trauma admissions during 1994 through 1999, being admitted to the intensive care unit (ICU). It is therefore crucial for critical care practitioners to be familiar with the care of trauma patients. Although many of the principles used to treat other critically ill patients apply, there are several conditions that are unique to trauma. This chapter will cover the pathophysiology, evaluation, and treatment of these conditions. Injuries to the brain and spinal cord as well as cervical spine clearance are covered in Chapter 34.

II. **Trauma evaluation.** The initial evaluation of the injured patient has been standardized by the American College of Surgeons as part of the Advanced Trauma Life Support (ATLS) course. This course covers the primary and secondary surveys used in the initial evaluation; however, an additional tertiary survey is often required within 24 hours of the injury.

   A. **Primary survey (ABCs).** This is a quick examination that aims to identify the most immediately life-threatening injuries.

   1. **Airway with C-spine control:** evaluation of airway patency, quality of both air exchange and voice, presence of stridor or foreign bodies; identification of airway compromise or the potential for progressive airway loss; if necessary, establishment of a definitive and secure airway.

   2. **Breathing:** examination of gas ventilation by evaluating the respiratory rate and pattern, chest wall movement, breath sounds, and oxygen saturation; identification of tracheal deviation, distension of neck veins, presence of cyanosis and/or chest wall injuries; diagnosis and treatment of tension or open pneumothorax, flail chest, or massive hemothorax.

   3. **Circulation:** assessment of the hemodynamic status by examining the mental status, quality of pulses, blood pressure, and skin color; identification and control of external hemorrhage, establishment of vascular access, and electrocardiogram monitoring.

    4. Disability (neurologic evaluation): examination of pupil size and reactivity, movement, and gross sensation in all extremities as well as the level of consciousness using either the **AVPU scale** (Alert; responds to Vocal stimuli; responds to Painful stimuli; or Unresponsive to all stimuli) or the **Glasgow Coma Scale.**

    5. Exposure/environmental control: undressing the patient for full evaluation while preventing hypothermia.

B. Secondary survey. This is a head-to-toe examination that includes the back and spine.

    1. Brief history: AMPLE (Allergies, Medications, Past Illnesses, Last meal, Events related to injury).

    2. Laboratory studies, including a type and screen or type and cross blood sample as indicated.

    3. Imaging, including FAST (Focused Abdominal Sonogram for Trauma) and plain films of chest and pelvis; computed tomography of head, c-spine, chest, abdomen, and pelvis as indicated by identified injuries or the potential for injuries based on the mechanism of trauma; plain films of injured extremities.

    4. Secondary survey may be delayed until injuries identified in the primary survey are addressed or until after the operating room in unstable patients.

C. Tertiary survey

    1. Complete and repeat primary and secondary surveys within 24 hours to assess for occult or missed injuries.

    2. Unrecognized injuries may occur in up to 65% of patients and are clinically significant in 15%.

    3. Especially important in ICU patients, who often cannot voice their complaints and symptoms.

III. Damage control surgery

A. Introduction. Thirty years ago, severely injured trauma patients who required surgery were often taken for one definitive operation. The objectives during this operation were to obtain definitive hemostasis, control enteric contamination with bowel resection and anastomosis, and repair all other injuries. Prolonged operative times were customary for patients with multiple injuries. Unfortunately, many patients died from a progressive intraoperative deterioration marked by the **lethal triad** of hypothermia, coagulopathy, and acidosis. In recent years, there has been a new approach to these patients with the use of damage control or stage laparotomy. The goal of this operation is not to serve as the definitive therapy, but instead to control or at least reduce bleeding and enteric contamination. The patient is then resuscitated in the ICU with the goals of restoring physiologic reserve and avoiding the lethal triad. The patient is subsequently brought back to the operating room, sometimes on several occasions, for further therapy. The critical care team must therefore be ready to address the lethal triad to allow for as early as possible definitive repair of injuries.

B. **Hypothermia.** Studies have shown that trauma patients with core temperatures of less than 32°C have 100% mortality. In trauma patients, hypothermia occurs not only from severe heat loss to the environment, but also from diminished heat production. Oxygen consumption is required for body heat generation, and therefore less heat is produced during shock. Hypothermia has an inhibitory effect on both the coagulation cascade and platelet function that is underestimated by the usual laboratory tests. This occurs because most laboratories rewarm the plasma to 37°C before measuring clotting times. External rewarming techniques such as blankets or convective hot air can help to decrease heat loss, but are not very efficient in transferring heat back to the patient. Pleural or peritoneal lavage with warm fluid can result in significant heat transfer, but large amounts of fluid are required. Administration of warm intravenous fluids and especially rewarming blood products, which are stored at 4°C, is critical. Cardiopulmonary bypass and continuous arteriovenous rewarming are the most rapid methods available.

C. **Coagulopathy.** In addition to the effects of hypothermia, trauma patients can also develop clotting factor depletion leading to a consumption coagulopathy and activation of fibrinolysis. Shock itself can lead to a dilutional thrombocytopenia that is independent of blood loss. Treatment should begin with transfusions of fresh-frozen plasma, clotting factors, and platelets. However, focus should be on rewarming the patient and reversing the underlying shock state. One should not rely on conventional coagulation tests not only for the reasons mentioned previously, but also because these tests take time to perform. In some cases of severely bleeding trauma patients, the entire blood volume can be replaced before the results of the laboratory tests come back.

D. **Acidosis.** Hypovolemic shock can cause a decrease in oxygen consumption and a persistent metabolic acidosis. This in turn can lead to decreased cardiac output, hypotension, and arrhythmias, further worsening the shock state. Failure to timely resuscitate the patient and correct the acidosis leads to a higher incidence of multisystem organ failure and death.

IV. **Abdominal compartment syndrome**

A. **Introduction/definition.** Although commonly associated with damage control laparotomy, abdominal compartment syndrome (ACS) is not uniquely associated with trauma. It can be seen in patients with ruptured abdominal aortic aneurysms, pancreatitis, neoplasms, massive ascites, liver transplantation, retroperitoneal hemorrhage, pneumoperitoneum, massive fluid resuscitation, or circumferential abdominal burns. ACS is defined as elevated intraabdominal pressure (IAP) associated with organ dysfunction. Normal IAP is atmospheric pressure. The level at which IAP causes ACS is not well defined, but pressure above 15 mm Hg is associated with physiologic changes.

B. **Pathophysiology.** ACS causes many derangements in normal physiology.

1. **Cardiac** output is decreased secondary to decreased venous return from the inferior vena cava. Extracardiac intrathoracic pressure also increases and impairs ventricular diastolic filling. Systemic vascular resistance is elevated from arteriolar vasoconstriction and IAP. The stroke volume and cardiac output are therefore further decreased. Central venous pressure and pulmonary artery wedge pressure are both elevated. Cardiac imaging will reveal a small but hyperdynamic left ventricle.

2. **Pulmonary.** The lungs are compressed by the elevated diaphragms, causing reduced total lung capacity, functional residual capacity, and residual volume. Pulmonary compliance is reduced and airway pressures are increased. Pulmonary vascular resistance can also increase, causing hypoxemia from ventilation/perfusion mismatch.

3. **Renal.** Renal perfusion and glomerular filtration progressively decrease as IAP increases. A decline in urine output occurs with oliguria at IAP of 15 to 20 mm Hg, and anuria occurs at IAP greater than 30 mm Hg. This occurs not only at the prerenal level secondary to the decreased cardiac output, but also at the renal level. Compression of the renal parenchyma decreases renal blood flow by compression of renal arterioles and veins. Elevated levels of renin, antidiuretic hormone, and aldosterone further contribute to the low urine output.

4. **Abdominal viscera.** Perfusion to all abdominal viscera is compromised. This can lead to abnormalities in gut mucosal barrier function and bacterial translocation.

5. **Central nervous system.** Increased IAP can also cause an elevation in intracranial pressure and a decrease in cerebral perfusion. This is thought to be related to elevations in central venous and pleural pressures.

C. **Evaluation.** IAP can be measured directly by placing a catheter in the peritoneal cavity. An indirect method measures the pressure in an abdominal organ, most commonly the bladder or the stomach. The easiest method is to instill 100 ml of sterile saline into the bladder via a Foley catheter connected to a T-connector. The catheter is then clamped and intravesical pressure can be measured using a pressure transducer or a manometer connected to the other arm of the T-connector. The symphysis pubis is used as a zero reference point. One should remember to convert from mm H_2O to mm Hg as needed.

D. Treatment. The treatment of IAP and ACS is to reduce the mass of the intraabdominal contents by removal of peritoneal blood, foreign bodies such as laparotomy pads, fluid, tumor, and so on or by simply opening the abdomen. Treatment should be instituted on an urgent basis. Relief of elevated pressure should produce almost an immediate improvement in cardiopulmonary parameters. Renal and visceral impairments will improve as long as irreversible ischemic damage had not already occurred. Most of the time, the abdomen cannot be closed without tension and it is left open until the primary intraabdominal problem(s) resolve. This usually occurs from a few days to several weeks later. In the interim, a wide variety of prosthetic materials such as silo or plastic drapes can be used to achieve temporary closure.

V. Crush injury/syndrome

A. Pathophysiology. Traumatic injury often causes muscle and soft tissue crush injury. If severe enough, this can manifest as the crush syndrome, which is defined as a systemic manifestation of muscle cell damage resulting from pressure or crushing. The natural history of untreated crush syndrome is characterized by systemic hypotension, circulatory shock, muscle swelling, and acute myoglobinuric renal failure. On a cellular level, muscle cells become stretched and their sarcolemmal membranes become more permeable. This releases myoglobin, phosphate, potassium, and urate into the circulation and also lets water, sodium, and calcium into the cell. The cells then become swollen and sequester fluid. This leads to intravascular volume depletion and hypovolemic shock. Cardiovascular compromise can also occur from electrolyte disturbances. Renal failure occurs not only from decreased renal blood flow secondary to the shock state, but also from the released nephrotoxic elements. Myoglobin, urate, and phosphate can precipitate in distal convoluted tubules and form tubular casts. Myoglobin may also cause oxidation injury to the kidney.

B. Evaluation. Patients with crush injury should have creatine kinase (CK) levels determined periodically. Peak CK level has been shown to correlate with the development of renal failure, with the highest risk in patients with CK levels greater than 75,000.

C. Management. After the initial trauma evaluation, patient with crush injury should have a urinary catheter placed to measure hourly urine production. As mentioned previously, CK and electrolytes should be measured periodically. Central venous pressure and arterial blood pressure measurements may be required. The patient should be volume resuscitated. The quantity and type of fluid to be given have been subject to debate.

Potassium-containing solutions have a theoretical potential to worsen hyperkalemia and therefore should be avoided. **Normal saline** has been used exclusively or alternated with 5% dextrose in water to decrease the sodium load. The reported recommended amount of fluid has varied from 200 to 1,500 ml/h, but most likely should be targeted to a urine output of more than 1 ml/kg/h. Invasive monitoring of CVP or stroke volume may be helpful in estimating the necessary resuscitation volume. Alkalinization of urine has also been shown to increase the solubility of myoglobin and promote its excretion. This may also help to prevent oxidative damage. Urine pH should be maintained above 6.5 by either 50 mmol bicarbonate boluses or by adding it to the fluid regiment. Some authors also advocate adding **mannitol** to the isotonic volume resuscitation to force an osmotic diuresis; however, the evidence to support this is not complete. It should be used at a dose of 1 to 2 g/kg over the first 4 hours as 20% solution with a maximum dose of 200 g/d. It should not be given to patients who are already anuric.

D. **Compartment syndrome** is a potential complication of crush injury. It can also be seen in skeletal trauma, in ischemia-reperfusion injury, due to iatrogenic causes, and in other conditions. It is caused by an increase in the intracompartmental pressure (ICP), which leads to compression of the venous outflow. This causes an increase in hydrostatic pressure that further increases ICP and leads to a vicious circle. Eventually the arterial inflow is also affected, leading to muscle and nerve ischemia and tissue necrosis.

1. **Signs and symptoms.** Compartment syndrome is marked by pain (out of proportion to injury) and paresthesias. On exam, one notes a tense, swollen compartment, sensory loss, especially loss of two-point discrimination, and pain on passive movement of the muscle. Loss of pulses is a late sign. Unfortunately, most of these can not be easily assessed in the sedated ICU patient. All extremities at risk should therefore be monitored. ICP should be measured in unconscious patients or conscious patients with equivocal signs for suspected compartment syndrome. Awake patients with unequivocal signs should proceed directly to fasciotomy. The normal ICP is between 0 and 8 mm Hg in resting muscle. The critical pressure for diagnosis of compartment syndrome is undefined. Some studies have shown that pressure greater than 30 mm Hg for 6 to 8 hours leads to irreversible damage. Others have suggested using a difference between the diastolic pressure and ICP of less than 30 mm Hg as a threshold. Lower thresholds obviously lead to a higher level of unnecessary fasciotomies.

2. **Treatment.** The primary treatment is by decompression with fasciotomies of all compartments in the

affected extremity. Some groups have suggested the use of mannitol in borderline cases to decrease the ICP and avoid unnecessary surgery and its attended complications. The fasciotomy wounds are usually left to heal by secondary intention or undergo delayed skin closure several days after decompression. Hyperbaric oxygen has been used as an adjunct to help with wound healing, but no controlled studies have demonstrated its efficacy.

VI. Management of blunt injury to liver and spleen

   A. Introduction: Similar to the advances in damage control surgery, the management of solid-organ injury has evolved over the last decade. Presence of blood in the intraperitoneal space, usually detected by diagnostic peritoneal lavage (DPL), used to be an automatic trigger for exploratory laparotomy. This led to a significant number of nontherapeutic laparotomies and their accompanied complications as well as an increase in postsplenectomy sepsis after unnecessary splenectomies. However, starting first with the pediatric trauma population, there has been a gradual shift toward nonoperative management of a select group of patients with both liver and spleen injuries (Table 33-1). Recent consensus from the Eastern Association for the Surgery of Trauma has concluded that although there is insufficient level I evidence, there is sufficient class II data to support the nonoperative management of blunt hepatic and splenic injuries in hemodynamically stable patients.

   B. Evaluation/management: Most trauma centers now use the FAST exam instead of DPL to evaluate for the presence of intraperitoneal blood. Hemodynamically unstable patients with a positive exam should undergo operative exploration. Stable patients with a positive FAST exam should undergo computed tomography (CT) of the abdomen with oral and intravenous contrast to further identify and assess the severity of injury. However, although important, the grade of injury and the degree of hemoperitoneum cannot fully predict the outcome of nonoperative management. The hemodynamic status of the patient is the most reliable

Table 33-1. Criteria for nonoperative management of solid-organ injury

Hemodynamic stability
Documentation of injury by computed tomography scan
No active contrast extravasation or pooling on computed
   tomography scan
Absence of other injuries requiring laparotomy
Absence of ongoing blood transfusion requirement or a persistently
   decreasing hematocrit that is not explained by other
   non-abdominal injuries
Ability to perform serial abdominal exams

Table 33-2. American Association for the Surgery of Trauma hepatic injury scale

Grade		Injury Description
I	Hematoma	Subcapsular, nonexpanding, <10% surface area
	Laceration	Capsular, nonbleeding, <1 cm depth
II	Hematoma	Subcapsular, nonexpanding, 10%–50% surface area
		Intraparenchymal, nonexpanding, <2 cm diameter
	Laceration	Capsular, active bleeding, 1–3 cm depth, <10 cm length
III	Hematoma	Subcapsular, expanding, or >50% surface area
		Ruptured subcapsular with active bleeding
		Intraparenchymal >2 cm diameter or expanding
	Laceration	>3 cm depth
IV	Hematoma	Ruptured central hematoma with active bleeding
	Laceration	25%–50% of lobe parenchymal disruption
V	Hematoma	>50% of lobe parenchymal disruption
	Laceration	Venous disruption: major hepatic veins, retrohepatic inferior vena cava
VI	Hepatic avulsion	

criterion for deciding on operative versus nonoperative management. Another predictor is contrast pooling or active contrast extravasation on CT, which indicates active bleeding. CT scans can, however, miss hollow viscous injury in 2% to 15% of patients. Angiography has been increasingly used to both diagnose and treat (by embolization) bleeding in both hepatic and splenic injuries.

C. **Liver.** The liver is the most commonly injured abdominal organ in both penetrating and blunt trauma (Table 33-2). The incidence of rebleeding following hepatic injury is less than 3% of all patients managed nonoperatively. In addition, if bleeding reoccurs, it does not follow the pattern of catastrophic bleeding that can be associated with splenic injuries. Transfusion requirement has been shown to be actually higher in operative cases than in nonoperative ones. Other potential complications include liver abscess and biliary tract injury with bilomas and hemobilia. These are rare and will usually manifest by physical signs and symptoms.

D. Spleen. Splenic injuries can be treated nonoperatively in 60% to 70% of children and about 50% of adults. In contrast to hepatic trauma, the failure rate is higher, at 5% to 10%, and bleeding can occur at a significant pace, potentially causing hemodynamic instability. Most often it reoccurs hours to days after injury, but has been reported up to several weeks later. A second peak in frequency occurs around 7 days after injury. Patients with splenic injuries should have frequent hematocrit checks. A continued transfusion requirement may indicate the need for an operation or angiography and embolization. Patients who undergo splenectomy may have a transient thrombocytosis of 600,000 to 1,000,000. Aspirin is recommended if the count is higher than 750,000 to try minimize thrombosis. Patients should also be vaccinated against *Pneumococcus, Haemophilus influenzae,* and *Meningococcus,* although the timing of vaccination is controversial. Some groups advocate immediate postoperative vaccination (because trauma patients do not always reliably return for follow-up), whereas others prefer to wait 2 weeks. Antibiotics for these patients should probably be given at first signs of infection and with invasive procedures rather than as a daily prophylactic dose.

E. Follow-up. Patients with both hepatic and splenic trauma should have serial abdominal exams and hematocrit checks. Follow-up CT scans are not routinely indicated unless there is a change in clinical status or an unexplained drop in hematocrit, which may represent ongoing bleeding. There is no evidence that bed rest is necessary; however, the time to resuming normal activity is variable and depends on the extent and severity of injury.

VII. Myocardial injury

A. Penetrating. The treatment of penetrating myocardial injury, which is mostly operative, is beyond the scope of this chapter. Any penetrating injury to the so-called "precordial box" should be suspected of having injured the heart until proven otherwise. The "box" encompasses the area between the mid-clavicular lines laterally, superior to the costal margins, and inferior to the clavicles. Because of its location, the right ventricle is at the greatest risk of injury. Stab wounds more commonly present with tamponade, whereas gunshot wounds tend to create larger defects and present with bleeding and hypovolemic shock.

1. Evaluation. Patients may or may not present with the classic Beck's triad of pericardial tamponade (muffled heart sounds, hypotension, and distended neck veins). The most important presentation is that of a hemodynamically unstable patient with a wound in the appropriate area. Hemodynamically stable patients should undergo echocardiography to assess for pericardial fluid. If the results are equivocal, a subxiphoid pericardial window should be performed in the operating room.

2. **Treatment.** Resuscitation should utilize the ATLS guidelines with volume resuscitation via large-bore intravenous lines. Stable patients with positive pericardial fluid should be expeditiously transported to the operating room. Unstable or borderline patients should undergo an emergent thoracotomy to relieve tamponade and then be transported to the operating room. Even though pericardiocentesis has no role in the diagnosis of tamponade because of a high false-negative rate, it can have a therapeutic role in a setting where thoracotomy cannot be performed expeditiously.

B. **Blunt cardiac injury** (BCI), formerly referred to as cardiac contusion, a term that has fallen out of favor, continues to be a controversial topic (Fig. 33-1). The overall incidence varies from 8% to 71% of all patients with blunt chest trauma. This wide variation is due to a lack of both a diagnostic gold standard and a uniform definition. It can encompass a variety of injuries, including myonecrosis, valvular disruption, coronary artery dissection, and/or thrombosis. It is most commonly caused by motor vehicle accidents and results from a direct blow to the chest or from rapid deceleration. Other causes include falls, sport injuries, and blast injuries.

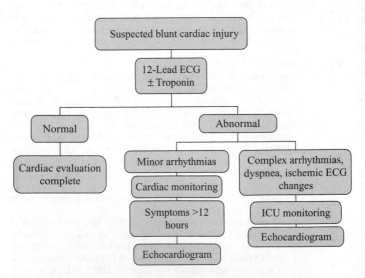

Fig. 33-1. Evaluation of suspected blunt cardiac injury. ECG, electrocardiogram; ICU, intensive care unit.

1. **Signs and symptoms.** Unfortunately, BCI has few reliable signs and symptoms. Many patients will have evidence of external chest trauma, and chest pain is a common complaint in trauma patients. One must therefore maintain a high index of suspicion in patients with an appropriate mechanism of injury or in patients who have an inappropriate cardiovascular response to the level of their injury.

2. **Evaluation.** All patients with suspected BCI should have a 12-lead electrocardiogram (ECG) performed on admission. Studies have shown that ECG has a negative predictive value of greater than 95%, and the risk of significant BCI that requires treatment with a normal ECG is small. Some studies have even suggested that the workup can be safely terminated at this point. If the ECG is abnormal (arrhythmia, ST changes, ischemia, heart block, etc.), the patient should be admitted for continuous ECG monitoring for 24 to 48 hours. Patients who complain of dyspnea or have ischemic ECGs or complex arrhythmias (atrial fibrillation, multifocal premature ventricular contractions, or conduction delays) should be admitted to the ICU. Measurement of cardiac enzymes is controversial. Creatine kinase can be nonspecifically elevated in trauma patients from skeletal muscle injury. Recent studies have also reported a low sensitivity and specificity of the CK-MB fraction. Measurements of troponins I and T have shown an improved specificity but not sensitivity. Several investigators reported that a normal troponin value in combination with a normal ECG is a good indicator for absence of cardiac injury. The ideal timing for measuring troponin has not been determined. Laboratory tests drawn shortly after the injury may not be reliable, and a second set may need to be repeated in 4 to 6 hours. **Echocardiogram,** either transthoracic or transesophageal, should not be used for primary screening in hemodynamically stable patients. Instead, it should be used as a complementary test in those with abnormal results on physical exam and in those with persistent symptoms for more than 12 hours or in hemodynamically unstable patients. Although more risky and more operator dependent, transesophageal echocardiography has been shown to more accurately diagnose BCI and to be safe in the evaluation of trauma patients.

3. **Treatment.** BCI is managed mostly symptomatically in hemodynamically stable patients. Pain control should be optimized and serum electrolytes corrected. If there is evidence of pericardial fluid on echocardiogram and the clinical picture is consistent with tamponade, the patient should have a subxiphoid pericardiotomy in the operating room or an anterolateral thoracotomy if in extremis.

Severe cardiac dyskinesis may require inotropes and/or intraaortic balloon pump.

VIII. Traumatic aortic disruption (TAD) is the second-most-common cause of death after motor vehicle accidents. It has also been described in other accidents that involve sudden deceleration of the body and/or chest compression. Most commonly it occurs at the aortic isthmus (90%), which is the most proximal portion of the descending thoracic aorta just distal to the origin of the left subclavian artery. This part of the aorta is relatively fixed to the main pulmonary artery by the ligamentum arteriosum, whereas the above aortic arch and the distal aorta are free to move. This can cause sheer stress leading to rupture. Other postulated mechanisms of injury include compression of the vessel between bony structures or profound intraluminal hypertension. Transection may be partial thickness, similar to a tear in aortic dissection, or full thickness and equivalent to a ruptured aneurysm. In both cases, permissive hypotension and minimization of changes in blood pressure over time (dP/dt) should be utilized.

A. Evaluation. TAD should be suspected in any patient with severe head trauma, multiple extremity fractures, multiple rib fractures, and/or a mechanism of injury that involves rapid deceleration. Symptoms are nonspecific, with chest pain, back pain and dyspnea being the most frequent. Physical findings are also nonspecific. External chest trauma is evident in 70% to 90% of patients. Less than one-third of patients will have unequal pulses or blood pressures in extremities. Evaluation should begin with a chest x-ray. TAD is associated with a widening of the mediastinum, with a ratio greater than 0.28 of mediastinal width to chest width at the aortic knob. Other potential findings include loss of the aortic knob, depression of left main bronchus, lateral deviation of the trachea, apical pleural hematoma, and left hemothorax. Nevertheless, a normal chest x-ray does not rule out the diagnosis of TAD. Angiography continues to be the gold standard. However, it has been replaced at most centers with helical CT scan as a primary screening test. The CT scan can show either the absence of a mediastinal hematoma, thus ruling out TAD, or clear signs of disruption. An equivocal situation can occur with an isolated mediastinal hematoma without other signs of aortic injury. These patients should undergo aortogram to further evaluate the aorta. Transesophageal echocardiogram has been evaluated as a potential tool for screening for TAD. However, it cannot always adequately visualize the aortic arch and distal ascending aorta. In addition, it is operator dependent, and few centers have experience with it in aortic trauma.

B. Treatment. Initial resuscitation follows ATLS guidelines. However, aggressive volume resuscitation is limited to maintaining systolic blood pressure around 100 mm Hg. Pharmacologic therapy to limit dP/dt (shear stress of the vessel wall) should be initiated as soon as the diagnosis is suspected, even before the full diagnostic studies, to reduce the chance of rupture during these tests. Invasive hemodynamic monitoring should be instituted with a right radial a-line. Intravenous β-blockade with **labetalol** or **propranolol** should be used. **Sodium nitroprusside** should be used as a secondary agent once the use of β-blockers is limited by bradycardia. Adequate analgesia and sedation are also important. Prompt surgical therapy is probably the best approach, although recent reports have shown that it is not as urgent as previously thought as long as the blood pressure is well controlled. Operative treatment may be delayed in multitrauma patients while other injuries are being stabilized. External fixation is used to stabilize pelvic and extremity fractures. Operative head injury or unstable intraabdominal injuries must be addressed. A subset of patients who are elderly or have comorbidities that prohibit emergency thoracic surgery such as sepsis, extensive burns, or severe central nervous injury may be managed medically with strict antihypertensive therapy that is transitioned from parenteral to enteral. There are several different techniques for operative repair. Postoperative complications include acute respiratory distress syndrome, need for prolonged ventilatory support, multisystem organ failure, renal insufficiency, and paraplegia.

SELECTED REFERENCES

American College of Surgeons, Committee on Trauma. *Advanced trauma life support for Doctors: ATLS*, 6th ed. Chicago: American College of Surgeons, 1997.

Cardarelli MG. The management of traumatic aortic rupture. *Adv Surg* 2003;37:123–37.

Eastern Association for the Surgery of Trauma Practice Management Guidelines. Available at www.east.org.

Mattox KL, Feliciano DV, Moore EE. *Trauma*, 4th ed. Stamford, CT: Appleton & Lange, 2000.

Sheridan RL, Massachusetts General Hospital. *The trauma handbook of the Massachusetts General Hospital*. Philadelphia: Lippincott Williams & Wilkins, 2004.

Neurotrauma

Neeraj Badjatia, Brian Hoh, and
Lee H. Schwamm.

I. Head injury

  A. **Epidemiology.** Traumatic brain injury (TBI) accounts
  for approximately 40% of all deaths from acute injuries
  in the United States. Annually, 200,000 victims of TBI
  need hospitalization, and 1.74 million persons sustain
  mild TBI requiring a physician visit or temporary disability of at least 1 day. The mortality rate for deaths outside
  the hospital is approximately 17 per 100,000 people, and
  for patients who are hospitalized is approximately 6 per
  100,000 people. Motor vehicle collisions and firearms mis-
  sile injuries remain the top causes of TBI in the United
  States.

  B. **Classification.** Categorization of TBI is based on the
  mechanism that leads to the injury, clinical severity, and
  radiographic appearance of the type of head injury.

   1. Understanding the mechanism is important in determining the potential types of injuries that may have
   occurred.

      a. **Blunt** injury usually occurs from motor vehicle col-
      lisions and falls. When the brain (within the skull)
      is moving and strikes a stationary object, the pre-
      dominant site of brain injury is contracoup (e.g.,
      skull vs. dashboard). When the brain is station-
      ary and is struck by a moving object, the predom-
      inant injury is coup (e.g., brain vs. baseball bat).
      These events transfer mechanical and thermal en-
      ergy to the brain and spine, causing primary brain
      injury.

      b. **Penetrating** injuries occur with missile (e.g., gun-
      shot) or knife wounds. They may produce imme-
      diate direct vascular compromise or mass lesions,
      such as hematoma or foreign body, that further in-
      jure the brain.

   2. **Clinical** classification is based on the **Glasgow Coma
   Scale (GCS)** (Table 34-1), which is a simple, reproducible, and widely accepted measure of brain dysfunction. Any alteration of consciousness in the setting of
   even minor trauma should raise the suspicion of TBI
   and prompt neurologic evaluation, especially in the elderly or anticoagulated patient. Frequent reevaluation
   of neurologic function is essential because early detection of secondary brain injury offers the best hope
   of preventing permanent neurologic dysfunction and
   should guide subsequent management.

      a. Mild: GCS of 14 to 15. Loss of consciousness, if
      present, is brief (<5 minutes). It requires close

Table 34-1. The Glasgow Coma Scale

Category	Score
Best motor response	
Obeys	6
Localizes	5
Withdraws	4
Abnormal flexion	3
Extensor response	2
None	1
Verbal response	
Oriented	5
Confused	4
Inappropriate words	3
Incomprehensible sounds	2
None	1
Eye opening	
Spontaneously	4
To speech	3
To pain	2
None	1

The Glasgow Coma Scale expresses a patient's level of consciousness by assessing motor response, verbal response, and eye opening. The individual scores for each of the three components are added to obtain a summary score. A fully alert and oriented patient would receive a score of 15. A flaccid patient with no eye opening or verbal response would receive a score of 3.

neurologic monitoring, but usually not in the intensive care unit (ICU).
- **b.** Moderate: GCS of 9 to 13. These patients have a mixed prognosis.
- **c.** Severe: GCS of 8 or less. Virtually all of these patients require ICU admission as well as intracranial pressure (ICP) monitoring.
3. **Radiographic.** Brain imaging helps to distinguish cases that require immediate surgical intervention from those that do not, and may identify those whose protracted recovery requires early tracheostomy and gastrostomy. The Marshall classification (Table 34-2) of initial computed tomography (CT) scan appearance categorizes patient with **diffuse axonal injury (DAI),** a pattern due to acceleration and deceleration injury across the brain as shear forces are applied during the moment of impact. This is a diffuse, nonfocal pattern of injury for which early surgical treatment is not indicated unless intractable ICP develops. CT may reveal only mild injury with loss of gray–white differentiation, ventricular compression, and small intraventricular blood, or severe, high-impact injury with multifocal contusions, edema, effacement of the basilar cisterns, and brainstem compression.

Table 34-2. The Marshall computed tomography grading system and relationship to mortality in traumatic brain injury

Injury Grade	Computed Tomography Appearance	Mortality (%)
I	Normal computed tomography scan	9.6
II	Cisterns present: shift <5 mm	13.5
III	Cisterns compressed/absent: shift <5mm	34
IV	Cisterns compressed/absent: shift >5mm	56.2

    a. The initial CT scan appearance is often in stark contrast to the poor clinical grade, and early magnetic resonance (MR) may show better the diffuse nature of the injury. Signs suggestive of DAI in the CT scans include punctuate hemorrhages in the periventricular white matter, corpus callosum, and brainstem, traumatic subarachnoid hemorrhage, and intraventricular hemorrhage as well as tissue tear hemorrhages. MR may show T2, diffusion-weighted imaging (DWI) hyperintense, and apparent diffusion coefficient (ADC) hypointense lesions, as well as gradient-echo evidence of microscopic hemorrhages.

C. Initial assessment

    1. History. A detailed account of the events leading up to the traumatic injury should be elicited from the emergency medical personnel and any bystanders who may have been present.

        a. An account of the **mechanism of injury** (e.g., speed of motor vehicular collision, use of seatbelt, and height of fall) are useful in determining the potential for the existence of blunt or penetrating injuries as well as for additional cerebrovascular or spinal cord trauma.

        b. Initial neurologic assessment done by the emergency medical personnel at the scene is very important. The initial GCS as well as any signs of poor prognosis such as deterioration in consciousness, pupillary asymmetry, decerebrate posturing, or occurrence of seizures should be noted.

        c. Details pertaining to **neurologic symptoms** should be elicited from those patients able to provide a history. Symptoms important to note include the presence of focal head, neck, or spine pain, changes in vision or hearing, focal motor weakness, and loss of sensation in the extremities.

    2. Physical examination

        a. Vital signs. Changes in respiratory pattern accompanied by hypertension and bradycardia (Cushing's reflex) are a sign of brain herniation. Atrial tachydysrhythmias and ventricular ectopy can occur, especially when intracranial hemorrhage is present. Pulmonary edema may occur and is probably due to pulmonary capillary fracture during the intense sympathetic outflow induced by intracranial hypertension. A variety of respiratory pattern disturbances can evolve, including changes in rate (bradypnea, tachypnea), rhythm (apneustic, ataxic, agonal, Cheyne-Stokes, apneic), or minute ventilation (hyperventilation, hypoventilation). Profound hypotension refractory to volume resuscitation is usually not encountered with isolated brain injury, and may be a sign of hemodynamic shock secondary to unsuspected cervical spinal cord injury.

b. Inspection. Periorbital ("raccoon") or retroauricular ("battle") hematomas, auditory canal blood, and otorhinorrhea are signs of basal skull fracture. Scalp lacerations should be noted but never probed because this can foster further injury and promote infection. These injuries are best evaluated with dedicated radiographic imaging of the skull either by computed tomography or plain film of the skull.

c. Level of consciousness is incorporated into the initial GCS assessment. Descriptive assessments of response to verbal and noxious stimuli are much more informative than the use of terminology referring to coma, stupor, or obtundation.

d. Cranial nerve assessments should focus on traumatic cranial neuropathies or signs consistent with brainstem injury.

e. Motor exam should focus on pattern weakness or asymmetry that may help with localization.

f. Sensory exam is of utility when assessing for a possible spinal cord injury.

3. **Brain imaging** has revolutionized management of TBI. It is useful to divide patients on presentation into three categories: those who require immediate neurosurgical intervention, intensive care management, or focused observation. Availability of CT in the emergency department permits rapid diagnosis of intracerebral hemorrhage (ICH), subdural hematoma (SDH) or epidural hematoma (EDH), subarachnoid hemorrhage (SAH), hydrocephalus, depressed skull fracture, and focal contusions and shortens the time to necessary neurosurgical intervention. In addition, newer techniques allow for noninvasive measures of cerebral blood flow, cerebral blood volume, and early ischemic tissue changes and help to increase understanding of the pathophysiology of TBI.

4. **Impaired autoregulation** of cerebral blood flow (CBF) in TBI. In the early hours after injury, CBF falls to critically low levels and is uncoupled from metabolic demand, which remains normal or elevated. This may cause widespread ischemic infarction and contribute

to subsequent cytotoxic edema and increased ICP, resulting in a poor outcome. Autoregulation of CBF responds to changes in pressure, blood viscosity, and probably some markers of metabolic activity to keep blood flow constant. Cerebrovascular reactivity is a different mechanism by which changes in cerebrovascular resistance (CVR) occur in response to changes in carbon dioxide pressure (PCO_2). This reactivity is often disordered in TBI, and may be heterogeneously distributed in different brain regions, with areas of both increased and decreased reactivity. Because the degree of vasoconstriction to hypocapnia is highly variable and perhaps also regional within the injured brain, it is possible to increase regional ischemia through excessive vasoconstriction even at relatively modest reductions in PCO_2. This may occur in the setting of seemingly beneficial reductions in ICP. There is no easy method for monitoring the adequacy of CBF at the bedside during hyperventilation, but indirect assessment of cerebral oxygenation may provide some information.

- **D. Increased ICP** is a frequent sequela of TBI and greatly increases its morbidity and mortality. Several different approaches are available to permit continuous monitoring of ICP.

  1. **Indications for ICP monitoring** include decreasing level of consciousness, risk of undetectable rise in ICP (e.g., paralyzed patient, intraoperative setting), and need to perform maneuvers that will likely increase ICP in vulnerable patients (e.g., clearance of pulmonary secretions, medications, positioning). All TBI patients **with a GCS of 8 or less after initial resuscitation should have an ICP monitor** placed (Fig. 34-1).

     a. **Interpretation of ICP measurements.** Elevation of ICP should prompt urgent evaluation. It is generally due to mass lesions, hydrocephalus, brain edema, or increased cerebral blood volume. The ICP waveform typically shows pressure variations within each cardiac and respiratory cycle (Fig. 34-2). The amplitude of the ICP waveform variation associated with cardiac pulsation normally is 1 mm Hg and increases with increasing ICP. Heterogeneity of intracranial pressure may exist within the cranial vault, especially above compared to below the tentorium.

     b. **Pressure waves** are rhythmic variations in ICP described as **A, B,** and **C** waves (Fig. 34-3). Only **A** waves are clinically significant; these are 50- to 100-mm Hg waves lasting 5 to 20 minutes. When sustained, they are called **plateau waves** and are often associated with clinical deterioration. Plateau waves can arise spontaneously or be precipitated by hemodynamic fluctuations or nursing procedures. The **B** waves are sharper, 50-mm Hg waves

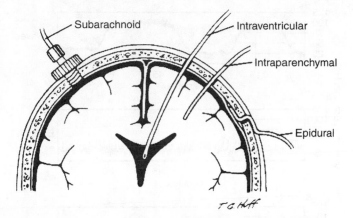

Fig. 34-1. Illustration of four different methods for transducing intracranial pressure. (From Lee KR, Hoff JT. Intracranial pressure. In: Youmans JR, ed. *Neurological surgery*, 4th ed. Philadelphia: WB Saunders, 1996:505. With permission.)

occurring at about 1-minute intervals. They can be associated with normal sleep or pathologically decreased levels of consciousness occurring at both high and normal ICP. The **C** waves are waves of less than 20 mm Hg occurring about six times per minute and may indicate decreased intracranial compliance. They usually occur in the presence of elevated ICP.

2. **Hydrocephalus** and **brain herniation** are common sequela of raised ICP after TBI.

   a. Communicating **hydrocephalus** is frequently due to the presence of blood products that cause an

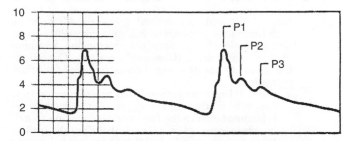

Fig. 34-2. Morphology of the intracranial pressure (ICP) waveform in the setting of normal intracranial pressure and compliance. The ICP waveform shows pressure variations within each cardiac and respiratory cycle. P1, P2, and P3 are cardiac pulsations. The units of measurement are millimeters of mercury. (From Lee KR, Hoff JT. Intracranial pressure. In: Youmans JR, ed. *Neurological surgery*, 4th ed. Philadelphia: WB Saunders, 1996:497. With permission.)

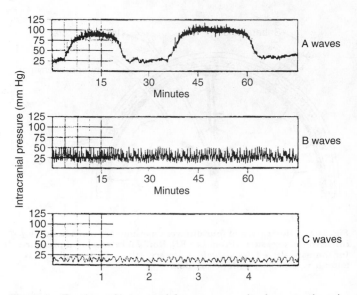

Fig. 34-3. Tracings of intracranial pressure monitoring over time. A waves, also described as "plateau waves," occur in the setting of very poor intracranial compliance. (From Lee KR, Hoff JT. Intracranial pressure. In: Youmans JR, ed. *Neurological surgery*, 4th ed. Philadelphia: WB Saunders, 1996:508. With permission.)

obstruction to flow of the cerebrospinal fluid (CSF) in the subarachnoid space and absorption of CSF through the arachnoid villi. Noncommunicating hydrocephalus often is caused by blood clot obstruction of blood flow at the fourth ventricle, cerebral aqueduct, third ventricle, or interventricular foramen.

3. **Brain herniation** is attributable to direct mechanical compression by an accumulating mass or to diffusely increased intracranial pressure. All patients with herniation syndromes will present with progressive somnolence and sudden hypertension accompanied by bradycardia **(Cushing's reflex).** The following types of supratentorial herniation syndromes are recognized:

   a. **Subfalcine herniation.** This most common type occurs when the cingulate gyrus of the frontal lobe is pushed beneath the falx cerebri when an expanding mass lesion causes a medial shift of the ipsilateral hemisphere. Clinical signs of increased tone or paresis in the contralateral leg may be present.

   b. **Central transtentorial herniation** is characterized by displacement of the basal nuclei and cerebral hemispheres downward while the diencephalon and adjacent midbrain are pushed through the tentorial notch. This usually occurs as a result of lesions lying toward the intracranial vertex or the frontal-occipital poles. Initial presentation will be an impairment of vertical gaze and bilateral extensor posturing.

c. **Uncal herniation.** This type of injury involves displacement of the medial edge of the uncus and the hippocampal gyrus medially and over the ipsilateral edge of the tentorium cerebelli foramen, causing compression of the midbrain, whereas the ipsilateral or contralateral third nerve may be stretched or compressed. Early in the course, patients will demonstrate asymmetric pupillary dilation **(anisocoria),** which will progress to marked ipsilateral pupillary dilation accompanied by contralateral hemiparesis. Occasionally, the hemiparesis is ipsilateral or the anisocoria is contralateral to the lesion, at which point these are considered falsely localizing signs.

d. **Upward cerebellar herniation.** This uncommon injury is marked by upward herniation of the vermis and cerebellar hemispheres through the tentorial opening, usually due to infratentorial space-occupying lesions (e.g., tumor, hematoma, edema). Imaging reveals effacement of the superior vermian cistern, compression of the fourth ventricle, and upward and forward displacement of the quadrigeminal plate, mesencephalon, and aqueduct, causing supratentorial hydrocephalus. If the condition is untreated, it will also compress the medulla, leading to bradycardia and respiratory arrest.

E. **ICP management**
   1. **Universal measures.** Regardless of the type or severity of injury, the common goal for all TBI patients is cardiopulmonary homeostasis and **hyperosmolar euvolemia** (also see Chapter 13). In addition to specific therapeutic options, there are some general measures that should be taken to minimize the occurrence of raised ICP or reduced cerebral perfusion pressure (CPP).

   a. Head positioning should be maintained at 30 to 45 degrees above horizontal and midline to best facilitate venous drainage. Elevation also causes reductions in cerebral mean arterial pressure (MAP) and may actually lower CPP. Because of this, systemic arterial pressure transducers should be zeroed at the level of the external auditory meatus whenever CPP is being controlled and the patient's head is elevated. Rotation of the head may impede venous drainage and increase ICP. Additionally, C-collars should be fitted so as not to obstruct venous outflow.

   b. **Seizure prophylaxis** with **phenytoin** for the first 7 days postinjury.

   c. **Monitoring** for raised **intrathoracic** and **intraabdominal pressures.**

2. **Adequate sedation and analgesia** are important first steps in managing raised ICP. Anesthetic agents that reduce ICP by primary reduction in cerebral metabolic rate (CMR) and subsequently CBF are not utilized for primary treatment of raised ICP. The goal is to achieve adequate control without obscuration of clinical examination. This is best accomplished with short-acting analgesics such as **morphine** sulfate, **fentanyl** citrate, and short-acting sedatives such as **propofol.**

3. **Positive end-expiratory pressure (PEEP)** may increase ICP in patients with compliant lungs. The hemodynamic effects of PEEP depend upon the resulting intrathoracic (or "pleural") pressure, which is a function of lung and chest wall compliance. Pulmonary parenchymal disease (e.g., pneumonia, aspiration, or acute respiratory distress syndrome) decreases pulmonary compliance and reduces the transmission of airway pressure, hence the hemodynamic effects of moderate levels (≤ 10 cm H_2O) of PEEP. Lungs with normal or increased compliance (e.g., emphysema) readily transmit airway pressure to the thorax; hence venous return and cardiac output may decrease when PEEP is applied.

4. **Hyperventilation** reduces ICP by vasoconstriction-induced alkalosis. The fall in ICP parallels the fall in CBV. Prolonged vasoconstriction results in reduction in CBF to ischemic levels. Effects are temporary, after which lower Pco_2 levels are required to achieve ICP control. Hence, arterial carbon dioxide ($Paco_2$) levels below 28 mm Hg are acceptable only as an emergency measure, for up to 30 minutes, until more definitive therapy is initiated.

5. **Osmotic agents** work by shifting fluid from edematous interstitial and intracellular spaces into the intravascular space.

   a. **Mannitol** is only indicated for ICP-directed care. The usual dose is 0.5 to 1.0 g/kg intravenously (IV) every 4 to 6 hours to reach an **osmotic gradient** of 10 to 20 mOsm (see Chapter 13). Osmotic gradients greater than 20 mOsm are associated with renal injury. Careful attention to intravascular volume status is necessary to maintain euvolemia. Although there is no value of Na or osmolality that is absolutely contraindicated, the effectiveness of osmolar therapy is diminished with serum Na concentration 160 mEq or greater or osmolality 320 mOsm or greater. Potential adverse effects include hyperosmotic prerenal failure, hypokalemia, dehydration, and hypotension.

   b. **Hypertonic saline** solutions are also effective osmotic agents, and are most often limited to cases where mannitol is contraindicated. Potential adverse effects include **central pontine myelinolysis,** seizures, congestive heart failure (CHF), hypokalemia, hyperchloremic acidosis, coagulopathy, phlebitis, and renal failure. Three percent NaCl, a 125- to 250-ml bolus every 6 hours or continuous infusion at 0.5 to 1.0 ml/kg/h, is targeted to the desired ICP. A 23.4% NaCl, 30-ml bolus every 6 hours is targeted to ICP. Hypertonic treatment should be held for serum Na concentration greater than 160 mEq/L.

   c. **Loop diuretics** such as **furosemide** (10–20 mg IV every 4 to 6 hours) may be useful for the subacute treatment of intracranial hypertension, possibly by decreasing vasogenic edema and CSF production. Potential adverse effects include hypovolemia, azotemia, metabolic alkalosis, electrolyte abnormalities, nephrotoxicity, and ototoxicity.

6. **Metabolic therapy.** Barbiturates are the primary agents utilized when initiating metabolic therapy. They reduce ICP by a reduction of cerebral metabolic rate for oxygen ($CMRO_2$) and secondarily by a reduction of cerebral blood flow and cerebral blood volume (CBV). Prolonged barbiturate therapy may result in serious side effects including hypotension due to vasodilation and cardiac suppression, gastric stasis, mucous plugging, immunosuppression, hypothermia, and prolonged coma.

   a. **Pentobarbital.** Loading dose is 3 to 5 mg/kg over 30 minutes, followed by a 50- to 200-mg IV bolus for raised ICP. Half-life is 15 to 48 hours (bolus). When assessing recovery from withdrawal of pentobarbital, pupillary responses recover first and motor responses last.

   b. **Thiopental.** A 250-mg IV bolus reduces ICP in seconds with duration of only 15 to 20 minutes. Multiple repeated doses significantly prolong its half-life.

7. **Surgical intervention**

   a. **Cerebrospinal fluid drainage** is achieved with an external ventriculostomy and is the most reliable method of assessing global ICP. Indications for drainage include hydrocephalus or extensive intraventricular hemorrhage (IVH), and this can be considered as the first line of therapy for raised ICP management. There is up to a 6% to 10% risk of infection.

   b. **Craniectomy** is considered for patients failing maximal medical therapy (see Table 34-1); however, recent clinical studies indicate this may be considered as part of the initial management of raised ICP.

8. Corticosteroids have no role in reducing ICP secondary to isolated head injury.

F. Maintenance of **normal physiologic parameters**

1. The presence of **hypotension** (systolic blood pressure [SBP] <80 mm Hg) at any time during the prehospital phase, at admission, intraoperatively, or in the intensive care unit has been shown to be an independent

predictor of poor outcome. The most common cause of hypotension in these patients once they reach the intensive care unit is underresuscitation. The goal is therefore to maintain a normal blood pressure (SBP > 90 mm Hg) primarily with volume resuscitation and occasionally with vasopressors.

2. **Hypoxia** worsens oxygen delivery to the brain, leading to cerebral ischemia and potentially increasing ICP secondary to a compensatory vasodilation and increase in cerebral blood volume. There is no established optimal goal arterial oxygen pressure (PaO_2); however, we attempt to maintain PaO_2 greater than 80 mm Hg, and saturated oxygen pressure (SaO_2) greater than 95%.

3. **Hyperthermia** increases cerebral metabolic rate by 5% to 7% per 1°C and ICP by 3 to 4 mm Hg per 1°C and should be treated vigorously with acetaminophen and, if necessary, surface or intravascular cooling. Moreover, fever significantly increases metabolic rate, excitatory neurotransmitter release, and neuronal injury. Induced hypothermia is not recommended, but shivering should be avoided because it increases temperature and CO_2 production. The goal is to maintain **normothermia** (37°C).

4. **Hyperglycemia** increases tissue acidosis and cerebral edema in and around injured tissue by acting as an osmotic agent. Moreover, it can impair endogenous antiinflammatory mechanisms of repair. The goal of care should be to attain normoglycemia (80–120 mg/dl) with the use of continuous insulin infusions.

G. **Surgical management**
   1. **Subdural hematoma (SDH).** The causative injury is commonly due to tearing of bridging veins between the surface of the brain and the dura matter. It is often associated with underlying cerebral contusion. The classic CT appearance is that of a crescent-shaped hyperdensity around the brain. Small SDH (<1 cm) may be closely monitored or evacuated via a burr hole. Larger lesions most often require evacuation via craniotomy and, depending on degree of underlying brain injury, even hemicraniectomy (Table 34-3).
   2. **Epidural hematoma.** The causative injury is arterial, and patients classically present with an initial, brief loss of consciousness, then a lucid period that may last several hours prior to progressive neurologic deterioration and signs of transtentorial herniation.

II. **ICU Management of traumatic spinal cord injury**
   A. **Epidemiology**
      1. Approximately 11,000 to 14,000 spinal cord injuries (SCIs) occur in North America each year. It is estimated that 53% of those occur among individuals in the 16- to 30-year age group, of which 80% are male.
      2. The most frequent neurologic injury is incomplete tetraplegia (31%), followed by complete paraplegia (27%), incomplete paraplegia (20%), and complete tetraplegia (19%). The majority (about 90%) of all

Table 34-3. Guidelines for posttrauma craniectomy

Age <55 years (relative indication)
Nonfatal primary brain injury
Asymmetric or focal brain swelling on computed tomography scan
Refractory intracranial hypertension
Failed maximal medical therapy ± cerebrospinal fluid drainage
Prior to utilization of barbiturates

persons with SCI are discharged to a private, noninstitutional residence (in most cases their homes before injury).

3. Despite education efforts and model trauma systems, many patients experience significant and preventable secondary neurologic and hemodynamic injury during the course of their acute and subacute care. It is estimated that 3% to 25% of SCIs occur after the initial traumatic insult, either during transit or early in the course of management.

B. **Initial management**
   1. **Spine immobilization**
      a. The American College of Surgeons recommends for preadmission transport a hard backboard, rigid cervical collar, lateral support devices, and tape or straps to secure the patient, collar, and lateral support devices to the backboard.
      b. Patients should be removed from hard backboard as soon as safely possible due to the significant association between the duration on a backboard and development of pressure sores.
      c. Although the technique of log-rolling has been called into question due to possible significant lateral motion produced in the lumbar spine, it remains the recommended way to move patients at risk of spine injury.
   2. **Clinical assessment**
      a. There are many different neurologic assessment and functional outcome scales for spinal cord injury. The representative motor functions of the spinal roots are shown in Table 34-4.
      b. The Guidelines for the Management of Acute Cervical Spine and Spinal Cord Injuries by the Section on Disorders of the Spine and Peripheral Nerves of the American Association of Neurological Surgeons and the Congress of Neurological Surgeons recommends the American Spinal Injury Association (ASIA) scale, which combines motor, sensory, and functional assessment (Fig. 34-4).
   3. **Radiographic assessment**
      a. **No radiographic assessment** of the cervical spine is necessary in the asymptomatic patient (i.e., a neurologically normal patient who is not intoxicated and is without neck pain, midline tenderness,

Table 34-4.   Representative motor functions of spinal roots

Spinal Root(s)	Representative Motor Function
C3-C4	Diaphragm function (phrenic nerve)
C5	Shoulder adduction
C5-C6	Elbow flexion (biceps, brachialis)
C7	Elbow extension (triceps)
C8-T1	Hand grip (finger flexors), finger adduction, oculosympathetics
T2-T12	Expiration (intercostal muscles)
L1-L2	Hip flexion (iliopsoas)
L2-L4	Knee extension (quadriceps)
L5-S1	Knee flexion (hamstrings)

or an associated injury that is distracting to the patient). This recommendation is based on clinical investigations in nearly 40,000 patients, and the combined negative predictive value of cervical spine radiographic assessment for a significant cervical spine injury in these studies was virtually 100%.

   b. A three-view cervical spine series (anteroposterior, lateral, and odontoid views), supplemented with CT should be performed in all **symptomatic patients** to further define areas that are suspicious or not well visualized on the plain cervical x-rays. The negative predictive value for cervical spine injury using a combination of three-view cervical spine series plus CT is between 99% and 100%.

   c. In **awake** patients with neck pain or tenderness and **normal** cervical spine x-rays (including supplemental CT as necessary), cervical spine immobilization can be discontinued after obtaining **either:**

     (1) Normal and adequate dynamic flexion/extension films; **or**

     (2) A normal magnetic resonance imaging study within 48 hours of injury.

   d. In **obtunded** patients with **normal** cervical spine x-rays (including supplemental CT as necessary), cervical spine immobilization may be discontinued after obtaining **either:**

     (1) Dynamic flexion/extension films performed under fluoroscopic guidance;

     (2) A normal magnetic resonance imaging study within 48 hours of injury; **or**

     (3) At the discretion of the treating physician.

Although there is a risk of undetected cervical spinal ligamentous injuries, the incidence in obtunded patients with normal cervical spine x-rays is less than 1%.

ASIA IMPAIRMENT SCALE

☐ **A = Complete:** No motor or sensory function is preserved in the sacral segments S4-S5.

☐ **B = Incomplete:** Sensory but not motor function is preserved below the neurological level and includes the sacral segments S4-S5.

☐ **C = Incomplete:** Motor function is preserved below the neurological level, and more than half of key muscles below the neurological level have a muscle grade less than 3.

☐ **D = Incomplete:** Motor function is preserved below the neurological level, and at least half of key muscles below the neurological level have a muscle grade of 3 or more.

☐ **E = Normal:** Motor and sensory function are normal.

CLINICAL SYNDROMES

☐ Central Cord
☐ Brown-Sequard
☐ Anterior Cord
☐ Conus Medullaris
☐ Cauda Equina

Fig. 34-4. The American Spinal Injury Association (ASIA) spinal cord injury scale and worksheet. (*continued*)

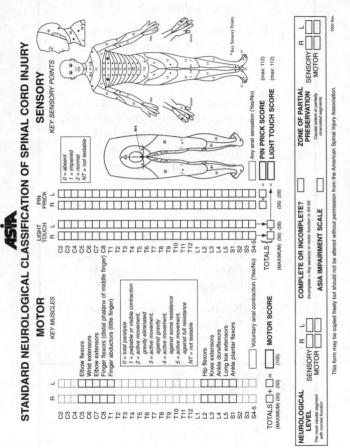

Fig. 34-4. (continued).

C. Intensive care monitoring. Patients with significant SCI should be acutely managed in an ICU for the following reasons:

1. The major causes of death in SCI are aspiration and shock.

2. In the pathophysiology of SCI, spinal cord ischemia is the most important factor resulting in neurologic deficit after primary injury. Appropriate resuscitation is essential to preserving neurologic function.

3. Respiratory insufficiency and pulmonary dysfunction are common in SCI patients and can cause hypoxemia, which can exacerbate spinal cord ischemia.

D. Therapeutic interventions

1. **Methylprednisolone.** The National Acute Spinal Cord Injury Study trial demonstrated that SCI patients who received high-dose methylprednisolone (30-mg/kg bolus followed by 5.4-mg/kg/h infusion for 23 hours) within 8 hours of injury had a significantly better improvement in motor function and sensation at 6-month follow-up than those who received placebo or naloxone. Because other studies have failed to consistently demonstrate a significant clinical benefit, this protocol should be reserved for patients within 8 hours of SCI.

2. **Hemodynamics**

   a. **Hypotension** contributes to secondary injury and worse neurologic outcome after SCI by further reducing spinal cord blood flow and perfusion. SCI patients are at risk for hypotension, cardiac dysrhythmias, reduced peripheral vascular resistance, and reduced cardiac output due to disruption of autonomic pathways. National guidelines recommend that **hypotension** (SBP <90 mm Hg) be avoided and corrected as soon as possible after acute SCI, and maintenance of MAP at 85 to 90 mm Hg for the first 7 days after acute SCI to improve spinal cord perfusion.

   b. Aggressive efforts should be utilized to support arterial pressure with crystalloid as a first agent, followed by colloid if the hematocrit is low or crystalloid is ineffective as a volume expander.

   c. **Neurogenic shock** secondary to SCI is manifested by the triad of hypotension, bradycardia, and hypothermia, and tends to occur more commonly in midthoracic injuries and above. The unopposed vagal tone from functional sympathectomy produces a decrease in vascular resistance and decreased cardiac output. It is differentiated from purely hypovolemic shock by the presence of bradycardia. Neurogenic shock should be considered in patients with suboptimal arterial pressure despite adequate fluid resuscitation. In such cases, the low-tone state can usually be treated with alpha-agonists; the need for addition of beta-agonists other than for bradycardia should raise suspicions for an occult cardiovascular insult. Flaccid paraparesis with sacral dysfunction (e.g., hypotonic bowel, bladder, bulbocavernosus reflex) may last several hours to days until the reflex arcs below the level of the injury are restored.

3. **Nutritional support.** Acute SCI is associated with hypermetabolism, and patients are at risk for negative nitrogen balance and severe malnutrition leading to increased susceptibility to infection, impaired wound healing, and difficulty weaning from mechanical ventilation. Enteral full-caloric, high-nitrogen nutritional support is recommended for SCI patients with adequate gastrointestinal function. Parenteral nutrition should be considered for those with prolonged ileus or other barriers to adequate enteral nutrition.

4. **Prevention of deep venous thrombosis (DVT) and thromboembolism**
   a. SCI patients are at high risk for the development of DVT, with a reported occurrence of 7% to 62%.
   b. Adjusted-dose heparin or low-molecular-weight heparin prophylaxis significantly decreases the incidence of thromboembolism compared to low-dose unfractionated heparin.
   c. Though less effective, pneumatic compression also significantly reduces the incidence of thromboembolic events, especially in combination with antithrombotic agents.
   d. Rotating beds in the first 10 days after acute SCI has been shown to decrease the incidence of DVT and may help to prevent decubitus ulceration.
   e. Placement of prophylactic inferior vena cava filters has been reported to reduce the incidence of pulmonary embolism, with an 81% 1-year patency rate, and should be performed in patients who do not respond to or are not candidates for anticoagulation therapy.

III. **Determination of death using brain criteria**
   A. The medical and legal communities have indicated that locally acceptable guidelines are to be used for the diagnosis of death. **Brain death** is defined as the irreversible loss of the clinical function of the whole brain, including the brainstem. Brain death from primary neurologic disease usually is caused by severe head injury or aneurysmal subarachnoid hemorrhage. Hypoxic-ischemic brain insults and fulminant hepatic failure also may result in irreversible loss of brain function. Brain death must be understood to be no different than a diagnosis of death made by other criteria. Guidelines do not replace the physician's judgment in individual cases because brain death is a clinical diagnosis. It is imperative to distinguish brain death from a **persistent vegetative state** (i.e., absence of cerebral function with preserved vital functions). Diagnostic criteria for the **clinical diagnosis** of brain death

in adults, adapted from those used at the Massachusetts General Hospital, are listed in what follows. Other institutions may have different criteria.

B. Brain death is the absence of clinical whole-brain function when the proximate cause is known and demonstrably irreversible. **Prerequisites** include the following:

1. Clinical or neuroimaging evidence of an acute central nervous system catastrophe.
2. Exclusion of complicating medical conditions that may confound clinical assessment (e.g., severe electrolyte, acid-base, or endocrine disturbance).
3. Toxicology screening with demonstrated barbiturate level less than 10 μg/ml and no evidence of drug intoxication or poisoning.
4. Demonstrated absence of pharmacologic neuromuscular blockade.
5. Core temperature 32°C (90°F) or greater.
6. In the presence of confounding variables, brain death may still be determined with the aid of **ancillary tests** (see later discussion).
7. A **period of observation** of at least 24 hours without clinical neurologic change is necessary if the cause of the coma is unknown.

C. Clinical syndrome. The three cardinal findings in brain death are coma or unresponsiveness, absence of brainstem reflexes, and apnea.

1. **Coma or unresponsiveness** as determined by the absence of any cerebrally mediated motor response to pain in all extremities (nail-bed pressure and supraorbital pressure).
2. **Absence of brainstem reflexes** (all those listed as follows):
   a. Pupils:
      (1) No response to bright light.
      (2) Size: from midposition (4 mm) to dilated (9 mm).
   b. Ocular movement:
      (1) No oculocephalic reflex (tested only when fractures and instability of the cervical spine are absent).
      (2) No deviation of the eyes to irrigation in each ear with 30 to 50 ml of ice water (observe for 1 minute after each irrigation and at least 5 minutes between testing on each side).
   c. Facial motor response to stimulation:
      (1) No corneal reflex to touch with a cotton swab.
      (2) No jaw reflex.
      (3) No facial grimacing to deep pressure on nail bed, supraorbital ridge, or temporomandibular joint.
   d. Pharyngeal and tracheal reflexes:
      (1) No response to stimulation of the posterior pharynx with tongue blade.
      (2) No coughing or significant bradyarrhythmia to bronchial suctioning.

3. **Apnea:** Apnea testing may be performed as follows:
   a. **Prerequisites:**
      (1) Core temperature 36.5°C (97°F) or greater, if possible.
      (2) Systolic blood pressure 90 mm Hg or greater, if possible.
      (3) Corrected diabetes insipidus or positive fluid balance in the last 6 hours.
      (4) $PaCO_2$ normal or 40 mm Hg or greater.
      (5) Arterial pH normal (7.35–7.45), if possible. Adjusting the ventilator to obtain a normal arterial pH and $PaCO_2$ prior to initiating the test minimizes time off the ventilator and decreases the risk of hypoxia or severe acidosis.
      (6) Preoxygenation with 100% inspired oxygen (FiO_2) for 5 minutes or to a PaO_2 of 200 mm Hg or greater, if possible.
   b. **Connect a pulse oximeter.** Attach a catheter to an oxygen source and deliver **100% O_2 at 8 to 10 L/min** via the endotracheal tube to the level of the carina immediately after disconnecting the ventilator. Because most ventilators do not supply a steady flow of oxygen unless the ventilator is cycling, in general, it is not adequate to leave the patient attached to the ventilator during the test.
   c. **Observe closely for respiratory movements** (defined as abdominal or chest excursions that produce adequate tidal volumes). Chest wall excursions secondary to cardiac pulsations are not considered respiratory efforts. Arterial pH usually decreases by 0.02 unit per minute of apnea.
   d. **Measure PaO_2, $PaCO_2$, and arterial pH** after approximately 8 minutes and reconnect to the ventilator. The apnea test must be terminated if the patient becomes cyanotic or hypotensive (see later discussion).
   e. **If respiratory movements are absent** and the final arterial blood gas analysis shows:
      (1) An arterial pH of 7.30 or less (from a patient with pretest pH ≥ 7.40); **or**
      (2) A $PaCO_2$ of 60 mm Hg or greater; **or**
      (3) $PaCO_2$ increasing 20 mm Hg over the pretest baseline;
      (4) **Then apnea has been demonstrated,** supporting the diagnosis of brain death.
   f. **If respiratory movements are observed or the blood gas criteria are not met,** the apnea test result is negative. If during testing the patient becomes cyanotic, the SBP becomes 90 mm Hg or less, the pulse oximeter indicates significant oxygen desaturation, or cardiac dysrhythmias develop, then immediately draw an arterial blood sample and reconnect the ventilator. If the blood gas values meet the foregoing criteria (see section **V.C.3.e**), then

apnea has been demonstrated. If the blood gas values do not meet the criteria, the apnea test is indeterminate and additional confirmatory testing is necessary.

D. Pitfalls in the diagnosis of brain death. The following conditions may interfere with the clinical diagnosis of brain death, so that the diagnosis cannot be made with certainty on clinical grounds alone. In such cases, confirmatory tests are recommended.

1. Severe facial trauma.
2. Preexisting pupillary abnormalities.
3. Toxic levels of any sedative drugs, aminoglycosides, tricyclic antidepressants, anticholinergics, antiepileptic drugs, chemotherapeutic agents, or neuromuscular blocking agents.
4. Sleep apnea or severe pulmonary disease resulting in severe chronic retention of CO_2.

E. Clinical observations still compatible with the diagnosis of brain death. These manifestations are seen occasionally and should not be misinterpreted as evidence for brainstem function.

1. Spontaneous "spinal" movements of limbs (not to be confused with pathologic flexion or extension response).
2. Respiratory-like movements (shoulder elevation and adduction, back arching, intercostal expansion without significant tidal volumes).
3. Sweating, blushing, tachycardia.
4. Normal blood pressure in the absence of pharmacologic support.
5. Absence of diabetes insipidus (i.e., normal osmolar control mechanism).
6. Deep tendon reflexes, triple flexion responses, or Babinski's reflex.

F. Confirmatory laboratory tests supporting the diagnosis of brain death. Brain death is a clinical diagnosis. Repeat clinical evaluation 6 hours later should be considered, but this interval is arbitrary. A confirmatory test is not mandatory but can be used as supportive data in those patients in whom specific components of clinical testing cannot be reliably performed or evaluated. Remember to write down the name of the physician interpreting the ancillary tests because this will be needed in the Declaration of Death note.

1. **Conventional angiography:** no intracerebral filling at the level of the carotid bifurcation or circle of Willis is observed. The external carotid circulation is patent, and filling of the superior sagittal sinus may be delayed.
2. **Electroencephalography:** no electrocerebral activity is present for at least 30 minutes of recording that adheres to the minimal technical criteria for electroencephalogram (EEG) recording in suspected brain death as adopted by the American Electroencephalographic Society, including 16-channel EEG

instruments. It should include the absence of nonartefactual activity and there should be no change with auditory, visual, or painful stimulation. Electrocardiographic artifact should be visible. There is no need for the patient to be normothermic, but core body temperature should be above 90°F. If an EEG is obtained, the absence of EEG activity should be confirmed by a neurologist prior to the declaration of brain death. This should be noted in the patient's medical record.

3. **Transcranial Doppler ultrasonography**
   a. Small systolic peaks in early systole occurring without diastolic flow or with reverberating flow are indicative of very high vascular resistance associated with greatly increased intracranial pressure and lack of tissue blood flow.
   b. Previously documented Doppler signals are lost. Because 10% of patients may not have temporal windows that permit insonation, however, the **initial** absence of Doppler signals cannot be interpreted as consistent with brain death.

4. **Technetium-99m** hexamethylpropyleneamineoxime (HMPAO) brain scan. No uptake of isotope in brain parenchyma ("hollow skull phenomenon") occurs, as interpreted by a nuclear medicine physician.

5. **Somatosensory-evoked potentials:** The N20-P22 response with median nerve stimulation is absent bilaterally. The recordings should adhere to the minimal technical criteria for somatosensory-evoked potentials recording in suspected brain death as adopted by the American Electroencephalographic Society.

G. **Medical record documentation.** The declaration of death by brain criteria should be documented in the medical record in a manner similar to any other declaration of death and include the following:

1. The time of declaration and name of the attending **neurosurgeon** or **neurologist** declaring brain death.
2. Etiology and irreversibility of condition.
3. Absence of brain stem reflexes.
4. Absence of motor response to pain.
5. Absence of respiration with $PaCO_{22}$ 60 mm Hg or greater.
6. Justification for confirmatory testing if indicated, and results of confirmatory test(s) if performed, with the name of the physician responsible for interpretation
7. Results of repeat neurologic examinations, if performed.
8. Indication that the medical examiner was contacted, if appropriate.

SELECTED REFERENCES

American College of Surgeons, Committee on Trauma. Spine and spinal cord trauma. In: *Advanced trauma life support program for doctors: ATLS*, 6th ed. Chicago: American College of Surgeons, 1997:215–242.

An appraisal of the criteria of cerebral death: a summary statement: A collaborative study. *JAMA* 1977;237:982–986.

Bracken MB, Shepard MJ, Collins WF, et al. A randomized, controlled trial of methylprednisolone or naloxone in the treatment of acute spinal-cord injury. Results of the Second National Acute Spinal Cord Injury Study. *N Engl J Med* 1990;322:1405–1411.

Chestnut RM. Emegency management of spinal cord injury. In: Narayan RK, Wilberger JE, Povlishock JT, eds. *Neurotrauma.* New York: McGraw-Hill, 1996:1121–1138.

Geerts WH, Code KI, Jay RM, et al. A prospective study of venous thromboembolism after major trauma. *N Engl J Med* 1994;331: 1601–1606.

Geisler FH, Coleman WP, Grieco G, et al. The Sygen Multicenter Acute Spinal Cord Injury Study. *Spine* 2001;26(24 Suppl):S78–S98.

Green D, Lee MY, Ito VY, et al. Fixed- vs adjusted-dose heparin in the prophylaxis of thromboembolism in spinal cord injury. *JAMA* 1988;260:1255–1258.

Grady PA, Blaumanis OR. Physiologic parameters of the Cushing reflex. *Surg Neurol* 1988;29:454–461.

Hoffman JR, Mower WR, Wolfson AB, et al. Validity of a set of clinical criteria to rule out injury to the cervical spine in patients with blunt trauma: National Emergency X-radiography Utilization Study Group. *N Engl J Med* 2000;343:94–99.

Lundberg N, Troupp H, Lorin H. Continuous recording and control of ventricular fluid pressure in neurosurgical practice. *Acta Psychiatr Neurol Scand* 1960;36(Suppl 149):1–193.

Marshall LF, Marshall SB, Eisenberg HM, et al. A new classification of head injury based on computerized tomography. *J Neurosurg* 1991;75(Suppl):S14–S20.

Narayan R, Polvishock J, Wilberger J, eds. *Neurotrauma.* New York: McGraw-Hill, 1996.

Robertson CS. Management of cerebral perfusion pressure after traumatic brain injury. *Anesthesiology* 2001;95:1513–1517.

Rosner MJ, Becker DP. Origin and evolution of plateau waves. *J Neurosurg* 1984;60:312–324.

Rosner MJ, Coley I. Cerebral perfusion pressure: a hemodynamic mechanism of mannitol and the postmannitol hemogram. *Neurosurgery* 1987;21:147–156.

Schaefer PW, Huisman TA, Sorensen AG, et al. Diffusion-weighted MR imaging in closed head injury: high correlation with initial Glasgow Coma Scale score and score on modified Rankin scale at discharge. *Radiology* 2004;233:58–66.

Section on Disorders of the Spine and Peripheral Nerves of the American Association of Neurological Surgeons and the Congress of Neurological Surgeons. Guidelines for the management of acute cervical spine and spinal cord injuries. *Neurosurgery* 2002;50(3):S1–S199.

Tator CH, Rowland DW, Schwartz MI, et al. Management of acute spinal cord injuries. *Can J Surg* 1984;27:289–293, 296.

Vale FL, Burns J, Jackson AB, et al. Combined medical and surgical treatment after acute spinal cord injury: results of a prospective pilot study to assess the merits of aggressive medical resuscitation and blood pressure management. *J Neurosurg* 1997;87:239–246.

Wijdicks EFM, ed. *Brain death.* Philadelphia: Lippincott Williams & Wilkins, 2001.

The Burned Patient

Rob Sheridan and Loreta Grecu

I. **Introduction**
   A. **Background.** The prognosis for burn patients, both for survival and for quality of life, has improved dramatically over the last 20 years. This change began with a realization that the natural history of burns can be changed by prompt surgery, the objective of which is to remove deep wounds and achieve immediate biologic closure prior to the inevitable development of wound sepsis. To support a patient with a serious burn through the physiologic trial of staged wound closure requires sophisticated critical care; many aspects are unique to the **burn unit.** This chapter presents these techniques in a concise format.
   B. **The role of intensive care in management of burns** is to bring a patient from a tragic injury to the optimal outcome: total reintegration into family, community, school, and workplace.
   C. **Overall management strategy.** Patients with large burns typically present with a deep wound associated with pain, impending sepsis, and potentially progressive multiorgan dysfunction. Immediate needs must be met, but a specific overall plan of care must also be generated. An organized plan of care can be viewed as having four phases (Table 35-1). The **initial evaluation and resuscitation phase,** from days 1 though 3, requires that an accurate fluid resuscitation be performed while the patient is thoroughly evaluated for other injuries and comorbid conditions. The second phase, **initial wound excision and biologic closure,** includes a series of staged operations that are completed during the first few days after injury. The third phase, **definitive wound closure,** involves replacement of temporary wound covers with definitive covers and closure and acute reconstruction of areas of small surface but high complexity, such as the face and hands. The final stage is **rehabilitation.** Although rehabilitation begins early, it becomes involved and time consuming toward the end of the acute hospital stay.
II. **Physiologic implications of burn injury**
   A. Successfully resuscitated burn patients manifest a sequence of **predictable physiologic changes** (Table 35-2).
      1. **Early ebb phase and later hyperdynamic phase.** The ebb phase relates to a period of hours to a day after injury in which there is a relative hypodynamic state, which needs to be supported in

Table 35-1. Phases of burn care

Phase	Objectives	Time Period
Initial evaluation and resuscitation	Accurate fluid resuscitation and thorough evaluation	0–72 hours
Initial wound excision and biologic closure	Exactly identify and remove all full-thickness wounds and achieve biologic closure	Days 1–7
Definitive wound closure	Replace temporary with definitive covers and close small complex wounds	Day 7–week 6
Rehabilitation, reconstruction, and reintegration	Initially, to maintain range of motion; reduce edema; subsequently, to strengthen and facilitate return to home, work, school	Day 1 through discharge

the resuscitation period. The flow phase relates to the subsequent predictable development of high cardiac output, low peripheral vascular tone, fever, and muscle catabolism that becomes particularly exaggerated in patients with large burns.

2. **Physiology of the resuscitation period.** Unique to a patient suffering a serious burn is a massive diffuse capillary leak, believed to be secondary

Table 35-2. Predictable physiologic changes in burn patients

Period	Physiologic Changes	Clinical Implications
Resuscitation period (day 0–3)	Massive capillary leak	Closely monitor fluid resuscitation
Postresuscitation period (day 3 until 95% definitive wound closure)	Hyperdynamic and catabolic state with high risk of infection	Remove and close wounds to avoid sepsis; nutritional support is essential
Recovery period (95% wound closure until 1 year after injury)	Continued catabolic state and risk of non-wound septic events	Anticipate and treat complications; nutritional support is essential

to wound-released mediators, which results in the vascular extravasation of fluids, electrolytes, and moderate-sized colloid molecules. Burn patients initially require a massive fluid resuscitation. Formulas have been developed over the last 40 years that attempt to predict resuscitation volume requirements based on body weight or body surface area and burn size. Multiple other variables, however, affect resuscitation requirements, including delay until resuscitation, inhalation injury, and the depth and vapor transmission characteristics of the wound itself. Not surprisingly, no formula has yet been developed that accurately predicts volume requirements in all patients. Inaccurate volume administration is associated with substantial morbidity. It is therefore essential that burn resuscitations be guided by hourly reevaluation of resuscitation endpoints, the formula serving only to help to determine initial volume infusion rates and to roughly predict overall requirements.

3. **Postresuscitation physiology.** In patients who are successfully resuscitated, volume requirements abruptly decline 18 to 24 hours after injury as the diffuse capillary leak predictably abates. Subsequently, a diffuse inflammatory state evolves that is characterized by a hyperdynamic circulation, fever, and massively increased protein catabolism. Release of poorly characterized inflammatory mediators, the counterregulatory hormones cortisol, catecholamines, and glucagon, bacteria and their byproducts from the wound and a compromised gastrointestinal barrier, pain, and infection are thought responsible for these changes.

B. **Physiologic support.** The metabolic stress associated with a large burn is enormous. Support includes accurate fluid repletion, provision of an adequate quantity and quality of substrate, control of environmental temperature, prompt removal of nonviable tissue with physiologic wound closure, support of the gastrointestinal barrier, and proper management of pain and anxiety. A critical component is support of **body temperature.** Burn patients have enormous evaporative water and energy losses if they are maintained in the typical cool, dry air of a general hospital. Burn units and operating rooms need to be engineered to maintain high ambient temperatures and humidity to avoid hypothermia.

III. **Initial evaluation**

The initial management of a seriously burned patient is usually not completed prior to arrival in the intensive care unit. Each of these patients should be approached as a potential polytrauma patient. The evaluation follows the primary and secondary survey format of Advanced Trauma Life Support (ATLS; see also Chapter 33).

A. **The primary survey**
   1. **Airway evaluation and protection.** The patency and security of the airway must be established because progressive mucosal edema can compromise airway patency over the first few postinjury hours. This is especially true of young children because airway resistance varies inversely with the fourth power of the airway radius. It is very important to evaluate a patient with burns as soon as he or she arrives in the institution for swelling of the tongue, face, eyes, neck, airway, presence of soot or other foreign body in the airway, impairment in gas exchange, the extent of the burns, and the presence of associated injuries. One should know the mechanism of injury—a thermal burn, electrical burn, or other toxic substances inhaled in the process, such as carbon monoxide—because the mechanism may change the management in terms of securing the airway. It is important to discuss the care of the patient with a surgeon specialized in treating burn patients and to decide together whether observation and a conservative approach is appropriate at this time or whether one should proceed with intubation of the trachea. Endotracheal intubation should be performed immediately if progressive airway edema is suspected. Facial and airway edema makes the burn patient's airway among the most challenging to manage. The method of intubation depends on whether the airway swelling has started. If the intubation is done prophylactically, direct laryngoscopy is generally a safe and adequate maneuver. If the patient's airway is already swollen or some difficulty is anticipated, extra help should be available and an awake fiberoptic intubation should be considered. It is important to have a surgeon present who can skillfully perform a cricothyroidotomy if needed. Once position of the endotracheal tube is confirmed, properly securing the tube is critical because inadvertent extubation in the patient with a burned, swollen face and airway is potentially lethal. A harness system using umbilical ties is recommended.
   2. **Vascular access and initial fluid support.** Reliable vascular access is essential. This usually requires central venous access, although the placement of central lines is most safely performed after immediate postburn hypovolemia has been corrected by volume administration.
   3. **Multiple trauma issues.** Each of these patients must be approached as a polytrauma patient because other injuries are common. Key issues in the trauma patient are outlined in Chapter 33.
B. **Burn-specific secondary survey.** (see Table 35-3).

Table 35-3. The burn-specific secondary survey

System	Important Considerations
History	1. Mechanism of injury, closed-space exposure, extrication time, delay in seeking attention, fluid given during transport and prior illnesses and injuries.
Head, ears, eyes, nose, throat	1. The globes should be examined and corneal epithelium stained with fluorescein before adnexal swelling makes examination difficult. Adnexal swelling provides coverage and protection of the globe during the first days after injury. Tarsorrhaphy is virtually never indicated acutely.
	2. Corneal epithelial loss can be overt, giving a clouded appearance to the cornea, but is more often subtle, requiring fluorescein staining for documentation. Topical ophthalmic antibiotics constitute optimal initial treatment.
	3. Signs of airway involvement include perioral and intraoral burns or carbonaceous material and progressive hoarseness.
	4. Hot liquid can be aspirated in conjunction with a facial scald injury and result in acute airway compromise requiring urgent intubation.
	5. Endotracheal tube security is crucial and is best maintained with an umbilical tape harness, rather than adhesive tape, on the burned face.
Neck	1. The radiographic evaluation is driven by the mechanism of injury.
	2. Rarely, in patients with very deep burns, neck escharotomies are needed to facilitate venous drainage of the head.
Cardiac	1. The cardiac rhythm should be monitored for 24–72 hours in those with electrical injury.
	2. Patients with or at high risk for coronary artery disease may suffer an ischemic event with the hemodynamic stress associated with the burn injury and should be appropriately monitored.
Pulmonary	1. Ensure that inflating pressures are less than 40 cm H_2O by performing chest escharotomies when needed.
	2. Severe inhalation injury may lead to sloughing of endobronchial mucosa and thick bronchial secretions that can occlude the endotracheal tube; one should be prepared for sudden endotracheal tube occlusions.
Vascular	1. The perfusion of burned extremities should be monitored by serial examinations. Indications for escharotomy include decreasing

(continued)

Table 35-3. The burn-specific secondary survey, *Continued*

System	Important Considerations
	temperature, increasing consistency, slowed capillary refill, and diminished Doppler flow in the digital vessels.
	2. Fasciotomy is indicated after electrical or deep thermal injury when distal flow is compromised on clinical examination. Compartment pressures can be helpful, but clinically worrisome extremities should be decompressed regardless of compartment pressure readings.
Abdomen	1. Nasogastric tubes should be in place and their function verified, particularly prior to air transport in unpressurized helicopters.
	2. An inappropriate resuscitative volume requirement may be a sign of an occult intraabdominal injury.
	3. Torso escharotomies may be required to facilitate ventilation in the presence of deep circumferential abdominal wall burns.
	4. Immediate ulcer prophylaxis is indicated in all patients with serious burns.
Genitourinary	1. Bladder catheterization facilitates using urinary output as a resuscitation endpoint.
	2. Ensure that the foreskin is reduced over the bladder catheter after insertion.
Neurologic	1. Early neurologic evaluation is important because the patient's sensorium is often progressively compromised by medication or hemodynamic instability during the hours after injury. This may require computed tomography scanning in those with a mechanism of injury consistent with head trauma.
Extremities	1. Extremities that are at risk for ischemia, particularly those with circumferential thermal burns or those with electrical injury, should be promptly decompressed by escharotomy and/or fasciotomy. Limbs at risk should be dressed so they can be frequently examined.
	2. The need for escharotomy usually becomes evident during the early hours of resuscitation. Many escharotomies can be delayed until transport has been effected if transport times will not extend beyond 6 hours postinjury.
	3. Burned extremities should be elevated and splinted in a position of function.
Wound	1. Wounds, although often underestimated in depth and overestimated in size on initial examination, should be evaluated for size,

(continued)

Table 35-3. The burn-specific secondary survey, *Continued*

System	Important Considerations
	depth, and the presence of circumferential components.
Laboratory	1. Arterial blood gas analysis is important when airway compromise or inhalation injury is present.
	2. A normal admission carboxyhemoglobin concentration does not eliminate the possibility of a significant exposure because the half-life of carboxyhemoglobin is 30–40 minutes in those effectively ventilated with 100% oxygen.
	3. Baseline hemoglobin and electrolytes can be helpful later during resuscitation.
	4. Urinalysis for occult blood should be performed in patients with deep thermal or electrical injuries.
Electrical	1. Monitor cardiac rhythm in high-voltage (>1,000 V) or intermediate-voltage (>220 V) exposures for 24–72 hours.
	2. Low- and intermediate-voltage exposures can cause locally destructive injuries, but rarely result in systemic sequelae.
	3. After high-voltage exposures, delayed neurologic and ocular sequelae can occur, so a carefully documented neurologic and ocular examination is an important part of the initial assessment.
	4. Injured extremities should be serially evaluated for intracompartmental edema and promptly decompressed when it develops.
	5. Bladder catheters should be placed in all patients suffering high-voltage exposure to document the presence or absence of pigmenturia.
Chemical	1. Irrigate wounds with tap water for at least 30 minutes. Irrigate the globe with isotonic crystalloid solution. Blepharospasm may require ocular anesthetic administration.
	2. Exposures to hydrofluoric acid may be complicated by life-threatening hypocalcemia, particularly exposures to concentrated or anhydrous solutions. Such patients should have serum calcium closely monitored and supplemented. Subeschar injection of a 10% calcium gluconate solution is appropriate after exposure to highly concentrated or anhydrous solutions.
Tar	1. Tar should be initially cooled with tap water irrigation and later removed with a lipophilic solvent.

Adapted from Sheridan RL, Tompkins RG. Burns. In: Greenfield LJ, Mulholland MW, Oldham KT, et al., eds. *Surgery: scientific principles and practice.* Philadelphia: Lippincott Williams & Wilkins, 1996:422–438.

1. **History.** The initial evaluation is the best time to elicit important points of medical history and mechanism of injury. These data should be actively sought from emergency personnel and family members because access to these individuals and their information often is transient. Important points include details of the injury mechanism, initial neurologic status, extrication time, and tetanus immune status.

2. **Burn-specific systematic physical examination.** Burn and trauma patients require a comprehensive physical assessment at the time of their initial admission. Several aspects of this physical assessment are unique to burn patients.

    a. **Head, eyes, ears, nose, and throat.** The head should be inspected for trauma. Pressure on the burned occiput should be avoided. The globes should be inspected prior to the development of massive adnexal edema that can severely limit an adequate examination. Serious burns of the globe are generally apparent by a clouded appearance of the cornea. More-subtle injuries are detectable after fluorescein staining. Adnexal burns are noted, but acute tarsorrhapy is virtually never indicated. Ear burns are noted; pressure is avoided on the burned auricle, and topical **mafenide acetate** is applied. Finally, signs of inhalation injury, such as carbonaceous debris and singed vibrissae, are noted on examination of the nose and throat. Devices used to secure the nasogastric and endotracheal tubes are adjusted to that they do not apply pressure on the nasal septum.

    b. **Neurologic.** Assess the patient for central nervous system trauma. Imaging of the head and spine is indicated depending on the mechanism of injury (Chapter 34). Pain and anxiety management is ideally begun during the initial evaluation. In paralyzed or obtunded patients, it is important that there is no pressure on peripheral nerves, so that neuropathies are avoided. Finally, those burned in structural fires should be assessed for **carbon monoxide (CO) exposure** by history, neurologic examination, and carboxyhemoglobin level because selected patients with significant exposures may benefit from hyperbaric oxygen (HBO) treatment. (see also Chapter 31).

    c. **The neck** should be assessed for trauma, based on mechanism of injury. This is particularly important in those suffering high-voltage injuries. Extremely deep circumferential neck burns may require escharotomy to facilitate normal venous drainage of the head.

    d. **The chest** should be assessed for bilateral air movement and compliance. Deep eschar should be sectioned if it interferes with ventilation. Escharotomy is best done, bilaterally if needed, along the anterolateral chest wall.

  e. **Cardiovascular system.** Most patients initially are hypovolemic and respond favorably to volume administration. Occasionally, patients with massive burns will have an element of primary myocardial dysfunction. These patients, identified with invasive monitoring, will benefit from the administration of β-adrenergic agonists such as **dobutamine** and **dopamine.**

  f. **Genitourinary system.** In males, foreskin retracted over the glans should be reduced after catheterization of the bladder so that progressive edema does not result in acute paraphimosis. Occasionally, a deeply burned foreskin must be sectioned to permit bladder catheterization.

  g. **Musculoskeletal system.** Burned extremities must be assessed for other trauma and monitored for adequacy of perfusion. It can sometimes be difficult to identify fractures in this setting, so liberal use of radiography is appropriate. Fractured and burned extremities are initially stabilized with external splints. Progressive edema during resuscitation can result in the late development of profound limb ischemia, secondary to swelling within circumferential eschar or inelastic muscle compartments. Extremity perfusion should be monitored throughout the resuscitation period.

3. **Initial wound evaluation and management.** Wounds are assessed for extent, using a Lund-Browder or other burn diagram (see Fig. 35-1); depth, using the practiced examiner's eye; and the presence of circumferential components, which may require decompression to assure adequate perfusion.

4. **Laboratory values and radiographs.** Little laboratory evaluation is required beyond routine electrolyte and hematologic testing except for carboxyhemoglobin and arterial blood gas determinations in the proper clinical setting. Chest radiographs are appropriate to ensure proper placement of resuscitative lines and the absence of chest trauma. Inhalation injuries rarely cause early radiographic changes. The mechanism of injury will dictate the need for other radiographs.

5. **Possibility of abuse.** All patients should be screened for abuse as the injury mechanism. Approximately 20% of burns in young children are reported to state authorities for investigation, but abuse occurs in all age groups. Often this determination is not made until the patient has been admitted to the burn unit. The entire team must consider this possibility and file any suspicious case with appropriate state agencies. Careful and complete

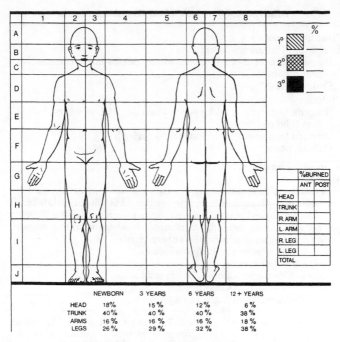

	NEWBORN	3 YEARS	6 YEARS	12 + YEARS
HEAD	18%	15%	12%	6%
TRUNK	40%	40%	40%	38%
ARMS	16%	16%	16%	18%
LEGS	26%	29%	32%	38%

Fig. 35-1. Example of one of the many age-specific burn diagrams available for facilitating accurate estimation of the extent of a burn, compensating for the varying anthropometrics among age groups.

documentation of the circumstances and physical characteristics of the injury is essential. Photographic documentation is ideal.

IV. Resuscitation

A. Physiology of the immediate postburn period. For perhaps as long as an hour after an extensive burn, patients experience little derangement in intravascular volume, which explains the common observation that, after even massive injuries, patients can be quite alert for the first postinjury hour. As wound-released mediators are absorbed into the systemic circulation and as stress- and pain-triggered hormonal release occurs, a diffuse loss of capillary integrity occurs that results in the extravasation of fluids, electrolytes, and even moderate-sized colloid molecules. For unknown reasons, this leak abates between 18 and 24 hours later in those successfully resuscitated. An increased leak can be seen in those whose resuscitations are delayed, which is thought to be due to the systemic release of reactive oxygen species formed upon reperfusion of marginally perfused tissues.

Table 35-4. The modified Brooke formula

First 24 hours
Adults and Children >10 kg:
  Ringer's lactate: 2–4 ml/kg per % burn per 24 hours (first half in
    first 8 hours)
  Colloid: none
Children <10 kg:
  Ringer's lactate: 2–3 ml/kg per % burn per 24 hours (first half in
    first 8 hours)
  Ringer's lactate with 5% dextrose: 4 ml/kg/h
  Colloid: none

Second 24 hours
All patients:
  Crystalloid: To maintain urine output; if silver nitrate is used,
    sodium leeching will mandate continued isotonic crystalloid; if
    another topical is used, free water requirement is significant;
    serum sodium should be monitored closely; nutritional support
    should begin, ideally by the enteral route.
  Colloid (5% albumin in Ringer's lactate):
    0%–30% burn: none
    30%–50% burn: 0.3 ml/kg/% burn/24 h
    50%–70% burn: 0.4 ml/kg/% burn/24 h
    >70% burn: 0.5 ml/kg/% burn/24 h

Adapted from Sheridan RL, Tompkins RG. Burns. In: Greenfield LJ, Mulholland MW, Oldham KT, et al., eds. *Surgery: scientific principles and practice.*
Philadelphia: Lippincott Williams & Wilkins, 1996:422–438.

  B. Formulas have been developed over the last 40 years
    that attempt to predict resuscitation volume require-
    ments. The multiple variables that impact resuscita-
    tion requirements render all such formulas inherently
    inaccurate. One such consensus formula is the modified
    Brooke formula, which is summarized in Table 35-4.
  C. Monitoring. Inaccurate volume administration is as-
    sociated with substantial morbidity. Burn resuscita-
    tions must be guided by hourly reevaluation of resusci-
    tation endpoints, which are summarized in Table 35-5.
    Oxygen delivery and consumption determinations have
    been advocated as guides to the adequacy of burn resus-
    citation, but there are no compelling data to suggest
    such information provides clinically relevant guidance
    in this setting.
  **D. Recognition and management of resuscitation
    problems.** The volume of infusate required by patients
    with large injuries can be enormous. It is essential to
    promptly recognize when resuscitation is not proceed-
    ing as it should and what to do if this is found to be
    the case. At any point during resuscitation, the total
    24-hour volume can be predicted based on the known
    volume infused so far and the current rate of infusion.
    If this number exceeds 6 ml/kg per percentage of burn

Table 35-5. Age-specific resuscitation endpoints

Endpoint	Target
Sensorium	Comfortable, arousable
Urine output	Infants: 1–2 ml/kg/h
	Children: 0.5–1 ml/kg/h
	All others: 0.5 ml/kg/h
Base deficit	Less than 2
Systolic pressure	Infants: 60–70 mm Hg
	Children: 70–90 + (twice age in years) mm Hg
	Adolescents and adults: 90–120 mm Hg

Adapted from Sheridan RL, Tompkins RG. Burns. In: Greenfield LJ, Mulholland MW, Oldham KT, eds. *Surgery: scientific principles and practice.* Philadelphia: Lippincott Williams & Wilkins, 1996:422–438.
Note: Resuscitation endpoints should be assessed regularly throughout burn resuscitation and infusions adjusted up or down in 10% to 20% increments to meet the needs of the individual patient.

per 24 hours, it is likely that the resuscitation is not proceeding optimally. At this point one can consider the use of low-dose dopamine, colloid administration, or the placement of a pulmonary artery catheter to gather additional information regarding the adequacy of ventricular filling and myocardial contractility. This is particularly important in older patients whose underlying cardiac disease is unmasked by the stress of burn resuscitation.

V. Neurologic issues that must be commonly addressed are pain and anxiety management, care of the exposed eye globe, and peripheral neuropathies.

A. Uncontrolled pain and anxiety have adverse physiologic as well as psychological sequelae. Both can contribute to the development of posttraumatic stress syndrome.

1. In the past, inadequate pain management occurred because the extraordinary opiate doses required to adequately address pain in the seriously burned patient inspired fear of respiratory depression, addiction, and litigation among providers of burn care.

2. The opiate tolerance that rapidly develops in patients with large open wounds can be remarkable. Despite this, addiction is rare; opiate requirements rapidly decrease after wound closure. In fact, the best way to manage pain in burn patients is with prompt biologic closure of their wounds.

3. Successful management is greatly aided by an organized pharmacologic guideline supplemented with nonpharmacologic measures. A combination of benzodiazepines and opiates can be used to decrease overall dose requirements (see Chapters 5 and 6).

B. Ocular exposure. Commonly, progressive contraction of the burned eyelids and periocular skin results in exposure of the globe. This predictably results in desiccation of the globe, which is followed by keratitis, ulceration, and globe-threatening infection. Frequent lubrication of the exposed globe with hourly application of ocular lubricant, and surgically releasing the eyelid in those who do not rapidly respond help to prevent these sequelae.

C. **Peripheral neuropathies** can be seen in burn patients because of direct thermal damage to peripheral nerves or because of one of the many metabolic derangements that these patients can suffer. Many peripheral neuropathies can be avoided. Diligent monitoring of extremity perfusion will avoid the morbidity of constricting eschar and missed compartment syndromes. Proper application of well-fitting splints will avoid pressure-induced neuropathies. Careful positioning of deeply sedated or anesthetized patients will avoid traction and pressure injuries.

VI. **Pulmonary issues**

A. **Airway issues.** The critical importance of initial airway evaluation and proper control has been reviewed in section **III.A.1.** This need continues throughout the period of intubation. The security of the endotracheal tube should be regularly verified, and ICU personnel should be drilled and equipped to deal with sudden airway emergencies. If there is only concern for inhalational injury, the patients can be extubated after the fiberoptic evaluation of the airway and the regression of airway edema if there is no concern for development of complications such as the acute respiratory distress syndrome. If the airway injury is not the major concern but the patient requires frequent courses of operating room treatments for debridement or the dressing changes are very painful, the ICU physicians may decide to maintain the endotracheal intubation for the duration of treatment and evaluate for possible tracheostomy.

B. **Inhalation injury**

1. **Diagnosis.** Inhalation injury is a clinical diagnosis based on a history of closed-space exposure, presence of singed nasal vibrissae, and carbonaceous sputum. Fiberoptic bronchoscopy facilitates diagnosis in equivocal cases and may help to document laryngeal edema. Such information is useful when making decisions regarding preemptive intubation for evolving upper airway edema. When the airway edema seems to have decreased, it is important to evaluate the airway before proceeding with extubation with a fiberoptic scope because it may help with the decision-making process and may decrease the risk of reintubation.

2. **Clinical consequences and management.** Five events with major clinical implications occur predictably in patients with inhalation injury.

a. **Acute upper airway obstruction** is anticipated and managed with endotracheal intubation.

b. **Bronchospasm** from aerosolized irritants is a common occurrence during the first 24 to 48 hours, particularly in young children. This is managed with inhaled β_2-adrenergic agonists (see Chapter 21). Some children will require intravenous bronchodilators such as terbutaline or **low-dose epinephrine infusions** and occasionally steroids. Ventilatory strategies should be designed to minimize auto–positive end-expiratory pressure (auto-PEEP).

c. **Small-airway obstruction** occurs as necrotic endobronchial debris sloughs, and complicates clearance of secretions. Small endotracheal tubes can become suddenly occluded, and it is important to be prepared to evaluate and respond to a sudden deterioration of the patient-ventilator unit. Therapeutic bronchoscopy facilitates clearance of the airways.

d. **Respiratory infection** develops in 30% to 50% of patients with inhalation injury. Differentiating between pneumonia and tracheobronchitis (purulent infection of the denuded tracheobronchial tree) is often difficult, but generally of little clinical consequence. A patient with newly purulent sputum, fever, and impaired gas exchange should be treated with antibiotics according to the results of cultures. Secretion clearance is a particularly important component of management because inhalation injury to bronchial mucosa greatly impairs mucociliary clearance.

e. **Respiratory failure** is common in those sustaining inhalation injury, and is managed as outlined in Chapters 5 and 20. It is not uncommon that some of these patients, especially some with extensive burns, may develop acute respiratory distress syndrome (ARDS), so they will require a special ventilatory management with decreased tidal volumes and permissive hypercapnia and daily evaluation with chest radiography.

3. **CO exposure** is common in patients injured in structural fires. Many are obtunded from a combination of CO, anoxia, and hypotension. HBO therapy has been proposed as a means of improving the prognosis of those suffering serious CO exposures, but its use remains controversial (see also Chapter 31). The question of whom to treat in the hyperbaric chamber commonly arises on a busy burn service.

a. **Physiology.** CO avidly binds and inactivates heme-containing enzymes, particularly hemoglobin and the cytochromes. The formation of carboxyhemoglobin results in an acute physiologic anemia, much like an isovolemic hemodilution. Because a carboxyhemoglobin concentration of 50% is physiologically similar to a 50% isovolemic hemodilution, the routine occurrence of unconsciousness at this level of carboxyhemoglobin makes it clear that other mechanisms are involved in the pathophysiology of CO injury. It is likely that CO binding to the cytochrome system in the mitochondria and interfering with oxygen utilization is more toxic than CO binding to hemoglobin. For unknown reasons, between 5% and 20% of patients with serious CO exposures have been reported to develop delayed neurologic sequelae.

  b. **Management options.** These patients can be managed with 100% isobaric oxygen or with hyperbaric oxygen. If serious exposure has occurred, manifested by overt neurologic impairment or a high carboxyhemoglobin level, then hyperbaric oxygen treatment is probably warranted if it can be administered safely.

  c. **HBO treatment** regimens vary, but an exposure to 3 atmospheres for 90 minutes with three 10-minute "air breaks" is typical. An air break refers to the breathing of pressurized room air rather than pressurized oxygen, which decreases the incidence of seizures from oxygen toxicity. Because treatment is generally in a monoplace chamber, unstable patients are suboptimal candidates. Other relative contraindications are wheezing or air trapping, which increases the risk of pneumothorax, and high fever, which increases the risk of seizures. Prior to placement in the chamber, endotracheal tube balloons should be filled with saline to avoid balloon compression and associated air leaks. Myringotomies are required in intubated patients.

  d. **Cyanide exposure** is often detectable in patients extricated from structural fires, but is rarely of the severity to justify the risk of treatment with amyl nitrate and sodium thiosulfate.

VII. **Gastrointestinal issues**

  A. **Ulcer prophylaxis.** Until the routine use of prophylactic therapies, burn patients had a virulent ulcer diathesis ("Curling's ulcer") that was a common cause of death. Ulceration is believed to be secondary to periods of reduced splanchnic blood flow. It is advisable to treat most patients with serious burns with empirical histamine-receptor blockers and antacids (see Chapter 26). Although it is unclear when to stop prophylactic therapy, most would agree that patients with closed wounds who are tolerating tube feedings are at low enough risk that this therapy can be stopped.

B. **Nutritional support.** Burn patients have predictable and protracted needs for supplemental protein and caloric support; which needs to be accurate because both under- and over-feeding have adverse sequelae (see Chapter 9).

1. **Routes and timing.** Intragastric continuous tube feedings are ideal and usually successful. Tube feedings are begun at a low rate during resuscitation. Initially, a sump nasogastric tube is used so that gastric residuals can be used to help determine tolerance of the feedings. Parenteral nutrition is used if tube feedings are not tolerated. Highly catabolic burn patients tolerate prolonged periods of fasting very poorly.

2. **Nutritional targets** in severely injured burned patients remain controversial. The many formulas propagated to predict these requirements vary widely in their predictions. The current consensus is that protein needs are about 2.5 gm/kg/d and caloric needs are between 1.5 and 1.7 times a calculated basal metabolic rate, or 1.3 to 1. 5 times a measured resting energy expenditure.

3. **Monitoring.** Substrate support needs to be titrated to nutritional endpoints during a lengthy burn hospitalization if the complications of over- or underfeeding are to be avoided. Regular physical examination, quality of wound healing, nitrogen balance, and indirect calorimetry are all useful in this regard. The combination of a highly catabolic state, the critical need to heal extensive wounds, and the length of time that support is required make monitoring and adjustment of nutritional support particularly important in patients with extensive burns.

VIII. **Infectious disease issues**

A. **Wound topical care.** The best way of avoiding wound sepsis is through **prompt excision and closure of deep wounds.** Topical antimicrobial agents are an adjunct in this regard, slowing the inevitable occurrence of wound sepsis in deep wounds and minimizing desiccation and colonization of healing wounds. There are several agents in wide general use; the most common are itemized in Table 35-6.

B. **Antibiotic use.** Burn physiology includes the routine occurrence of moderate fever, which is not necessarily a sign of infection. When unexpected fever occurs, a complete physical assessment is done, wounds are inspected for evidence of sepsis, directed labs and radiographs are taken, and cultures of blood, urine, and sputum are sent. If the patient appears unstable, empirical broad-spectrum coverage is reasonable pending return of culture data (Chapters 11 and 28). If no infectious focus is identified, then antibiotics are stopped. It is critically important that deteriorating burn patients be compulsively evaluated for occult foci of infection to

Table 35-6. Common topical antimicrobial agents employed in burn wound management

Silver sulfadiazine	Painless on application, fair to poor eschar penetration, no metabolic side effects, broad antibacterial spectrum
Mafenide acetate	Painful on application, excellent eschar penetration, carbonic anhydrase inhibitor, broad antibacterial spectrum
0.5% Silver nitrate	Painless on application, poor eschar penetration, leeches electrolytes, broad spectrum (including fungi)

allow prompt treatment prior to the development of systemic sepsis.

   C. Infection control issues. Proper infection control practices are of particular importance to avoid cross-contamination of vulnerable patients with these organisms. Universal precautions and compulsory hand washing are essential components of practice (Chapter 12).

   D. Recognition and management of burn complications. Successful management of burned patients requires that a predictable series of complications are appropriately treated as the burn wound is progressively closed. Table 35-7 summarizes such complications.

IX. Rehabilitation efforts in the burn unit. Rehabilitation efforts begin as soon as the patient is stabilized and proceed throughout critical illness.

   A. Physical and occupational therapists play important roles in the burn ICU. Initially, twice-daily passive ranging of all joints and static antideformity positioning is begun to prevent the development of contractures.

   B. Perioperative therapy. Physical and occupational therapists should be informed of the sequence of planned operations and the modifications of therapy plans that these imply. Therapists should be encouraged to range patients under anesthesia in conjunction with planned operations and to fabricate custom face molds and splints in the operating room, particularly in children, who often poorly tolerate these activities when awake.

X. Intraoperative support
Burn patients must undergo staged excision and closure of their wounds even if they are critically ill; not to do so will render them even sicker. Close communication between the ICU and operating room teams is essential.

   A. Transport to and from the operating room must be carefully planned. Operating rooms must be maintained hot and humid to minimize the occurrence of hypothermia in exposed burn patients. Intraoperative hypothermia is poorly tolerated, causes coagulopathy, and increases bleeding.

Table 35-7. Systematic reassessment of seriously ill burn patients

System	Complication
Neurologic	1. *Delirium* occurs in up to 30% of patients and generally resolves with supportive therapy. 2. *Seizures* may result from hyponatremia or abrupt benzodiazepine withdrawal. 3. *Peripheral nerve injuries* occur from direct thermal injury, compression from compartment syndrome or overlying inelastic eschar, major metabolic disturbances, or improper splinting techniques. 4. *Delayed peripheral nerve and spinal cord deficits* develop weeks or months after high-voltage injury secondary to small-vessel injury and demyelinization.
Renal	1. *Early acute renal failure* follows inadequate perfusion during resuscitation or myoglobinuria. 2. *Late renal failure* complicates sepsis, multiorgan failure, or the use of nephrotoxic agents.
Adrenal	1. *Acute adrenal insufficiency* secondary to hemorrhage into the gland presents with hypotension, fever, hyponatremia, and hyperkalemia.
Cardiovascular	1. *Endocarditis and suppurative thrombophlebitis* typically present with fever and bacteremia without signs of local infection. 2. *Hypertension* occurs in up to 20% of children and is best managed with β-adrenergic blockers. 3. *Venous thromboembolic complications* are so infrequent in patients with large burns that routine prophylaxis is not recommended.
Pulmonary	1. *Carbon monoxide intoxication* is best managed acutely with effective ventilation with pure oxygen and can be associated with delayed neurologic sequelae. 2. *Pneumonia* may occur with or without antecedent inhalation injury and is treated with pulmonary toilet and antibiotics. 3. *Respiratory failure* may occur early postinjury secondary to inhalation of noxious chemicals or later in the course secondary to sepsis or pneumonia.
Hematologic	1. *Neutropenia and thrombocytopenia* as well as *disseminated intravascular coagulation* are common indicators of impending sepsis and should prompt appropriate investigations.

(continued)

Table 35-7. Systematic reassessment of seriously ill burn patients *Continued*

	2. *Global immunologic deficits* associated with burn injury contribute to a high rate of infectious complications.
Otologic	1. *Auricular chondritis* secondary to bacterial invasion of cartilage results in rapid loss of viable tissue and is prevented by the routine use of topical mafenide acetate.
	2. *Sinusitis and otitis media* can be caused by transnasal instrumentation and are treated by relocation of tubes, antibiotics, and surgical drainage.
	3. *Complications of endotracheal intubation* include nasal alar and septal necrosis, vocal cord erosions and ulcerations, tracheal stenosis, and tracheoesophageal and tracheo-innominate artery fistulae. Such complications are minimized by compulsory attention to tube position and cuff pressures and avoidance of oversized tubes.
Enteric	1. *Hepatic dysfunction,* secondary to transient hepatic blood flow deficits and manifested as transaminase elevations, is common and resolves with volume repletion; late hepatic failure may complicate sepsis and multiorgan failure.
	2. *Pancreatitis,* beginning with enzyme elevation and ileus and progressing through hemorrhagic pancreatitis, is generally coincident with splanchnic flow deficits early and sepsis-induced organ failures later in the course.
	3. *Acalculous cholecystitis* can present as sepsis without localized symptoms, accompanied by rising cholestatic chemistries; ultrasound-guided bedside percutaneous cholecystostomy is indicated in unstable patients.
	4. *Gastroduodenal ulceration* secondary to splanchnic flow deficits is extremely common and often life threatening if proper ulcer prophylaxis is not administered.
	5. *Intestinal ischemia,* which can progress to infarction, is secondary to inadequate resuscitation.
Ophthalmic	1. *Ectropia,* from progressive contraction of burned ocular adnexae, results in exposure of the globe. This requires acute eyelid release. Tarsorrhaphy is rarely helpful.
	2. *Corneal ulceration,* which develops after initial epithelial injury or later exposure secondary to ectropion, can progress to full thickness corneal destruction if secondary infection

(continued)

**Table 35-7. Systematic reassessment
of seriously ill burn patients** *Continued*

	occurs. This is prevented by careful globe lubrication with topical antibiotics in the former case and acute lid release in the latter.
	3 *Symblepharon*, or scarring of the lid to the denuded conjunctiva following chemical burns, and corneal epithelial defects complicating toxic epidermal necrolysis are prevented by daily examination and adhesion disruption with a fine glass rod.
Genitourinary	1. *Urinary tract infections* are minimized by maintaining indwelling bladder catheters only when absolutely required, and are treated with appropriate antibiotics. Neither catheterization nor colonic diversion is necessarily required for management of perineal and genital burns.
	2. *Candida cystitis* occurs in those patients treated with bladder catheters and broad-spectrum antibiotics. Catheter change and amphotericin irrigation for 5 days is generally successful. If infections are recurrent, the upper urinary tracts should be screened ultrasonographically.
Musculoskeletal	1. *Burned exposed bone* is generally debrided until viable cortical bone is reached, which is then allowed to granulate and is autografted.
	2. *Fractured and burned extremities* are best immobilized with external fixators while overlying burns are grafted. Burn patients with coincident fractures in unburned extremities benefit from prompt internal fixation.
	3. *Heterotopic ossification* develops weeks after injury, most commonly around deeply burned major joints such as the triceps tendon, and presents with pain and decreased range of motion. Most patients respond to physical therapy, but some require excision of heterotopic bone to achieve full function.
Soft tissue	1. *Hypertrophic scar formation* is a major cause of long-term functional and cosmetic deformities of burn patients. This poorly understood process is heralded by an increase in neovascularity between 9 and 13 weeks after epithelialization. Management options include grafting of deep dermal and full-thickness wounds, compression garments, judicious steroid injections, topical silicone products, and scar release and resurfacing procedures.

Adapted from Sheridan RL, Tompkins RG. Burns. In: Greenfield LJ, Mulholland MW, Oldham KT, et al., eds. *Surgery: scientific principles and practice.* Philadelphia: Lippincott Williams & Wilkins, 1996:422–438.

B. **Intraoperative critical care and communication.**
   Critical care must proceed during surgery. The surgical and anesthesia teams must be in constant communication so that each knows what the other is
   doing, blood replacement can be appropriate, and
   extension of the operation can be thoughtfully considered.

XI. **Special considerations**
   A. **Electrical injury**
      1. Patients exposed to low and intermediate voltages
         may have severe local wounds, but rarely suffer sys-
         temic consequences.
      2. Patients exposed to high voltages commonly suf-
         fer compartment syndromes, myocardial injury, frac-
         tures of the long bones and axial spine, and free pig-
         ment in the plasma that may cause renal failure if
         not promptly cleared.
      3. Patients suffering high-voltage injuries should re-
         ceive cardiac monitoring, radiographic clearance of
         the spine, and examination of the urine for myo-
         globin. Fluid resuscitation initially is based on burn
         size, but this generally does not correlate well with
         deep tissue injury, so resuscitations need to be
         closely monitored and adjusted. Muscle compart-
         ments at risk should be closely monitored by serial
         physical examinations; they should be decompressed
         in the operating room when an evolving compart-
         ment syndrome is suspected. Wounds are debrided
         and closed with a combination of skin grafts and
         flaps.
   B. **Tar injury**
      1. Numerous thermoplastic road materials are the
         source of occupational injury. They are highly vis-
         cous and heated to between 300°F and 700°F.
      2. The wounds should be immediately cooled by tap
         water irrigation. Resuscitation is based on burn
         size and monitored. Wounds are dressed in a
         lipophilic solvent and then debrided, excised, and
         grafted. The underlying wounds are generally quite
         deep.
   C. **Cold injury**
      1. Soft tissue necrosis from cold injury is often man-
         aged in the burn unit. Wound care is conservative
         until the extent of irreversible soft tissue necrosis is
         apparent; this often requires several weeks if not
         months. When definitely demarcated, surgical de-
         bridement, excision, and reconstruction or closure
         are carried out if needed, with lesser injuries often
         healing without need for surgery.
      2. Cold-injured patients may manifest all the problems
         of systemic **hypothermia** when they present, and
         should be managed accordingly (see Chapter 32).
   D. **Chemical injury**
      1. Patients can be exposed to a variety of chemicals,
         which are often heated. It is important to consider

the thermal, local chemical, and systemic chemical effects.

2. Consultation with **poison control information centers** for guidance regarding systemic effects is extremely useful. Most agents can be washed off with tap water (see Chapter 31).

   a. **Alkaline substances** may take longer than the traditional 30 minutes. When the soapy feel that these alkalis typically impart to the gloved finger is gone or when litmus paper applied to the wound shows a neutral pH, irrigation can be stopped.

   b. Concentrated **hydrofluoric acid** exposure will cause dangerous hypocalcemia, and subeschar injection of 10% calcium gluconate and emergent wound excision may be appropriate.

   c. **Elemental metals** should be covered with oil, and **white phosphorus** should be covered in saline to prevent secondary ignition.

E. **Toxic epidermal necrolysis (TENS)**

1. TENS is a diffuse process in which the epidermal-dermal bonding is acutely compromised. Patients commonly present with a drug exposure preceding the illness and develop both a **cutaneous** and a **visceral** wound.

2. This disease is similar in presentation to a total-body second-degree burn. With good wound care, most patients will heal the cutaneous wound without the need for surgery. Involvement of the aerodigestive tract mucosa may lead to sepsis and organ failures, particularly if septic complications are not promptly recognized and treated.

F. **Purpura fulminans (PF)**

1. PF is a complication of meningococcal sepsis in which extensive soft tissue necrosis and, commonly, organ failures occur. It is believed to be secondary to a transient hypercoagulable state that occurs early in the primary septicemic event.

2. These patients often present with sepsis-associated organ failures and extensive deep wounds. Both should be managed concurrently because the wounds are prone to infection if not promptly excised and closed.

G. **Soft tissue infections**

1. Patients with soft tissue infections share many characteristics of burn patients. Accurate classification of serious soft tissue infections is difficult, but all are approached in the same general fashion.

2. These patients need to go directly to the operating room. The operative goal is exposure of the infection so that its anatomic extent can be accurately described and its microbiology determined by culture, Gram's stain, and biopsy. Debridement under general anesthesia is repeated until infection is controlled, and the wounds are then closed or grafted. Broad-spectrum, and then focused, antibiotics

Table 35-8. Burn/polytrauma patients: conflicting priorities

Area of Conflict	Consensus Resolution
Neurologic	
Patients with burns and head injuries must have cerebral edema controlled during resuscitation; pressure monitors increase risk of infection.	A very tightly controlled resuscitation with short-term placement of indicated pressure monitors with antibiotic coverage.
Chest	
Patients with blunt chest injuries and overlying burns may require chest tubes through burned areas with risk of empyema and difficulty closing the tract.	Use of a long subcutaneous tunnel to decrease trouble closing the tract and remove tubes as soon as possible to decrease empyema risk.
Abdomen	
Blunt abdominal injuries may be hard to detect if there is an overlying burn. There is a high incidence of wound dehiscence operating through a burned abdominal wall.	Liberal use of imaging to detect occult injuries. Routine use of retention sutures after laparotomy.
Orthopedic	
Optimal management of a fracture may be compromised by an overlying burn	Most such extremities are best managed with prompt excision and grafting of the wound with external fracture fixation.

are important adjuncts. Some patients, particularly those with clostridial infection, may benefit from adjunctive HBO, but prompt surgery is the primary therapeutic modality.

H. The burned polytrauma patient. Burn care priorities frequently conflict with orthopedic, neurosurgical, and other priorities. Thoughtful resolution of these differences is an important part of successful management (see Table 35-8). These situations commonly require a great deal of judgment and liberal consultation.

SELECTED REFERENCES

Rabban J, Blair J, Rosen C, et al. Mechanisms of pediatric electrical injury: new implications for product safety and prevention. *Arch Pediatr Adolesc Med* 1997;151:696–700.

Goldstein AM, Weber JM, Sheridan RL. Femoral venous catheterization is safe in burned children: an analysis of 224 catheters. *J Pediatr* 1997;3:442–446.

Prelack K, Cunningham J, Sheridan RL, et al. Energy provided and protein provisions for thermally injured children revisited: an outcome-based approach for determining requirements. *J Burn Care Rehabil* 1997;10:177–182.

Sheridan RL. The seriously burned child: resuscitation through reintegration. Part 1. *Curr Prob Pediatr* 1998;28(4):105–127.

Sheridan RL. The seriously burned child: resuscitation through reintegration. Part 2. *Curr Prob Pediatr* 1998;28(5):139–167.

Sheridan RL, Hinson M, Blanquierre M, et al. Development of a pediatric burn pain and anxiety management program. *J Burn Care Rehabil* 1997;18:455–459.

Sheridan RL, Prelack K, Cunningham JJ. Physiologic hypoalbuminemia is well tolerated by severely burned children. *J Trauma* 1997;43:448–452.

Sheridan RL, Tompkins RG, Burke JF. Management of burn wounds with prompt excision and immediate closure. *J Intensive Care Med* 1994;9:6–19.

Sheridan RL, Weber JM, Benjamin J, et al. Control of methicillin resistant *Staphylococcus aureus* in a pediatric burn unit. *Am J Infect Control* 1994;22:340–345.

Vascular Surgery

Lee V. Wesner and Rae M. Allain

I. **General considerations.** The vascular surgical patient represents many challenges to both the anesthesiologist and postoperative care providers. In addition to the inherent risks of major vascular surgery, these patients often have significant comorbidities. Common coexisting diseases include hypertension, coronary artery disease (CAD), chronic obstructive pulmonary disease (COPD), diabetes mellitus (DM), and chronic renal insufficiency. The presence or absence of these conditions may influence the decision to proceed with elective vascular procedures. The reader is referred to the corresponding chapters for a more detailed discussion of these comorbidities.

II. **Carotid artery stenosis.** Interventions to correct carotid artery stenosis are performed very frequently, second only to interventions to correct CAD.

   A. **Carotid endarterectomy (CEA)** has been traditionally performed in both symptomatic patients and asymptomatic patients having greater than 70% stenosis involving the carotid bifurcation.

   1. CEA has been demonstrated to be superior to conservative medical therapy in preventing fatal, disabling, and nondisabling stroke in multiple trials.

   2. The surgery may be performed under either general or regional anesthesia

   3. Methods of monitoring cerebral perfusion during CEA include continuous electroencephalogram (EEG), jugular venous O_2 saturation, evoked potentials, and serial neurologic examination (in the awake patient).

   4. **Perioperative complications**

   a. **Cardiac complications** are the leading cause of postoperative mortality in patients undergoing CEA, resulting in approximately 50% of total deaths. Myocardial infarction is most common on postoperative days 2 to 3. The incidence of fatal myocardial events has been decreased somewhat by the expanding use of pre- and perioperative beta-blockade.

   b. **Neurologic complications** include ischemic events, which may be either embolic or hemorrhagic in origin. A new deficit present in the immediate postoperative period represents a surgical emergency and may prompt diagnostic angiographic studies or reexploration.

   c. **Airway compromise** resulting in respiratory failure may be the result of a rapidly expanding wound hematoma with tracheal compression. Postoperative bleeding may be more likely in patients who have received potent antiplatelet agents or warfarin in the preoperative period. Recurrent laryngeal nerve injury may result in vocal cord paralysis and/or increased risk of aspiration. If airway loss is imminent, **endotracheal intubation** should be performed immediately regardless of the etiology, and subsequent therapy should be dictated by specific circumstances.

d. Respiratory difficulties may be encountered due to ablation of the carotid body. Loss of chemoreceptor function will result in decreased responsiveness to hypoxia and may result in hypercarbia with subsequent narcosis. Oxygen saturation should be monitored carefully for a minimum of 24 hours postoperatively. The risks of hypoxia and hypercarbia are higher in patients who have previously undergone contralateral carotid endarterectomy.

e. Manipulation of the carotid sinus frequently results in **bradyarrhythmias,** and postoperative hypotension is often seen secondary to the sinus sensing higher intraarterial pressures after removal of the atherosclerotic plaque.

f. Hypertension may been seen secondary to an exacerbation of preexisting hypertension, a response to denervation of the carotid sinus, incisional pain, bladder distention secondary to intravenous (IV) fluid administration, or as a sympathetic response to hypercarbia. Aggressive management of hypertension is recommended to decrease stress on fresh surgical anastomotic sites as well as to avoid neurologic complications such as cerebral edema.

g. Postendarterectomy hyperperfusion syndrome occurs secondary to a profound increase in ipsilateral perfusion following CEA. Longstanding decreased cerebral blood flow (CBF) leads to impaired autoregulation. The subsequent increase in CBF can lead to cerebral edema or even intracranial hemorrhage in severe cases.

B. Carotid artery stenting has gained popularity in recent years as an alternative to CEA.

1. The fundamental rationale for carotid stenting is the relief of arterial obstruction as opposed to removal of a dynamic disease process as with CEA.

2. Early use of carotid artery stenting was limited by risks of compression of the stent as well as embolization of plaque debris to the brain secondary to manipulation of atheroma.

3. Crush-resistant stents and emboli-protection devices have been developed to address these problems. Modern devices include an ultrasmall guide wire of 0.04 cm diameter and an expandable filter basket with a pore size of approximately 100 μm.

4. Recent evidence suggests that carotid stenting may be comparable to CEA in terms of rates of ipsilateral stroke, myocardial infarction, and death. However, because patients who are stented typically receive potent antiplatelet drugs (e.g., clopidogrel), results may be biased.

5. Stenting may be the preferred option in patients for whom surgery poses a high risk or those who have co-existing conditions that would prohibit them from being surgical candidates. The increased complexity of these patients may put them at higher risk of aforementioned complications depending on individual circumstances.

III. **Thoracic aortic aneurysm (TAA)** is the primary indication for procedures on the thoracic aorta. The incidence is approximately 10.4 per 100,000 person-years and is rising, likely due to an aging population with its associated increased risk.

A. The distribution of TAA etiology is approximately 80% degenerative (also termed atherosclerotic), 15% to 20% due to chronic dissection (including those with familial connective tissue disease), 2% infectious, and 1% to 2% resulting from aortitis.

1. Atherosclerotic vascular disease is commonly associated with TAA, although a causative role in the pathophysiology is not clearly established.

2. Some connective tissue diseases (e.g., Marfan's syndrome, Ehlers-Danlos syndrome) weaken the medial layer of the aorta, leading to aneurysm formation. In addition, a familial form of aortic aneurysmal disease has been identified with histopathology showing cystic medial degeneration of the aortic wall, similar to that seen in Marfan's syndrome.

3. Aneurysm characteristics that increase risk for rupture include size, dissection, extension, and rate of expansion.

4. Patient factors that increase rupture risk include hypertension, smoking, COPD, renal insufficiency, aneurysm symptoms, and female gender.

B. TAAs are described according to the Crawford classification system (Fig. 36-1).

1. **Type I** originates in the proximal descending thoracic aorta distal to the left subclavian artery and extends to the upper abdominal aorta, ending proximal to the renal arteries.

2. **Type II** originates in the proximal descending thoracic aorta distal to the left subclavian artery and extends to the abdominal aorta, ending below the renal arteries.

3. **Type III** originates in the mid-descending thoracic aorta at the level of the sixth intercostal space and extends to the abdominal aorta, ending below the renal arteries.

4. **Type IV** is a total abdominal aneurysm, originating superior to the celiac axis and extending to the distal abdominal aorta.

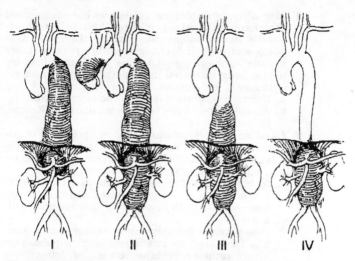

Fig. 36-1. The Crawford classification of thoracoabdominal aortic aneurysms. (From Morrissey NJ, Hollier LH. Anatomic exposures in thoracoabdominal aortic surgery. *Semin Vasc Surg* 2000;13:283–289, with permission.)

C. **Surgical resection of TAA** most often occurs in patients with significant medical comorbidities.
1. Hypertension is nearly universal
2. Renovascular occlusive disease occurs in one-third of these patients, with 25% presenting with a serum creatinine of 1.8 mg/dl or greater. To avoid the risk of contrast-induced nephropathy (CIN), contrast studies should be minimized in patients with any degree of renal insufficiency.
3. COPD is frequently encountered. Approximately 30% of patients present with moderately compromised pulmonary function, with 15% having severe COPD and a forced expiratory volume in 1 second (FEV_1) less than 50% of the predicted value.
D. Size criteria for TAA repair are not as clearly defined as those for abdominal aortic aneurysm (AAA) repair.
1. In general, aneurysms of types I through III that are greater than or equal to 6 cm in diameter should be considered for elective repair.
2. A threshold diameter of 5.0 cm or greater may be used for rapidly expanding aneurysms, patients with Marfan's syndrome, or in cases of chronic aortic dissection due to the increased risk for rupture.
3. Approximately 25% of patients will be treated in urgent or emergent circumstances, with half of this group presenting with frank rupture.
E. **Complications** associated with open TAA repair

1. **Mortality.** Multiple large case series have determined that the overall mortality of open TAA repair is approximately 10% (intraoperatively and in the first 30 days postoperatively). Independent predictors of mortality include advanced age, baseline renal or pulmonary insufficiency, increased intraoperative transfusion requirements, and nonelective operation.
   a. Emergent operation doubles the mortality rate.
   b. Approximately 50% of deaths are due to multiorgan failure.
2. **Cardiac complications** occur in up to 15% of patients and include myocardial infarction, dysrhythmias, prolonged inotropic requirement, tamponade requiring drainage, or congestive heart failure.
   a. Mobilization of "third-space" fluids on postoperative days 2 to 3 may precipitate intravascular volume overload with resultant congestive heart failure (CHF).
   b. Postoperative hemodynamic management is usually facilitated by monitoring with a pulmonary artery catheter or other means of determining cardiac preload and contractile function (e.g., the PiCCO monitor, continuous echocardiography; see Chapter 2). Baseline hemodynamic values in the operating room are useful benchmarks to guide postoperative care.
3. **Pulmonary complications** are the most common source of postoperative morbidity in TAA patients, occurring in up to 40% of cases.
   a. A history of heavy cigarette smoking is common in this patient population with resultant COPD.
   b. Diaphragmatic dysfunction is often seen due to surgical manipulation or division in order to ensure adequate exposure to the aneurysm sac.
      i. Radial division of the diaphragm, although providing rapid, direct, and uncompromised aortic access, also results in paralysis of the left hemidiaphragm.
      ii. Circumferential division is time consuming and less hemostatic but spares the phrenic nerve.
      iii. Partial diaphragm division under the costal margin with aortic hiatal dissection will preserve the phrenic nerve as well and may be optimal in patients with evidence of significant preoperative pulmonary compromise.
   c. Surgical trauma to the left lung is often seen in patients with proximal thoracic origin of TAA. The injury is exaggerated in patients having adhesions between the aneurysmal sac and the lung, where intraoperative dissection commonly results in frank bleeding from the left lung. These patients require vigorous suctioning of blood and clots from the endotracheal tube postoperatively and may benefit from fiberoptic bronchoscopy for pulmonary toilet.

    d. Left lung collapse during the surgical procedure may result in a reperfusion injury to the left lung following reexpansion and volutrauma to the right lung during one-lung ventilation.

    e. Pneumothorax and hemothorax are so common that tube thoracostomy at the conclusion of the procedure is standard technique.

4. Postoperative renal failure is generally defined as a doubling of the baseline creatinine level or an increase in the serum creatinine to greater than or equal to 3 mg/dl.

    a. The incidence is 15% to 20% of patients, with 2% to 5% requiring dialysis.

    b. Development of renal failure is associated with a grave prognosis because mortality is increased by 5- to 10-fold. About one-third of patients who develop renal failure die perioperatively.

    c. Risk factors include baseline renal dysfunction, prolonged intraoperative ischemic time (>30 minutes), and prolonged intraoperative hypotension.

    d. The surgical approach to renal arterial revascularization and minimization of ischemic damage is critical.

        i. Renal artery side arms are often incorporated into the primary aortic graft when the potential for correction of flow-limiting renovascular lesions exists.

        ii. Cold renal perfusion is recommended intraoperatively when access to the renal ostia is safe. This may be accomplished by direct instillation of renal preservation solution (4°C lactated Ringer's solution with 25 g/L mannitol and 1 g/L methylprednisolone) into the renal artery ostia once the aorta is open (see Fig. 36-2A).

    e. The etiology of postoperative renal failure may be multifactorial.

        i. Preoperative diagnostic imaging studies with iodinated contrast, especially in cases of emergent operation, may result in CIN (see Chapter 24).

        ii. Aortic cross-clamping above the level of the renal arteries results in ischemic damage.

        iii. Atheromatous embolization related to aortic cross-clamping or dissection of diseased vascular segments may cause renal arterial obstruction.

        iv. If a renal arterial bypass is employed, kinking of the graft may occur with the return to normal anatomic position following retroperitoneal repair.

        v. Perioperative hemodynamic instability may result in renal hypoperfusion.

5. Mesenteric ischemia with resultant ischemic colitis is seen in approximately 2% of patients.

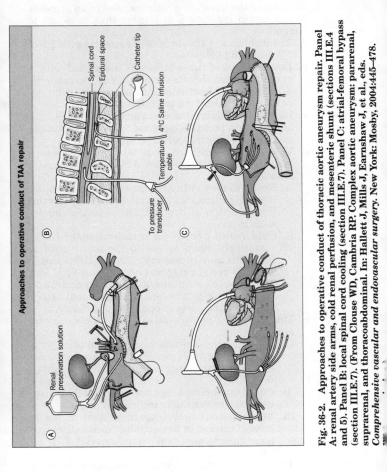

Fig. 36-2. Approaches to operative conduct of thoracic aortic aneurysm repair. Panel A: renal artery side arms, cold renal perfusion, and mesenteric shunt (sections III.E.4 and 5). Panel B: local spinal cord cooling (section III.E.7). Panel C: atrial-femoral bypass (section III.E.7). (From Clouse WD, Cambria RP. Complex aortic aneurysm: pararenal, suprarenal, and thoracoabdominal. In: Hallett J, Mills J, Earnshaw J, et al., eds. *Comprehensive vascular and endovascular surgery.* New York: Mosby, 2004:445–478.

a. Sacrifice/ligation of the inferior mesenteric artery in the absence of adequate collateral flow is thought to be the precipitating factor. This complication is seen almost exclusively in aneurysmal reconstruction and rarely in aortoocclusive disease.

b. Supraceliac clamping with consequent bowel and hepatic ischemia may precipitate a coagulopathy.

c. The surgical plan may include the use of an **in-line mesenteric shunt** to minimize ischemic time to the liver and gut (see Fig. 36-2A).

  i. Prior to aortic cross-clamping, a side arm is sewn into the main aortic graft slightly distal to the area of the proximal anastomosis.

  ii. Once the proximal aortic anastomosis is complete, the cross-clamp is moved onto the graft distal to the sidearm.

  iii. An arterial perfusion cannula is attached to the side-arm graft and antegrade pulsatile perfusion is subsequently established to either the celiac or the superior mesenteric artery (SMA) while the more distal aortic reconstruction takes place.

  iv. Once the mesenteric vessels are incorporated into the main aortic graft, the arterial perfusion cannula is removed and the side arm is ligated.

6. Bleeding and coagulation disorders

a. From 2% to 5% of TAA patients experience postoperative bleeding.

b. The operative transfusion requirement has been shown to correlate with perioperative mortality.

c. Massive resuscitation from intraoperative hemorrhage may result in a wide variety of complications including dilutional thrombocytopenia, hypothermia, disseminated intravascular coagulation (DIC), and hypocalcemia (see Chapter 10).

d. Postoperative care to treat hypothermia and coagulopathic bleeding may include the use of fluid warming devices, forced hot air systems, and increased ambient temperature.

e. The use of autotransfusion or a "cell saver" system may significantly decrease the need for transfusion of banked packed red blood cells (PRBCs) because up to 50% of blood turnover during TAA resection may be returned to the patient via these methods.

f. Minimizing mesenteric ischemia is also critical to avoiding coagulopathic bleeding.

g. Postoperative thrombocytopenia is a common finding that may result from dilution following resuscitation or consumption in the case of ongoing bleeding. In the absence of these findings, however, thrombocytopenia may be explained by platelet adhesion to or activation by the Dacron aortic graft, especially in the case of extensive aortic replacement. Less commonly, heparin-induced thrombocytopenia may be the etiology, especially in cases where the platelet count fails to normalize while the patient is receiving heparin (e.g., in the form of heparin flushes, subcutaneous heparin for deep venous thrombosis [DVT] prophylaxis) or when accompanied by evidence of vascular thrombosis (see Chapter 10).

7. **Paraplegia and spinal cord ischemia (SCI)** is perhaps the most feared and devastating nonfatal complication of TAA repair, with some clinical manifestation apparent in up to 20% of patients. When diagnosed immediately following the surgical procedure, the etiology is likely ischemic injury due to aortic cross-clamping or sacrifice of critical intercostal vessels supplying the spinal cord. A postoperative, delayed-onset injury may also occur in the intensive care unit (ICU) and is theorized to be caused by reperfusion injury or tenuous collateral blood supply to the spinal cord.

   a. The thoracolumbar watershed region is at the highest risk for development of ischemia because it is typically supplied by a single artery.

   b. Seventy percent of deficits are immediate, with the remainder occurring in a delayed fashion hours or even weeks postoperatively.

   c. Independent correlates of SCI include types I and II TAA, aneurysm rupture, prolonged duration of aortic cross-clamp, sacrifice of "critical" T8-L1 intercostal vessels, and prolonged intraoperative hypotension.

      i. Emergency surgery results in a threefold increase in rate of SCI.

      ii. Oversewing of intercostal arteries is associated with a 10-fold increase in the rate of SCI in types I and II TAA repair.

   d. Several techniques have been advocated for decreasing the incidence of perioperative SCI. Efforts to prevent SCI are divided between preservation of spinal cord perfusion and use of neuroprotective adjuncts to increase spinal cord tolerance to ischemia (systemic/regional hypothermia and pharmacologic agents).

      i. **Reimplantation of intercostal arteries** in the critical T8-L1 aortic segment is performed whenever feasible, and every effort is made to minimize ischemic cross-clamp time.

      ii. **Local spinal cord cooling** (see Fig. 36-2B) is a method employed at the Massachusetts General Hospital that employs an iced saline epidural infusion system to provide moderate hypothermia to the spinal cord during the critical cross-clamp period.

         (a) An epidural catheter is first inserted in the T12-L1 interspace. A separate intrathecal catheter is placed in the low lumbar region to monitor cerebrospinal (CSF) temperature and pressure as well as to provide a mechanism for draining CSF via active or passive means.

(b) Epidural cooling is initiated early in the course of the procedure so that the target temperature ($25°C–27°C$) is reached immediately prior to the aortic cross-clamp placement. Cooling is then continued until the critical intercostal vessels have been incorporated into the graft.

(c) Postoperatively, the intrathecal catheter is placed to drainage at 13 cm H_2O for 48 to 72 hours while careful clinical neurologic exams of the lower extremities are serially performed.

(d) Following extubation, the epidural catheter may be employed for postoperative analgesia, although its location is too low for ideal analgesic purposes.

(e) Data from MGH suggest that in patients with types I through III TAA, use of regional epidural cooling may reduce the risk of SCI from 20% to 10.6% of patients. Results, however, have not been verified in other centers.

iii. **Atrial-femoral or partial left heart bypass** (**LHB;** see Fig. 36-2C):

(a) A drainage cannula is inserted into the left atrium (usually via the left inferior pulmonary vein) and the return cannula is usually placed in the left femoral artery.

(b) Distal aortic perfusion allows reduction of ischemic times to the spinal cord and viscera because their vascular beds are perfused during construction of the proximal aortic anastomosis.

(c) LHB may decrease the incidence of complete paraplegia from 13% to 4.5% according to one large series of 1,400 patients.

(d) Atrial-femoral bypass also provides easily titratable unloading of the left ventricle, which may be desirable in patients with significant valvular or left heart dysfunction.

iv. **CSF drainage** is also commonly employed as a protective measure against SCI, although evidence of its benefit is largely from animal data or nonrandomized trials in humans.

(a) The exact mechanism of beneficial action of CSF drainage is unclear, but animal studies show that placement of a proximal thoracic aortic cross-clamp increases CSF pressure. Because perfusion pressure to the spinal cord is dependent upon the arterial inflow pressure less the CSF pressure (analogous to the situation of elevated intracranial pressure), CSF drainage is believed to increase perfusion pressure to the spinal cord by decreasing the CSF pressure. Another theory holds that CSF drainage is beneficial because it removes deleterious excitatory neurotransmitters that accumulate in the CSF during the ischemic period.

(b) Most sources target passive drainage of CSF to a pressure less than 10 mm Hg perioperatively.

(c) Duration of maintenance of CSF drainage is controversial, although many experts advocate continuing drainage for 48 to 72 hours postoperatively to cover the time course of maximal edema of the spinal cord.

(d) Anecdotal reports suggest that immediate CSF drainage (including in some cases active aspiration) may be successful in reversing the phenomenon of delayed neurologic deficit, which often manifests postoperatively in the ICU.

(e) Adverse effects of CSF drainage may occur, including subdural hematoma, precipitated by tearing of bridging dural veins secondary to increased tension.

e. **The delayed-onset neurologic deficit** is increasingly recognized in distinction from immediate SCI; this may be due to improved intraoperative techniques for protecting the spinal cord. Anecdotal reports suggest a temporal relationship to periods of hypotension, often occurring in the intensive care unit. For this reason, hemodynamic stability with the avoidance of extremes of both hyper- and *hypo*tension should be a steadfast goal in the postoperative management of these patients. Use of short-acting vasoactive medications is advisable for hemodynamic control in the first 48 to 72 postoperative hours. In the Massachusetts General Hospital experience and in anecdotal reports, delayed neurologic deficit may be reversed with induced hypertension (to a level congruous with the surgeon's confidence in the vascular anastomoses) while CSF drainage is being considered and, if feasible, initiated.

f. It should be recognized that postoperative paraplegia may be due to compressive **hematoma** of the spinal cord. Clinicians must have a high index of suspicion for possible spinal or epidural hematoma as the causative factor for postoperative paralysis, especially in cases where neuraxial catheters have been placed with subsequent coagulopathy related to the surgical procedure. When suspicion is high, immediate diagnostic imaging should be obtained followed by surgical decompression if indicated.

F. **Endovascular stenting of thoracic aneurysms** has seen tremendous growth in the last decade. At the time of publication, only one thoracic aortic stent device is approved for use in the U.S. by the Food and Drug Administration. However, significant clinical experience with the use of endovascular stents for the thoracic aorta has been gained in Europe, and the experience there predicts the safety and durability of this new modality. In particular, endovascular stent repair appears to offer a substantially reduced morbidity and mortality when compared to open TAA repair.

1. The majority of uncomplicated elective stent graft TAA repairs will not require postoperative critical care.
2. **Procedural complications** may merit treatment in a critical care unit.
   a. Intraoperative **positioning error of the stent graft** or graft migration may result in occlusion of the celiac, superior mesenteric, or renal artery with consequent visceral ischemia. Limb ischemia may also occur if the stent occludes flow to the iliac or femoral arteries. Urgent operative correction may be required.
   b. The risk of **stroke** (approximately 0.5%–2%) appears higher than with open repair and is due to wire or catheter manipulation of diseased aortic segments resulting in embolization of atherosclerotic debris.
   c. **Spinal cord ischemia** with resultant paraplegia, although reduced in incidence (1%–4%), is not eliminated with endovascular stent grafting and is attributable to coverage of critical intercostal arteries by the stent.
   d. Rare **operative catastrophe** (aneurysm rupture, injury to major arterial access vessels) may result in emergent conversion to open repair with its associated complications.
   e. **Endoleak** is the term used to describe the continued entry of blood into the aneurysm sac following endovascular stent placement. It may be discovered immediately intraoperatively or later on radiographic follow-up. The importance of endoleak lies in the ongoing potential for aneurysm rupture.
3. Expanded use of endovascular stent grafts in emergent/urgent situations (e.g., ruptured, leaking, or rapidly expanding TAA) may result in the admission of these patients to a critical care unit postoperatively.
4. Case reports of endovascular stent repair of traumatic aortic pseudoaneurysms are accumulating, suggesting that this less invasive approach may be the repair of choice in the patient with multiple blunt traumatic injuries.
5. **Contrast-induced nephropathy (CIN)** is a major source of concern in patients undergoing endovascular procedures. CIN is typically defined as an increase in serum creatinine of 25% or more from baseline within 24 to 96 hours following contrast exposure. The incidence of CIN accounts for more than 10% of

hospital-acquired renal failure and is a leading cause of acute renal failure. Several methods have been evaluated for decreasing the incidence of CIN.

   a. Hydration with 154 mEq/L of **sodium bicarbonate** (3 ml/kg/h for 1 hour prior to contrast exposure followed by 1 ml/kg/h for 6 hours after the procedure) has been shown to be more effective than hydration with sodium chloride in prevention of CIN. The theorized mechanism of protection involves scavenging of free radicals by the bicarbonate as well as disruption of oxygen radical creation.

   b. Fenoldopam mesylate is a specific agonist of the dopamine-1 receptor that produces systemic, peripheral, and renal arterial vasodilation and has been shown to increase renal plasma flow in patients with and without chronic renal insufficiency.

      i. Initial reports in anesthetized canine models as well as small observational studies suggested that fenoldopam's increased renal blood flow might decrease the incidence of CIN.

      ii. However, a recent large scale placebo-controlled trial has failed to demonstrate any benefit in the prevention of CIN.

   c. *N*-**Acetylcysteine** has also been proposed as a therapeutic option for reducing CIN. When it was given in oral doses of 600 mg twice daily 1 day prior to and on the day of exposure to radiocontrast media, initial data suggested a moderate decrease in rates of CIN. Follow-up studies, however, have produced mixed results with respect to diminished incidence of CIN. Nevertheless, given the lack of deleterious side effects attributable to *N*-acetylcysteine, some intensivists (including ourselves) routinely prescribe the drug prior to contrast administration in at-risk patients.

IV. Thoracic aortic dissection is less common than TAA, with an estimated incidence of 5 to 30 cases per million people per year. A classic symptom of dissection is the sudden onset of chest/back pain, which is often accompanied by symptoms of organ hypoperfusion (e.g., syncope, abdominal pain, leg weakness) due to involvement of side branches of the aorta.

  A. Risk factors for aortic dissection include specific connective tissue diseases (e.g., Marfan's syndrome, Ehlers-Danlos syndrome), hereditary aortic disease predisposing to aneurysm and dissection, long-standing hypertension, cocaine use, and iatrogenic injury to the aortic wall (e.g., clamp or cannulation site trauma).

  B. Early mortality from acute dissection is high, with approximately 20% of patients dying before admission to a hospital. Death is usually caused by the following factors:

   1. Aortic rupture.

   2. Cardiac failure due to dissection involving the pericardium with resultant tamponade; the coronary

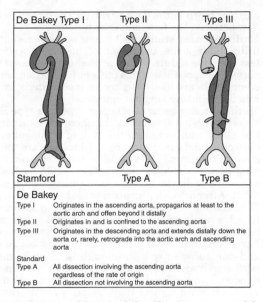

De Bakey Type I	Type II	Type III
Stamford	Type A	Type B

De Bakey

Type I	Originates in the ascending aorta, propagarios at least to the aortic arch and offen beyond it distally
Type II	Originates in and is confined to the ascending aorta
Type III	Originates in the descending aorta and extends distally down the aorta or, rarely, retrograde into the aortic arch and ascending aorta

Standard

Type A	All dissection involving the ascending aorta regardless of the rate of origin
Type B	All dissection not involving the ascending aorta

Fig. 36-3. DeBakey and Stanford classification systems of thoracic aortic dissection. (From Nienaber CA, Eagle KA. Aortic dissection: new frontiers in diagnosis and management. Part I: from etiology to diagnostic strategies. *Circulation* 2003;108:628–635. With permission.)

arteries, leading to myocardial ischemia; or the aortic valve leaflets, causing acute, severe aortic regurgitation.

C. The two major **classification systems** of thoracic aortic dissection, **DeBakey** and **Stanford,** are depicted in Fig. 36-3. The classification is important to both treatment and outcome.

D. **Stanford type A** dissection is a surgical emergency, except in the rare case where concurrent injury poses a contraindication to cardiopulmonary bypass and/or anticoagulation. This usually occurs in patients who have suffered a stroke (often as a result of the dissection) or traumatic brain injury. Early diagnosis of type A dissection is crucial because the mortality rate is 1% to 2% per hour after symptom onset.

E. **Stanford type B** dissections have a better outcome, with an estimated 30-day mortality rate of 10% in uncomplicated cases. Medical management of type B dissections is standard due to the lack of outcome superiority of surgery. Surgical intervention, however, is indicated in cases of compromised perfusion to vital organs (e.g., kidneys, bowel) or limbs with resultant ischemia. This usually occurs when an intimal flap obstructs flow to the celiac, superior mesenteric, or renal artery. The surgical plan may involve replacement of a portion of the dissected aorta or a procedure ("fenestration") designed to connect flow between the false and true lumens.

F. Endovascular stent graft placement has recently been utilized for acute treatment of aortic dissection. The less invasive nature of this procedure compared to open surgery is appealing in this patient population, and, thus, stent grafts are likely to play an increasingly important role in the future surgical approach.

G. Medical management of either type A or type B dissections is targeted at reducing the shear force (dP/dt) across the aortic wall to reduce the risk of propagation of the dissection and aortic rupture. **β-blockers** are the cornerstone of treatment and should be initiated prior to beginning pure vasodilator therapy (e.g., **SNP, hydralazine**) to avoid a reflex tachycardia and consequent increase in dP/dt. After achieving an acceptable heart rate (e.g., 55 to 65 beats/min), a vasodilator may be initiated if necessary to achieve an acceptable mean arterial blood pressure (e.g., 50–65 mm Hg). The balance between an acceptably low mean arterial blood pressure to avoid aortic rupture and one sufficiently high enough to provide end-organ perfusion may be precarious due to long-standing hypertension with a shifted autoregulatory mechanism.

1. Heart rate control may be achieved intravenously with esmolol, metoprolol, or propranolol. **Labetolol** offers the advantage of both heart rate control and blood pressure lowering via alpha-adrenergic blocker effect.

2. Blood pressure control may be achieved with intravenous infusion of **nitroglycerin, SNP, fenoldopam**, or some combination thereof.

V. Abdominal aortic aneurysm (AAA) occurs in 5% to 7% of people older than the age of 60 years. The risk of rupture risk is directly related to the aneurysm size, so that elective repair is usually recommended for patients who are surgical candidates when aneurysm diameter equals or exceeds 5.5 cm. The advent of endovascular stent repair of AAA (see later discussion) has expanded the pool of patients who are surgical candidates.

A. The perioperative mortality of elective open AAA repair is 4%.

1. Two major predictors of mortality following elective open AAA repair are increased baseline creatinine and poor preoperative lung function.

2. The majority of deaths, however, are due to cardiac complications (myocardial infarction, lethal arrhythmia, CHF).

3. Potential complications associated with open abdominal aortic aneurysm repair are similar to those of TAA repair (see section **III.E**), although they occur at a lower rate for specific entities (e.g., SCI).

B. Endovascular repair of AAA has been shown to have an operative mortality of approximately 1.5% in several large series. Uncomplicated elective repairs usually do not require postoperative treatment in the critical care

unit. Complications that may result in transfer to the ICU
are similar to those seen in stent graft repair of TAA (see
section **III.F.2**), except that the risk of stroke and SCI is
rare.

VI. Peripheral vascular procedures

A. Patients who are admitted to the ICU following peripheral revascularization procedures (e.g., femoral to
popliteal bypass graft) usually are suffering from complications of comorbid conditions. These may include myocardial ischemia, dysrhythmias, or CHF. Complications
of diabetes (e.g., diabetic ketoacidosis, renal failure) are
also common indications for postoperative critical care.
Treatment of these patients is targeted to the comorbid disease, and the reader is directed to the appropriate
chapter for management.

B. Severe peripheral vascular disease with ischemia, ulceration, and infection may rarely result in development of a
"septic limb" with all the associated sequelae of sepsis.
These patients are best managed by emergent amputation of the affected extremity and treatment with broad-
spectrum antimicrobials until tailored according to operative cultures.

C. Occlusion of peripheral vascular grafts due to thrombosis
or mechanical mishap may lead to limb ischemia causing
severe pain. Prolonged ischemia may lead to muscle
death, elevated creatine phosphokinases levels causing rhabdomyolysis, and even compartment syndrome.
Treatment options include surgical exploration, pharmacologic thrombolysis with intraarterial catheters directed
at the site of clot, and amputation.

D. **Repeated or unexplained graft thromboses** merit an
investigation for possible acquired or inherited hypercoagulable state.

SELECTED REFERENCES

Brady AR, Fowkes FGR, Greenhalgh RM, et al. Risk factors for postoperative death following elective surgical repair of abdominal aortic aneurysm: results from the UK Small Aneurysm Trial. *Br J
Surg* 2000;87:742–749.

Cambria RP, Clouse WD, Davison JK, et al. Thoracoabdominal aneurysm repair: results with 337 operations performed over a 15-
year interval. *Ann Surg* 2002;236:471–479.

Coselli JS, LeMaire SA, Conklin LD, et al. Morbidity and mortality after extent II thoracoabdominal aortic aneurysm repair. *Ann
Thorac Surg* 2002;73:1107–1116.

Gorham TJ, Taylor J, Raptis S. Endovascular treatment of abdominal
aortic aneurysm. *Br J Surg* 2004;91:815–827.

Hallett JW. *Comprehensive vascular and endovascular surgery*.
St. Louis, MO: Mosby, 2003.

Kshirsagar AV, Poole C, Mottl A, et al. *N*-Acetylcysteine for the prevention of radiocontrast induced nephropathy: a meta-analysis of
prospective controlled trials. *J Am Soc Nephrol* 2004;15:761–769.

Khan IA, Nair CK. Clinical, diagnostic, and management perspectives of aortic dissection. *Chest* 2002;122:311–328.

Lee WA, Carter JW, Upchurch G, et al. Perioperative outcomes after open and endovascular repair of intact abdominal aortic aneurysms in the United States during 2001. *J Vasc Surg* 2004;39:491–496.

Ling E, Arellano R. Systematic overview of the evidence supporting the use of cerebrospinal fluid drainage in thoracoabdominal aneurysm surgery for prevention of paraplegia. *Anesthesiology* 2000;93:1115–1122.

Merten GJ, Burgess WM, Gray LV, et al. Prevention of contrast-induced nephropathy with sodium bicarbonate. A randomized controlled trial. *JAMA* 2004;291:2328–2334.

Murakami H, Yoshida K, Hino Y, et al. Complications of cerebrospinal fluid drainage in thoracoabdominal aortic aneurysm repair. *J Vasc Surg* 2004;39:243–245.

Prinssen M, Verhoeven ELG, Buth J, et al. A randomized trial comparing conventional and endovascular repair of abdominal aortic aneurysms. *N Engl J Med* 2004;351:1607–1618.

Rectenwald JE, Huber TS, Martin TD, et al. Functional outcome after thoracoabdominal aortic aneurysm repair. *J Vasc Surg* 2002; 35:640–647.

Rutherford RB, Krupski WC. Current status of open versus endovascular stent-graft repair of abdominal aortic aneurysm. *J Vasc Surg* 2004;39:1129–1139.

Stone GW, McCullough PA, Tumlin JA, et al. Fenoldopam mesylate for the prevention of contrast-induced nephropathy. A randomized controlled trial. *JAMA* 2003;290:2284–2291.

The EVAR Trial Participants. Comparison of endovascular aneurysm repair with open repair in patients with abdominal aortic aneurysm (EVAR Trial 1), 30-day operative mortality results: randomised controlled trial. *Lancet* 2004;364:843–848.

Yadav JS, Wholey MH, Kuntz RE, et al. Protected carotid artery stenting versus endarterectomy in high risk patients. *N Engl J Med* 2004;351:1493–1501.

Thoracic Surgery

Kristopher Davignon and Kenneth L. Haspel

I. Introduction

Thoracic surgery patients often need intensive care unit (ICU) level care in the immediate postoperative period. Intrathoracic procedures are associated with considerable cardiopulmonary dysfunction, resulting in significant patient morbidity and mortality if not managed appropriately and in a timely fashion. ICU monitoring allows full implementation of analgesia, monitoring for dysrhythmias and myocardial ischemia, as well as prompt recognition and treatment of respiratory compromise.

II. General considerations

A. **Preoperative pulmonary function tests (PFTs)** are often obtained to determine whether the patient is a candidate for resection. Indications and use of PFTs are described in detail in Chapter 3 of *Anesthesia Procedures of the Massachusetts General Hospital*, 6th edition. Although there is not a direct relationship between the degree of impairment noted on preoperative PFTs and the rate of postoperative respiratory complications, PFTs may provide a helpful baseline reference when managing patients with postoperative respiratory failure.

B. **Postoperative analgesia** is important in the management of the post-thoracotomy patient. Without adequate pain control, patients cannot deep breathe or cough, and are prone to developing atelectasis, respiratory acidosis, and hypoxemia.

   1. **Epidural analgesia** is the preferred method of pain management at our institution for the thoracotomy patient. Epidural analgesia may be provided with local anesthetic, a narcotic, or, most commonly, a combination of both. A low concentration of local anesthetic (**0.1% bupivacaine**) with a low-dose narcotic (**2 μg/ml fentanyl** or **20 μg/ml hydromorphone**) is commonly used. Choice of epidural narcotic is often based on lipophilicity. The more lipophilic the narcotic, the less it spreads along the epidural space. This results in less sedation, but also less analgesia at dermatomes far from the tip of the epidural catheter.

   2. **Intercostal nerve blocks** may be useful for patients with contraindications to epidural analgesia. Duration of action and multiple injections are the primary limitations to the utility of intercostal blocks.

   3. **Nonsteroidal antiinflammatory agents** (NSAIDs) are useful adjuncts to either epidural or parenteral narcotics. **Ketorolac** offers high-grade analgesia without respiratory depression. All NSAIDs (see

Appendix 1 to this handbook) should be used cautiously in patients with renal dysfunction, patients with gastritis, and those who are prone to bleeding.

4. **Parenteral opioids** are effective analgesics. However, they also cause respiratory depression and thus must be used cautiously in the thoracic surgery patient. **Patient-controlled analgesia (PCA)** has been shown to be superior to nurse-administered analgesia and to be safe in selected thoracic surgery patients.

C. **Atrial dysrhythmias** are common following thoracotomy. They are often self-limited and result primarily from surgical manipulation of the heart and pulmonary veins and its associated irritation. These patients also have risk factors for other etiologies of atrial dysrhythmias. Common associated etiologies include myocardial ischemia, pulmonary embolism, electrolyte imbalances, fluid overload, hypoxemia, acidosis, pulmonary infections, mechanical irritation from invasive monitors, and pneumothorax. If an underlying cause cannot be found and corrected, the management often rests on rate control and consideration of cardioversion. **Beta-blockers** and **calcium-channel blockers** are first-line drugs for rate control. **Amiodarone** is effective for rate control and possibly cardioversion, but care must be taken because pulmonary fibrosis can be a devastating complication.

D. **Ventilatory dysfunction** is common postoperatively in the thoracic patient. Prolonged lung collapse during surgery may cause interstitial edema and inflammation; thoracotomy incisions are associated with splinting and poor inspiratory effort. This may result in decreased tidal volume as well as decreased functional residual capacity (FRC). Poor cough may further promote atelectasis, resulting in poor gas exchange and a decrease in FRC. General considerations on ventilatory management of patients with acute respiratory failure are discussed in Chapters 5 and 20. Specific considerations for ventilatory management of the postoperative thoracic patient vary significantly for the various procedures, and are outlined later.

E. **Postoperative fluid management** can be challenging for the intensivist. Strategies are quite different for the variety of thoracic surgical procedures and are discussed individually in subsequent sections.

III. **Specific surgical procedures**
A. **Pulmonary resection.** ICU admission following a lung resection is determined by a combination of factors, including primarily the extent of the procedure, the preexisting respiratory and cardiac conditions, and, occasionally, unexpected intraoperative events.

1. **Post-pneumonectomy pulmonary edema** (PPE) is a severe complication of major lung resections (almost exclusively pneumonectomies) associated with a high mortality. PPE is a form of acute lung injury/acute respiratory distress syndrome (see Chapter 20), which develops 48 to 72 hours following an often

otherwise uneventful pneumonectomy and rapidly requires high levels of ventilatory and hemodynamic support. The role of intravenous fluids in causing or exacerbating this problem is controversial. Proposed mechanisms for PPE include disruption of the thoracic lymphatic drainage and increased hydrostatic pressure secondary to the relative increase in cardiac output being delivered to the remaining lung. The incidence of PPE is higher with right-sided pneumonectomy. It seems to occur with low pulmonary artery occlusion pressures and despite very cautious restriction of intravenous fluids administration. When PPE develops, no particular therapeutic measure—including diuresis, corticosteroids, and inhaled nitric oxide—has been proven to make a difference. We generally employ a strategy of fluid restriction, hemodynamic support and "lung-protective" mechanical ventilation as outlined in Chapter 20.

2. **Post-pneumonectomy syndrome** is characterized by extreme shifts and rotation of the mediastinum after pneumonectomy. This results in proximal airway obstruction and air trapping leading to dyspnea. Diagnosis is usually made by a combination of chest radiograph, chest computed tomography (CT), echocardiogram, PFTs, and flexible bronchoscopy. Treatment is surgical and consists of implantation of saline-filled prosthesis (such as breast implants) into the vacant pleural cavity.

3. **Ventilatory management** postoperatively is rarely necessary; **the goal is extubation at the completion of the surgery.** This is ideal for reducing stress on new suture lines as well as for reducing the incidence of postoperative respiratory infections.

   a. **Noninvasive positive-pressure ventilation (NPPV)** has been demonstrated to be effective in treating acute respiratory failure following lung resections. It is important to realize that NPPV is merely a bridge while other therapies are begun to improve the underlying cause of hypoxemia or hypercapnia. Prolonged use of NPPV increases the risk of aspiration and fatigue; after 24 to 48 hours of NPPV, its benefits and risks as an alternative to tracheal intubation must be reconsidered.

   b. **Chronic obstructive pulmonary disease (COPD)** is very common in patients undergoing lung resection. Treatment of acute respiratory failure following lung resection often has all the implications of treatment of exacerbation of COPD. Ventilatory management in patients with COPD is discussed in Chapters 5 and 21.

4. **Lung volume reduction surgery.** Patients with COPD/emphysema with life-limiting dyspnea who have been maximally medically managed may be candidates for volume reduction surgery. The resection of overinflated areas of the lung may improve both gas

exchange and respiratory mechanics, leading to significant clinical improvement. Preoperative selection of the most appropriate surgical candidates seems to be key to postoperative success of this procedure.

   a. Mechanical ventilation in the postoperative period should be avoided if possible.

   b. Auto–positive end-expiratory pressure (auto-PEEP) and air trapping are common problems in patients after this surgery.

B. Airway surgery. Tracheal resection and reconstruction is performed for tracheal stenosis, tracheal disruption, and tumor removal. Postoperatively, these patients require time in an experienced critical care environment for monitoring of their tenuous airway. Their early recovery is characterized by a fine balance between the need for analgesia and anxiolysis and the need to promote effective cough and airway clearance. It is important that this early recovery period (24–48 hours) occur in a location where staff are highly skilled in airway management in general and of these patients in particular.

C. Esophageal surgery is most often a resection for tumor. There are three common surgical approaches to the esophagus: the left thoracoabdominal approach, the right thoracotomy and upper laparotomy approach (Ivor-Lewis), and the transhiatal approach, which involves an abdominal incision and a neck incision, blunt dissection of the esophagus, and an anastomosis in the neck. The first two approaches, which allow the best intraoperative exposure and staging of the tumor, are also the most disruptive in terms of intraoperative tissue dissection and trauma, the need for one-lung ventilation, and postoperative fluid management, respiratory insufficiency, and pain.

   1. Fluid management for esophageal surgeries is quite different than that for pulmonary resections. Patients who have undergone esophageal surgery appear more like patients who have undergone major abdominal gastrointestinal surgery. They tend to have a large volume requirement in the first 1 to 2 postoperative days and then begin to diurese in the subsequent days. There is little concern for pulmonary edema, assuming normal left ventricular function.

   2. Ventilatory management in patients following esophageal surgery revolves around the upper airway. Esophageal surgery is often lengthy and in the lateral decubitus position, and large volumes of crystalloid are administered. This combination may result in swelling of the upper airway and the need for postoperative intubation. Esophageal surgery often requires one-lung ventilation for periods of time. This results in significant postoperative atelectasis and alveolar dysfunction resulting in abnormal gas exchange. This is coupled with the general respiratory dysfunction associated with thoracotomies that was outlined previously. At Massachusetts General Hospital, patients undergoing eshopagogastrectomy are extubated at the end of the procedure if the case was less than 8 hours in duration, there is no excessive airway edema noted, oxygenation and ventilation were not an issue during the procedure, and analgesia was accomplished with a thoracic epidural. **Aspiration of gastric contents** is an ever-present risk in patients who have recently undergone esophageal surgery, and care must be taken to avoid this complication. The patient's head should be elevated greater than 30 degrees, and gastric acid suppressive agents should be used. A nasogastric tube is inserted at the time of surgery and must be carefully managed. This provides decompression of the anastomosis.

D. **Mediastinal surgery.** The most common causes of mediastinal masses are **lymphomas** and **thymomas,** both located in the anterior mediastinum. If the mass is mobile, it can completely obstruct the airway in certain positions (usually supine) or if muscular tone is lost (anesthesia or muscle relaxants). A flow-volume loop can aid in diagnosis of the mobile anterior mediastinal mass (Fig. 37-1). If the airway becomes obstructed, positive pressure in addition to changes in position (lateral or prone) may be helpful. Skilled professionals in the operating room or a location with equivalent equipment and staff should obtain control of the airway for these patients.

E. **Lung transplant** surgery. See Chapter 39.

IV. **Thoracic surgical emergencies/complications**

A. **Tracheal disruption** is most commonly caused by trauma. Trauma may be the result of blunt injury,

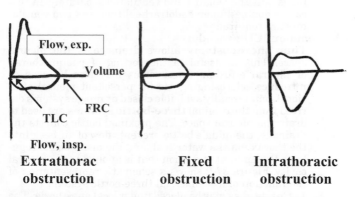

Fig. 37-1. Flow-volume loops obtained starting from functional residual capacity (FRC) and inspiring to total lung capacity (TLC) as indicated by the arrows. Inspiration is by convention from right to left and in the bottom part of the loop. Exp., expiratory; insp., inspiratory.

penetrating injury, or inappropriate airway manipulation, that is, iatrogenic.

1. **Spontaneous breathing** should be maintained if possible until the airway can be secured distal to the tracheal injury. Positive-pressure ventilation will likely exacerbate pneumothorax or pneumomediastinum. **Securing the airway** is most definitive if done in conjunction with bronchoscopy. This will allow demonstration that the lesion has been excluded. After control of the airway is established, repair of the tracheal lesion may be undertaken.

B. **Pulmonary hemorrhage/hemoptysis** has many etiologies, including pulmonary artery rupture from trauma or from right heart catheterization with a pulmonary artery catheter. Occasionally, erosion into a pulmonary artery from a tumor, abscess, or suture line may occur, or aortobronchial fistula can develop from similar pathophysiologic processes. Tumor, pneumonia, abscess, and vasculitis may also cause hemoptysis, although these processes are often less emergent in their presentation.

1. **Airway suctioning** and **intubation** must occur expeditiously.
2. **Bronchoscopy** to identify a source allows diagnosis and therapeutic maneuvers. If a unilateral source can be identified, lung isolation should be considered.
3. **Surgery** or **angiographic embolization** often provides definitive treatment.

C. **Bronchopleural fistulas (BPFs)** can occur after pulmonary resection. BPF can be a difficult process to manage, in particular with regard to mechanical ventilation. Volume-cycled ventilatory modes are necessary to provide a constant minute ventilation. Measured tidal volumes by the ventilator will significantly underestimate the true volumes being delivered. Occasionally, the two lungs must be isolated and ventilated separately. In this case a double-lumen endotracheal tube and two ventilators are required.

V. **Common ICU procedures**

A. **Tube thoracostomy** allows drainage of the pleural space. This is useful in the setting of pneumothorax or pleural effusion. Chest tubes may also be used to introduce sclerosing agents for persistent pleural effusion. Commercially available closed drainage systems derived from the original **three-bottle systems** are used to drain the pleural space. The proximal bottle collects the drainage, the middle bottle prevents flow of air back into the thorax via the water seal, and the distal bottle regulates the amount of suction that is applied to the pleural cavity. Figure 37-2 shows a schematic representation of the function of a commercial three-bottle system.

1. Chest tubes may be placed under local anesthesia. The chest tube is inserted above the rib (to avoid the neurovascular bundle) and most often directed apically.
2. Generally, chest tubes are initially placed to 20-cm H_2O suction (except to drain the empty pleural cavity

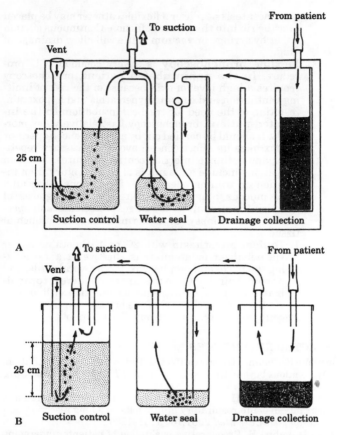

A

B

Fig. 37-2. Chest tube drainage system. A. A commercial apparatus. The proximal chamber is for pleural drainage, the middle chamber (the water seal) prevents air or fluid from being driven into the thorax), and the distal chamber regulates the level of suction. B. A traditional "three-bottle" system show for comparison.

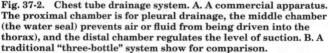

following a pneumonectomy). When no air leak is detected, often the chest tube can be left only on water seal. Once the drainage is minimal (usually <150 ml over 24 hours) and there is no pneumothorax and no air leak, the chest tube should be removed.

3. Complications of tube thoracostomy include intraparenchymal placement of the tube, with consequent possible lung contusion, hemorrhage, and BPF, hemothorax from injury to intercostals vessels, and subcutaneous emphysema.

B. Thoracentesis will allow drainage of a pleural effusion either diagnostically or therapeutically. Most often, thoracentesis is done under ultrasound guidance. Either a thoracentesis needle or a flexible catheter may be placed over the rib into the pleural effusion. Continuous suction either by syringe or vacuum bottle will allow drainage of fluid.

C. **Flexible bronchoscopy** is a very common ICU procedure. **In the nonintubated patient,** bronchoscopy requires a high level of skill because of the risk of limiting ventilation and causing hypercarbia and hypoxemia, resulting in the need for tracheal intubation. **In the intubated patient,** bronchoscopy has relatively low morbidity. It should be carried out by an experienced operator to maximize its effectiveness, avoid unnecessary repetitions, and optimize infection control measures. Common indications include a diagnosis of airway injury from inhalation or trauma, clearance of secretions (especially large mucous plugs causing atelectasis), diagnosis of infection (bronchoalveolar lavage, protected brush specimens), and biopsy of abnormal lung or bronchial tissue.

1. **Topical anesthesia** with 2% or 4% lidocaine either via nebulizer or atomizer is effective at anesthetizing the naso- and oropharynx, larynx, vocal cords, and proximal airway. Once the airway is entered, **topicalization** continues with further injection of lidocaine via the suction channel of the bronchoscope.

D. **Percutaneous tracheostomy.** See Chapter 4.

SELECTED REFERENCES

Adoumie R, Shennib H, Brown R, et al. Differential lung ventilation. Applications beyond the operating room. *J Thorac Cardiovasc Surg* 1993;105:229–233.

Auriant I, Jallot A, Herve P, et al. Noninvasive ventilation reduces mortality in acute respiratory failure following lung resection. *Am J Respir Crit Care Med* 2001;164:1231–1235.

Datta D, Lahiri B. Preoperative evaluation of patients undergoing lung resection surgery. *Chest* 2003;123:2096–2103.

Enzinger PC, Mayer RJ. Esophageal cancer. *N Engl J Med* 2003;349: 2241–2252.

Grillo HC, Shepard JO, Mathisen DJ, et al. Postpneumonectomy syndromes: diagnosis, management, and results. *Ann Thorac Surg* 1992;54:638–651.

Hulscher JBF, Van Sandick JW, de Boer AG, et al. Extended transthoracic resection compared with limited transhiatal resection for adenocarcinoma of the esophagus. *N Engl J Med* 2002;347: 1662–1669.

Slinger PD. Perioperative fluid management for thoracic surgery: The puzzle of postpneumonectomy pulmonary edema. *J Cardiothorac Vasc Anesth* 1998;9:442–451.

Spira A, Ettinger DS. Multidisciplinary management of lung cancer. *N Engl J Med* 2004;350:379–392.

Cardiac Surgery

Michael G. Fitzsimons and
Thomas E. MacGillivray

I. Management of postoperative cardiac surgical patients has changed due to administrative drives to decrease the period of postoperative intubation, intensive care unit (ICU) length of stay, hospital stay, and mortality. Anesthetic techniques and critical care management are evolving accordingly.

   A. Preoperative identification of individuals who are at increased risk of perioperative morbidity/mortality remains difficult. Several patient characteristics, however, define a group at increased risk of having postoperative complications and a prolonged ICU stay.

      1. Severe myocardial dysfunction is associated with renal insufficiency and gastrointestinal (GI) complications. Preoperative cardiogenic shock is the greatest risk factor for morbidity and mortality.

      2. Renal dysfunction is associated with higher mortality and longer ICU stay.

      3. Older age is associated with a higher rate of renal failure and postoperative neurologic and GI dysfunction.

      4. Prior cardiac surgery. "Re-do" cardiac surgery is associated with higher rates of renal failure, GI complications, and mortality. Additionally, these patients are less likely to be candidates for early extubation due to longer periods of cardiopulmonary bypass (CPB).

      5. Emergency surgery is consistently associated with poorer outcomes.

      6. Type of surgery. Traditionally, coronary artery bypass grafting (CABG) procedures were associated with less complicated courses than valve procedures. However, patients who are now undergoing CABG are older and with more comorbidities. Patients undergoing CABG and valve repair or multivalve repair tend to have an even higher morbidity.

   B. Intraoperative events often foretell the problems a patient will manifest in the ICU.

      1. Myocardial ischemia may occur in the pre-CPB period, manifested by ventricular dysfunction and arrhythmias. Options for treatment include rapid institution of CPB with immediate revascularization and placement of an intraaortic balloon pump (IABP). **Myocardial protection** during the CPB period includes anterograde and retrograde cardioplegia and attempts to minimize the ischemic period. Advanced myocardial protection strategies have significantly decreased the incidence of postcardiotomy cardiogenic shock.

2. **Dysrhythmias** are common in the post-CPB period. Early dysrhythmias may include atrial fibrillation (AF), premature atrial contractions (PACs), premature ventricular contractions (PVCs), ventricular tachycardia, and heart block. Initial attempts at correction of common electrolyte abnormalities, pacing, or antiarrhythmics such as β-**blockers** and **amiodarone** are warranted.

3. **Bleeding** is common in the immediate post-CPB period. Prior to transport to ICU, the anesthesiologist should be aware of the amount of bleeding from pleural and mediastinal drainage systems. The use of ε-**aminocaproic acid** (Amicar) or **aprotinin** (Trasylol) should be recorded. Because cardiac patients commonly receive transfusions, any problems encountered should be noted in detail including hypotension, pulmonary edema, and fever.

II. **Postoperative care of the routine cardiac surgical patient.** Cardiac surgery lends itself to standardization of postoperative care. Many intensive care units have formalized protocols. The different procedures are usually followed by a typical pattern of recovery. Patients who have isolated coronary disease and few other medical problems may be managed using a **"fast-track"** approach. Their anesthetic is tailored for early awakening so that rapid extubation (<4 hours) may be possible. This approach appears to be safe for selected patients and does not appear to increase morbidity or mortality for patients who fail early tracheal extubation.

A. **ICU admission.** The anesthesia team is responsible for the patient from transport to the ICU until a full report is given to the ICU team and the patient is considered to be stable from a surgical standpoint.

1. **Monitoring during transport** should include systemic and central pressures as were used intraoperatively—arterial line, pulmonary artery (PA), or central venous pressure (CVP) line—in addition to the electrocardiogram (ECG) and hemoglobin oxygen saturation (SpO_2). If pacing is required, it is generally in an asynchronous mode.

2. **Adequate oxygenation and ventilation** should be assured prior to and during transfer because secretions, edema, and tube position might impair gas exchange. A portable mechanical ventilator is very useful in complex patients.

3. Any **vasopressors, inotropic agents,** and **vasodilators** should be continued.

4. **A full report** should be given by the anesthesiologist to the ICU team. The report should include medical history, outpatient medications, preoperative events with pertinent cardiac data, intraoperative events, including hemodynamic, respiratory, and metabolic data, vasoactive drugs, last dose of muscle relaxant, anticipated time of emergence from anesthesia, and plan for resuscitation and extubation. The short-term

plans regarding hemodynamic management, weaning of mechanical ventilation, sedation, and so on should be discussed with the ICU team prior to handing off the patient.

B. Cardiovascular dysfunction and instability are common in the immediate postoperative period. Generally these issues can be divided into five parameters: preload, contractility, afterload, heart rate, and heart rhythm (see also Chapters 1, 2, and 8).

1. **Preload.** Hypovolemia is common on arrival to the ICU. Ongoing bleeding from chest tubes and third spacing due to the systemic inflammatory response from CPB contribute. Replacement with crystalloid may contribute to further total body fluid overload. Crystalloids, colloids, and blood products as dictated by coagulation studies may adequately replace volume. Frequently, coagulation studies may be abnormal in the early postoperative period without significant bleeding. Transfusion may not be necessary to correct this.

2. **Contractility.** The vast majority of patients experience some degree of acute myocardial dysfunction in the immediate post-CPB period, generally defined as a cardiac index less than 2.2 $L/min/m^2$. This manifests as decreased stroke volume despite adequate ventricular filling pressures and mean arterial pressure (see also Chapter 1). Studies have shown that the degree of myocardial dysfunction is greater in patients with poorer preoperative function and continues for a longer period in those patients. The dysfunction is also independent of CPB times, number of grafts placed, or preoperative medications, such as nitrates, calcium-channel blockers, and β-blockers.

3. **Afterload** may be low in the immediate postoperative period due to the systemic inflammatory response generated during the period of CPB. If there is adequate volume resuscitation and acceptable myocardial function, vasopressors in the form of α-agonists **(phenylephrine),** mixed agonists **(dopamine, norepinephrine),** or **vasopressin** may be used to achieve an acceptable mean arterial pressure and to assure adequate myocardial perfusion (see also Chapter 8). Occasionally, patients may be hypertensive or require strict limits on mean arterial pressure due to suture line bleeding, which would require the continuous infusion of antihypertensive medications such as **sodium nitroprusside** (Nipride).

4. **Heart rate.** Sinus bradycardia, junctional bradycardia, or idioventricular rhythm, and heart block are frequently encountered after CPB. Epicardial pacing wires are generally placed by the surgeon and exit the chest wall. Ideally, atrial pacing to take advantage of improved ventricular filling is preferred. Atrioventricular (AV) sequential pacing or ventricular pacing may

be utilized in the absence of organized atrial activity. Atrial pacing at rates between 85 and 100 beats per minute can improve myocardial contraction, "systolic potentiation," and increase cardiac output.

5. **Rhythm.** Dysrhythmias are frequently encountered in the cardiac surgery patient. Many are benign; often they can contribute to a reduced cardiac output and limit effectiveness of other therapies, such as IABP. Electrolyte abnormalities, surgical trauma, and myocardial ischemia should be considered. Medications are a common contributing factor and include exogenous catecholamines (**dobutamine, dopamine, and inhaled β-agonists**) or physiologic rebound from preoperative withdrawal of α-agonists (**clonidine**) or β-**blockers.**

   a. **Ventricular arrhythmias.** PVCs are the most common of the dysrhythmias encountered in the cardiac surgery patient and are generally benign. PVCs occurring at a frequency greater than 6 per minute or in triplets require treatment. Simple maneuvers include correction of electrolytes or pacing at a rate greater than the patient's native rate. PVCs during AV sequential pacing may respond to shortening of the AV interval to 100 to 150 msec.

   b. **Supraventricular arrhythmias. Atrial fibrillation (AF)** is common in the postoperative period, occurring in more than one-third of patients undergoing CABG surgery and perhaps even more after valve surgery. Risk factors include increased age, chronic lung disease, and a previous history of AF. These patients are at a higher risk of subsequent cognitive changes, renal dysfunction, and infection. **Early cardioversion** may convert the patient to sinus rhythm, but the addition of a β-blocker or **amiodarone** is generally indicated. **Atrial flutter** is treated in a similar manner. Atrial flutter may also respond to overdrive atrial pacing followed by a reduction in the pacing rate. AF lasting longer than 36 hours or paroxysmal AF requires anticoagulation.

   c. **Nodal rhythms** are generally tolerated well, except in patients with a noncompliant left ventricle (aortic stenosis, hypertrophic obstructive cardiomyopathy, long-standing hypertension). Junctional tachycardia may occur in patients with surgery in the region of the bundle of His. Treatment is geared toward restoring sinus rhythm. **Sympathomimetic drugs** such as dopamine, isoproterenol, dobutamine, and norepinephrine may increase rate. **AV sequential pacing** just above the intrinsic junctional rate may improve AV synchrony and increase cardiac output. Junctional bradycardia can generally be treated by pacing.

   d. **Heart block.** First-degree AV block is common and usually self-limiting. Third-degree AV block can occur transiently intraoperatively after myocardial reperfusion, and usually resolves in the early postoperative period. Patients with baseline conduction abnormalities (bundle-branch and fascicular blocks) and patients undergoing intracardiac procedures near the conduction system (aortic valve, tricuspid valve, ventricular septal defect repair) are at risk for persistent conduction blocks requiring permanent implanted pacemakers.

C. **Pulmonary function and ventilator weaning** (see also Chapter 23). Although a number of patients are now extubated immediately after cardiac surgical procedures, many are still transported to the ICU intubated. Spontaneous ventilation returns as patients rewarm and relaxants and narcotics are metabolized. Most cardiac surgical ICUs have a standardized ventilator weaning protocol. The transition from controlled mechanical ventilation to spontaneous ventilation to extubation may place additional stress on the patient. Elimination of positive-pressure ventilation may increase venous return and challenge a heart with marginal function. Hemodynamics must be monitored closely during this period.

D. **Electrolytes and fluid balance** (also see Chapter 7). Most stable cardiac surgical patients will be somewhat hypovolemic but also have increased extravascular fluid manifested as diffuse edema. Common electrolyte and metabolic abnormalities seen in the immediate postoperative period include the following:

1. **Hypomagnesemia** may contribute to dysrhythmias. Generally, serum levels less than 2 mg/dl are corrected with magnesium sulfate 1 to 2 g intravenously (IV).

2. **Hypocalcemia.** Virtually all vasopressors and inotropic agents affect calcium homeostasis. Cardioplegic solutions result in abnormal myocardial potassium homeostasis in the early reperfusion period. Intravenous calcium administration increases ventricular stroke volume and offsets the adverse effects of hyperkalemia. Although systolic function improves, diastolic function may suffer with calcium administration. Additionally, the administration of calcium chloride may increase the risk of postoperative acute pancreatitis (see section **III.H**).

3. **Hypophosphatemia** is common in the postoperative period and may be associated with an increased incidence of complications such as weakness leading to prolonged duration of mechanical ventilation, the need for cardioactive drugs, and longer hospital stay. Hypophosphatemia results in impaired high-energy phosphate stores and contributes to muscle weakness, but the benefit of replacement in the cardiac surgical patient is unclear.

4. **Hypokalemia** contributes to dysrhythmias commonly encountered in the ICU. ECG findings of hypokalemia include prolongation of the PR interval and QRS widening along with ST-segment depression

and T-wave peaking. Treatment is generally indicated when the potassium level is less than 4 mEq/L.

5. **Hyperglycemia** (see also Chapter 27). The benefits of aggressive control of hyperglycemia in the postoperative cardiac surgical patient are recognized. Efforts to control glucose between 80 and 110 mg/dl with continual insulin infusion should be undertaken although the risk of hypoglycemia needs to be recognized and closely monitored.

E. **Lines and drains.** Patients will generally arrive from the operating room with pleural drains, mediastinal drains, pulmonary artery catheters, pacing wires, and peripheral IV access.

1. **Pleural and mediastinal drains** are placed to prevent the collection of blood in the pleural or mediastinal space, prevent tamponade, and allow monitoring for ongoing blood loss. Indications for reexploration include drainage greater than 500 ml in 1 hour, 400 ml/h for 2 hours, 300 ml/h for 3 hours, or 200 ml/h for 4 hours. Any new-onset rapid bleeding needs to be addressed immediately. Coagulopathy should be aggressively treated. Most drains are removed within 24 hours to decrease the risk of infection, and antibiotics are continued until this time.

2. **PA catheters.** The admission chest radiogram must be checked for proper positioning of the PA catheter. Displacement is common in transit, and in the setting of coagulopathy, hypothermia, and pulmonary hypertension, pulmonary artery injury may be more common.

3. **Left atrial lines** are sometimes placed directly for monitoring when the pulmonary artery catheter is not an adequate reflection of left ventricular end-diastolic pressure (pulmonary hypertension, severe pulmonary disease with high left atrial pressures, and heart transplants).

III. **Postoperative complications**

A. **Bleeding** is a common problem following cardiac surgery. **Factors associated with excessive postoperative blood loss** include prolonged duration of CPB, lower pre-CPB heparin dose, lower core temperature in the ICU, combined procedures, older age, "re-do" procedures, increased volume in salvaged red cells administered, and abnormal laboratory coagulation results. The increasing use of preoperative anticoagulation and platelet inhibitors such as **glycoprotein IIb/IIIa** inhibitors, **aspirin,** 3-hydroxy-3-methylglutaryl coenzyme A (HMG-CoA) reductase inhibitors, and **argatroban** may also contribute. The common causes include the following:

1. **Surgical.** Pleural and mediastinal drains usually produce less than 100 ml/h of blood. Greater amounts should trigger an intervention, for example, tighter blood pressure control, empiric additional protamine, positive end-expiratory pressure (PEEP), patient warming, rechecking coagulation parameters, and a

chest radiogram to rule out pleural accumulation of blood.

2. **Coagulopathy.** Elevated activated clotting time (ACT), partial thromboplastin time (PTT), or quantitative heparin assay suggests inadequate heparin neutralization, sometimes referred to as "heparin rebound"; this may be treated by the slow administration of additional protamine (25 mg/h).

3. **Platelet abnormalities.** Qualitative or quantitative platelet problems often contribute to bleeding. Although platelets may be present in sufficient number to begin hemostasis, function may not be adequate due to the presence of aspirin, dipyridamole, and other antiplatelet agents. Platelet transfusion may be considered even with a count greater than 100,000/mm^3 in a patient who continues to bleed after anatomic, anticoagulant, or clotting factor abnormalities have been corrected or ruled out. It needs to be recognized that cardiac surgical patients who receive platelets have a higher rate of infection, stroke, vasopressor use, respiratory medication use, and death.

4. **Clotting factor deficiency.** Levels of clotting factors fall rapidly during CPB. Most levels remain above 30% of normal and do not contribute significantly to increased bleeding. Plasma products are often empirically transfused in the operating room. In the ICU, however, fresh-frozen plasma (FFP) and cryoprecipitate transfusions should be guided by appropriate coagulation studies.

5. **Other considerations**
   a. **Desmopressin acetate (DDAVP)** is known to increase plasma factor VIII and von Willebrand's factor levels and may be an effective treatment of platelet dysfunction of various etiologies. The standard dose is 0.3 μg/kg administered over 30 minutes (see also Chapter 10). Adverse effects include hypotension, tachycardia, and hyponatremia due to water retention.
   b. **PEEP** is touted as a way to decrease blood loss in post-CABG patients. The proposed mechanism of action is through the tamponade of venous bleeding by the expanded lung. Although PEEP is still used by many surgeons, the majority of studies have not shown benefit.
   c. **Antifibrinolytics,** including **aprotinin** (Trasylol) and ε-**aminocaproic acid** (Amicar) (see section **I.B.3**), may decrease blood loss when administered prior to initiation of CPB. The utility of postoperative administration is unclear.
   d. **Blood pressure control** is very important **to prevent bleeding** in the postoperative cardiac patient. Deliberate reduction of a patient's blood pressure below his or her normal baseline is occasionally employed. However, this practice carries a substantial risk of unrecognized hypoperfusion

of other organs, and postoperative hypotension has been shown to increase the incidence of complications.

B. **Myocardial dysfunction** evidenced by a low cardiac output (usually considered as a cardiac index <2.2 L/min/m^2) is common in the cardiac surgical ICU (see section **II.B**). Those patients with preoperative depressed ventricular function (ejection fraction [EF] $<40\%$) are more likely to manifest problems. Post-CPB, the myocardium is generally poorly compliant, and the response to volume in the form of crystalloid or colloid is relatively flat once a certain filling pressure is reached—PA occlusion pressure (PAOP) or left atrial pressure. Ventricular filling or preload, adequate heart rate, and rhythm should be optimized by measurements, physical examination, echocardiography, or chest radiogram. Other causes of apparent postoperative myocardial dysfunction may include cardiac tamponade, pneumothorax, acidosis, and ischemia and should be ruled out. Once these measures have been addressed, pharmacologic or mechanical interventions are indicated.

1. **Catecholamines** and **sympathomimetic agents** (see also Chapter 8) commonly used in the cardiac surgical patient include **epinephrine, norepinephrine, dopamine,** and **dobutamine.** Isoproterenol is still occasionally used in heart transplant patient due to its exquisite positive chronotropic effect.

   a. **Epinephrine** increases heart rate, contractility, and peripheral vascular resistance but at the expense of increased dysrhythmias.

   b. **Norepinephrine** generally increases mean arterial pressure with minimal increase in heart rate.

   c. **Dopamine** increases contractility and cardiac output in the setting of myocardial dysfunction at medium-range doses. At high doses, α effects predominate, increasing blood pressure. Dysrhythmias are common.

   d. **Dobutamine** can increase inotropy and chronotopy with minimal change in peripheral vascular resistance.

   e. **Isoproterenol** increases contractility, heart rate, and cardiac output. It may also act as a bronchodilator.

2. **Phosphodiesterase inhibitors** such as **milrinone** (see Chapter 8) increase myocardial contractility with afterload reduction and an ultimate increase in cardiac output. The beneficial effects on myocardial performance may require support with a vasopressor.

3. **Vasopressin** (see Chapters 8, 11, and 14) is a vasoconstrictor, and is potentially useful in those patients with post–cardiopulmonary bypass vasodilatory shock who do not respond to catecholamines. These patients are generally those with poor preoperative ejection fractions or preoperative use of angiotensin-converting-enzyme inhibitors (ACEIs). Vasopressin is most

effective in patients with adequate output with vasodilation. The use of vasopressin in patients with low-output states is associated with poor outcomes.

4. **Mechanical support.** The use of an IABP may be indicated in patients with myocardial dysfunction. Indications for placement of an IABP prior to cardiac surgery generally include severe preoperative left ventricular dysfunction (cardiac index <1.8 L/m/m^2), ongoing ischemia or angina despite medical management, mitral regurgitation, or postinfarction ventricular septal defect. An IABP may be useful on separation from CPB when the cardiac output is severely depressed despite optimal medical management. The effects of an IABP include **augmentation of diastolic blood pressure** (thus increasing coronary perfusion), **decrease in systolic blood pressure** (reducing impedance to ejection), heart rate, PAOP, left ventricular wall stress, and an increase in cardiac output. **Implantable left** and **right ventricular assist devices (VADs)** are mechanical pumps that are used to assume the function of damaged myocardium. These are placed in the operating room and may serve as a bridge to recovery of function or transplant. Common problems include bleeding, right-sided heart failure, thromboembolism, infection, and device malfunction.

C. **Pulmonary dysfunction** is defined as the need for mechanical ventilation for more than 48 hours; it complicates the postoperative course of 8% of cardiac surgery patients. The etiology of respiratory failure in the postoperative patient is multifactorial but can generally be divided into abnormal gas exchange and poor lung mechanics. The contribution of cardiopulmonary bypass itself is unclear because abnormalities also occur after off-pump coronary artery bypass grafting. Several factors that are known to contribute to postoperative pulmonary dysfunction include the following:

1. Atelectasis secondary to prolonged CPB.
2. Complement and neutrophil activation during CPB may cause acute lung injury (ALI) via cytokines, interleukins, neutrophil elastase, and tumor necrosis factor.
3. Hypoperfusion can produce pulmonary ischemia, gut ischemia, and endotoxin translocation, which may contribute to ALI.
4. High left atrial pressures in the patient with poor cardiac function can contribute to hydrostatic pulmonary edema.
5. Intraoperative trauma may cause phrenic nerve dysfunction.
6. Pleural effusions can decrease pulmonary compliance and increase work of breathing.

The emphasis on "fast-track" cardiac surgery has resulted in anesthetic techniques tailored toward early extubation. Studies have shown that patients extubated early have shorter ICU, hospital stays, no difference in pain scores or opioid use, and ambulate earlier. Patients extubated early also have less atelectasis and require less fluid. Early extubation has also been shown to be feasible and to result in decreased mean length of stay even among the elderly population, without an increased rate of reintubation. Additional benefits to early extubation include improved ciliary action, less need for sedation, decreased risk of nosocomial pneumonia, and perhaps better hemodynamic stability.

D. **Acute renal failure** occurs in up to 3% to 4% of cardiac surgical patients. The development of acute renal failure results in an increase in ICU and hospital stay, particularly if renal replacement therapy is needed. Mortality is greater than 40% in those patients who develop acute renal failure and up to 63% in those requiring renal replacement therapy. Preoperative risk factors include increased age, female gender, preoperative renal dysfunction (creatinine >1.4 mg/dl), low ejection fraction, diabetes mellitus, chronic obstructive pulmonary disease, and prior cardiac surgery. Intraoperative risk factors include mitral valve surgery, need for intraaortic balloon counterpulsation, emergency surgery, and longer duration of CPB. Early institution of continuous renal replacement therapy is indicated for impending renal failure and volume overload.

E. **Neurologic complications** occur in 3% of cardiac surgical patients. Older age may increase the incidence to 10%. Traditionally, it was felt that lower rates occurred in closed cardiac cases such as coronary artery bypass grafting, whereas higher rates occurred in open procedures such as valve replacement. This may not be the case because a recent study found the lowest rate of neurologic complications in single-valve procedures. The highest incidence occurs with **advanced age, diabetes mellitus,** and **preexisting cerebral vascular disease.** Intraoperative events such as macroemboli from air, fat, and atheromatous disease and CPB, along with hypoperfusion, are the primary causes. Up to 43% of patients may have a delayed onset of cerebral symptoms, suggesting that postoperative factors play an important role. Those caring for the cardiac surgical patient should closely watch hemodynamics and neurologic changes. Hypotension, hypoxemia, hypercarbia, hyperglycemia, and hyperthermia should be avoided to limit secondary cerebral injury.

F. **GI complications** include GI bleeding, acute pancreatitis, bowel infarction or perforation, acute cholecystitis, and liver dysfunction. They occur in about 5% of patients, and increase the mortality in cardiac surgical patients six- to sevenfold. Adverse GI outcomes also increase ICU length of stay, hospital stay, and cost of care. Preoperative factors associated with an increased incidence of GI complications include age greater than 75 years, preoperative congestive heart failure, right heart dysfunction, tricuspid valve disease, EF less than 40%, increased total bilirubin (>1.2 mg/dl), thrombocytopenia, prolonged PTT, prior cardiovascular surgery, and combined cardiac surgical procedures. Intraoperative factors associated with adverse outcomes include prolonged CPB times (>100 minutes), prolonged aortic occlusion (>55 minutes), hypotension, circulatory failure, need for pharmacologic support, and transfusion of red blood cells. Postoperative **acute pancreatitis** is indicated by abdominal distention and hypoactive bowel sounds in the setting of increased pancreatic enzymes. Excessive administration of calcium chloride is an independent risk factor for pancreatitis. Splanchnic hypoperfusion is the likely cause of such complications.

   G. **Cardiac tamponade** occurs in about 1% of postoperative cardiac patients. Tamponade decreases stroke volume by compression and consequent underfilling of the ventricles. Tamponade can occur with mediastinal drains still in place, even in the patient whose pericardium was left open. The diagnosis of tamponade may be quite difficult in the postoperative cardiac surgery patient. The classic diagnostic signs of tachycardia, low cardiac output, elevation and equalization of filling pressures, exaggerated blood pressure response to positive-pressure ventilation, and widened mediastinum by chest radiograph may not be present, and even classic echocardiographic criteria may be insensitive to postoperative tamponade. Tamponade also has been described to occur as late as several weeks postoperatively. A patient who deteriorates for unclear reasons may require operative exploration of the mediastinum.

   H. **Readmission** to the ICU deserves special mention as a complication. The high mortality rate (~35%) of these patients warrants aggressive initial recognition of the complication that lead to the readmission and its appropriate management.

IV. **Special considerations**
   A. **Minimally invasive surgery and off-pump cardiopulmonary bypass.** Minimally invasive cardiac surgery is rapidly gaining ground for patients with both coronary artery disease and valvular heart disease, although the exact definition of minimally invasive is uncertain. Some define surgery on a beating heart as minimally invasive, whereas others define those procedures requiring video assistance and closed-chest CPB as minimal. Off-pump cardiac artery bypass (OP-CAB), minimally invasive direct coronary artery bypass (MIDCAB), and endoscopic atraumatic coronary artery bypass grafting (endo-CAB) have all been developed in an attempt to improve cost effectiveness, avoid or limit CPB times, avoid aortic manipulation, and extend indications for surgery in patients who would otherwise not be considered candidates. Changes in surgical, anesthetic, and ICU management have been developed. Comparisons between minithoracotomy and conventional sternotomy for valve surgeries have shown that the complexity of the surgical approach with minithoracotomy results in an increase in

operating room time, cardiopulmonary bypass times, aortic cross-clamp time, and total blood loss. Additionally, graft patency has been a concern when exposure is other than a full sternotomy. The platelet dysfunction seen after CPB and full heparinization may not be present, and this may be detrimental to graft patency. A likely advantage is the fact that, in general, cardiac biomarker release after OP-CAB is less than after procedures requiring full CPB.

B. **Transesophageal echocardiography (TEE) in the cardiac surgical intensive care unit** (see Chapter 2). Transthoracic echocardiography (TTE, see Chapter 2) is sometimes limited in the ICU due to surgical dressings, tapes, tubes, subcutaneous emphysema, obesity, COPD, mechanical ventilation, poor positioning, or pneumomediastinum. Three primary indications for TEE in the ICU patient are hypoxemia, shock, and endocarditis.

1. **Hypoxemia.** TEE is generally more sensitive than transthoracic echocardiography in detecting the presence of a patent foramen ovale (PFO), atrial septal defect (ASD), or ventricular septal defect (VSD) as a cause of shunt resulting in hypoxemia.

2. **Causes of hypotension and hemodynamic instability.** TEE can be used for detecting the presence of large pulmonary emboli and a cause of right heart failure and hypotension. TEE can also evaluate the presence of valvular disorders. TEE is especially valuable in the diagnosis of post-cardiac surgery tamponade. In addition, ascending and descending aortic dissection can be accurately diagnosed.

3. **Endocarditis.** If endocarditis is still suspected despite a normal or limited TTE, TEE may be more sensitive in the evaluation for vegetations and abscess.

C. **Pain management** remains a challenge in some postoperative cardiac surgical patients especially in the setting of pressures to limit time to extubation, ICU stay, and hospital stay. A full review of techniques for postoperative pain control is beyond the scope of this chapter; we will discuss two relevant modalities:

1. **Thoracic epidural analgesia (TEA)** has been suggested as a technique for postoperative pain relief in cardiac surgical patients. Major concerns to wide implementation are questions about its actual effectiveness, the time to placement, and the risk of epidural hematoma in the setting of **full systemic anticoagulation.** The complication of an epidural hematoma after TEA in cardiac surgery has been reported but is extremely rare. TEA should be considered as an option in patients with ongoing myocardial ischemia and anticipated incomplete surgical revascularization, tenuous pulmonary function, and chronic opioid dependency. Placement of the epidural catheter should precede systemic heparinization by at least 1 hour. Normal neurologic function should be documented after placement as well as in the postoperative period. Catheter

removal, at which time up to 40% of epidural hematomas occur, should only be done in the setting of acceptable coagulation profile.

2. **Nonsteroidal antiinflammatory drugs (NSAIDs)** are nonspecific inhibitors of the cyclooxygenase pathway involved in the production of prostaglandins. Reluctance is commonly encountered in using these drugs in the cardiac surgical population due to concerns about gastrointestinal injury, renal complications, and platelet dysfunction. Administration of rectal **indomethacin** can reduce opiate requirements. Recent evidence of serious cardiovascular toxicity has led to the **discontinuation or serious warnings on the use of selective cyclooxygenase-2 inhibitors.** Intravenous **ketorolac** (15–30 mg IV) is commonly used in cardiac surgical patients, and appears to be safe in the absence of excessive bleeding, GI disorders, diabetes mellitus, and renal insufficiency.

3. **Dexmedetomidine** is an α_2-agonist commonly used in the general ICU patient, but rarely used in the cardiac surgical patient. When compared with a propofol-based sedation regimen, those patients receiving dexmedetomidine required less morphine, antiemetics, and NSAIDs. Hypotension and bradycardia may occur.

SELECTED REFERENCES

Ahlgren E, Aren C. Cerebral complications after coronary artery bypass and heart valve surgery: risk factors and onset of symptoms. *J Cardiothorac Vasc Anesth* 1998;12:270–273.

Argenziano M, Chen JM, Choudhri AF, et al. Management of vasodilatory shock after cardiac surgery: identification of predisposing factors and use of a novel pressor agent. *J Thorac Cardiovasc Surg* 1998;116:973–980.

Bove T, Calabro MG, Landoni G, et al. The incidence and risk of acute renal failure after cardiac surgery. *J Cardiothorac Vasc Anesth* 2004;18:442–445.

Despotis GJ, Filos KS, Zoys TN, et al. Factors associated with excessive postoperative blood loss and hemostatic transfusion requirements: a multivariate analysis in cardiac surgical patients. *Anesth Analg* 1996;82:13–21.

Fillinger MP, Yeager MP, Dodds TM, et al. Epidural anesthesia and analgesia: effects on recovery from cardiac surgery. *J Cardiothorac Vasc Anesth* 2002;16:15–20.

Johnson D, Thomson D, Mycyk T, et al. Respiratory outcomes with early extubation after coronary artery bypass surgery. *J Cardiothorac Vasc Anesth* 1997;11:474–480.

Kern MJ. Intra-aortic balloon counterpulsation. *Coron Artery Dis* 1991;2:649–658.

Levy JH, Buckley MJ, D'Ambra MN, et al. Symposium: pharmacologic control of bleeding in patients undergoing open heart surgery. *Contemp Surg* 1996;48:175–188.

Mangano D. Biventricular function after myocardial revascularization in humans: deterioration and recovery patterns during the first 24 hours. *Anesthesiology* 1985;62:571–577.

Mathew JP, Fontes ML, Tudor IC, et al. A multicenter risk index for atrial fibrillation after cardiac surgery. *JAMA* 2004;291:1720–1729.

McSweeney ME, Garwood S, Levin J, et al., Adverse gastrointestinal complications after cardiopulmonary bypass: can outcome be predicted from preoperative risk factors? *Anesth Analg* 2004;98:1610–1617.

Ng CSH, Wan S, Yim APC, et al. Pulmonary dysfunction after cardiac surgery. *Chest* 121;4:1269–1277.

Pastor MC, Sanchez MJ, Casas MA, et al. Thoracic epidural analgesia in coronary artery bypass graft surgery: seven years' experience. *J Cardiothorac Vasc Anesth* 2003;17:154–159.

Ryan TA, Rady MY, Bashour CA, et al. Predictors of outcome in cardiac surgical patients with prolonged intensive care stay. *Chest* 1997;112:1035–1042.

Slama MA, Novara A, Van De Putte P, et al. Diagnostic and therapeutic implications of transesophageal echocardiography in medical ICU patients with unexplained shock, hypoxemia, or suspected endocarditis. *Intensive Care Med* 1996;22:916–922.

Speiss BD, Royston D, Levy JH, et al. Platelet transfusions during coronary artery bypass graft surgery are associated with serious outcomes. *Transfusion* 2004;44:1143–1148.

Liver, Kidney, and Lung Transplantation

Michael G. Fitzsimons
and Andrew M. Cameron

I. **Principles of care for transplant patients**
   A. **Time course.** The complex clinical picture of transplant patients (Table 39-1) may be simplified by considering time periods that emphasize different issues:
   1. **First 7 days: donor and recipient surgery.** As a rule, the allograft is the organ most affected by hemodynamic perturbations, so that good allograft function will almost always lead to swift clinical improvement. Allograft dysfunction, on the other hand, requires sorting out the contribution of the recipient's preoperative status and intraoperative course, the quality of the donor organ, and the possibility of technical complications.
   2. **After 1 week: acute rejection.** Because of the numerous steps in the complex cascade leading to full T-cell differentiation, clinically detectable acute rejection does not usually occur until 1 week after implantation. As long as technical complications have been ruled out, organ dysfunction at that point is usually attributed to rejection and is treated empirically with increased immunosuppression.
   3. **After 6 months: chronic issues.** The risk of opportunistic infections increases with the degree of recipient immunosuppression (see Chapter 11). Thus, these infections are more typical in the late postoperative period, especially if repeated bouts of rejection have required multiple courses of heightened immunosuppression. Late allograft dysfunction raises the specter of disease recurrence or chronic rejection, both of which may lead to steadily worsening allograft failure and will be unresponsive to increased immunosuppression.
   B. **Immunosuppression.** Administration of any immunosuppressive agent is invariably limited by side effects. By combining different agents, it is possible to increase immunosuppression while limiting troublesome side effects. For this reason, most whole-organ transplant patients receive either double or triple (two- or three-drug) immunosuppression.
   1. **Calcineurin inhibitors. Cyclosporine** (Sandimmune, Neoral, Gengraf) and **tacrolimus** (Prograf) specifically target the activation of T lymphocytes (the immune cells principally responsible for rejection). Calcineurin inhibitors are the core of most current immunosuppressive protocols. Either one may be started

Table 39-1. Factors affecting the transplant recipient's postoperative course

Underlying preoperative organ failure
Quality of the donor allograft
Intraoperative hemodynamics
Technical complications
Rejection
Immunosuppression
Adverse drug reaction
Disease recurrence

perioperatively and then taken orally as long-term maintenance. Both are nephrotoxic and require careful adjustment based on blood levels. Other side effects include hypertension, hyperkalemia, hyperglycemia (especially in patients on high-dose steroids), neurotoxicity (seizures and tremors), and hyperuricemia (gout).

2. **Antilymphocyte antibody agents. OKT3** (Muromonab), **antithymocyte globulin** (ATG or thymoglobulin), **basiliximab** (Simulect), **and daclizumab** (Zenapax) also target T cells, but can only be given intravenously. The antibody-based agents are used for induction of immunosuppression, for treating steroid-resistant acute rejection, and as part of newer "tolerance"-inducing protocols. Multiple courses are often ineffective and can become dangerous. In patients with postoperative renal failure, cyclosporine or tacrolimus may be discontinued, with OKT3 or ATG being substituted for equivalent, but nonnephrotoxic, immunosuppression. This simplifies the early postoperative management, but expends an important therapeutic option, which may then be unavailable to treat subsequent resistant rejection later in the postoperative course.

3. **Antimetabolite agents. Mycophenolate** (Cellcept) **and azathioprine** (Imuran) inhibit DNA or RNA synthesis and therefore block active lymphocyte proliferation. Dose reduction may be required if leukopenia, thrombocytopenia, or anemia occurs.

4. **Corticosteroids** provide relatively nonspecific immunosuppression. High-dose intravenous **methylprednisolone** typically is initiated on the day of transplantation and reduced over the next 4 to 5 days to a maintenance level. When feeding resumes, oral **prednisone** is substituted. If rejection occurs, high-dose methylprednisolone boluses (500 mg intravenously [IV] every day for 2 days) are given as initial treatment. Once they are receiving corticosteroids, patients require stress dose supplementation for major procedures. Intravenous **hydrocortisone** (100 mg IV every 8 hours) is given on the day of surgery and

tapered over 3 days. During this time, maintenance immunosuppression is continued with either oral prednisone or intravenous methylprednisolone (see equivalency table in Chapter 27). Patients on high-dose steroids may develop hyperglycemia and gastrointestinal bleeding, which may be mitigated by prophylactic histamine-2 (H_2) blockers.

5. **Efforts to wean immunosuppressive agents.** In addition to ongoing research efforts directed at the generation of true "transplantation tolerance" or specific immunologic nonreactivity toward the donor organ, there are clinical protocols for the reduction of traditional triple-drug immunosuppression down to monotherapy. These protocols often include recipient pretreatment with T-cell–depleting antibody reagents and seek to rapidly exclude steroids from the regimen. These protocols may begin with only daily calcineurin-inhibitor monotherapy and progress to dose reduction to a once-weekly dose.

6. **Drug interactions.** The transplant patient's complex drug regimen should constantly be reevaluated and simplified. This approach will improve compliance and avoid potentially catastrophic and sometimes unpredictable drug interactions. In particular, the addition of new medications to an immunosuppressive regimen should be carefully considered. For example, **allopurinol,** if administered in combination with azathioprine, may precipitate life-threatening leukopenia. Numerous medications (e.g., **sucralfate, verapamil,** and **erythromycin**) may alter cyclosporine absorption and thus precipitate rejection or toxicity.

C. **Infections**

1. **Prophylactic strategies.** Different types of infections occur at predictable times in the postoperative course, leading to corresponding prophylactic strategies (see Chapter 11). Long-term, low-dose **trimethoprim-sulfa** effectively prevents *Pneumocystis* infections. During periods of heightened immunosuppression, **ganciclovir** or **acyclovir** is added to lower the incidence of cytomegalovirus (CMV) and Epstein-Barr virus (EBV) infections. Because invasive procedures increase the risk of bacterial infections, systemic antibiotics are administered during the perioperative period and prior to cholangiograms or percutaneous biopsies.

2. **Preventative measures** include minimizing immunosuppression, avoiding endotracheal intubation and intravascular catheters, and correcting malnutrition. Evaluation of possible hematomas, abscesses, or fluid collections should be pursued by serial ultrasound or computed tomography (CT), and appropriate drainage should be expeditiously undertaken. Because immunosuppression blunts the usual signs of inflammation, an aggressive **surveillance** and diagnostic approach is crucial, with routine cultures

(e.g., biweekly cultures of sputum, urine, bile, and wound drainage) and daily chest radiographs while the recipient is receiving mechanical ventilation.

II. Liver transplantation

A. The indications

for liver transplant include virtually any disease leading to progressive, irreversible liver disease and may be divided into acute or chronic processes. Characteristics of acute liver failure are detailed in Chapter 25. Disorders may be grouped according to features that will affect the postoperative course:

1. **Chronic and progressive liver cirrhosis.** Liver fibrosis and disorganized regeneration, as it occurs in cirrhosis, impedes portal blood flow, with resultant portal hypertension (ascites, bleeding varices, and thrombocytopenia from hypersplenism). Multiple venous collaterals develop throughout the abdomen, increasing the likelihood of major perioperative blood loss and hemodynamic instability.

2. **Chronic hepatocyte failure.** Patients eventually develop hepatocyte failure leading to encephalopathy, fatigue, jaundice, and coagulopathy. The encephalopathy is a metabolic phenomenon that is reversible with transplantation. Such patients tend to be debilitated and malnourished. Poor healing, susceptibility to infection, and a prolonged recovery can be predicted.

3. **Acute fulminant hepatic failure.** These patients are technically straightforward and do very well with a timely allograft, but may develop fatal cerebral edema with resultant elevated intracerebral pressure. Perioperative intracerebral pressure monitoring is often helpful, as are head CT scans.

4. **Liver failure with preserved hepatocyte function.** In these individuals, the pathologic process in the biliary tree is either too diffuse or too complex, or the predicted resultant hepatic reserve too compromised, for conventional surgery (e.g., **biliary atresia, sclerosing cholangitis, primary biliary cirrhosis**). Transplantation in these patients is technically straightforward, and they do very well in the perioperative period.

B. Donor allograft

1. **Donor.** The likelihood of early allograft failure is correlated with donor characteristics (obesity, prolonged ICU stay, malnutrition, terminal hypotension, and fatty liver changes). Although the characteristics of the "ideal donor" are well described, there has been increasing use of "marginal" or suboptimal donor grafts in the United States. This practice has been a response to the insufficient supply of needed donor organs and has had a proportionate impact on recipient performance in the postoperative period. In many cases, recipients who are unlikely to receive organs because of severe illness may receive marginal grafts as an alternative to dying without a transplant.

2. **Efforts to increase organ availability.** In addition to the use of marginal donors, other efforts to increase the number of available organs include the use of **donors after cardiac death** (DCD), splitting cadaveric grafts for two recipients, and the use of living donors. DCD liver grafts probably give inferior overall graft and patient survival, whereas grafts from living donors function well but place additional risk on the healthy donor. Splitting of well-chosen cadaveric organs for an adult–child recipient pair with one member critically ill has shown very promising results.

3. **Preservation.** Prolonged ischemia time is also correlated with allograft dysfunction. During procurement, the donor allograft is flushed with University of Wisconsin (UW) solution and stored on ice until transplantation. This cold ischemia time usually is limited to 12 to 15 hours, and to less in marginal donor livers.

C. **Recipient operation**

1. **Native hepatectomy.** The coagulopathy of end-stage liver disease and the multiple venous collaterals of portal hypertension can lead to **massive blood loss,** which is directly correlated with postoperative morbidity and mortality. Therefore, this phase of the transplant procedure is often the most technically difficult. Once the liver is removed, patients frequently develop a **metabolic acidosis,** requiring correction to prepare for reperfusion. Overcorrection with sodium bicarbonate, however, may lead to severe postoperative **metabolic alkalosis.** This phenomenon results from the metabolism of the **citrate** administered with transfused blood products to bicarbonate by a functioning allograft.

2. **Donor liver implantation** includes either a traditional technique of venous anastomoses at the supra- and infrahepatic vena cava or, if the "piggy-back" technique is employed, sparing of the recipient inferior vena cava (IVC), oversewing of the donor infrahepatic IVC, and anastomosis of the donor suprahepatic IVC to the recipient IVC in an end-to-side fashion. This is followed by portal vein, hepatic artery, and bile duct anastomoses (either a choledocho-choledochostomy or Roux-en-Y choledocho-jejunostomy). A biliary stent or T-tube may be placed across the anastomosis and exits percutaneously. Drains are also placed in the supra- and infrahepatic spaces.

3. **Reperfusion of the allograft,** usually within 60 minutes of warm ischemia time, returns a sudden bolus of cold, hyperkalemic, acidotic blood from the lower body and liver and may cause severe **pulmonary artery vasoconstriction** with resultant hypotension and possible dysrhythmia ("reperfusion phenomenon"). Reperfusion of the ischemic liver may also precipitate accelerated **fibrinolysis.** Aggressive

replacement of coagulation factors and antifibrinolytic agent administration (see Chapter 10) may be required to achieve hemostasis.

D. Posttransplant management

1. **General care.** In addition to routine physical exam (checking mental status, abdomen, wound, and peritoneal and biliary drains) and invasive monitoring, evaluation includes serial laboratory studies, and Doppler ultrasound examination in the first 48 hours to screen for hepatic artery thrombosis (see later discussion). Maintenance intravenous fluids should always contain dextrose to avoid depletion of glycogen stores in the liver. Patients often tolerate sips by 24 to 48 hours after surgery, although feeding is resumed cautiously in patients with a Roux-en-Y choledochojejunostomy. On the fifth postoperative day, a cholangiogram is obtained if a biliary tube was placed, after which the biliary stent or T-tube is clamped for increasing periods of time, with full clamping usually achieved by the tenth postoperative day.

2. **Cardiovascular**

   a. **Hemodynamics.** The high cardiac output and low peripheral vascular resistance typical of end-stage liver disease commonly persist into the early postoperative period, so that inotropic agents are rarely required in liver transplant recipients.

   b. **Hypotension.** The usual first therapeutic response is volume administration. Excessively high central venous pressures should be avoided because transmission back to the hepatic sinusoids may exacerbate allograft edema already present from reperfusion injury. If hypotension persists without detectable hypovolemia or cardiac dysfunction, sepsis should be suspected, blood cultures obtained, and empiric antibiotic therapy initiated. The use of prostaglandin E infusion to improve portal vein flow may contribute iatrogenically to postoperative hypotension.

   c. **Hypertension.** Because of the increased risks of cerebral edema, hemorrhage, and seizures, sustained hypertension requires aggressive treatment.

3. **Respiratory.** In the presence of good graft function, successful endotracheal extubation usually can be accomplished within 12 to 48 hours, but may be delayed by right diaphragmatic paralysis from intraoperative placement of the suprahepatic vascular clamp and by metabolic alkalosis (see earlier discussion). "Fast-track" extubation at the end of uneventful orthotopic liver transplants is becoming the norm at high-volume centers.

4. **Renal.** Most liver allograft recipients develop mild postoperative renal dysfunction because of preexisting renal insufficiency, intraoperative caval occlusion, bleeding and hypotension, postimplantation hepatic allograft dysfunction, and nephrotoxic drugs such

as cyclosporine and tacrolimus. Other nephrotoxic drugs, such as aminoglycosides, should be avoided. **Prostaglandin E$_1$** may have a beneficial effect on the liver recipient's renal function during the early postoperative period. Other patients whose preoperative renal dysfunction is a result of their liver failure (i.e., those with the hepatorenal syndrome) will show posttransplant improvement. If postoperative oliguria persists despite optimized hemodynamics, a nonnephrotoxic antibody immunosuppressant is substituted for tacrolimus or cyclosporine. With this approach, dialysis usually can be avoided. **Continuous venovenous hemofiltration** (see Chapter 24) is preferred if renal replacement therapy is indicated. Dialysis should be used with extreme caution because rapid osmotic shifts may worsen the brain swelling already present in patients with hepatic failure. In patients whose renal dysfunction progresses to the need for dialysis, mortality rates may be as great as 90%.

5. **Hematology.** Leukopenia and thrombocytopenia secondary to hypersplenism typically persist into the early postoperative period, sometimes requiring a dose reduction of azathioprine if part of the immunosuppressive regimen. If the white blood cell count falls below 1,500/mm^3, **granulocyte colony-stimulating factor** (filgrastim) can be administered to decrease the incidence of postoperative infections. The postoperative hematocrit is maintained in the range of 25% to 30% because higher values may be associated with hepatic artery thrombosis. Fibrinogen levels are likewise monitored, and lower levels may require continuation of antifibrinolytic agents into the postoperative period. The likelihood of significant postoperative bleeding is related directly to the degree of intraoperative bleeding and the quality of immediate allograft function. If major blood loss persists despite reversal of coagulopathy, surgical reexploration is indicated. Even in patients whose early bleeding stops, reexploration may be indicated to evacuate clot, which may otherwise become secondarily infected.

E. **Allograft dysfunction** (Fig. 39-1)

1. **Primary graft nonfunction (PGNF),** defined as initial poor hepatic allograft function, occurs in about 10% of recipients, and has a greater than 80% mortality without retransplantation.

a. PGNF must be differentiated from the reversible preservation injury that is frequently noted in the first two postoperative days. Preservation injury is typically associated with a serum glutamic-oxaloacetic transaminase (SGOT) peak below 2,000 U/L and rapid clinical improvement. Technical problems with any of the vascular anastomoses must be ruled out as well and is typically done with abdominal ultrasound (see later discussion). In contrast, PGNF is associated with a marked

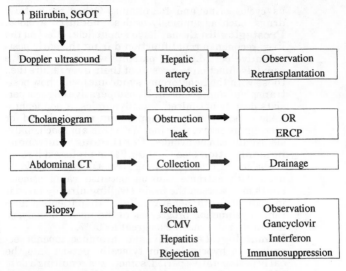

Fig. 39-1. Liver allograft dysfunction. CMV, cytomegalovirus; CT, computed tomography; ERCP, endoscopic retrograde cholangiopancreatography; SGOT, serum glutamic-oxaloacetic transaminase.

elevation of bilirubin and transaminases (e.g., SGOT >2,000 U/L), persistent hepatic encephalopathy, minimal bile output (<30–60 ml/day, often colorless or white), uncorrectable coagulopathy, and profound hypoglycemia.

    b. **Treatment** consists of early prostaglandin E_1 infusion, intensive support, and retransplantation.

2. **Acute rejection.** Both acute rejection and acute viral hepatitis (B, C) or CMV may be heralded by a bilirubin and transaminase elevation. Acute rejection is uncommon following liver transplantation, but can occur during the first or second postoperative weeks, whereas hepatitis more commonly occurs later. A percutaneous biopsy may be necessary to establish the correct diagnosis. Approximately two-thirds of patients suffer a rejection episode; of these, two-thirds respond to steroid boluses. Most of the remainder respond to antibody-based therapy. Retransplantation is rarely required due to uncontrolled rejection.

3. **Technical complications**
    a. **Hepatic artery thrombosis (HAT)** is more common in pediatric recipients, especially those with small or multiple allograft arteries. Presentation varies: Approximately one-third demonstrate acute hepatic failure, with marked elevation of transaminases (SGOT 2,000–10,000 U/L), or bile duct leak

because the hepatic artery is the sole blood supply to the bile ducts; one-third have recurrent septic episodes with or without hepatic abscess; and one-third are asymptomatic with the diagnosis an incidental finding. Late sequelae of HAT may include biliary dysfunction or ductal stricture. Doppler ultrasound is used liberally to screen for HAT, whereas an arteriogram may be required to confirm the diagnosis. Treatment options depend on the presentation, and include retransplantation, reoperation, selective urokinase injection, and no treatment.

b. **Bile duct complications** may be detected by the appearance of bile in a drain or an unexplained rise in serum bilirubin. Endoscopic retrograde cholangiopancreatography (see Chapter 26) or reexploration may be required.

c. **Other complications,** such as portal vein or vena cava thrombosis, manifested by ascites accumulation or variceal bleeding or detected by radiographic studies, are exceedingly rare. Treatment options usually include medical support, radiologic intervention, and operative correction.

III. **Renal transplantation**

A. **Indications.** A 1998 consensus conference regarding placement of patients on the United Network for Organ Sharing cadaveric renal transplant waiting list determined that, to be listed, an adult candidate for placement should have **progressive renal disease and a glomerular filtration rate (GFR) less than 18 ml/min.** The most common indications for renal transplantation include **chronic glomerulonephritis, diabetic nephropathy, chronic pyelonephritis, malignant nephrosclerosis,** and **polycystic kidney** disease.

B. **Renal transplant recipients** are at significant risk for cardiovascular complications. Diabetes is the most common indication for renal transplantation, and hypertension and hypercholesterolemia often complicate renal failure. Cardiovascular complications are nevertheless relatively rare in the immediate postoperative period because aggressive pretransplant screening and preoperative treatment of occult coronary artery disease is the rule. Long-term recipients, however, are at higher risk for cardiovascular complications.

C. **Donor allograft.** Adverse donor characteristics, such as advanced age, terminal or prolonged hypotension, and the need for vasopressors, are highly correlated with posttransplant acute tubular necrosis (ATN). Nevertheless, as long as the allograft has reasonable underlying parenchyma (established by biopsy), recovery may be expected. Excessive prolonged cold ischemia time, associated with shipping of renal grafts longer distances and the use of DCD donors, can also contribute to poor intra- and postoperative graft function. Delayed allograft function is much easier to manage in kidney recipients than in liver recipients because of the availability of dialysis. Acute tubular necrosis is extremely rare in living donor recipients. Though efforts at HLA matching have proven successful in lengthening the half-life of well-matched renal allografts, no difference in perioperative immunosuppression or performance is expected.

D. Recipient operation. The allograft is implanted in the pelvis, with the renal artery and vein sewn into the corresponding iliac vessels. If the ureter is implanted into the bladder, a Foley catheter should be left in place for 5 days to prevent bladder distention and resultant anastomotic strain. On the other hand, if an uretero-ureterostomy is constructed (after a native nephrectomy), prolonged catheter bladder drainage is not required. In either case, a Jackson-Pratt drain is left in place at the site of the ureteral anastomoses.

E. Immediate postoperative course
1. Immediate allograft function is heralded by a massive diuresis necessitating aggressive fluid replacement (e.g., per-hour rate equal to the previous hour's urine output in ml plus 30 ml, limited to 400 ml/h) and diligent electrolyte monitoring.
2. Oliguria in the early postoperative course is usually due to reversible ATN, but technical complications must be excluded (see Fig. 39-2).

F. Late course. Elevated creatinine (see Fig. 39-3) leads to a decision about whether to reduce the dose of a nephrotoxic immunosuppressant (cyclosporine or tacrolimus) or to increase immunosuppression in an attempt to treat rejection. A biopsy often is required to clarify the situation.

G. Complications. The most common vascular complication following kidney transplant is renal artery stenosis, often associated with rejection involving the renal artery and manifesting as severe hypertension. Treatment may

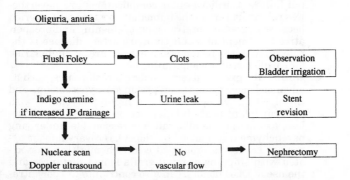

Fig. 39-2. Oliguria in the immediate postoperative period. JP, Jackson-Pratt.

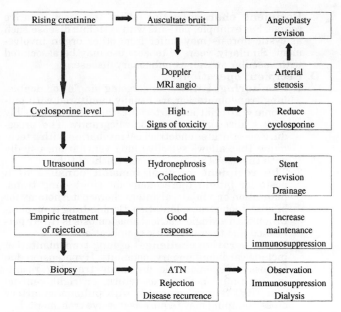

Fig. 39-3. Rising creatinine in a renal allograft recipient. ATN, acute tubular necrosis; MRI, magnetic resonance imaging.

be surgical or via percutaneous balloon-based techniques. Urologic complications include leak from the bladder closure or ureteral anastomosis, and ureteral obstruction. Lymphocele of the transplant bed can be avoided with careful ligation of the surrounding lymphatics during recipient preparation.

IV. **Lung transplantation**

  A. **Indications** include end-stage chronic obstructive pulmonary disease (**COPD), cystic fibrosis, pulmonary fibrosis, alpha-1-antitrypsin deficiency, sarcoidosis, bronchiectasis, lymphangioleiomytosis,** and **occupational lung diseases.** Candidates have end-stage pulmonary disease with an estimated survival of 2 to 3 years without transplantation.

  B. **Donor organs.** Improved organ preservation and perioperative management have expanded the pool of potential donor organs, but **the lung remains more susceptible to ischemic injury than any other transplanted organ.** Ischemic time for lung transplantation should be limited to 4 to 6 hours; lungs from older donors are less tolerant of long ischemic times than those from younger donors. **Living related lung donation** (with two donors each donating a lung lobe) is a real option, which is exercised with increasing frequency in experienced centers. DCD has also been performed for lung transplantation.

C. **Recipient characteristics** affect the postoperative course. For example, patients with systemic disease such as cystic fibrosis may suffer from other organ involvement. Similarly, years of tobacco use may be associated with vascular as well as pulmonary disease.

D. **Recipient operation:**

1. **Monitoring.** Patients undergoing single- or double-lung transplantation are usually monitored with pulmonary arterial and arterial catheters and possibly with transesophageal echocardiography. The procedure necessitates endotracheal intubation with a technique that allows selective lung ventilation, usually with the use of a double-lumen tracheal tube.

2. **The recipient surgical incision consists of a** posterior lateral thoracotomy for single-lung transplantation or a bilateral antero-thoracosternotomy for bilateral-lobe transplantation. Double-lung transplantation with a single tracheal anastomosis is rarely performed due to anastomotic complications.

3. **Intraoperative challenges** of lung transplantation include cardiopulmonary instability. Hypotension due to loss of sympathetic drive, air trapping resulting in diminished venous return, or right ventricular (RV) failure associated with pulmonary artery cross-clamping may require aggressive treatment. Hypercapnia and hypoxemia during the procedure are common problems. Pulmonary arterial hypertension may warrant treatment with vasodilators, including **prostaglandin E$_1$** infusion or **nitroglycerin,** but systemic hypotension may limit the efficacy of these drugs. Inhaled **nitric oxide,** a selective pulmonary artery vasodilator, may be preferred. Continued RV dysfunction despite vasodilators requires cardiopulmonary bypass (CPB), with resultant requirement for systemic anticoagulation and potential bleeding complications. Once the donor lung is implanted, reperfusion pulmonary edema is common and frequently refractory to treatment with positive end-respiratory pressure (PEEP). In this circumstance, treatment with pulmonary vasodilators may again be considered.

E. **Postoperative management**

1. **General.** Postoperative issues in the lung transplant patient generally involve management of respiratory status, hemodynamics, prevention and treatment of infection, continuation of immunosuppressive regimen, and pain control.

2. **Respiratory management.** The goal of postoperative respiratory management in the lung transplant patient is to achieve adequate oxygenation and ventilation while avoiding oxygen toxicity and barotrauma. PEEP is generally added to a level of 5 to 10 cm H_2O to help decrease the fraction of inspired oxygen as low as possible. Limiting tidal volume and peak airway pressures to less than 40 cm H_2O is thought to decrease barotrauma and bronchial anastomotic

complication. Pulmonary reimplantation response is a phenomenon of noncardiogenic pulmonary edema lasting up to 3 weeks and requiring ventilatory support, but is generally associated with a good prognosis. Following extubation, lung transplant patients demonstrate a hypoventilatory response to hypercapnia, but the etiology is not fully delineated.

3. **Hemodynamic management.** Postoperative hemodynamic management of the lung transplant patient is a fine balance between adequate volume for vital organ function and prevention of additional pulmonary edema, and, thus, monitoring with a pulmonary artery (PA) catheter may facilitate management. Hemorrhage is more common following transplantation in which CPB was utilized. CPB may also increase postoperative transfusion requirement, intubation duration, and overall hospital stay. Pulmonary hypertension is common in the immediate postoperative period; patients may benefit from treatment with inhaled nitric oxide to decrease PA pressures without systemic hypotension.

4. **Pain management** generally involves either systemic opioids or epidural analgesia. Those with chronic respiratory failure due to either COPD or cystic fibrosis may be particularly susceptible to the development of hypercapnia when treated with systemic opioids. Although epidural opioids may also cause hypercapnia, equivalent analgesia may generally be achieved with a significantly lower opioid dose. Epidural analgesia may decrease times to extubation and discharge from the ICU.

5. **Immunosuppression.** Most centers initiate immunosuppression in the operating room. Almost all protocols include a nonspecific antiinflammatory corticosteroid. Side effects of corticosteroids such as hyperglycemia and myopathy must be considered. A calcineurin inhibitor such as **cyclosporine** is generally initiated as well. Side effects include nephrotoxicity, hypertension, and neurotoxicity. **Tacrolimus** (FK 506) has essentially the same mechanism of action as cyclosporine but is more effective in preventing acute rejection. Tacrolimus does have higher rates of neurotoxicity, nephrotoxicity, and new-onset diabetes. **Azathioprine** or **mycophenolate,** both of which inhibit lymphocyte proliferation, may be adjunct immunosuppressant agents. Toxicities include leukopenia, hepatitis, and cholestasis. Finally, antilymphocyte preparations such as polyclonal **antilymphocyte globulin, ATG,** and **OKT3** may be initiated.

6. **Infections** (see also Chapter 11). Immunosuppression increases the transplant recipient's incidence of both bacterial and viral infection. Early infections tend to be bacterial, with gram-negative organisms predominating. **Cytomegalovirus** is the most common early viral infection and may be due to reactivation

of an infection in a seropositive recipient (secondary) or, more commonly, new infection in a seronegative recipient from the seropositive donor organ (primary). The most serious manifestation of CMV is pneumonitis or pneumonia; treatment is with **ganciclovir,** which, when given prophylactically, may decrease the incidence. *Aspergillus fumigatus* is the most common fungal infection, with a peak incidence within the first 2 months. Manifestations include ulcerations, pseudomembranes, and tracheobronchitis.

7. **Rejection.** Hyperacute, acute, and chronic rejection may be encountered in the intensive care unit. Hyperacute rejection is extremely uncommon, occurring within the first minutes to hours after transplantation, and is almost universally fatal. It is due to preformed antibodies against HLA and ABO antigens and may be confused with ischemia-reperfusion injury. Acute rejection occurs within the first 3 to 6 months. Symptoms of acute rejection include fever, cough, dyspnea, and anorexia. Decreases in pulmonary spirometry or diffusion capacity may aid the diagnosis, which requires biopsy for confirmation. Treatment of acute rejection consists of a course of high-dose steroids and elimination of other causes of symptoms. Chronic rejection occurs generally between 6 and 12 months and is characterized by airflow limitation primarily due to fibroproliferation in the small airways manifesting as bronchiolitis obliterans. Treatment includes corticosteroids and immunosuppressants, but mortality remains high despite treatment.

SELECTED REFERENCES

Abt PL, Desai NM, Crawford MD, et al. Survival following liver transplantation from non-heart-beating donors. *Ann Surg* 2004;239:87–92.

Arcasoy SM, Kotloff RM. Lung transplantation. *N Engl J Med* 1999;340:1081–1091.

Busutill RW, Klintmaim GB. *Transplantation of the liver.* Philadelphia: WB Saunders, 1996.

Busuttil RW, Shaked A, Millis JM, et al. One thousand liver transplants. The lessons learned. *Ann Surg* 1994;219:490–497.

Consensus conference on standardized listing criteria for renal transplant candidates. *Transplantation* 1998;66:962.

DeMeo DL, Ginns LC. Clinical status of lung transplantation. *Transplantation* 2001;72:1713–1724.

Findlay JY, Jankowski CJ, Vasdeve GM, et al. Fast track anesthesia for liver transplantation reduces postoperative ventilation time but not intensive care unit stay. *Liver Transpl* 2002;8:670–675.

Gerstenkorn C. Non-heart-beating donors: renewed source of organs for renal transplantation during the twenty-first century. *World J Surg* 2003;27:489–493.

Ghobrial RM, Busuttil RW. Future of adult living donor liver transplantation. *Liver Transpl* 2003;9:S73–S79.

Organ Procurement and Transplantation web site. Available at www.optn.org.

Ploeg RJ, D'Alessandro AM, Knechtle SJ, et al. Risk factors for primary dysfunction after liver transplantation—a multivariate analysis. *Transplantation* 1993;55:807–813.

Renz JF, Emond JC, Yersiz H, et al. Split-liver transplantation in the United States: outcomes of a national survey. *Ann Surg* 2004; 239:172–181.

Singh H, Bossard FR. Perioperative anaesthetic considerations for patients undergoing lung transplantation. *Can J Anaesth* 1997;44: 284–299.

Sleiman C, Mal H, Fournier M, et al. Pulmonary reimplantation response in single-lung transplantation. *Eur Respir J* 1995;8:5–9.

Sollinger HW, Knechtl SJ, Reed A, et al. Experience with 100 consecutive simultaneous kidney-pancreas transplants with bladder drainage. *Ann Surg* 1991;214:703–711.

Starzl TE, Murase N, Abu-Elmagd K, et al. Tolerogenic immunosuppression for organ transplantation. *Lancet* 2003;361:1502–1510.

Tolkoff RN, Rubin RH. The infectious disease problems of the diabetic renal transplant recipient. *Infect Dis Clin North Am* 1995;9:117–130.

Tzakis AG, Gordon RD, Shaw BW Jr, et al. Clinical presentation of hepatic artery thrombosis after liver transplantation in the cyclosporin era. *Transplantation* 1985;40:667–671.

40

Critical Care Aspects of Obesity and Bariatric Surgery

Timothy A. Jackson and Jean Kwo

I. **Introduction.** Obesity is a disorder of energy balance. It is derived from the Latin word *obesus,* which means fattened by eating. Obesity has reached epidemic proportions in the United States, with an age-adjusted prevalence of 30.5% in adults.

II. **The body mass index (BMI)** reflects the relative amount of fat tissue. It is calculated as

$$BMI = Weight\ (kg)/Height\ (m)^2$$

Patients are considered overweight if their BMI is greater than 25 and obese if their BMI is greater than 30 (Table 40-1).

III. **Physiologic changes associated with obesity.** The care of the obese patient in the intensive care unit (ICU) is challenging not only because of the patient's size, but also because of the significant number of obesity-associated pathophysiologic changes that increase morbidity and mortality and influence postoperative care. Of particular importance are the interrelated changes that occur in the cardiovascular and respiratory systems.

A. **Cardiovascular changes**

1. **Heart failure**

a. Excess adipose tissue and increased loading of supporting muscle and bone **elevate metabolic demand.**

b. Circulating blood volume and cardiac output (stroke volume) increase to meet this demand. The increased blood volume results in increased ventricular wall stress eventually leading to left ventricular enlargement. This, coupled with hypertension, causes eccentric **left ventricular hypertrophy.**

c. The resulting systolic and diastolic dysfunction, coupled with ischemic heart disease, can lead to **left ventricular failure.**

d. Hypoxemia and hypercapnia, as well as left ventricular failure, contribute to pulmonary arterial hypertension and **right ventricular failure.**

e. The incidence and severity of heart failure is correlated with BMI.

f. Cor adiposum, or fatty infiltration of the heart, as a cause of failure is no longer considered a valid pathologic entity.

2. **Hypertension** is the most common overweight- and obesity-related health condition. Blood pressure values closely correlate with BMI.

Table 40-1. **Body mass index and weight classification**

Body Mass Index	Classification
18.5–24.9	Healthy weight
25–29.9	Overweight
30–34.9	Class I (moderate) obesity
35–39.9	Class II (severe) obesity
≥40, or 35 with comorbidities	Class III (morbid) obesity

3. **Coronary artery disease.** Hypertension, hyper-cholesterolemia, and type 2 diabetes mellitus are all significantly correlated with obesity and are all risk factors for the development of atherosclerosis. Obesity is an independent risk factor for coronary artery disease.

4. **Dysrhythmias.** Hypoxemia, hypercapnia, electrolyte abnormalities, coronary artery disease, increased circulating catecholamines, heart failure, and fatty infiltration of the conduction system predispose the obese patient to cardiac dysrhythmias. The obese are at risk for sudden cardiac death.

5. **Valvular heart disorders**
    a. Patients who used the appetite suppressants **dexfenfluramine** or **fenfluramine** for more than 4 months are at an increased risk for cardiac valve disorders, particularly aortic regurgitation. These medications have been off the market since 1997.
    b. The mechanism of injury is postulated to be potentiation of serotonin-mediated valvular injury similar to that seen in patients with carcinoid syndrome or those taking ergot preparations.
    c. Though no cases have been reported with appetite suppressant and antidepressant serotonin-reuptake inhibitors, caution may be warranted in patients taking these medications.

B. **Respiratory system changes**
    1. **Respiratory compliance** (see also Chapter 3)
        a. Obesity is associated with a decreased compliance of the respiratory system.
        b. Adipose tissue within the thoracic cage, diaphragm, and abdomen coupled with an exaggerated thoracic kyphosis and lumbar lordosis decrease chest wall compliance.
        c. Increased pulmonary blood volume (from increased circulating blood volume) and closure of dependent airways decrease pulmonary parenchymal compliance.
        d. The obese abdomen restricts diaphragm descent, especially in the supine position.
        e. **Pulmonary function testing** may reflect these changes with decreased expiratory reserve volume,

inspiratory capacity, vital capacity, and functional residual capacity (FRC).

   f. Both obesity and anesthesia are associated with a **reduction in FRC.** In the supine position, FRC may fall within the closing volume, resulting in airway closure, ventilation-perfusion mismatch, and hypoxemia during normal tidal volume ventilation.

2. Respiratory insufficiency

   a. Oxygen consumption and carbon dioxide production are increased due to the elevated metabolic demand.

   b. Maintaining eucapnia requires increased minute ventilation and increased work of breathing.

   c. Hypoxemia due to ventilation-perfusion mismatch, intrapulmonary shunt, and coexisting respiratory disease results in respiratory insufficiency.

3. Obstructive sleep apnea (OSA) and obesity hypoventilation syndrome (OHS)

   a. Obesity is a risk factor for **OSA,** which is characterized by frequent episodes of apnea or hypopnea, snoring, excessive daytime sleepiness, and psychological changes.

   b. OSA is associated with increased cardiovascular morbidity and mortality.

   c. OSA may lead to **OHS,** which is characterized by central apneic episodes resulting in sustained hypercarbia and hypoxemia.

   d. The presence of **polycythemia** suggests long-standing hypoxemia.

   e. Long-standing hypoxemia and hypercarbia from **OSA and OHS** can lead to **pulmonary artery hypertension** and eventually right ventricular failure.

C. Other pathophysiologic changes

1. Gastrointestinal

   a. Obesity is associated with increased gastric volume, diaphragmatic hernia, and gastroesophageal reflux.

   b. However, there are no data to suggest that the obese are at increased risk for aspiration pneumonitis.

2. Hepatobiliary

   a. Abnormalities in lipid and cholesterol metabolism lead to fatty infiltration of the liver.

   b. Although fatty liver disease is generally benign, in some cases it can lead to cirrhosis, liver failure, or hepatocellular carcinoma.

   c. Risk factors for progression of disease include age greater than 45 years, BMI greater than 30, type 2 diabetes mellitus, alanine transaminase/aspartate aminotransferase ratio greater than 1, and female gender.

   d. Obese individuals are also at risk for **cholelithiasis,** especially with rapid weight loss after gastric bypass surgery.

3. Renal
  a. Glomerular sclerosis and nephron loss from increased GFR (from increased circulating blood volume and cardiac output), hypertension, and type 2 diabetes mellitus lead to chronic renal insufficiency and failure.
  b. Renal dysfunction leads to sodium retention, hypervolemia, and hypertension, causing additional glomerular damage.

4. Hematologic
  a. Obesity is associated with a **hypercoagulable state** with impaired fibrinolysis.
  b. Chronic hypoxemia causes **polycythemia**
  c. Vena cava compression and immobility lead to venous engorgement and stasis. These changes increase the risk of **deep venous thrombosis** (DVT) and **thromboembolism.**

5. Endocrine. Obesity is associated with hyperglycemia, insulin resistance, and hyperinsulinemia resulting in **type 2 diabetes mellitus.**

6. Metabolic syndrome
  a. The metabolic syndrome is defined by the presence of three or more of the following: abdominal obesity, high triglyceride level, low high-density-lipoprotein cholesterol level, hypertension, and/or high fasting plasma glucose level.
  b. Its incidence increases with waist circumference and BMI.
  c. This cluster of coronary artery disease risk factors has in common insulin resistance and is likely due to obesity and/or an inherited genetic defect.

7. Immunologic
  a. Excess adipose tissue is associated with the presence of **inflammatory cytokines** such as tumor necrosis factor-α and interleukin-6 and markers of inflammation such as C-reactive protein.
  b. Obesity is considered a low-grade inflammatory condition associated with **immunosuppression.**

8. Integument. Obese individuals are predisposed to intertriginous dermatitis.

9. Psychological. Obese individuals are at risk for depression and poor self-esteem.

IV. Bariatric surgery. Surgical treatment for obesity is gaining in popularity and is the most effective treatment for weight loss. Selection criteria for bariatric surgery include class III (morbid) obesity, failure of nonsurgical attempts at weight loss, absence of endocrine disorders that cause obesity, and psychological stability. Surgery is most effective when accompanied by pre- and postoperative comprehensive therapy to modify eating and exercise behavior.

A. Surgical approach. Several types of bariatric surgery exist, including gastric restrictive (stapled gastroplasty, gastric banding, and Roux-en-Y gastric bypass) and malabsorptive (biliopancreatic bypass) operations (Figs. 40-1 and 40-2).

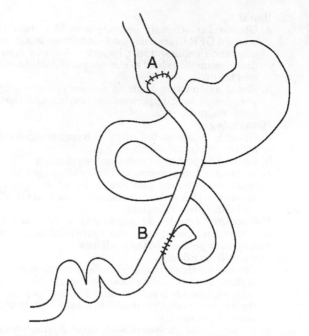

Fig. 40-1. Types of bariatric surgery. Roux-en-Y gastric bypass. A
15- to 30 ml gastric pouch is formed and anastomosed to the proximal
jejunum (A). A jejuno-jejunostomy is formed distally (B). (From
Ogunnaike BO, Jones SB, Jones DB, et al. Anesthetic considerations
for bariatric surgery. *Anesth Analg* 2002;95:1793–1805. With
permission.)

1. The **roux-en-Y gastric bypass** is the most commonly
   performed type of bariatric surgery and is often performed laparoscopically. Advantages of laparoscopy include less blood loss, shorter length of hospitalization,
   faster recovery, and a reduction in wound-related complications.
B. **Complications** (Table 40-2).
   1. **Risks**
      a. Procedural complexity, patient's age, degree of obe-
         sity, and coexisting medical conditions affect risk of
         perioperative complications.
      b. Patients with respiratory insufficiency, venous sta-
         sis, higher BMI, male gender, diabetes, cardiovas-
         cular disease, or those experiencing intraoperative
         complications are at higher risk for postoperative
         complications and should be considered for triage to
         an ICU.
   2. **DVT and pulmonary embolism (PE)** (Chapter
      22) occur in approximately 2.4% to 4.5% of patients

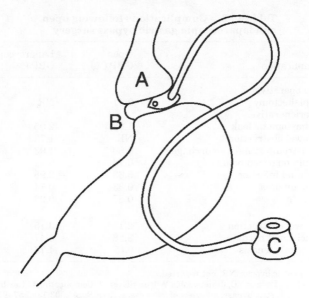

Fig. 40-2. Adjustable gastric banding. An adjustable, inflatable band (B) is placed around the proximal stomach (A) to limit oral intake. Saline is injected or removed through a needle port (C) to vary the size of the band. (From Ogunnaike BO, Jones SB, Jones DB, et al. Anesthetic considerations for bariatric surgery. *Anesth Analg* **2002;95:1793–1805. With permission.)**

undergoing bariatric surgery. The risk of DVT and PE in the obese patient having nonmalignant abdominal surgery is twice that of the lean patient.

3. Obese patients are at risk of postoperative **respiratory failure** due to respiratory muscle insufficiency, OSA, and OHS.

4. **Poor wound healing** in the obese leads to anastomotic breakdown and gastrointestinal leaks, stomal stenosis and/or obstruction, and bleeding.

5. The most frequent perioperative complication associated with both laparoscopic and open gastric bypass is **wound infection.**

6. The most frequent late complication after laparoscopic gastric bypass is anastomotic stomal stenosis, and that after open gastric bypass is incisional hernia.

7. **Perioperative mortality** associated with bariatric surgery is approximately 0.5%.

8. **Critical illness** in the obese patient carries **higher morbidity** than in the lean patient. Fortunately, less than 20% of patients who undergo gastric bypass surgery require to admission to the ICU.

Table 40-2. Complications following open and laparoscopic gastric bypass surgery

Complication	Open GBP (%)	Laparoscopic GBP (%)
Intraoperative		
Splenectomy	0.41	NR
Perioperative		
Anastomotic leak	1.68	2.05
Bowel obstruction	NR	1.73
Gastrointestinal hemorrhage	0.60	1.93
Pulmonary embolus	0.78	0.41
Wound infection	6.63	2.98
Pneumonia	0.33	0.14
Death	0.87	0.23
Late		
Bowel obstruction	2.11	3.15
Incisional hernia	8.58	0.47
Stomal stenosis	0.67	4.73

GBP, gastric bypass; NR, not reported.
Table from Podnos YD, Jimenez JC, Wilson SE, et al. Complications after laparoscopic gastric bypass: a review of 3464 cases. *Arch Surg* 2003;138:957–961. With permission.

V. Postoperative care. Postoperative intensive care of the bariatric surgical patient is challenging not only because of the technical difficulties encountered while caring for the obese, but also because of the significant number of preexisting medical conditions.

   A. Airway management

   1. Hospitalized obese are at increased risk of developing respiratory complications. Acute postoperative pulmonary events are twice as likely in the obese.

   2. Studies show that **high Mallampati score and large neck circumference** (see Chapter 4) but neither obesity nor BMI predict difficulty with laryngoscopy and intubation.

   a. Placing the patient in a "sniff" position by placing bolsters under the patient's head, neck, and shoulders or alternatively by placing the bed in moderate reverse Trendelenburg can improve the view of the glottic opening during intubation.

   3. Because emergent reintubation may be necessary, extubation should be planned when **adequate personnel and appropriate airway adjuncts** are available.

   B. Respiratory failure

   1. Mechanical ventilation

   a. To avoid lung injury during mechanical ventilation, initial **tidal volumes** should be based on ideal body weight instead of total body weight. Tidal volumes can then be adjusted aiming for a reasonable inspiratory pressure limit (keeping in mind decreased chest wall compliance) and arterial partial pressure of carbon dioxide (see Chapter 20).

  b. Positive end-respiratory pressure (PEEP) may be used to prevent airway closure, atelectasis, and shunt.

2. **Weaning** from mechanical ventilation (see Chapter 23) may be difficult due to lack of pulmonary reserve, warranting the consideration of an **early tracheostomy.**

  a. Tracheostomy may be surgically difficult to achieve due to the increased amount of pretracheal tissue and anatomic distortions.

  b. Patients with a substantial amount of pretracheal tissue may need a **custom-made tracheostomy tube** because a standard tracheostomy may not fit properly.

  c. A tracheostomy tube with an adjustable flange (Rusch, Bivona) may be used temporarily until the custom-made tracheostomy tube is available.

C. **Hemodynamic monitoring.** Due to preexisting cardiovascular comorbidities, the critically ill obese patient is often a candidate for invasive hemodynamic monitoring (see Chapter 1).

1. An **arterial catheter** provides more reliable blood pressure measurement due to the difficulty in obtaining an optimal fit with the noninvasive blood pressure cuff.

2. **Central venous and pulmonary artery catheterization** may aid in evaluation of volume status and cardiac function in the setting of preexisting cardiovascular abnormalities (increased intravascular volume, hypertension, heart failure, ischemic heart disease, etc.) and renal insufficiency.

D. **Vascular access**

1. Excessive subcutaneous tissue may obscure landmarks and make **access technically difficult.** Ultrasound guidance may be helpful in identifying blood vessels.

2. Intertriginous dermatitis in the femoral crease may preclude placement of femoral venous and arterial catheters.

3. Despite the technical challenges, the rate of **line-associated complications** is not significantly increased in the obese.

E. **Postoperative analgesia**

1. **Ventilatory depression** is an important concern in the obese (especially in those with preexisting OSA or OSH).

2. **Opioids** should be given intravenously and not intramuscularly or subcutaneously because these routes may result in unreliable plasma levels. The initial dose for **patient-controlled analgesia** should be

based on ideal body weight and carefully titrated thereafter.

3. **Epidural** infusion of opioids and local anesthetic may provide effective analgesia.

   a. **Epidural placement** may be technically challenging due to obscurity of the usual bony landmarks as well as difficulty in placing the patient in the optimal position.

   b. **Catheter maintenance** in the epidural space may prove difficult due to the thick layer of subcutaneous tissue between the point of surface and ligament contact.

   c. **Local anesthetic** volume should be reduced by 20% to 25% because the volume of the epidural space is reduced by fatty infiltration and venous engorgement from increased intraabdominal pressure.

   d. **Analgesic adjuncts** such as nonsteroidal antiinflammatory agents should be utilized unless contraindicated.

F. Pharmacology

1. Little information exists regarding the **pharmacokinetics** and **pharmacodynamics** of drugs in obese individuals. Alteration in distribution, binding, and elimination necessitates titration of dose based on clinical endpoints and serum concentrations as opposed to weight.

2. Obesity decreases the enzymatic activity of cytochrome P-450. Steatosis and/or biliary dysfunction may decrease hepatic metabolism and clearance.

3. Increased circulating blood volume increases the initial **volume of distribution** for a given drug.

4. **Renal clearance** may be increased in the setting of elevated glomerular filtration rate (GFR) from increased circulating blood volume and cardiac output. Alternatively, chronic renal insufficiency and reduced GFR may decrease renal clearance.

5. **Plasma protein binding** is affected by increased concentrations of alpha-1 acid glycoprotein and hyperlipidemia.

6. **Drug dosing** is complicated. Some suggest dosing drugs based on ideal body weight or ideal body weight plus some fraction of the difference between total body weight and ideal body weight.

7. A sensible approach is to use short-acting, readily titratable drugs such as **propofol** and **fentanyl** and muscle relaxants with predictable kinetics such as *cis*-**atracurium**.

8. **Specific drugs**

   a. **Succinylcholine** dosing should be based on total body weight when used for rapid-sequence induction.

   b. **Desflurane** anesthesia is associated with faster immediate and intermediate postoperative recovery after general anesthesia than propofol or isoflurane in morbidly obese patients.

   c. The volume of distribution of certain **antibiotics** (namely **vancomycin** and **aminoglycosides**) correlates with total body weight and thus should be dosed accordingly.

   d. **Sedatives** may have a prolonged effect in the obese patient.

      (1) **Midazolam** has a prolonged effect due to accumulation in adipose tissue and inhibition of cytochrome P-450 3A4 by other drugs and/or obesity.

      (2) **Fentanyl,** but not morphine, shows a cumulative effect after prolonged use in the obese.

   e. Drugs with narrow **therapeutic indices** such as **aminophylline, aminoglycosides,** and **digoxin** may become toxic if dosed based on weight.

G. **Wound infection** is twice as common in the obese due to several factors.

   1. The thick, hypovascular adipose layer provides a rich **substrate for bacterial growth.**

   2. Hyperglycemia as well as chronic inflammation and immunosuppression lead to **impaired neutrophil migration and activation.**

   3. **Anastomotic leak** complicates approximately 1% to 2% of cases of bariatric surgery. Signs and symptoms include persistent fever, abdominal pain, leukocytosis, left shoulder pain, anxiety, hiccups, isolated left pleural effusion, persistent tachycardia, and tachypnea. Early recognition of this potentially devastating complication is a necessity. Antibiotic management of wound infections is discussed in Chapter 28.

H. **Skin**

   1. **Thorough assessment and monitoring** of skin integrity is very important in the obese.

   2. Multiple deep skin folds harbor moisture and bacteria and are commonly infected with fungus. Frequent washing with thorough drying and application of an antifungal powder may prevent skin-related complications.

   3. Large, open wounds are effectively treated with **vacuum-assisted closure.**

 I. **Deep venous thrombosis prophylaxis** (see also Chapter 12) should be started preoperatively and continued through the perioperative period with subcutaneous heparin or low-molecular-weight heparin, serial compression devices, and, when indicated, inferior vena cava filter.

 J. **Nutrition** (see also Chapter 9)

   1. During periods of metabolic stress, the obese are unable to mobilize their fat stores. Reliance on carbohydrates to fuel gluconeogenesis accelerates protein catabolism and increases the risk of **protein malnutrition.**

2. **Nutritional support** in the form of enteral or parenteral nutrition in the critically ill obese is a necessity.
3. In the absence of indirect calorimetry, patients should receive 20 to 30 kcal/kg of ideal body weight per day. Nitrogen balance should be maintained by providing 1.5 to 2.0 g/kg of ideal body weight of protein.
4. The Roux-en-Y gastric bypass procedure typically does not lead to malnutrition. However, other malabsorptive procedures may lead to bacterial overgrowth and protein calorie malnutrition.
5. Steatorrhea may cause a fat-soluble **vitamin deficiency.**
6. Gastrectomy may lead to an **acquired intrinsic factor/B_{12} deficiency** and iron-deficiency anemia.

K. **Elimination**
1. A **Foley catheter** should be placed until the patient can control micturition.
2. **Fecal incontinence** appliances often fail to fit properly, which may lead to soiling and infection. Rectal tubes are an option but may cause rectal necrosis. When used, the balloon should be deflated every 2 hours for 15 minutes.

L. **Equipment.** The standard ICU bed may not be adequate for the obese patient. **Special bariatric beds** are available with an 850-lb weight limit, a low air loss treatment surface, built-in scale, chair egress, rotational therapy, and percussion option.

SELECTED REFERENCES

Adams JP, Murphy PG. Obesity in anaesthesia and intensive care. *Br J Anaesth* 2000; 85:91–108.

Brolin RE. Bariatric surgery and long-term control of morbid obesity. *JAMA* 2002; 288:2793–2796.

Buchwald H. Overview of bariatric surgery. *J Am Coll Surg* 2002; 194: 367–375.

Cheymol G. Effects of obesity on pharmokinetics: implications for drug therapy. *Clin Pharmacokinet* 2000; 39:215–231.

Flegal KM, Carroll MD, Ogden CL, et al. Prevalence and trends in obesity among US adults, 1999–2000. *JAMA* 2002; 288:1723–1727.

Gastrointestinal surgery for severe obesity: National Institutes of Health Consensus Development Conference Statement. *Am J Clin Nutr* 1992; 55:615S–619S.

Hall JE, Crook ED, Jones DW, et al. Mechanisms of obesity-associated cardiovascular and renal disease. *Am J Med Sci* 2002; 324:127–137.

Koenig SM. Pulmonary complications of obesity. *Am J Med Sci* 2001; 321:249–279.

Levi D, Goodman ER, Patel M, et al. Critical care of the obese and bariatric surgical patient. *Crit Care Clin* 2003; 19:11–32.

Marik P, Varon J. The obese patient in the ICU. *Chest* 1998; 113:492–498.

Podnos YD, Jimenez JC, Wilson SE, et al. Complications after laparoscopic gastric bypass: a review of 3464 cases. *Arch Surg* 2003; 138:957–961.

Shenkman Z, Shir Y, Brodsky JB. Perioperative management of the obese patient. *Br J Anaesth* 1993; 70:349–359.

Obstetrics and Gynecology

Jason P. Jenkins and Kevin C. Dennehy

I. **Introduction.** The obstetric patient population is mostly a healthy one, but several conditions contracted during pregnancy are associated with significant morbidity and mortality. The gynecologic patient population represents extremes of age and often has significant comorbid disease. This chapter primarily discusses obstetric illnesses and, when appropriate, critical care of the gynecologic patient.

II. **Hyperemesis gravidarum** is characterized by excessive nausea and vomiting, not related to other pathology, that occurs for the first time before the 20th week of gestation and is severe enough to cause weight loss, dehydration, and electrolyte and acid/base disturbances. It can result in oliguria, ketonuria, hypochloremic metabolic alkalosis, and hemoconcentration. Rarely, confusion, coma, and death from hepatorenal failure will occur if appropriate treatment is not instituted.

A. **The incidence** of hyperemesis gravidarum varies from 0.3% to 1.5% of pregnancies. The disorder is self-limiting; it does not extend beyond the duration of the pregnancy, but can recur in subsequent pregnancies; its cause is unknown.

B. **Liver function tests** may also be abnormal, with the alkaline phosphatase being increased above the normal elevation expected during pregnancy. Bilirubin and aminotransferases may also be mildly elevated. Serum levels of 5'-nucleotidase and gamma-glutamyl transpeptidase should remain normal in the absence of liver disease.

C. **Other conditions** that may mimic hyperemesis gravidarum (e.g., peptic ulcer disease, intestinal obstruction, cholecystitis, intracranial pathology, genitourinary pathology, drug toxicity, and hydatidiform mole) should be excluded.

D. **Treatment** is aimed initially at correcting fluid and electrolyte abnormalities, followed by insulin administration for patients suffering from diabetic ketoacidosis.

E. **Antiemetic medications** may be administered during the first trimester after carefully weighing the risk of teratogenic drug effects against the adverse consequences of maternal dehydration, ketosis, and malnutrition on the fetus. A partial list of medications used to safely treat hyperemesis gravidarum, with their Food and Drug Administration pregnancy categorization in parentheses, includes **cylcizine** (B), **meclizine** (B), **diphenhydramine** (B in first trimester), and the serotonin 5-HT3 receptor antagonists (B) such as **ondansetron. Ginger** may also be somewhat helpful in alleviating symptoms, but concerns exist regarding its thromboxane synthetase inhibition, affecting sex-steroid differentiation and testosterone-receptor binding.

F. **Nutritional support** includes adequate calories, vitamins, especially thiamine to prevent the development of Wernicke-Korsakoff disease, and trace elements. Enteral feeding may work by preventing the mother from seeing or smelling food, but parenteral nutrition may be necessary.

III. **Preeclampsia and eclampsia**

A. **Preeclampsia** is characterized by hypertension (systolic blood pressure >140 mm Hg or >30 mm Hg above prepregnant values; diastolic blood pressure >90 mm Hg or >15 mm Hg above prepregnant values), proteinuria ($\geq$300 mg/24 h or $\geq$1+ on urine dipstick) and peripheral edema occurring usually after the 20th week of pregnancy. Hyperuricemia (serum urate >5.5 mg/dl) is present in almost all cases. **Severe preeclampsia** is characterized by a blood pressure of greater than 160/110 mm Hg, proteinuria ($\geq$5 g/24 h or $\geq$3+ on urine dipstick), oliguria (urine output <400 ml/24 h), epigastric or right upper quadrant pain, visual or cerebral disturbances, and, occasionally, pulmonary edema. **Eclampsia** is defined by the presence of seizures in a patient with preeclampsia. The cause of eclampsia is unknown. Immunologic incompatibility between the placenta and the maternal organs and a defect in trophoblastic invasion into the uterus have been postulated to produce an imbalance of placental prostaglandin release or nitric oxide synthesis. This results in endothelial dysfunction manifested as vasospasm, altered vascular permeability, and activation of the coagulation system.

B. **Effects on specific organ systems**

1. **Cardiovascular.** Total body water is increased, but intravascular volume may be reduced by 30% to 40%. Edema may complicate airway management. Central venous pressure is usually low. Myocardial function varies from hyperdynamic to depressed. A **pulmonary artery (PA) catheter** may be useful to monitor myocardial performance in patients developing left ventricular failure or pulmonary edema.

2. **Neurologic.** Seizure threshold is decreased and central nervous system (CNS) irritability is increased, presumably because of increased brain water, cerebral vasospasm, or thrombotic occlusion of the cerebral microcirculation. Hyperreflexic deep tendon reflexes are expected.

3. **Renal.** Injury to renal vascular endothelium results in proteinuria. Swelling of glomerular cells, termed "endotheliosis," results in a reduction in glomerular filtration and creatinine clearance.

4. **Hepatic** involvement can range from mild edema to periportal hemorrhages, subcapsular hematoma,

and, rarely, spontaneous hepatic rupture. Initial signs include epigastric tenderness with elevations in hepatic transaminase level and a reduction in synthetic function.

5. **Hematologic.** Increased platelet consumption causes **thrombocytopenia** (platelet count <150,000/mm³) in 15% of patients with preeclampsia. A qualitative defect in platelet function also may be present. A low-grade consumptive coagulopathy and primary fibrinolysis are common.

C. **Therapy**

1. **Goals**

   a. Control of hypertension and replacement of intravascular volume will reduce CNS irritability and improve organ perfusion.

   b. Eliminate the cause of the preeclampsia through delivery of the fetus. The timing of delivery depends on the clinical condition of the mother and the viability of the fetus. Provided hypotension is avoided, the antihypertensive agents mentioned in what follows provide good control of blood pressure with minimal effects on uterine blood flow.

2. **Pharmacologic therapy**

   a. **Magnesium sulfate** (loading dose of 2–4 g intravenously [IV] over 15 minutes followed by an infusion of 1–3 g/h) produces vasodilation and acts as an anticonvulsant. It is effective in preventing the recurrence of seizures in eclampsia and in seizure prophylaxis in preeclampsia. The infusion rate is reduced with renal insufficiency. The therapeutic range is a serum magnesium of 4 to 8 mEq/L. Levels of 7 to 10 mEq/L result in loss of deep tendon reflexes. Levels in excess of 10 mEq/L can produce respiratory depression and heart block. In case of an overdose, **calcium gluconate** administration will reverse the harmful skeletal muscle effects. Magnesium therapy is usually continued for 24 hours after delivery because eclampsia can develop in up to 20% of cases in the postpartum period.

   b. **Labetalol** (5–10 mg IV every 5–10 minutes or administered by IV infusion) produces combined α- and β-blockade, which rapidly reduces blood pressure and causes minimal reflex tachycardia.

   c. **Hydralazine** (5–10 mg IV every 15 minutes as needed) dilates arteriolar smooth muscle. The peak antihypertensive effect occurs in 10 to 20 minutes following IV administration. Reflex tachycardia and postural hypotension are common.

   d. **Sodium nitroprusside** is a fast-acting, direct vasodilator with a very short duration of action used to treat hypertensive crises. Because of concern regarding fetal cyanide toxicity (the fetal liver has less thiosulfate substrate for rhodanese detoxification of cyanide than the maternal liver), infusion duration should be limited to that time of immediate danger to the mother.

    e. Fenoldopam (0.03–1.0 μg/kg/min IV infusion) is a dopamine-1–receptor agonist with potent vasodilator and natriuretic properties indicated for the acute management of hypertensive crises. It does not cause cyanide toxicity but can cause reflex tachycardia, flushing, nausea, and vomiting.

IV. HELLP syndrome

A. HELLP syndrome is characterized by **hemolysis, elevated liver enzymes,** and **low platelets.** It usually occurs in association with preeclampsia, but can occur without hypertension and proteinuria. The cause is unknown. Intravascular platelet activation and microvascular endothelial damage are pathologic hallmarks.

    1. Symptoms include malaise, nausea, vomiting, and epigastric or right upper quadrant pain.

    2. Diagnosis relies on the demonstration of:

        a. An abnormal peripheral blood smear and an elevated bilirubin level (>1.2 mg/dl).

        b. Aspartate aminotransferase greater than 70 IU/L and lactate dehydrogenase greater than 600 IU/L.

        c. Platelet count less than 100,000/mm^3.

    3. Differential diagnosis includes hepatitis, gallbladder disease, acute fatty liver of pregnancy, and thrombotic thrombocytopenic purpura. All patients have evidence of diffuse intravascular coagulation (DIC). Severe DIC is extremely rare.

    4. Treatment is supportive along with immediate delivery. The abnormal laboratory values return to normal in 2 to 7 days. Maternal and fetal morbidity increase with increasing disease severity.

V. Acute fatty liver of pregnancy

A. This idiopathic condition is characterized by a short history of malaise, anorexia, persistent nausea or vomiting, heartburn, upper abdominal pain, mild jaundice, fevers, and hematemesis. Some patients will also have concomitant diabetes insipidus. This condition may be caused by a defect in mitochondrial β-oxidation of fatty acids causing microvesicular steatosis of the liver. The incidence has been reported to vary from 1 in 6,600 to 1 in 15,900 deliveries. Half of these patients are nulliparous, and the average maternal age is 27 years. The average gestation is 37.5 weeks, with a predominance of male fetuses (from 3:1 to 5:1) and an increased incidence with twins. The maternal and fetal mortality rates are 10% and 20%, respectively. Morbidity and mortality are caused by DIC with fibrin-induced organ dysfunction, gastrointestinal hemorrhage, renal failure, acute pancreatitis, and fulminant hepatic failure.

B. Laboratory findings include elevated transaminase, bilirubin, prothrombin time, partial thromboplastin time (PTT), blood urea nitrogen (BUN), creatinine, and white blood cell count; fibrinogen and glucose levels are decreased. Tests of acute or chronic viral hepatitis should be performed to exclude an infectious cause. The gallbladder should be imaged to exclude choledocholithiasis. A liver biopsy can be helpful in the diagnosis of questionable cases, but should be considered carefully if coagulation studies are abnormal.

C. **Delivery of the fetus** is necessary to halt progression of the condition. Although most patients do not develop problems with excess bleeding, occasionally hemorrhage can be severe. Laboratory values return toward normal values 5 to 7 days following delivery.

VI. **Acute respiratory distress syndrome (ARDS) in pregnancy**

A. **ARDS** is described in Chapter 20.

B. **Common causes** of ARDS during pregnancy include infections (e.g., urinary tract infections, viral causes, endometritis, amnionitis), preeclampsia or eclampsia, acute fatty liver of pregnancy, tocolytic therapy with beta-agonists, aspiration during anesthesia, and massive hemorrhage.

C. **The clinical course** is variable. **Increased intraabdominal pressures** during pregnancy will be transmitted to the diaphragm and reduce thoracic compliance and functional residual capacity. The physiologic anemia of pregnancy and reduced venous return (caused by inferior vena caval compression) can reduce oxygen delivery to peripheral tissues.

D. **Pulmonary and hemodynamic management** goals and techniques are generally as outlined in Chapters 8 and 20. Of note, little information is available regarding the use of prone positioning during pregnancy as a ventilatory strategy to improve matching of ventilation to perfusion. The use of vasoactive drugs also has not been extensively studied in pregnancy. α-adrenergic agonists can decrease uteroplacental blood flow but may be necessary to treat maternal hypotension. Extracorporeal lung support and inhaled nitric oxide (Chapter 20) may be useful adjunctive therapies in selected patients.

E. **Obstetric management.** The timing and the route of neonatal delivery are determined on an individual basis. The mother should be monitored for signs of active labor and the fetus for signs of fetal distress. If delivery is indicated, some authors recommend vaginal delivery and reserve cesarean section for obstetric indications. Successful vaginal deliveries during mechanical ventilation for ARDS have been reported.

F. **Morbidity in the parturient with acute respiratory failure** is significant. A prolonged course of mechanical ventilation, however, does not imply increased maternal mortality. In one series, 6 of 9 mothers intubated for more than 40 days survived.

VII. **Asthma**

A. **Asthma** continues to be a cause of maternal mortality. Because of its prevalence in the general population (approximately 9%), it is the most common respiratory complaint in pregnancy (approximately 6%). It is characterized by reversible airway obstruction, airway inflammation, and increased bronchial smooth muscle reactivity to a variety of stimuli (Chapter 21).

B. **Treatment of the asthmatic parturient** is the same as for the nonpregnant patient. Inhaled β-adrenergic agonists, anticholinergics, corticosteroids, and sodium cromoglycate, oral corticosteroids, and leukotriene inhibitors have all been used during pregnancy. The effect of these drugs on the fetus is less than the resultant effects of inadequately treated asthma.

Approximately 10% of asthmatic patients will have an exacerbation of their asthma during labor. Supplemental doses of corticosteroids (hydrocortisone 50–100 mg every 8 hours during labor) should be administered to those who have been receiving steroids. Prostaglandin $F_{2\alpha}$ causes bronchoconstriction and should be avoided as a treatment for uterine atony.

C. **The overall perinatal prognosis** is comparable to that of the nonasthmatic population if asthma is well managed. Patients with moderate or severe asthma do, however, have an increased rate of cesarean delivery.

VIII. **Diabetic ketoacidosis (DKA)**

A. **DKA** is characterized by insulin deficiency, hyperglycemia, acidosis, and dehydration (Chapter 27). Early and frequent antenatal screening for diabetes mellitus has reduced the morbidity associated with the development of DKA during pregnancy. The fetal mortality was as high as 90% prior to 1975, but more recently is reported to be 35%.

B. **The cause** of the adverse effects of DKA on the fetus is unknown. Maternal dehydration and acidosis can cause fetal hypoxia through impaired uterine blood flow. Maternal hypokalemia can cause fetal cardiac dysrhythmias. The relative catabolic state that exists during pregnancy results in relative hypoglycemia, hypoinsulinemia, hyperketonemia, and protein catabolism. Therefore, DKA can develop at lower serum glucose levels than it does in the nonpregnant diabetic patient.

C. **Clinical features** of DKA are the same in the pregnant patient as the nonpregnant patient; they range from vomiting, polyuria, and polydypsia to disorientation and coma.

D. **Laboratory abnormalities** include hyperglycemia, acidosis (arterial pH <7.3, serum HCO_3 <15 mEq/L, with an anion gap >12 mEq/L), and ketonemia. Serum osmolality and plasma glucose values, although variable, usually are greater than 280 mOsm/kg and greater than 300 mg/dl, respectively.

E. **Management.** Baseline laboratory data including complete blood count, electrolytes, serum creatinine, BUN, serum phosphorus, and serum magnesium should be obtained. A **source of infection** should be sought and

Table 41-1. Management of diabetic ketoacidosis in pregnancy

1. Admit to an intensive care unit
2. Position the patient with left lateral tilt and monitor the fetal heart rate
3. Ensure airway protection if the patient is comatose
4. Ensure adequate oxygenation
5. Obtain baseline lab data
6. Place central venous and arterial lines as indicated
7. Monitor urine output
8. Search for the source of infection (blood, urine cultures)

appropriate cultures should be done. Antibiotic therapy is directed toward a specific source or begun empirically if infection is suspected. General management following admission to an intensive care unit (ICU) is detailed in Table 41-1 (also see Chapter 27). Specific measures concerning fluid, electrolyte, and insulin administration are detailed in Table 41-2. Maintaining a target blood glucose between 80 and 110 mg/dl may reduce morbidity

Table 41-2. Correction of metabolic abnormalities associated with diabetic ketoacidosis in pregnancy

Fluids
1. Administer 0.9% saline at 1 L/h for the first 1–2 hours
2. Administer 0.45% saline at 1 L/h for the first 1–2 hours if Na^+ >155 mEq/L, serum osmolality >320 mOsm/kg, or pH <7.0
3. Administer 0.45% saline at 250–400 ml/h after the first 1–2 hours of fluid replacement
4. Add 5% dextrose to fluids and reduce infusion to 150 ml/h as serum glucose reaches 200 mg/dl

Insulin
1. Administer an intravenous loading dose of 0.4 IU/kg regular insulin
2. Administer continuous infusion at 6–10 IU/h
3. Double the infusion rate if there is no response within 1 hour
4. Decrease the infusion to 1–2 IU/h as serum glucose decreases to 250 mg/dl
5. Continue the infusion at reduced rate for 12–24 h after diabetic ketoacidosis has resolved

Potassium
1. Administer KCl at 40 mEq/h if serum potassium <3.0 mEq/L
2. Administer KCl at 20 mEq/h if serum potassium is normal
3. Withhold KCl if serum potassium ≥6 mEq/L
4. Monitor electrocardiogram if oliguric

Bicarbonate
1. Add 100 ml of 8.4% $NaHCO_3$ to each liter of 0.45% saline if pH <7.0; solution approaches isotonicity

and mortality in critically ill patients, but the effect of this strategy in pregnant diabetics has not been tested.

F. Obstetric management. Preterm contractions and abnormal fetal biophysical profiles can revert to normal following treatment of the underlying maternal condition. Magnesium should be used for tocolysis if necessary. β-adrenergic agonists promote glycogenolysis and lipolysis and can aggravate the DKA. Corticosteroids administered to promote fetal lung maturity can have similar adverse effects. Maternal stabilization with the fetus *in utero* is probably the best course. An emergency cesarean section offers minimal benefit to the fetus and exposes the parturient to the increased risks of an operative delivery.

IX. Cardiovascular disease (see also Chapter 18)

A. Valvular heart disease

1. **Severe or critical aortic stenosis (AS)** has been reported to result in a maternal mortality rate of 17%.

   a. It is recommended that these patients undergo corrective surgery prior to becoming pregnant.

   b. Percutaneous balloon valvuloplasty may be necessary during pregnancy or postpartum.

   c. Antibiotic prophylaxis should be administered during labor and delivery.

2. **Aortic regurgitation (AR)** is more common in women of childbearing age than AS; 75% of cases are caused by previous rheumatic fever.

   a. Acute AR can follow rupture of the valvular apparatus caused by endocarditis, trauma, or aortic dissection from cystic medial necrosis of the aorta. The result is an increase in left ventricular end-diastolic volume and left ventricular end-diastolic pressure with left ventricular failure and eventual development of pulmonary edema. If this occurs acutely, emergency surgery may be necessary to save the life of the mother.

   b. Antibiotic prophylaxis should be administered during labor and delivery.

   c. Treatment with digoxin, salt restriction, and diuretics may be necessary during pregnancy and continued into the postpartum period.

3. **Severe mitral stenosis** is common following rheumatic fever. Approximately 90% of pregnant women who have rheumatic heart disease have mitral stenosis.

   a. **Beta-blocker administration** has been shown to reduce the incidence of maternal pulmonary edema without adverse effect on the fetus or neonate.

   b. The *autotransfusion* that occurs at delivery can result in severe volume overload and pulmonary edema. Intravenous nitroglycerin and diuresis may attenuate these rapid changes. However, because of the fixed nature of blood flow from the left atrium to the left ventricle, hypovolemia and reduced venous return including aortocaval compression must be prevented.

c. Those patients with mitral stenosis who are asymptomatic prior to becoming pregnant usually tolerate pregnancy well. Those with preexisting pulmonary edema have a higher incidence of mortality during or after pregnancy.

d. **Closed mitral valvotomy or balloon valvuloplasty** may be necessary during pregnancy and is performed if maternal symptoms warrant. Mortality rate is approximately 2% to 3% following valvotomy. It is a palliative procedure that may allow completion of the pregnancy.

e. **Antibiotic prophylaxis** should be administered during labor and delivery.

4. **Mitral regurgitation (MR)** can occur secondary to rheumatic heart disease, myxomatous degeneration, congenital causes, endocarditis, hypertrophic cardiomyopathy, trauma, or, occasionally, following spontaneous chordal rupture. Mortality related to MR is low in pregnancy unless MS coexists. Chronic, severe MR results in increased left atrial pressure. Antibiotic prophylaxis should be administered during labor and delivery.

5. **Mitral valve prolapse** appears to be well tolerated during pregnancy with no increased risk of obstetric or fetal complications. MR can occur, however, and require treatment. Antibiotic prophylaxis should also be administered.

6. **Prosthetic cardiac valves** are associated with special risks during pregnancy.

a. Despite the replacement of a malfunctioning heart valve with a mechanical or bioprosthetic valve, some degree of myocardial, valvular, or pulmonary dysfunction usually persists.

b. **Thromboembolic phenomena** are a concern. All obstetric patients with mechanical valves and those with bioprosthetic valves who are also in atrial fibrillation or have demonstrated thromboembolism should receive anticoagulation.

c. Women with **porcine heterograft valves** and no risk factors do not require anticoagulation. For this reason, porcine heterografts are considered the best choice for valve replacement in women of childbearing age, although these valves can fail earlier than mechanical valves.

d. **Warfarin** is teratogenic and should not be administered during pregnancy.

e. **Endocarditis** is a potentially serious problem for the obstetric patient with a prosthetic valve. She should receive antibiotic prophylaxis for any genitourinary procedure performed during pregnancy.

7. **Cardiopulmonary bypass (CPB)** occasionally is necessary for progressive heart failure secondary to valve dysfunction, prosthetic valve failure, trauma, massive pulmonary embolism, or coronary revascularization. These cases are rare. Maternal mortality is reportedly less than 5%. Fetal mortality, however, is 30% to 50%, which is thought to be related to the preexisting condition of the mother and the abnormal blood flow and hypothermia associated with CPB. Should CPB be necessary shortly after vaginal delivery or cesarean section, the anticoagulation can cause profuse bleeding from the surgical site or the site of placental implantation. Inhibition of fibrinolysis using aprotinin has been reported to reduce bleeding complications associated with CPB in the early puerperium.

B. **Congenital heart disease** (see also Chapter 38):
   1. Women born with congenital heart disease frequently survive to childbearing age.
      a. **Common congenital lesions** include left-to-right shunts, tetralogy of Fallot (TOF), and coarctation of the aorta.
      b. **Left-to-right intracardiac shunting** can occur via an atrial septal defect (ASD), a ventricular defect (VSD), or a patent ductus arteriosus (PDA).
      c. **De-airing of all intravenous lines** and injections must be ensured in congenital lesions with a shunt.
      d. **Shunt reversal and paradoxical embolism** can occur in association with straining at delivery or with the reduction in systemic vascular resistance (SVR) following regional blockade. Mild degrees of shunting are generally well tolerated, and mortality in this group is less than 1%.
   2. **TOF** involves a VSD, right ventricular hypertrophy, right ventricular outflow tract (RVOT) obstruction, and an aorta that overrides the right and left ventricles. Very few of these women survive to childbearing age without surgical correction. Correction usually involves closure of the VSD and widening of the RVOT. Reduction in SVR will increase the right-to-left shunting. The mortality rate in corrected TOF is less than 1%, but is 5% to 15% if the TOF has not been corrected.
   3. **Uncorrected coarctation of the aorta** places patients at risk for left ventricular failure, aortic rupture or dissection, and endocarditis during pregnancy. The mortality rate in this group is 5% to 15%. The coarctation is usually located just distal to the left subclavian artery, and patients will have a gradient between blood pressure measured in the upper and lower limbs. Fetal mortality approaches 20%.
      a. The condition is associated with intracranial aneurysms and bicuspid aortic valves.

   b. Invasive monitoring proximal and distal to the coarctation will allow measurement of uterine perfusion pressure and maintenance of the pre-existing gradient if interventions are planned.

   c. Antibiotic prophylaxis should be administered.

C. Coronary artery disease (see also Chapter 17)

   1. The risk of myocardial infarction (MI) during pregnancy has been estimated to be between 1 per 10,000 and 1.5 per 100,000 deliveries. Most occur in the third trimester. The incidence of MI in this patient population appears to be increasing along with mean maternal age. More than half of women suffering an MI during pregnancy are of age at least 35 years.

   2. Approximate occurrences of MI are 40% secondary to coronary atherosclerosis; 10% from coronary aneurysms or obstruction; 30% to 40% from coronary thrombosis; and 10% in those with normal coronary arteries. Smoking and cocaine use are significant cofactors. The mortality rate is approximately 30%, with the greatest risk of death occurring immediately following infarction and if the MI occurs around the time of delivery. An MI occurring in association with severe preeclampsia is associated with a particularly poor prognosis.

   3. Investigations should include serial electrocardiograms (ECGs), cardiac enzymes, tests of coagulation, full blood count, BUN, creatinine level, and electrolytes. An echocardiogram can be useful for establishing ventricular and valvular function. Cardiac catheterization may demonstrate a coronary lesion and be followed by percutaneous transluminal coronary angioplasty (PTCA) or coronary bypass grafting.

   4. Systemic thrombolytic therapy has been associated with significant maternal bleeding, premature labor, and dysfunctional uterine contractions. Little or no information is available on the use of intracoronary lytic therapy, dipyridamole, aspirin, or clopidogrel administration following MI in the pregnant patient. The use of inotropes and an intraaortic balloon pump may be necessary.

   5. Adjunctive therapy includes administration of β-blockers, heparin, nitroglycerin, and oxygen, and lateral uterine displacement. The timing and method of delivery should be determined on a case-by-case basis.

D. Pulmonary hypertension is present when the mean pulmonary artery pressure is greater than 25 mm Hg.

   1. Primary pulmonary hypertension (PPH) is a progressively fatal disease of unknown cause. Estimates of the incidence of PPH range from 1 to 2 per million of the general population. The pathophysiology involves pulmonary vasoconstriction, vascular wall remodeling, and thrombosis, leading to right ventricular failure (RVF) and death. RVF can rapidly ensue when pregnancy-induced increases of blood volume and cardiac output are superimposed on pre-existing PPH.

a. Diagnosis is based on the demonstration of elevated pulmonary artery pressures by cardiac catheterization or echocardiography.

b. Management should be individualized in each case and a multidisciplinary team approach adopted. It has been suggested that these patients be admitted to the hospital 4 to 8 weeks before delivery. **Oxygen,** either continuous or for a few hours each day and at night, has been recommended. **Anticoagulation** with either subcutaneous or IV heparin may prevent pulmonary emboli (PE). Minute PE can be fatal in established pulmonary hypertension. **Specific pulmonary vasodilator therapy** has been attempted. High-dose calcium-channel blockade (20 mg of nifedipine orally every hour until an effect is seen); **inhaled nitric oxide** at 20 to 80 ppm; and inhaled, subcutaneous (SQ) or IV prostacyclin can be useful if the patient has some reversibility of pulmonary vasoconstriction. Newer phosphodiesterase inhibitors (e.g., **sildenafil**), which act by enhancing nitric oxide-dependent cGMP-mediated pulmonary vasodilation, are being investigated. **Bosentan,** a new endothelin-receptor antagonist, is unfortunately contraindicated in pregnancy due to teratogenicity. Monitoring with a **PA catheter** is useful for determining the effects of drug administration. **Systemic arterial pressure** should be maintained greater than PA pressure to ensure adequate coronary perfusion of the right ventricle. Heart-lung or lung transplantation should be considered early in those patients who do not respond to pulmonary vasodilator therapy and urgently in those with critically low cardiac output. End-stage right ventricular failure usually does not respond well to inotrope administration.

2. Secondary pulmonary hypertension can develop from long-standing mitral valve disease, Eisenmenger's syndrome, or untreated ASD, VSD, PDA, or TOF. The mortality rate in these patients is 25% to 50%. Causes of death include embolism, dysrhythmia, right ventricular failure, myocardial infarction, and hypotension.

E. Peripartum cardiomyopathy is characterized by heart failure of unknown etiology but may be due to myocarditis arising from an infectious, autoimmune, or idiopathic process. Its incidence is 1 in 1,300 to 1 in 15,000 pregnancies, most commonly in obese, black, multiparous women of age greater than 30 years. It is estimated that 250 to 1,350 women develop peripartum cardiomyopathy in the United States each year.

1. **Diagnosis** is based on evidence of left ventricular dysfunction (i.e., left ventricular ejection fraction <45%), symptoms of heart failure that manifest in the last month of pregnancy or within 5 months of delivery, and no other apparent cause of heart failure. These patients have an increased incidence of premature births and low-birth-weight babies.

2. **Treatment** involves fluid restriction, modest daily exercise, amlodipine, hydralazine, nitrates, digoxin, diuretics, α-blockers, angiotensin-converting-enzyme inhibitors or angiotensin II-receptor blockers, and anticoagulation. Low-dose β-blockers may be added postpartum, and inotropes may be considered for those unresponsive to other therapies. For those patients with progressive disease despite optimal medical management, cardiac transplantation may be necessary.

3. Interpretation of data from follow-up studies is difficult because of the small number of patients who develop peripartum cardiomyopathy. Some studies suggest that 50% of patients will have spontaneous resolution of their symptoms; others suggest that 93% have progressive or persistent cardiomyopathy with eventual death or transplant as an endpoint. Subsequent pregnancies in those who recover have been uneventful in 75% of cases and resulted in temporary deterioration in 25%. Subsequent pregnancies in those with persistent cardiomyopathy have resulted in death in up to 50% of these patients.

X. **Neurologic problems** (see also Chapter 29)

A. **Stroke.** The risk of stroke during pregnancy has been estimated at 5.6 per 100,000 deliveries. Ischemic and hemorrhagic strokes are responsible for approximately one-third and two-thirds of events, respectively. Transient ischemic attacks and cerebral infarction are five times more common during pregnancy and the early puerperium than in the nonpregnant patient.

1. **Common signs and symptoms** include severe headaches, weakness, aphasia, and visual disturbances. Evaluation should proceed urgently with computed tomography, angiography, or magnetic resonance imaging.

2. **Reversible causes** include carotid artery or cerebral venous thrombosis or a leaking aneurysm or arteriovenous (AV) malformation. These can be successfully treated surgically, or recanalization may be possible by using thrombolytics and interventional radiologic procedures. Surgical management of aneurysms, but not AV malformations, has been associated with significantly lower maternal and fetal mortality. Care is supportive, but there are case

reports of delivery by cesarean section at the time of aneurysm clipping.

3. The risk of **aneurysm** bleeding increases as pregnancy progresses. Some authors recommend urgent delivery should subarachnoid hemorrhage (SAH) occur during labor. Treatment of arterial spasm with nimodipine to prevent ischemic stroke following SAH has also been recommended. The prognosis following SAH is very serious, with maternal mortality rates as high as 80%.

B. **Status epilepticus** is characterized by a seizure lasting longer than 30 minutes or recurrent seizures without intervening recovery.

1. **Generalized tonic-clonic seizures** are those seen most commonly during pregnancy; however, petit mal and focal seizures of the temporal lobe and motor cortex status epilepticus also occur. Other causes, including eclampsia, encephalitis, meningitis, tumor, drug withdrawal, local anesthetic toxicity and intracranial hemorrhage, should be excluded.

2. When related to a preexisting epileptic focus, status epilepticus usually occurs in the second half of pregnancy and is associated with subtherapeutic levels of anticonvulsant drugs. Absorption of anticonvulsants falls, metabolism usually increases, and plasma protein binding falls, resulting in a decrease in total blood anticonvulsant levels and a lesser decrease in free, or unbound, drug. If possible, free drug levels should be monitored during pregnancy.

3. **Treatment goals** include (a) maintaining an adequate airway, (b) ensuring adequate oxygenation, (c) determining the cause of the seizure, and (d) stopping the seizure. The patient should be placed in the **lateral position** and supplemental oxygen administered. Further treatment of seizures is detailed in Chapter 29. Of note, valproate is categorized as class D in pregnancy and should be avoided if possible.

4. **The pharmacokinetics of phenytoin** loading in preeclamptic patients has been determined. Therapeutic free phenytoin levels can be achieved with a loading dose of 10 mg/kg initially, followed by 5 mg/kg 2 hours later.

5. **For intractable seizure activity,** electroencephalographic monitoring, suppression of seizure activity with high-dose barbiturates (20 mg/kg phenobarbital), tracheal intubation, and mechanical ventilation may be necessary.

XI. **Hematologic problems** (see also Chapters 12 and 22)

A. **Thromboembolic disease** is the leading cause of maternal mortality. Changes in the coagulation system during pregnancy result in a hypercoagulable state, but pregnant patients without risk factors have a low incidence of spontaneous venous thrombosis (0.5–3 per 1,000). The risk of recurrence has been reported to be between 7.5% and 12%.

1. **Risk factors** include increased age and parity, obesity, prolonged bed rest, surgery, acquired or congenital hypercoagulable states, and postphlebitic syndrome. The American College of Chest Physicians recommendations for antithrombotic therapy during pregnancy are listed in Table 41-3.

2. Controlled trials of thrombolytic therapy during pregnancy have not been performed. Use is generally restricted to hemodynamically unstable patients with acute PE or patients with extensive iliofemoral thrombosis and a low risk of bleeding. The risk of maternal hemorrhage is increased, and is greatest if these agents are given at the time of delivery. The pregnancy loss rate has been reported to be 5.8% following lytic therapy.

B. **Antepartum hemorrhage**

1. **Causes** of antepartum hemorrhage include the following:

   a. Placenta previa and vasa previa.

   b. Placental abruption.

   c. Uterine rupture.

2. The incidence of **placenta previa** is approximately 1 in 200 pregnancies. It is associated with multiparity, increased maternal age, previous cesarean section or uterine surgery, and previous placenta previa. Bleeding is painless and usually stops spontaneously on the first occasion. Subsequent hemorrhage can be more profuse and lead to shock. Up to 10% of patients have a coexisting placental abruption. Diagnosis is confirmed by ultrasound or, occasionally, a double set-up examination in which preparations are made for possible immediate delivery. Investigations include complete blood count, coagulation tests, and assessment of fetal lung maturity. Cross-matched blood should be available. Preparation should be made for a large-volume resuscitation because these patients can bleed spontaneously or secondary to placental incision during cesarean section and an increased risk of placenta accreta, increta, or percreta exists.

3. The cause of **placental abruption** (separation of the placenta before delivery) is unknown. Risk factors include hypertension, increased maternal age, tobacco and cocaine use, trauma, prolonged rupture of membranes, and history of previous abruption. The incidence is approximately 1% of pregnancies. The amount of vaginal bleeding can underestimate the true blood loss because a large hematoma may have formed at the placental site. Complications include fetal distress or death, shock, DIC, and acute renal failure.

4. **Uterine rupture** occurs following previous uterine surgery, trauma, inappropriate use of oxytocin; in grand multiparous patients; and secondary to tumors, uterine anomaly, and fetal macrosomia or malposition. Anterior rupture and extension into the

Table 41-3. The American College of Chest Physicians guidelines for antithrombotic therapy during pregnancy

Condition	Recommendation
Previous VTE prior to current pregnancy or thrombophilia with or without VTE	Surveillance, heparin (5,000 U SQ q12h or adjusted to an anti-Xa level of 0.1–0.3 U/ml), or prophylactic LMWH (dalteparin 5,000 U SQ q24h, or enoxaparin 40 mg SQ q24h to keep anti-Xa level 0.2–0.6 U/ml) throughout pregnancy followed by postpartum anticoagulation for 4–6 weeks. The indication for active prophylaxis is stronger in antithrombin-deficient women.
VTE or PE during current pregnancy	Adjusted-dose LMWH [weight adjusted, full treatment doses (e.g., dalteparin 200 U/kg q24h or enoxaparin 1 mg/kg q12h)] or heparin in full IV doses for 5–10 days, followed by q12h SQ injections to prolong 6-hour postinjection PTT into the therapeutic range and then held for delivery followed by postpartum anticoagulation for 6 weeks.
Planning pregnancy in patients who are being treated with long-term oral anticoagulants	Either heparin SQ q12h to prolong 6-hour postinjection PTT into the therapeutic range, or: Frequent pregnancy tests and substitute heparin (as above) for warfarin when pregnancy is achieved
Mechanical heart valves	Either heparin SQ q12h to prolong 6-hour postinjection PTT into therapeutic range, or LMWH to keep a 4-hour postinjection anti-Xa level at approximately1.0 U/ml, or: Adjusted-dose SQ heparin or LMWH as above until week 13, warfarin (target INR 2.5–3.0) until the middle of the third trimester, then restart SQ heparin or LMWH until delivery.
APLA and more than one previous pregnancy loss	Antepartum aspirin and heparin or LMWH as for previous DVT above.
APLA and no or one previous pregnancy loss	Either surveillance, aspirin 80–325 mg q24h, heparin 5,000 U SQ q12h, or prophylactic LMWH (dalteparin 5,000 U SQ q24h or enoxaparin 40 mg SQ q24h to keep anti-Xa level 0.2–0.6 U/ml).
APLA and previous venous thrombosis	Either heparin q12h SQ to prolong 6-hour postinjection PTT into the therapeutic range or LMWH to keep 4-hour postinjection anti-Xa level at approximately 1.0 U/ml. Resumption of long-term anticoagulation postpartum.

APLA, antiphospholipid antibodies; PTT, activated partial thromboplastin time; INR, International Normalized Ratio; LMWH, low-molecular-weight heparin; PE, pulmonary embolism; q12h, every 12 hours; q24h, every 24 hours; SQ, subcutaneous; VTE, venous thromboembolism.
Adapted from Ginsberg JS, Greer I, Hirsh J. Use of antithrombotic agents during pregnancy. *Chest* 2001;119:122S–131S. With permission.

uterine vessels laterally results in massive hemorrhage. Uterine repair can be possible, but hysterectomy may be necessary.

C. Postpartum hemorrhage. Usual blood loss is 300 to 600 ml following vaginal delivery and 500 to 1,000 ml following cesarean section. Any bleeding in excess of this is considered postpartum hemorrhage.

1. **Primary postpartum hemorrhage** occurs in the first 24 hours following delivery. **Secondary postpartum hemorrhage** occurs after 24 hours to 6 weeks postpartum.

2. **Causes** include uterine atony, trauma, retained placenta; placenta accreta, increta, or percreta; and uterine inversion.

3. **Management** includes the ability to administer large-volume resuscitation, continual assessment of the effectiveness of transfusion by following the hematocrit and coagulation tests, and correction of the obstetric cause of the problem.

4. **Pharmacologic treatment of uterine atony** includes IV infusion of **oxytocin, ergometrine** (100–250 μg, usually administered intramuscularly [IM]) with preexisting hypertension being a relative contraindication, or 15-methyl **prostaglandin F$_{2\alpha}$** (250 μg administered intramyometrially or IM), which can cause or aggravate bronchospasm. Correction of obstetric cause usually requires surgery but can be amenable to radiologic embolization.

XII. Amniotic fluid embolism (AFE) has an incidence of approximately 3 per 100,000 live births. The mortality rate is as high as 80%, with most deaths occurring in the first few hours.

A. Clinical features consist of rapid onset of hypotension and dyspnea, followed by development of coagulopathy (probably from the presence of factor X activator, circulating trophoblast, or hemorrhage caused by uterine atony), seizures, and cardiopulmonary arrest.

B. The cause is unclear. IV injection of autologous amniotic fluid does not produce the syndrome, and the amount of particulate matter found in the pulmonary vasculature does not correlate with the severity of the presentation. Unidentified vasoactive substances that cause intense PA vasoconstriction and right ventricular failure may be present in amniotic fluid. Pulmonary hypertension is of short duration in those patients resuscitated from AFE because their PA pressures are near normal when monitoring begins.

C. Treatment involves aggressive resuscitation methods. Tracheal intubation, mechanical ventilation, and establishment of the ability to administer large volumes of IV fluids and blood products should be performed. Early consultation with a hematologist and the blood bank may facilitate treatment of the coagulopathy. Monitoring should include arterial and PA catheters or transesophageal echocardiography. Pulmonary vasodilators and inotropic support of the heart, including possible intraaortic balloon pump or cardiopulmonary bypass, may be necessary.

D. Other sequelae include neurologic injury, ARDS, acute renal failure, and hepatic failure. Successful pregnancies have been reported in two patients who survived AFE.

XIII. Infectious complications

A. Toxic shock syndrome (TSS) is caused by infection with *Staphylococcus (S.) aureus* and release of toxin from the bacteria. TSS can develop following postpartum infections, with the use of contraceptive sponges or diaphragms, or with the use of tampons during menstruation. The mortality rate approximates 2% to 3%.

1. **Clinical features of TSS** include a fever of 38.9°C or greater; diffuse, macular erythroderma; desquamation, particularly of the palms and soles 1 to 2 weeks after onset of the illness; and systemic hypotension. Evidence of other organ system involvement can include vomiting, diarrhea, mucous membrane hyperemia, myalgia with elevated creatine phosphokinase levels, and disorientation or alterations in level of consciousness. Progression to multiple-organ failure can occur with hepatic and renal dysfunction, thrombocytopenia, and ARDS.

2. **Diagnosis of TSS** is based on the constellation of signs and symptoms. No specific diagnostic test is available. Differentiation between TSS and **toxic epidermal necrolysis (TEN)** can be difficult. Examination of the roof of a bulla reveals only epidermal cell layers above the stratum granulosum, whereas in TEN the roof is composed of the entire epidermis. This distinction is important because glucocorticoid administration may offer benefits in TEN but can aggravate TSS.

3. **General principles of therapy** include removing all foreign bodies, draining accessible collections of pus, administering IV antimicrobials, and looking for metastatic foci of infection. The peak serum antibiotic level should be documented to be eight or more times the minimum inhibitory concentration of the organism in all severe infections. Until susceptibility data are available, the choice of antibiotic for severe infections should ensure activity against all strains of *S. aureus*. A reasonable choice would be to administer vancomycin (30 mg/kg/d) in three divided doses. If the organism is found to be β-lactamase negative, therapy can be changed to penicillin G or nafcillin or continued with vancomycin if the patient is allergic to penicillin.

B. Chorioamnionitis occurs in approximately 1% of all pregnancies. Clinical signs include temperature greater than 38°C, maternal or fetal tachycardia, and uterine tenderness with or without foul-smelling amniotic fluid.

Ascending infection from the maternal genital tract is the most common cause, but blood-borne spread via the placenta has also been implicated. The infection is usually polymicrobial, with bacteroides, group B *Streptococcus,* and *Escherichia (E.) coli* organisms predominating. Maternal bacteremia occurs in 10% of patients.

1. **Maternal complications** include postpartum infection, sepsis, postpartum hemorrhage, and death. **Neonatal complications** include pneumonia, meningitis, sepsis, and death.

2. **Treatment** is based on antepartum antibiotic administration and results in reduced maternal and neonatal morbidity when compared with postpartum antibiotic therapy. A combination of ampicillin and gentamicin is generally effective.

C. **Pyelonephritis** is common during pregnancy. Clinical features of acute pyelonephritis include fever, rigors, flank pain, dysuria, frequency, pyuria, and leukocytosis. Bacteremia is documented in 10% to 15% of cases. Common causative organisms include *E. coli, Klebsiella* spp, and *Proteus* spp. Pyelonephritis is associated with an increased risk of preterm labor and delivery and pulmonary injury leading to ARDS. Excessive fluid administration and the concomitant use of tocolytics are associated with pulmonary injury. Hospitalization and IV antibiotic therapy are usually required.

XIV. Miscellaneous

A. **Local anesthetic (LA) toxicity** following regional anesthesia in nonpregnant, adult patients is greatest depending on the type of regional block performed (e.g., caudal > supraclavicular brachial plexus > interscalene brachial plexus > axillary brachial plexus > epidural).

1. Total serum **bupivacaine** levels greater than 4 μg/ml and total serum **lidocaine** levels greater than 10 μg/ml have been associated with cardiac toxicity. The serum concentration of **ropivacaine** that produces toxic manifestations is similar to that of bupivacaine, but the dose required to produce these levels is 40% to 50% greater for ropivacaine, probably because of its shorter elimination half-life and faster clearance. LA toxicity is exacerbated by hypoxia, acidosis, hyponatremia, and hyperkalemia.

2. **The pregnant patient** is more susceptible to LA toxicity because of reduced levels of α_1-acid glycoprotein, which results in increased levels of free LA in the blood.

3. **Clinical features** are manifested sequentially by convulsions, hypotension, apnea, and, finally, circulatory collapse. Provisions for airway management and ventilation should be available should seizures occur.

4. **Therapy.** Should cardiovascular collapse occur, norepinephrine and epinephrine are the drugs indicated for resuscitation. Norepinephrine use can be associated with fewer ventricular dysrhythmias

following resuscitation. Various degrees of atrioventricular conduction blockade can persist following resuscitation as well as ventricular tachycardias resembling torsades de pointes; these may respond to atrial pacing. Return of spontaneous circulation following bupivacaine-induced cardiovascular collapse may require prolonged resuscitative efforts, and thus standard advanced cardiac life support should be continued for at least 45 minutes following arrest. **Phenytoin** (7 mg/kg) has been shown to be useful for the treatment of resistant ventricular dysrhythmias associated with bupivacaine toxicity in neonates. Lipid emulsions have shown promise in some studies. No single drug is optimal for treating the various manifestations of bupivacaine-induced cardiac toxicity. Most recommendations have been extrapolated from animal research. The optimal treatment of toxic manifestations is prevention. This can be achieved by administration of small, fractionated doses and attention to the total dose administered. Toxicity appears to be additive if a combination of local anesthetics is administered.

B. **Cardiopulmonary resuscitation (CPR)** (also see Chapter 14):

1. **Cardiac arrest** in the pregnant patient is a rare event, estimated to occur in 1 of 30,000 deliveries. The causes include amniotic fluid embolism, pulmonary embolism, eclampsia, drug toxicity, aortic dissection, trauma, and hemorrhage. Cardiopulmonary resuscitation should include early airway protection by endotracheal intubation.

2. **Major mechanical changes** secondary to the enlarging uterus and its contents produce alterations in cardiopulmonary physiology, with peak effects noted in the second and third trimesters. With the patient supine, the gravid uterus obstructs the inferior vena cava (IVC) in the later stages of pregnancy, impairing venous return and thereby reducing cardiac output. The uterus may be displaced to the left, reducing the obstructive effect of the gravid uterus on the IVC by providing 30 degrees of left lateral tilt of the abdomen. The compressive force that can be generated on the sternum during CPR at this angle is reduced to 80% of the force generated in the supine position.

3. **Cesarean delivery of the fetus** has been recommended if CPR has not been successful within the first 4 to 5 minutes. This recommendation is based on anecdotal case reports describing successful CPR following delivery of the near-term fetus. Neonatal survival following perimortem cesarean section has been quoted to be between 50% and 70%, with good neurologic outcome provided the delivery occurs within 5 minutes of maternal arrest. The lower limit of gestational age for the beneficial effect of emergent delivery of the fetus during CPR is unknown. A case

of resuscitative delivery at 32 weeks' gestation has been reported.

4. **Venous access** during CPR should be placed above the diaphragm.

5. **Emergent thoracotomy and open cardiac massage** has been advocated if no response occurs during closed-chest CPR.

C. **Supine hypotensive syndrome** is caused by aortocaval compression by the gravid uterus and must be considered when caring for the pregnant patient in the intensive care setting. In the supine position, both the IVC and the aorta are compressed by the uterus. Compression of the IVC by the gravid uterus is evident as early as 13 to 16 weeks' gestation. This results in reduced femoral artery pressures, increased femoral vein and IVC pressures, reduced venous return to the heart, reduced stroke volume and cardiac output, compensatory tachycardia, and hypotension. Uterine and lower extremity blood flow decreases. Proper positioning of the pregnant patient to maintain left lateral displacement of the uterus is mandatory.

D. **Anticoagulant therapy** during pregnancy is used for the treatment of acute thromboembolic events and for prophylaxis of patients with a history of thromboembolism or thrombosis, valvular heart disease, or antiphospholipid antibody syndrome. Prospective data regarding anticoagulant therapy in pregnancy is difficult to obtain because pregnant women are usually excluded from many prospective studies. Table 41-3 lists the recommendations of the American College of Chest Physicians (see Chapters 12 and 22).

1. **Warfarin (Coumadin)** crosses the placenta and has the potential to cause both bleeding and teratogenicity in the fetus. The rate of fetal loss from Warfarin use ranges from 8% to 50%. Treatment with Warfarin during pregnancy is usually restricted to patients with mechanical heart valves whose fetus is between 12 and 34 weeks of gestation. The significant failure rate of heparin anticoagulation must be balanced against the risk of increased bleeding during a traumatic delivery if the mother has been anticoagulated with Warfarin. The incidence of adverse outcomes is reported to be 16.9% with Warfarin compared with 3% with heparin. Warfarin can be given to lactating mothers because little or none diffuses into breast milk.

2. **Heparin** is the anticoagulant of choice during pregnancy because it is a large, charged molecule and does not cross the placenta. **Heparin requirements increase** during pregnancy because of increases in heparin-binding proteins, plasma volume, renal clearance, and degradation by the placenta. It is difficult, therefore, to maintain an anticoagulant effect with subcutaneous heparin administration

throughout the pregnancy. Doses as high as 20,000 units every 8 hours may be necessary to maintain a therapeutic (PTT level). Subcutaneous (SQ) administration of heparin via a programmable pump may prove beneficial, but further studies are needed.

3. **Low-molecular-weight heparin (LMWH)** is derived from standard heparin by either chemical or enzymatic depolymerization to yield fragments that are approximately one-third the size of heparin. The dose–response relationship of LMWH has been shown to be more predictable; however, anticoagulant activity may be monitored with postinjection anti-Xa levels. LMWH does not cross the placenta.

4. **Thrombolytic therapy** during pregnancy has been relatively contraindicated because of the concerns of maternal and fetal hemorrhage, particularly at delivery or within the first 1 to 2 weeks postpartum. Streptokinase and tissue plasminogen activator do not cross the placenta in animals. Although little is known about human placental transfer, these agents are not thought to be teratogenic. Preterm delivery and fetal loss are other concerns.

5. **The choice of anticoagulant therapy** is based on the indication.

   a. **Acute thromboembolism** requires IV heparin anticoagulation for 5 to 10 days, followed by SQ heparin to prolong the 6-hour postinjection PTT into the therapeutic range. Adjusted-dose LMWH may be used to keep a 4-hour postinjection anti-Xa level between 0.5 and 1.2 U/ml. Prophylaxis should be continued for 6 weeks into the postpartum period, during which warfarin can be administered.

   b. **Prophylaxis** for patients who have had a previous thromboembolic event is generally recommended, but treatment strategies proposed by the various working groups are contradictory. Patients with risk factors (e.g., a previous deep venous thrombosis, a positive family history of thrombosis, chronic venous insufficiency) should probably receive prophylaxis. Others can be monitored with periodic ultrasound surveillance of the deep veins. Heparin (7,500–10,000 U SQ twice daily during pregnancy and continued postpartum) can be used for prophylaxis. The PTT should be checked early in pregnancy to ensure that it is not excessively prolonged and later in pregnancy to ensure that it is sufficiently prolonged. The PTT can become significantly prolonged at term because of reduced heparinase activity from placental aging. LMWH may be used to keep a 4-hour postinjection anti-Xa level between 0.2 and 0.6 U/ml.

c. **Prophylaxis for patients with mechanical heart valves** can involve heparin or LMWH administration throughout the pregnancy. Warfarin can be substituted during the second and third trimesters and then replaced with heparin or LMWH at the time of delivery.

SELECTED REFERENCES

Barbour LA. Current concepts of anticoagulant therapy in pregnancy. *Obstet Gynecol Clin North Am* 1997;24:499–521.

Chien PFW, Khan KS, Arnott N. Magnesium sulphate in the treatment of eclampsia and preeclampsia: an overview of the evidence from randomised trials. *Br J Obstet Gynaecol* 1996;103:1085–1091.

Datta S. *Anesthetic and obstetric management of high-risk pregnancy*, 2nd ed. St. Louis, MO: Mosby, 1996.

Donaldson JO. Neurologic emergencies in pregnancy. *Obstet Gynecol Clin North Am* 1991;18:199–212.

Ginsberg JS, Greer I, Hirsh J. Use of antithrombotic agents during pregnancy. *Chest*. 2001;119:122S–131S.

Knox T, Olans L. Liver disease in pregnancy. *N Engl J Med* 1996; 335:569–576.

Sibai BM. Treatment of hypertension in pregnant women. *N Engl J Med* 1996;335:257–265.

Thornhill ML, Camann WR. Cardiovascular disease. In: Chestnut DH, ed. Obstetric anesthesia: principles and practice. St. Louis, MO: Mosby, 1994:746–779.

Veldtman GR, Connolly HM, Grogan M, et al. Outcome of pregnancy in women with Fallot's tetralogy. *J Am Coll Cardiol* 2003;41:490.

Weinberg G. Current concepts in resuscitation of patients with local anesthetic cardiac toxicity. *Reg Anes Pain Med* 2002;27:568–575.

Wood AJJ. Drugs in pregnancy. *N Engl J Med* 1998;338:1128–1137.

Appendices

Supplemental Drug Information

Robert K. Hallisey, Jr.

Abciximab (Reopro)

Indications	To prevent thrombus formation following percutaneous transluminal coronary angioplasty (PTCA) and following stent placement
Dosage	Bolus: 25 mg/kg administered 10–60 minutes prior to PTCA Maintenance dose: 0.125 μg/kg/min to max 10 μg/min for 12 hours postprocedure
Effect	Glycoprotein IIB/IIIA inhibitor, preventing platelet adhesion and aggregation
Onset	2 hours
Duration	2–4 hours for bleeding; up to 24 hours for platelet recovery
Comments	Anaphylaxis may occur; hypotension with bolus dose; bleeding complications and thrombocytopenia are common side effects

Acetazolamide (Diamox)

Indications	Metabolic alkalosis; alternative antiepileptic agent; increased intraocular and intracranial pressures
Dosage	125–500 mg IV over 1–2 minutes or PO not to exceed 2 g in 24 hours
Effect	Carbonic anhydrase inhibitor that increases the excretion of bicarbonate ions
Onset	IV: 2 minutes
Duration	Extended-release capsule: 18–24 hours Tablet: 8–12 hours IV: 4–5 hours
Clearance	From 70% to 100% excreted unchanged in the urine within 24 hours
Comments	May increase insulin requirements in diabetic patients and cause renal calculi in patients with past history of calcium stones; may cause hypokalemia, thrombocytopenia, aplastic anemia, increased urinary excretion of uric acid,

and hyperglycemia; initial dose may produce marked diuresis; tolerance to desired effects of acetazolamide occurs in 2–3 days; rare hypersensitivity reaction in patients with sulfa allergies

Acyclovir (Zovirax)

Indications	1. Treatment of initial and prophylaxis of recurrent mucosal and cutaneous herpes simplex (HSV-1 and HSV-2) infections
	2. HSV encephalitis
	3. Varicella-zoster infections
	4. Herpes zoster, genital herpes, and varicella-zoster infections in immunocompromised patients
Dosage	May vary with specific indication

Adult:
1. IV: 750 mg/m^2/d divided every 8 hours or 15 mg/kg/d divided every 8 hours for 5–10 days
2. IV: 1,500 mg/m^2/d divided every 8 hours or 30 mg/kg/d divided every 8 hours for 10 days
3. IV: 1,500 mg/m^2/d divided every 8 hours or 30 mg/kg/d divided every 8 hours for 5–10 days
   Oral: 600–800 mg/dose 5 times/d for 7–10 days or 1,000 mg every 6 hours for 5 days
4. IV: 7.5 mg/kg/dose every 8 hours
   Oral: 800 mg every 4 hours (5 times/d) for 7–10 days

Pediatric:
1. IV: 750 mg/m^2/d divided every 8 hours or 15 mg/kg/d divided every 8 hours for 5–10 days
2. IV: 1,500 mg/m^2/d divided every 8 hours or 30 mg/kg/d divided every 8 hours for 10 days
3. IV: 1,500 mg/m^2/d divided every 8 hours or 30 mg/kg/d divided every 8 hours for 5–10 days
   Oral: 10–20 mg/kg/dose (up to 800 mg) 4 times/d
4. IV: 7.5 mg/kg/dose every 8 hours
   Oral: 250–600 mg/m^2/dose 4–5 times/d

Neonate:
HSV infection:
IV: 1,500 mg/m^2/d divided every 8 hours or 30 mg/kg/d divided every 8 hours for 10–14 days

Effect	Antiviral; inhibits herpes DNA synthesis
Onset	Oral: within 1.5–2 hours
	IV: within 1 hour
Duration	Half-life:
	Neonates: 4 hours
	Children 1–12 years: 2–3 hours
	Adults: 3 hours

Clearance	Primary route is the kidney (30%–90% of a dose is excreted unchanged); hemodialysis removes ~60% of the dose, whereas while removal by peritoneal dialysis is to a much lesser extent
Comments	Dose should be reduced in patients with renal impairment; use with caution in patients with preexisting renal disease or in those receiving other nephrotoxic drugs concurrently; use with caution in patients with underlying neurologic abnormalities and in patients with serious renal, hepatic, or electrolyte abnormalities or substantial hypoxia

Adenosine (Adenocard)

Indications	Paroxysmal supraventricular tachycardia, Wolff-Parkinson-White syndrome
Dose	Adult: 6–12 mg IV bolus Pediatric: 50 μg/kg IV
Effect	Slow or temporary cessation of AV node conduction and conduction through reentrant pathways
Onset	Immediate
Duration	<10 seconds
Clearance	Red blood cell and endothelial cell metabolism
Comments	Its effects are antagonized by methylxanthines such as theophylline; adenosine is contraindicated in patients with high-degree heart block or sick sinus syndrome; hypotension can occur; not effective in atrial flutter or fibrillation; asystole for 3–6 seconds is not uncommon

Albuterol (Proventil, Ventolin)

Indications	Bronchospasm
Dose	Adult: Aerosolized: 2.5 mg in 3 ml of saline via nebulizer, 180 or 200 μg (two puffs) via inhaler Oral: 2.5 mg Pediatric: Oral: 0.1 mg/kg (syrup 2 mg/5 ml)
Effect	β_2-receptor agonist
Onset	Immediate
Duration	3–6 hours
Clearance	Hepatic metabolism; renal elimination.
Comments	Possible β-adrenergic overload, tachydysrhythmias

Aminocaproic acid (Amicar)

Indications	Hemorrhage due to fibrinolysis
Dosage	5 g/100–250 ml of NSS IV to load followed by 1-g/h infusion.
Effect	Stabilizes clot formation by inhibiting plasminogen activators and plasmin
Clearance	Primarily renal elimination
Comments	Contraindicated in disseminated intravascular coagulation

Aminophylline (theophylline ethylenediamine)

Indications	Bronchospasm, infant apnea
Dosage	Adult: Loading dose: 5.0 mg/kg IV at <25 mg/min Maintenance dose: 0.5–0.7 mg/kg/h IV; lower dose in elderly, congestive heart failure, hepatic disease Pediatric: 1 month–1 year: 0.16–0.7 mg/kg/h 1–9 years: 0.8 mg/kg/h
Effect	Inhibition of phosphodiesterase and adenosine antagonism, resulting in bronchodilation with positive inotropic and chronotropic effects
Onset	Rapid
Duration	6–12 hours
Clearance	Hepatic metabolism, renal elimination (10% unchanged)
Comments	May cause tachydysrhythmias; therapeutic concentration, 10–20 μg/ml; each mg/kg raises concentration approximately 2 μg/ml; aminophylline 100 mg = theophylline 80 mg

Amiodarone (Cordarone)

Indications	Refractory or recurrent ventricular tachycardia or ventricular fibrillation; rapid supraventricular arrhythmias, particularly atrial fibrillation
Dosage	Loading dose: 800–1,600 mg/d PO × 1–3 weeks, then 600–800 mg/d PO × 4 weeks Maintenance dose: PO: 100–400 mg/d

	IV: 150 mg over 10 minutes (15 mg/min), 360 mg over the next 6 hours (1 mg/min), then 540 mg over the next 18 hours (0.5 mg/min)
Effect	Depresses the sinoatrial node, prolongs the PR, QRS, and QT intervals, and produces α- and β-adrenergic blockade.
Onset	Oral: 2 days–3 months
Duration	Weeks to months
Clearance	Biliary elimination
Comments	May cause severe sinus bradycardia, ventricular dysrhythmias, AV block, liver and thyroid function test abnormalities, hepatitis, and cirrhosis; pulmonary fibrosis may follow long-term use; increases serum levels of digoxin, oral anticoagulants, diltiazem, quinidine, procainamide, and phenytoin

Aprotinin (Trasylol)

Indications	Prophylactic reduction in perioperative blood loss in patients undergoing cardiopulmonary bypass
Dosage	Supplied as 10,000 kallikrein inhibitor units (KIU)/ml or 1.4 mg/ml; test dose 1 ml followed by: Loading dose: 1–2 million KIU (100–200 ml) IV over 20–30 minutes "Pump prime": 1–2 million KIU Maintenance dose: 250,000–500,000 KIU/h (25–50 ml/h)
Effect	Protease inhibitor of trypsin, plasmin, and kallikrein; antifibrinolytic; protects glycoprotein Ib receptor on platelets during cardiopulmonary bypass
Clearance	Renal elimination
Comments	Rapid administration may cause transient hypotension; anaphylactic reaction in <0.5% of patients

Argatroban

Indications	Therapeutic anticoagulation in patients with strongly suspected or confirmed heparin-induced thrombocytopenia (HIT type II)
Dosage	0.5–2 μg/kg/min titrated to 1.5–3 times activated partial thromboplastin time (aPTT) control; do not exceed 10 μg/kg/min

Effect	Inhibitor of bound and soluble thrombin
Clearance	Hepatic
Comments	Discontinue and remove all heparin products, obtain a baseline aPTT prior to initiating therapy (except in cath lab); once a stable dose is achieved, draw aPTT every 24 hours; obtain order for each change in dose; there is no antidote or reversal agent for argatroban; the International Normalized Ratio and prothrombin time may also be elevated, but should not be considered monitoring parameters; administer via a dedicated line, argatroban is not compatible with other drugs

Atenolol (Tenormin)

Indications	Hypertension, angina, following myocardial infarction
Dosage	PO: 50–100 mg/d
	IV: 5 mg prn (not available in the United States)
Effect	β_1-selective adrenergic receptor blockade
Onset	PO: 30–60 minutes
	IV: 5 minutes
Duration	PO: >24 hours
	IV: 12–24 hours
Clearance	Renal, intestinal elimination unchanged
Comments	High doses block β_2-adrenergic receptors; relatively contraindicated in congestive heart failure, asthma, and heart block; caution in patients on calcium-channel blockers; rebound angina may occur with abrupt cessation

Atropine

Indications	1. Antisialagogue
	2. Bradycardia
Dosage	Adult:
	1. 0.2–0.4 mg IV
	2. 0.4–1.0 mg IV
	Pediatric:
	1. 0.01 mg/kg/dose IV/IM (<0.4 mg)
	2. 0.02 mg/kg/dose IV (<0.4 mg)
Effect	Competitive blockade of acetylcholine at muscarinic receptors
Onset	Rapid
Duration	Variable

Clearance   50%–70% hepatic metabolism, renal elimination
Comments   May cause tachydysrhythmias, AV dissociation, premature ventricular contractions, dry mouth, or urinary retention; CNS effects occur at high doses

Azathioprine (Imuran)

Indications
1. Adjunct for prevention of rejection in allotransplantation
2. Rheumatoid arthritis

Dosage   May vary with specific indication
Adult:
1. Renal transplantation:
   PO, IV: 200–300 mg/d to start
   Maintenance dose: 50–200 mg/d
2. Rheumatoid arthritis:
   PO: 50–100 mg/d for 6–8 weeks; increase by 0.5 mg/kg every 4 weeks until response or up to 200 mg/d
   Maintenance therapy: the lowest effective dose

Pediatric:
1. Renal transplantation:
   PO, IV: 3–5 mg/kg/d to start
   Maintenance dose: 1–3 mg/kg/d

Effect   Antimetabolite, immunosuppressant
Clearance   Extensively metabolized by hepatic xanthenes oxidase to 6-mercaptopurine (active)
Comments   Dose should be reduced for white blood cell count (WBC) <4,000 cells/mm^3 and/or held for WBC <3,000 cells/mm^3; azathioprine metabolism is competitively inhibited by allopurinol, and dose reduction is required; use with caution in patients with liver disease, renal impairment; chronic immunosuppression increases the risk of neoplasia; has mutagenic potential to both men and women and with possible hematologic toxicities

Bicarbonate, sodium

Indications   Metabolic acidosis
Dosage   IV dose in mEq NaHCO3 = Base deficit × Weight (kg) × 0.3 (subsequent doses titrated against patient's pH)

Effect	Metabolic acid neutralization
Onset	Rapid
Duration	Variable
Clearance	Plasma metabolism; pulmonary, renal elimination
Comments	May cause metabolic alkalosis, hypercarbia, hyperosmolality; may decrease cardiac output, systemic vascular resistance, and myocardial contractility; in neonates, may cause intraventricular hemorrhage; crosses placenta; an 8.4% solution is approximately 1.0 mEq/ml; a 4.2% solution is approximately 0.5 mEq/ml

Bumetanide (Bumex)

Indications	Edema, hypertension, intracranial hypertension
Dosage	0.5–1.0 mg IV, repeated to a maximum of 10 mg/d
Effect	Loop diuretic with principal effect on the ascending limb of the loop of Henle; causes increased excretion of Na+, K+, Cl⁻, and H_2O
Onset	Immediate, peak 15–30 minutes
Duration	2–4 hours
Clearance	Hepatic metabolism, 81% renal excretion (45% unchanged)
Comments	May cause electrolyte imbalance, dehydration, and deafness; patients who are allergic to sulfonamides may show hypersensitivity to bumetanide; effective in renal insufficiency

Calcium chloride, Calcium gluconate (Kalcinate)

Indications	Hypocalcemia, hyperkalemia, hypermagnesemia, severe hypotension
Dosage	Calcium chloride: 5–10 mg/kg IV prn (10% $CaCl_2$ = 13.6 mEq Ca^{2+}/10 ml and 273 mg Ca^{2+}) Calcium gluconate: 15–30 mg/kg IV prn (10% calcium gluconate = 4.5 mEq Ca^{2+}/10 ml and 93 mg Ca^{2+})
Effect	Maintenance of cell membrane integrity, muscular excitation–contraction coupling,

	glandular stimulation–secretion coupling, and enzyme function; increases blood pressure
Onset	Rapid
Duration	Variable
Clearance	Incorporated into muscle, bone, and other tissues; rapid onset; variable duration
Comments	May cause tachycardia, bradycardia, and dysrhythmia (especially with digitalis); CaCl should not be administered peripherally undiluted except in emergency situations; CaCl has three times more available elemental calcium

Captopril (Capoten)

Indications	Hypertension, congestive heart failure
Dosage	Loading dose: 12.5–25.0 mg PO 2–3 times/d Maintenance dose: 25–150 mg PO 2–3 times/d
Effect	Angiotensin I-converting-enzyme inhibition decreases angiotensin II and aldosterone levels; reduces both preload and afterload in patients with congestive heart failure
Onset	15–60 minutes, peak 60–90 minutes
Duration	4–6 hours
Clearance	Hepatic metabolism; 95% renal elimination (40%–50% unchanged)
Comments	Can be used in hypertensive emergency; may cause neutropenia, agranulocytosis, hypotension, or bronchospasm; avoid in pregnant patients; exaggerated response in renal artery stenosis and with diuretics

Chlorothiazide (Diuril)

Indications	Edema, heart failure, acute/chronic renal failure, hypertension
Dosage	Adult: 250–500 mg IV push at 50–100 mg/min, 2,000 mg maximum over 24 hours Pediatric: oral, 20 mg/kg/d in two divided doses every 12 hours
Effect	Thiazide diuretic
Onset	2 hours
Duration	Oral: 6–12 hours IV: ~2 hours
Clearance	Renal elimination

Comments	Enhances activity of antihypertensives, digoxin; may enhance activity of loop diuretics in renal failure; may increase insulin requirements in diabetic patients

Clonidine (Catapres)

Indications	Hypertension; adrenergic overload due to narcotic withdrawal
Dosage	0.1–1.2 mg/d PO in divided doses (2.4 mg/d maximum dose); also available as a transdermal patch delivering 0.1, 0.2, or 0.3 mg/d for 7 days
Effect	Central α_2-adrenergic agonist, resulting in decrease in systemic vascular resistance and heart rate
Onset	30–60 minutes, peak 2–4 hours
Duration	8 hours
Clearance	50% hepatic metabolism; elimination 20% biliary, 80% renal
Comments	Abrupt withdrawal may cause rebound hypertension or dysrhythmias; may cause drowsiness, nightmares, restlessness, anxiety, or depression; IV injection may cause transient peripheral α-adrenergic stimulation

Dalteparin (Fragmin)

Indications	1. DVT/PE prophylaxis
	2. Therapeutic anticoagulation for treatment or prevention of thrombosis
	3. Acute coronary syndrome
Dosage	1. 2,500–5,000 units SQ daily
	2. 100 units/kg SQ q12h
	3. 120 units/kg SQ q12h
Effect	Binds with antithrombin III, and accelerates inactivation of factors IIa (thrombin), Xa, IXa, XIa, and XIIa
Onset	2 hours
Duration	10–24 hours
Clearance	Renal
Comments	Therapeutic doses should be used with caution in patients with renal impairment; factor Xa levels are of little value in

determining therapeutic response;
incompletely and unpredictably reversed by
protamine; do not use in patients with
heparin-induced thrombocytopenia

Dantrolene (Dantrium)

Indications	Malignant hyperthermia, skeletal muscle spasticity
Dosage	Prophylactic treatment is generally not recommended; if signs of malignant hyperthermia develop: 3 mg/kg IV bolus; if syndrome persists after 30 minutes, repeat dose, up to 10 mg/kg
Effect	Reduction of Ca^{2+} release from sarcoplasmic reticulum
Onset	30 minutes
Duration	8 hours
Clearance	Hepatic metabolism; renal elimination
Comments	Mix 20 mg in 60 ml of sterile water; dissolves slowly into solution; may cause muscle weakness, gastrointestinal upset, drowsiness, sedation, or abnormal liver function (chronically); additive effect with neuromuscular blocking agents; tissue irritant

Desmopressin acetate (DDAVP)

Indications	Coagulation improvement in von Willebrand's disease, hemophilia A, renal failure; antidiuretic
Dosage	Adult:
	1. 0.3 μg/kg IV (diluted 50 ml NSS), infused over 15–30 minutes preoperatively and/or every 12–24 hours up to a maximum of 3 days
	2. 2–4 μg/d usually in two divided doses
	Pediatric: <10 kg: dilute adult dose in 10 ml of NSS >10 kg: see adult dose
Onset	Minutes; peak 15–30 minutes
Duration	3 hours for von Willebrand's disease, 4–24 hours for hemophilia A

Effect	Increases plasma levels of factor VIII activity by causing release of von Willebrand's factor from endothelial cells; increases renal water reabsorption
Clearance	Renal elimination
Comments	Chlorpropamide, carbamazepine, and clofibrate potentiate the antidiuretic effect; for bleeding diathesis, repeated doses will have diminished effect compared to initial dose

Dexamethasone (Decadron)

Indications	Cerebral edema from CNS tumors; airway edema
Dose	Loading dose: 10 mg IV Maintenance dose: 4 mg IV q6h (tapered over 6 days)
Onset	IV: immediate
Duration	IV: 4–6 hours up to 24 hours
Effect	Antiinflammatory and antiallergic effect; mineralocorticoid effect; stimulation of gluconeogenesis; inhibition of peripheral protein synthesis; membrane-stabilizing effect; has 25 times the glucocorticoid potency of hydrocortisone; minimal mineralocorticoid effect
Clearance	Primarily hepatic metabolism; renal elimination
Comments	May cause adrenocortical insufficiency (Addison's crisis) with abrupt withdrawal, delayed wound healing, CNS disturbances, osteoporosis, or electrolyte disturbances

Dexmedotomidine (Precedex)

Indications	Short-term use as a sedative for patients undergoing mechanical ventilation in the intensive care setting
Dosage	Loading infusion: 1 μ/kg over 10 minutes Maintenance dose: 0.2–0.7 μg/kg/h;
Effect	Selective α-2 adrenoreceptor agonist used for short-term therapy as a sedative for patients undergoing mechanical ventilation in the intensive care setting

Onset	30 minutes
Duration	Up to 4 hours
Clearance	Hepatic
Comments	Hypotension can occur in about 30% of patients; transient hypertension may be associated with bolus dosing; hypoxia can occur in nonventilated patients

Dextran 40 (Rheomacrodex)

Indications	Inhibition of platelet aggregation; improvement of blood flow in low-flow states (e.g., vascular surgery); intravascular volume expander
Dosage	Adult: Loading dose: 30–50 ml IV over 30 minutes Maintenance dose: 15–30 ml/h IV (10% solution) Pediatric: <20 ml/kg/24 h of 10% dextran
Effect	Immediate, short-lived plasma volume expansion; adsorption to RBC surface preventing RBC aggregation, decreasing blood viscosity and platelet adhesiveness
Onset	Rapid
Duration	4–8 hours
Clearance	100% renal elimination
Comments	Administer Promit (dextran monomer), 20 ml IV, prior to giving dextran 40 to minimize the risk of anaphylaxis; may cause volume overload, anaphylaxis, bleeding tendency, interference with blood cross-matching, or false elevation of blood sugar; can cause renal failure

Digoxin (Lanoxin)

Indications	Heart failure, tachydysrhythmias, atrial fibrillation, atrial flutter
Dosage	Adult: Loading dose: 0.5–1.0 mg/d IV or PO in divided doses Maintenance dose: 0.125–0.5 mg IV or PO daily

	Maintenance dose: 20%–35% of load daily (reduce in renal failure)
Effect	Increase in myocardial contractility; decrease in conduction in AV node and Purkinje fibers
Onset	15–30 minutes
Duration	2–6 days
Clearance	Renal elimination (50%–70% unchanged)
Comments	May cause gastrointestinal intolerance, blurred vision, ECG changes, or dysrhythmias; toxicity potentiated by hypokalemia, hypomagnesemia, hypercalcemia; cautious use in Wolff-Parkinson-White syndrome and with defibrillation; heart block potentiated by β-blockade and calcium-channel blockade

Diltiazem (Cardizem)

Indications	Angina pectoris, variant angina from coronary artery spasm, atrial fibrillation/flutter, paroxysmal supraventricular tachycardia, hypertension
Dosage	Loading dose: 0.25 mg/kg (~15–20 mg; maximum dose 25 mg) direct IV bolus over 2 minutes; for inadequate response an additional 0.35 mg/kg IV over 2 min (~25–30 mg) may be given 15 minutes after initial dose
	Maintenance dose: 10 mg/h (5 mg/h if hemodynamically unstable); titrate by 2.5 mg/h every 0.5–2 hours to achieve desired heart rate; recommended maximum 30 mg/h
	PO: 30–60 mg q6h
Effect	Calcium-channel antagonist that slows conduction through sinoatrial and AV nodes, dilates coronary and peripheral arterioles, and reduces myocardial contractility
Onset	IV: 1–3 minutes
	PO: 1–3 hours
Duration	IV: 1–3 hours
	PO: 4–24 hours
Clearance	Primarily hepatic metabolism; renal elimination
Comments	May cause hypotension, bradycardia, and heart block; may interact with β-blockers and digoxin to impair contractility; causes transiently elevated liver function tests; avoid use in patients with accessory tracts, AV block, IV β-blockers, or ventricular tachycardia

Diphenhydramine (Benadryl)

Indications	Allergic reactions, drug-induced extrapyramidal reactions, sedation
Dosage	Adult: 10–50 mg IV q6–8h
	Pediatric: 5.0 mg/kg/d IV in four divided doses (maximum 300 mg)
Effect	Antagonism of histamine action on H_1 receptors; anticholinergic; CNS depression
Onset	Rapid
Duration	4–6 hours
Clearance	Hepatic metabolism; renal excretion
Comments	May cause hypotension, tachycardia, dizziness, urinary retention, seizures; it should be administered IV or IM; do NOT administer subcutaneously

Dobutamine (Dobutrex)

Indications	Heart failure, hypotension
Dosage	Infusion mix: 250 mg in 250 ml of 5% D/W or NS
	Adult: start infusion at 2 μg/kg/min and titrate to effect
	Pediatric: 5–20 μg/kg/min
Effect	β_1-adrenergic agonist
Onset	1–2 minutes
Duration	<5 minutes
Clearance	Hepatic metabolism; renal elimination
Comments	May cause hypertension, hypotension, dysrhythmias, or myocardial ischemia; can increase ventricular rate in atrial fibrillation; doses >20 μg/kg have a high rate of cardiac dysrhythms

Dopamine (Intropin)

Indications	1. Hypotension, heart failure
	2. Oliguria
Dosage	Infusion mix: 200–800 mg in 250 ml of 5% D/W or NSS
	1. Infusion at 5–20 μg/kg/min IV, titrate to effect
	2. Infusion at 1–3 μg/kg/min IV
Effect	Dopaminergic, α and β-adrenergic agonist

Onset	5 minutes
Duration	<10 minutes
Clearance	75% metabolized in the liver, kidneys, and plasma by monoamine oxidase and catechol O-methyltransferase to inactive homovanillic acid
Comments	May cause hypertension, dysrhythmias, or myocardial ischemia; primarily dopaminergic effects (increased renal blood flow) at 1–5 μg/kg/min; primarily α- and β-adrenergic effects at $\geq$10 μg/kg/min; run via central line

Droperidol (Inapsine)

Indications	1. Nausea, vomiting
	2. Agitation, sedation, adjunct to anesthesia
Dose	Adult:
	1. 0.625–2.5 mg IV prn
	2. 2.5–10 mg IV prn
	Pediatric
	1. 0.05–0.06 mg/kg q4–6 h
Effect	Dopamine (δ_2)-receptor antagonist; apparent psychic indifference to environment, catatonia, antipsychotic, antiemetic
Onset	3–10 minutes
Duration	3–6 hours
Clearance	Hepatic metabolism; renal excretion
Comments	May cause anxiety, extrapyramidal reactions, or hypotension (from moderate α-adrenergic and dopaminergic antagonism); residual effects may persist $\geq$24 hours; Potentiates other CNS depressants; the drug should not be administered in men with QTc intervals >440 msec or in women with QTc intervals >450 msec; ECG monitoring should continue for 2–3 hours after completion of droperidol treatment; at-risk patients, according to the manufacturer, include those with congestive heart failure, bradycardia, cardiac hypertrophy, hypokalemia, or hypomagnesemia; also those using diuretics or other drugs known to cause QT-interval prolongation

Enalapril/enalaprilat (Vasotec)

Indications	Hypertension, congestive heart failure
Dosage	PO:
	Loading dose: 2.5–5.0 mg daily

	Maintenance dose: 10–40 mg daily
	IV: 0.125–5.0 mg q6h (as enalaprilat)
Effect	Angiotensin-converting-enzyme inhibitor; synergistic with diuretics
Onset	1 hour
Duration	6–24 hours
Clearance	Renal/fecal elimination; hepatic metabolism of enalapril to active metabolite (enalaprilat)
Comments	Hyperkalemia, increased renal blood flow, volume-responsive hypotension; subsequent doses are additive in effect; may cause angioedema, blood dyscrasia, cough, lithium toxicity, or worsening of renal impairment

Enoxaparin (Lovenox)

Indications	1. DVT/PE prophylaxis
	2. Therapeutic anticoagulation for treatment or prevention of thrombosis, acute coronary syndrome
Dosage	1. 30 mg SQ twice daily or 40 mg SQ daily
	2. 1 mg/kg SQ q12h
Effect	Binds with antithrombin III and accelerates inactivation of factors IIa (thrombin), Xa, IXa, XIa, and XIIa
Onset	2 hours
Duration	10–24 hours
Clearance	Renal
Comments	Therapeutic doses should be used with caution in patients with renal impairment; factor Xa levels are of little value in determining therapeutic response; incompletely and unpredictable reversed by protamine; do not use in patients with heparin-induced thrombocytopenia

Ephedrine

Indication	Hypotension
Dosage	5–50 mg IV prn
Effect	α- and β-adrenergic stimulation; norepinephrine release at sympathetic nerve endings
Onset	Rapid
Duration	1 hour
Clearance	Mostly renal elimination, unchanged
Comments	May cause hypertension, dysrhythmias, myocardial ischemia, CNS stimulation, decreased uterine

activity, or mild bronchodilation; avoid giving to patients taking monoamine oxidase inhibitors; minimal effect on uterine blood flow; tachyphylaxis with repeated dosing

Epinephrine (adrenaline)

Indications	1. Heart failure, hypotension, cardiac arrest
	2. Bronchospasm, anaphylaxis
Dosage	Infusion mix: 1 mg in 250 ml of 5% D/W or NSS
	Adult:
	1. 0.1–1 mg IV or (intracardiac) every 5 minutes prn; 1–3 mg intratracheal during CPR
	2. 0.1–0.5 mg SQ, 0.1–0.25 mg IV, or 0.25–1.5 μg/min IV infusion
	Pediatric:
	1. Neonates: 0.01–0.03 mg/kg every 3–5 minutes
	2. Children: 0.01 mg/kg IV or intratracheal q3–5h (up to 5 ml 1:10,000)
	3. 0.01 mg/kg IV up to 0.5 mg; 0.01 mg/kg SQ every 15 minutes by two doses up to 1 mg/dose
Onset	Rapid
Duration	1–2 minutes
Effect	α- and β-adrenergic agonist
Clearance	Monoamine oxidase/catechol O-methyltransferase metabolism
Comments	May cause hypertension, dysrhythmias, or myocardial ischemia; dysrhythmias potentiated by halothane; topical or local injection 1:80,000–1:500,000 causes vasoconstriction; crosses placenta

Epinephrine, racemic (Vaponefrin)

Indications	Airway edema, bronchospasm
Dosage	Adult: inhaled via nebulizer: 0.5 ml of 2.25% solution in 2.5–3.5 ml of NSS q1–4h prn
	Pediatric: inhaled via nebulizer: 0.5 ml of 2.25% solution in 2.5–3.5 ml of NSS q4h prn
Effect	Mucosal vasoconstriction; see also epinephrine
Clearance	Monoamine oxidase/catechol O-methyltransferase metabolism
Comments	See epinephrine

Ergonovine (Ergotrate)

Indication	Postpartum hemorrhage due to uterine atony
Dosage	For postpartum hemorrhage: IV (emergency only): 0.2 mg in 5 ml of NSS over ≥1 minute IM: 0.2 mg q2–4h prn for up to five doses; then PO: 0.2–0.4 mg q6–12h for 2 days or prn
Effect	Constriction of uterine and vascular smooth muscle
Onset	IV: 1 minute IM: 2–3 minutes PO: 6–15 minutes
Duration	IV: 45 minutes PO/IM: 3 hours
Clearance	Hepatic metabolism; renal elimination
Comments	May cause hypertension from systemic vasoconstriction (especially in eclampsia and hypertension), dysrhythmias, coronary spasm, uterine tetany, or gastrointestinal upset; IV route is only used in emergencies; overdose may cause convulsions or stroke

Esmolol (Brevibloc)

Indications	Supraventricular tachydysrhythmias, myocardial ischemia
Dosage	Start with 5–10 mg IV bolus and increase every 3 minutes prn to total 100–300 mg; infusion 1–15 mg/min
Effect	Selective β_1-adrenergic blockade
Onset	Rapid
Duration	10–20 minutes following discontinuation
Clearance	Degraded by RBC esterases; renal elimination
Comments	May cause bradycardia, AV conduction delay, hypotension, congestive heart failure; β_2 activity at high doses

Ethacrynic acid (Edecrin)

Indications	Edema, congestive heart failure, acute/chronic renal failure
Dosage	Adult: IV: 25–100 mg IV over 5–10 minutes; 24-hour cumulative dose: 400 mg Oral: 50–200 mg/d in one to two divided doses

Pediatric:
IV: 1 mg/kg/dose; repeat doses with caution due to potential for ototoxicity Oral: 25 mg/d to start, increase by 25 mg/d until response is obtained; maximum 3 mg/kg/d

Effect	Diuretic
Onset	IV: 5 minutes
	Oral: within 30 minutes
Duration	IV: 2 hours
	Oral: 12 hours
Clearance	Hepatically metabolized to active cysteine conjugate (35%–40%); 30%–60% excreted unchanged in bile and urine
Comments	May potentiate the activity of antihypertensives, neuromuscular blocking agents, and digoxin and increase insulin requirement in diabetic patients; oral preparations are not readily available; long-term therapy is generally not feasible

Famotidine (Pepcid)

Indications	Stress ulcer and aspiration prophylaxis; gastroesophageal reflux, gastric acid hypersecretion; gastrointestinal bleeding
Dosage	20 mg IV/PO q12h (dilute in 1–10 ml of 5% D/W or NSS)
Effect	Histamine-2 receptor antagonism with inhibition of gastric acid secretion
Onset	1 hour
Duration	8–12 hours
Clearance	30%–35% hepatic metabolism; 65%–70% renal elimination
Comments	May cause confusion; rapid IV administration may increase risk of cardiac arrhythmias and hypotension

Fenoldepam (Corlopam)

Indications	1. Hypertension
	2. Oliguria
Dosage	Adult
	1. Hypertension: initial, 0.03–0.1 μg/kg/min IV; increase every 15 minutes by 0.05–0.1 μg/kg/min based on response, maximum 1.6 μg/kg/min
	2. Oliguria: 0.03 μg/kg/min with no dose adjustments

	Pediatric
	1. Hypertension: initial, 0.2 μg/kg/min IV; increase in increments of up to 0.3–0.5 μg/kg/min every 20–30 minutes; doses >0.8 μg/kg/min have resulted in tachycardia with no observation of additional benefit
Effect	Selective δ-1 receptor agonist
Onset	15–30 minutes
Duration	Up to 4 hours
Clearance	Hepatic (insignificant)
Comments	Hypotension, increases in heart rate, and asymptomatic T-wave flattening on the electrocardiogram have been reported; other adverse effects include headache, dizziness, flushing, nausea and vomiting, and increases in portal pressure in cirrhotic patients

Filgrastim (G-CSF, granulocyte-colony stimulating factor, Neupogen)

Indications	Neutropenia secondary to immunosuppressive drug therapy
Dosage	Adult and pediatric: Initial dosing recommendation: 5 μg/kg/d administered SQ or IV Doses may be increased in increments of 5 μg/kg as titrated to patient response, according to the duration and severity of the absolute neutrophil count nadir
Effect	Promotes neutrophil production
Onset	Rapid elevation in neutrophil counts within the first 24 hours, reaching a plateau in 3–5 days
Duration	Absolute neutrophil count decreases by 50% within 2 days after discontinuing G-CSF; white counts return to the normal range in 4–7 days
Clearance	Systemically metabolized
Comments	Filgrastim dose should be adjusted to coincide with available single-use containers (300, 480 μg) whenever possible

Flumazenil (Romazicon)

Indication	1. Reversal of benzodiazepine sedation
	2. Benzodiazepine overdose
Dosage	1. 0.2–1.0 mg IV every 20 minutes at 0.2 mg/min
	2. 3–5 mg IV at 0.5 mg/min

Effect	Competitive antagonism of CNS benzodiazepine receptor
Onset	1–2 minutes
Duration	1–2 hours (dose dependent)
Clearance	100% hepatic metabolism; 90%–95% renal elimination of metabolite
Comments	Duration of action depends on dose and duration of action of benzodiazepine; flumazenil will reverse CNS sedation, but has little effect on respiratory (CO_2 dependent) drive; may induce CNS excitation including seizures, acute withdrawal, nausea, dizziness, agitation; does not reverse non–benzodiazepine-induced CNS depression

Folic acid (folacin, folate)

Indications	Megaloblastic and macrocytic anemias
Dosage	Adult:
	Oral, IM, IV, SQ:
	Initial dose: 1 mg/d
	Maintenance dose: 0.5 mg/d; pregnant and lactating women: 0.8 mg/d
	Pediatric:
	Oral, IM, IV, SQ:
	Initial dose: 1 mg/d
	Maintenance dose:
	1–10 years: 0.1–0.3 mg/d
	Infants: 15 μg/kg/d or 50 μg/d
Effect	Vitamin B complex substrate
Onset	Within 0.5–1 hour
Comments	Folic acid may alleviate the hematologic complications of pernicious anemia while allowing neurologic sequelae to occur; therefore, it should be administered with extreme caution to patients with undiagnosed anemia; may produce allergic reactions

Fondaparinux (Arixtra)

Indications	1. Prophylaxis of DVT and PE in orthopedic surgery and hip fractures
	2. Treatment of DVT and PE
Dosage	1. 1 2.5 mg SQ daily
	2. <50 kg: 5 mg SQ daily

	50–100 kg: 7.5 mg SQ daily
	>100 kg: 10 mg SQ daily
Effect	Anti-Xa pentasaccharide
Onset	60–90 minutes
Duration	17–21 hours
Clearance	Renal (avoid in patients with creatinine clearance <30 ml)
Comments	Renally excreted; does not cross-react with PF4 heparin antibodies

Furosemide (Lasix)

Indications	Edema, hypertension, renal failure, hypercalcemia
Dosage	Adult: 10–40 mg IV (initial dose, dose individualized) at a rate not to exceed 10 mg/min
	Pediatric: 1–2 mg/kg/d
Effect	Increase in excretion of Na^+, Cl^-, K^+, PO_4^{3-}, Ca^{2+}, and H_2O by inhibiting reabsorption in loop of Henle
Onset	5 minutes
Duration	6 hours
Clearance	Hepatic metabolism; 88% renal elimination
Comments	May cause electrolyte imbalance, dehydration, transient hypotension, deafness, hyperglycemia, or hyperuricemia; sulfa-allergic patients may exhibit hypersensitivity to furosemide

Ganciclovir (Cytovene)

Indications	Treatment of cytomegalovirus (CMV) retinitis in immunocompromised individuals; treatment of CMV colitis and pneumonitis
Dosage	Adult and pediatric:
	Initial: 5 mg/kg every 12 hours for 14–21 days
	Followed by 5 mg/kg/d as a single dose for the duration of patient's immunosuppression; adjust dose for renal impairment
Effect	Antiviral
Onset	Oral absorption increased with food
Duration	Half-life: 1.7–5.8 hours; increases with impaired renal function
Clearance	Majority (94%–99%) excreted unchanged drug in the urine
Comments	Dose adjustment or interruption of ganciclovir therapy may be necessary in patients with neutropenia and/or thrombocytopenia and patients with impaired renal function

Glucagon

Indications	Duodenal or choledochal relaxation
Dosage	0.25–0.5 mg IV every 20 minutes *prn*
Effect	Catecholamine release
Onset	45 seconds
Duration	9–25 minutes (dose dependent)
Clearance	Hepatic and renal proteolysis
Comments	May cause anaphylaxis, nausea, vomiting, hyperglycemia, or positive inotropic and chronotropic effects; high doses potentiate oral anticoagulants;

Glycopyrrolate (Robinul)

Indications	1. Decrease gastrointestinal motility, antisialagogue
	2. Bradycardia
Dosage	Adult:
	1. IV/IM/SQ: 0.1–0.2 mg: PO: 1–2 mg
	2. 0.1–0.2 mg/dose IV
	Pediatric: 0.004–0.008 mg/kg IV/IM up to 0.1 mg
Effect	See atropine
Onset	IV: 1–4 minutes
	IM: 30–45 minutes
Duration	IV: 2–4 hours
	IM: 2–7 hours
Clearance	Renal elimination
Comments	See atropine; doses do not cross blood–brain barrier or placenta; with less chronotropy than atropine; erratic oral absorption

Haloperidol (Haldol)

Indications	Psychosis, agitation, delirium
Dosage	0.5–2 mg IV prn (dose individualized)
Onset	IV peak effect <20 minutes
Duration	IV half-life 14 hours
Effect	Antipsychotic effects due to dopamine (D_2)-receptor antagonism; CNS depression
Clearance	Hepatic metabolism; renal/biliary elimination

Comments   May cause extrapyramidal reactions or very
mild α-adrenergic antagonism; may
precipitate neuroleptic malignant syndrome;
contraindicated in Parkinson's disease, toxic
CNS depression, coma

Heparin

Indications
1. Anticoagulation for thrombosis,
   thromboembolism
2. Cardiopulmonary bypass
3. Disseminated intravascular coagulation

Dosage   Adult:
1. Loading dose: 50–150 units/kg IV
   Maintenance dose: 15–25 units/kg/h IV;
   titrate dosage with partial thromboplastin
   time or activated clotting time
2. Loading dose: 300 units/kg IV.
   Maintenance dose: 100 units/kg/h IV;
   titrate with coagulation tests
3. Loading dose: 50–100 units/kg IV

Pediatric:
Loading dose: 50 units/kg IV
Maintenance dose: 15–25 units/kg/h IV;
titrate with coagulation tests

Effect   Potentiates action of antithrombin III;
blockade of conversion of prothrombin and
activation of other coagulation factors

Onset   IV: immediate
SQ: 1–2 hours

Duration   Half-life 1–6 hours; increases with dose

Clearance   Primarily by reticuloendothelial uptake,
hepatic biotransformation

Comments   May cause bleeding, thrombocytopenia,
allergic reactions, or diuresis (36–48 hours
after a large dose); half-life increased in renal
failure and decreased in thromboembolism
and liver disease; does not cross placenta;
reversed by protamine

Hydralazine (Apresoline)

Indication   Hypertension

Dosage   2.5–20.0 mg IV q4h or prn (dose
individualized)

Effect	Relaxation of vascular smooth muscle (arteriole > venule)
Onset	5–20 minutes, peak effect 10–80 minutes
Duration	2–6 hours
Clearance	Extensive hepatic metabolism; renal elimination
Comments	May cause hypotension (diastolic > systolic), reflex tachycardia, systemic lupus erythematosis syndrome, or Coombs'-positive hemolytic anemia; increases coronary, splanchnic, cerebral, and renal blood flows

Hydrocortisone (SoluCortef-see also Chapter 27 for comparison of various corticosteroids)

Indications	Adrenal insufficiency, inflammation and allergy, cerebral edema from CNS tumors, asthma
Dosage	Non–life-threatening conditions: 50–200 mg IV q2–10h prn Life-threatening conditions: 50 mg/kg IV over several minutes q4–24h not longer than 2–3 days
Effect	Antiinflammatory and antiallergic effect; mineralocorticoid effect; stimulation of gluconeogenesis; inhibition of peripheral protein synthesis; membrane-stabilizing effect
Onset	1 hour
Duration	6–8 hours (dose/route dependent)
Clearance	Hepatic metabolism; renal elimination
Comments	May cause adrenocortical insufficiency (Addison's crisis) with abrupt withdrawal, delayed wound healing, CNS disturbances, osteoporosis, or electrolyte disturbances

Hydroxyzine (Vistaril, Atarax)

Indications	Anxiety, nausea and vomiting, allergies, sedation
Dosage	PO: 25–200 mg q6–8h IM: 25–100 mg q4–6h Not an IV drug

Effect	Antagonism of histamine action on histamine-1 receptors, CNS depression, antiemetic
Onset	15–60 minutes
Duration	4–6 hours
Clearance	Hepatic (P-450) metabolism; renal elimination
Comments	May cause dry mouth; minimal cardiorespiratory depression; IV injection may cause thrombosis; crosses placenta

---

Insulin (see Chapter 27 for a comparison chart of various insulin formulations)

Indications	1.	Hyperglycemia
	2.	Diabetic ketoacidosis
Dosage	1.	Individualized: usually 5–10 units IV/SQ prn (regular insulin)
	2.	Loading dose: 10–20 units IV (regular insulin). Maintenance dose: 0.05–0.1 units/kg/h IV (regular insulin), titrated against plasma glucose level
Effect		Facilitation of glucose transport intracellularly; shift of K^+ and Mg^{2+} intracellular
Onset		SQ: insulin aspartate, lispro: rapid acting Regular: 30 minutes Semilente: 30 minutes NPH: 1–2 hours Lente: 1–4 hours PZI: 4–6 hours Ultralente: 4–6 hours
Duration		SQ: insulin aspartate: rapid acting Lispro: 60–90 minutes Regular: 5–7 hours Semilente: 12–16 hours NPH: 18–24 hours Lente: 18–28 hours PZI: 24–36 hours Ultralente: 30–36 hours
Clearance		Hepatic and renal metabolism; 30%–80% renal elimination; unchanged insulin is reabsorbed
Comments		May cause hypoglycemia, allergic reactions, or synthesis of insulin antibodies; may be absorbed by plastic in IV tubing; when initiating insulin therapy, use human rather than beef or pork insulin to minimize the development of antibodies

Isoproterenol (Isuprel)

Indications	Bradycardia
Dosage	2 μg/min titrated up to 10 μg/min of 20–200 μg/ml solution
Effect	β-adrenergic agonist; chronotropy, inotropy
Onset	Immediate
Duration	1 hour
Clearance	Hepatic and pulmonary metabolism; 40%–50% renal excretion unchanged
Comments	May cause dysrhythmias, myocardial ischemia, hypertension, or CNS excitation; tachyphylaxis after repeated inhaled doses

Isosorbide dinitrate (Isordil)

Indications	Angina, hypertension, myocardial infarction, congestive heart failure
Dosage	5–20 mg PO q6h
Effect	See nitroglycerin
Onset	15–40 minutes
Duration	4–6 hours
Clearance	Nearly 100% hepatic metabolism; renal elimination
Comments	See nitroglycerin; tolerance develops

Ketorolac (Toradol)

Indications	Nonsteroidal antiinflammatory analgesic drug (NSAID) for moderate pain; useful adjunct for severe pain when used with parenteral or epidural opioids
Dosage	PO: 10 mg q4–6h IM/IV: 30–60 mg, then 15–30 mg q6h
Effect	Limits prostaglandin synthesis by cyclooxygenase inhibition
Onset	30–60 minutes
Duration	4–6 hours
Clearance	<50% hepatic metabolism, renal metabolism; 91% renal elimination
Comments	Adverse effects are similar to those with other NSAIDs: peptic ulceration, bleeding, decreased renal blood flow; duration of treatment not to exceed 5 days

Labetalol (Normodyne, Trandate)

Indications	Hypertension, angina
Dosage	IV: 5- to 10-mg increments at 5-minute intervals, to 40–80 mg/dose
	Infusion: 5 mg/ml mix; start at 0.05 μg/kg/min
Effect	Selective α1-adrenergic blockade with nonselective β-adrenergic blockade; ratio of α/β blockade is 1:7
Onset	Minutes
Duration	2–12 hours
Clearance	Hepatic metabolism; renal elimination
Comments	May cause bradycardia, AV conduction delays, bronchospasm in asthmatics, and postural hypotension; crosses placenta

Levothyroxine (Synthroid)

Indications	Hypothyroidism
Dosage	Adjust according to individual requirements and response
	Adults:
	Oral: 0.1–0.2 mg/d
	IV: 75% of oral dose
	Pediatric:
	Oral:
	0–6 months: 25–50 μg/d or 8–10 μg/kg/d
	6–12 months: 50–75 μg/d or 6–8 μg/kg/d
	1–5 years: 75–100 μg/d or 5–6 μg/kg/d
	6–12 years: 100–150 μg/d or 4–5 μg/kg/d
	>12 years: >150 μg/d or 2–3 μg/kg/d
	IV: 75% of oral dose
Effect	Exogenous thyroxine
Onset	Oral: 3–5 days
	IV: within 6–8 hours
Duration	Peak effect at approximately 24 hours
Clearance	Metabolized in the liver to triiodothyronine (active); eliminated in feces and urine
Comments	Contraindicated with recent myocardial infarction or thyrotoxicosis, or uncorrected adrenal insufficiency; phenytoin may decrease levothyroxine levels; increases effects of oral anticoagulants; tricyclic antidepressants may increase toxic potential of both drugs; intravenous therapy can be given at three-fourths of the oral dose

Lidocaine (Xylocaine)

Indications	1. Ventricular dysrhythmias
	2. Cough suppression
	3. Local anesthesia
Dosage	Adult:
	1. Loading dose: 1 mg/kg IV × 2 (second dose 20–30 minutes after first dose) Maintenance dose: 15–50 μg/kg/min IV (1–4 mg/min)
	2. 1 mg/kg IV
	3. 5 mg/kg maximum dose for infiltration or conduction block
	Pediatric:
	1. Loading dose: 0.5–1 mg/kg IV (second dose 20–30 minutes after first dose) Maintenance dose: 15–50 μg/kg/min IV
Effect	Antiarrhythmic effect; sedation; neural blockade; decreased conductance of sodium channels
Onset	Rapid
Duration	5–20 minutes
Clearance	Hepatic metabolism to active/toxic metabolites; renal elimination (10% unchanged)
Comments	May cause dizziness, seizures, disorientation, heart block (with myocardial conduction defect), or hypotension; crosses placenta; therapeutic concentration is 1–5 mg/L; avoid in patients with Wolff-Parkinson-White syndrome

Lansoprazole (IV) (Prevacid)

Indications	1. Intravenous prevention of gastrointestinal bleeding following endoscopic treatment of bleeding ulcers and varices in patients who are unable to receive oral proton-pump inhibitors intolerant or refractory to IV histamine-2 antagonists
	2. Intravenous treatment of active gastrointestinal bleeding in patients who are unable to receive oral proton-pump inhibitors intolerant or refractory to IV histamine-2 antagonists
Dosage	1. 30 mg IV daily or twice daily

Effect	Selectively inhibits the parietal cell membrane enzyme H^+/K^+-ATPase proton pump
Onset	Peak concentrations obtained in 1–2 hours; complete antisecretory effects may take hours to days
Duration	Antisecretory effect up to 24 hours
Clearance	Nearly 100% hepatic metabolism; renal elimination

Magnesium sulfate

Indications	1. Preeclampsia/eclampsia 2. Hypomagnesemia 3. Polymorphic ventricular tachycardia (*torsades de pointes*)
Dosage	Adult: 1. Loading dose: 1–4 g (32 mEq) IV (10% or 20% solution) Maintenance dose: 1–3 ml/min (4 g/250 ml of 5% D/W or NSS) 2. 1 g (8 mEq) every 6 hours × four doses 3. 1–2 g in 10 ml of 5% D/W over 1–2 minutes; 5–10 g may be administered for refractory dysrhythmias
Effect	To replete serum magnesium; for the prevention and treatment of seizures or hyperreflexia associated with preeclampsia/eclampsia
Onset	Rapid
Duration	4–6 hours
Clearance	100% renal elimination for IV route
Comments	Potentiates neuromuscular blockade (both depolarizing and nondepolarizing agents); potentiates CNS effects of anesthetics, hypnotics, and opioids; toxicity occurs with serum concentration ≥ 10 mEq/L; avoid in patients with heart block; may alter cardiac conduction in digitalized patients; caution in patients with renal failure

Mannitol (Osmitrol)

Indications	1. Increased intracranial pressure 2. Oliguria, or anuria associated with acute renal injury

Dosage	Adult:
	1. 0.25–1.0 g/kg IV as 20% solution over 30–60 minutes (in an acute situation, can give a bolus of 1.25–25.0 g over 5–10 minutes)
	2. 0.2-g/kg test dose over 3–5 minutes, then 50–100 g IV over 30 minutes if adequate response
	Pediatric:
	1. 0.2-g/kg test dose, with maintenance of 2 g/kg over 30–60 minutes
Effect	Increase in serum osmolality, which reduces cerebral edema and lowers intracranial and intraocular pressure; also causes osmotic diuresis and transient expansion of intravascular volume
Onset	15 minutes
Duration	2–3 hours
Clearance	Renal elimination; onset 15 minutes, duration 2–3 hours
Comments	Rapid administration may cause vasodilation and hypotension; may worsen or cause pulmonary edema, intracranial hemorrhage, systemic hypertension, or rebound intracranial hypertension; hyponatremia common

Metaproterenol (Alupent)

Indication	Bronchospasm
Dosage	Inhaled (metered aerosol): 2–3 puffs (0.65 mg/puff) q3–4h prn (maximum 12 puffs/d)
	Inhaled intermittent positive-pressure breathing: 0.2–0.3 ml of 5% solution in 2.5 ml of NSS q4h
Effect	β-adrenergic stimulation (mostly β_2), resulting in bronchodilation
Onset	1–10 minutes
Duration	1–5 hours
Clearance	Hepatic/intestinal metabolism; renal elimination
Comments	May cause dysrhythmias, hypertension, CNS stimulation, nausea, vomiting, or inhibition of uterine contractions; tachyphylaxis can occur

Methylene blue

Indications	1. Surgical marker for genitourinary surgery
	2. Methemoglobinemia

Dosage	1. 100 mg (10 ml of 1% solution) IV
	2. 1–2 mg/kg IV of 1% solution over 10 minutes; repeat every 1 hour prn
Effect	Low dose promotes conversion of methemoglobin to hemoglobin; high dose promotes conversion of hemoglobin to methemoglobin;
Onset	Immediate
Clearance	Tissue reduction; urinary and biliary elimination
Comments	May cause RBC destruction (prolonged use), hypertension, bladder irritation, nausea, diaphoresis; may inhibit nitrate-induced coronary artery relaxation; interferes with pulse oximetry for 1–2 minutes; may cause hemolysis in patients with glucose-6-phosphate dehydrogenase deficiency

Methylergonovine (Methergine)

Indication	Postpartum hemorrhage
Dosage	IV (EMERGENCY ONLY, after delivery of placenta): 0.2 mg in 5 ml of NS/dose over ≥1 min.
	IM: 0.2 mg q2–4h prn (<5 doses)
	PO (after IM or IV doses): 0.2–0.4 mg q6–12h × 2–7 days
Onset	IV: immediate
	IM: 2–5 minutes (maximum response after 30 minutes)
	PO: 5–10 minutes
Duration	1–3 hours
Clearance	Hepatic metabolism; renal elimination
Comments	See ergonovine; hypertensive response is less marked than with ergonovine

Methylprednisolone (Solu–Medrol) (see Chapter 27 for a comparison of various corticosteroids)

Indications	See hydrocortisone
Dosage	Adult:
	For non–life-threatening conditions: 10–250 mg IV q4–24h (IV given over 1 minute)
	For life-threatening conditions: 100–250 mg IV q2–6h, or 30 mg/kg IV (given over 15 minutes) q4–6h

Pediatric:
For life-threatening conditions: no more than
0.5mg/kg/24 h

Effect   See hydrocortisone; has five times the
                  glucocorticoid potency of hydrocortisone; almost
                  no mineralocorticoid activity
Onset   Minutes
Duration   6 hours
Clearance   Hepatic metabolism; renal elimination
                  (dose/route dependent)
Comments   See hydrocortisone

Metoclopramide (Reglan)

Indications   Gastroesophageal reflux, diabetic gastroparesis,
                  premedication for patients needing pulmonary
                  aspiration prophylaxis, antiemetic
Dose   Adult:
                  IV: 10 mg
                  PO: 10 mg.
                  Pediatric: 0.1 mg/kg
Effect   Facilitates gastric emptying by increasing
                  gastrointestinal motility and lower esophageal
                  sphincter tone; antiemetic effects are secondary
                  to antagonism of central and peripheral
                  dopamine receptors
Onset   IV: 1–3 minutes
                  PO: 30–60 minutes to peak effect
Duration   IV, PO: 1–2 hours
Kinetics   Hepatic metabolism; renal elimination
Comments   Avoid in patients with gastrointestinal
                  obstruction, pheochromocytoma, and
                  Parkinson's disease; extrapyramidal reactions in
                  0.2%–1% of patients; may exacerbate depression

Metoprolol (Lopressor)

Indications   Hypertension, angina pectoris, dysrhythmia,
                  hypertrophic cardiomyopathy, myocardial
                  infarction, pheochromocytoma
Dosage   50–100 mg PO q6–24h
Effect β_1-adrenergic blockade (β_2-adrenergic
                  antagonism at high doses)
Onset   15 minutes
Duration   6 hours

Clearance	Hepatic metabolism, renal elimination
Comments	May cause bradycardia, bronchoconstriction (with doses >100 mg/d), dizziness, fatigue, insomnia; may increase risk of heart block; crosses placenta and blood–brain barrier

Milrinone (Primacor)

Indications	Congestive heart failure
Dosage	Infusion concentration: 100, 150, 200 μg/ml Loading dose: 50 μg/kg IV over 10 minutes Maintenance dose: titrate 0.375–0.750 μg/kg/min to effect
Effect	Phosphodiesterase inhibition causing positive inotropy, vasodilation
Onset	Immediate
Duration	2–3 hours
Clearance	Renal elimination.
Comments	Short-term therapy; may increase ventricular ectopy.

Nadolol (Corgard)

Indications	Angina pectoris, hypertension
Dosage	40–240 mg/d PO
Effect	Nonselective β-adrenergic blockade.
Onset	1–2 hours
Duration	>24 hours
Clearance	No hepatic metabolism; renal elimination
Comments	May cause severe bronchospasm in susceptible patients (see propranolol)

Naloxone (Narcan)

Indications	Reversal of systemic opioid effects
Dosage	Adult: 0.04- to 0.4-mg doses IV, titrated q2–3 min Pediatric: 1–10 μg/kg (in increments) IV q2–3 min (up to 0.4 mg)
Effect	Antagonism of opioid effects by competitive inhibition

Onset	Rapid
Duration	Dose dependent; lasting 20–60 minutes
Clearance	95% hepatic metabolism; primarily renal elimination
Comments	May cause reversal of analgesia, hypertension, dysrhythmias, rare pulmonary edema, delirium, or withdrawal syndrome (in opioid-dependent patients); renarcotization may occur because antagonist has short duration; caution in hepatic failure

Nifedipine (Procardia)

Indications	Coronary artery spasm, hypertension, myocardial ischemia
Dosage	PO: 10–40 mg thrice daily SL: 10–20 mg (extracted from capsule)
Effect	Blockade of slow calcium channels in heart; systemic and coronary vasodilation and increase in myocardial perfusion
Onset	PO: 20 minutes SL: 1–5 minutes
Duration	4–24 hours
Clearance	Hepatic metabolism
Comments	May cause reflex tachycardia, gastrointestinal upset, or mild negativeinotropic effects; little effect on automaticity and atrial conduction; may be useful in asymmetric septal hypertrophy; drug solution is light sensitive

Nitric oxide (Inomax)

Indications	Hypoxemic acute respiratory failure in term and near-term neonates
Dosage	1–40 ppm by continuous inhalation
Effect	Cyclic guanosine monophosphate–mediated pulmonary vasodilation of ventilated lung regions
Onset	5–10 minutes
Duration	Variable
Clearance	Bound to hemoglobin; metabolized to nitrates/nitrites
Comments	Not approved by Food and Drug Administration for adult use; off-label uses may include acute respiratory distress syndrome, cardiogenic shock, acute right ventricular failure,

post–lung or heart transplant
ischemia–reperfusion injury, and
post–cardiopulmonary bypass pulmonary
hypertension

Nitroglycerin

Indications	Angina pectoris, myocardial ischemia/infarction, hypertension, congestive heart failure, esophageal spasm
Dosage	IV infusion initially at 10 μg/min; titrate to effect; customary mix: 30–50 mg in 250 ml of 5% D/W or NSS SL: 0.15–0.6 mg/dose Topical: 2% ointment, 0.5–2.5 inches q6–8h
Effect	Smooth muscle relaxation by enzymatic release of nitric oxide, causing systemic, coronary, and pulmonary vasodilation (veins > arteries); bronchodilatation; biliary, gastrointestinal, and genitourinary tract relaxation
Onset	IV: 1–2 minutes SL: 1–3 minutes PO: 1 hour Topical: 30 minutes
Duration	IV: 10 minutes SL: 30–60 minutes PO: 8–12 hours Topical: 8–24 hours
Clearance	Nearly complete hepatic metabolism; renal elimination
Comments	May cause reflex tachycardia, hypotension, headache; tolerance with chronic use may be avoided with a 10- to 12-hour nitrate-free period; may be absorbed by plastic in IV tubing; may cause methemoglobinemia at very high doses

Nitroprusside (Nipride, Nitropress)

Indications	Hypertension, controlled hypotension, congestive heart failure
Dosage	IV: infusion initially at 0.1 μg/kg/min, then titrated against patient response to maximum 10 μg/kg/min (total dose <1.0–1.5 mg/kg over 2–3 hours); customary mix: 50 mg in 250 ml of 5% D/W or NS

Effect	Direct nitric oxide donor causing smooth muscle relaxation (arterial > venous)
Onset	1–2 minutes
Duration	1–10 minutes after stopping of infusion
Clearance	RBC and tissue metabolism; renal elimination
Comments	May cause excessive hypotension, reflex tachycardia; accumulation of cyanide with liver dysfunction; thiocyanate with kidney disfunction; cyanide/thiocyanate build-up with prolonged infusion; avoid with Leber's hereditary optic atrophy, tobacco amblyopia, hypothyroidism, or vitamin B_{12} deficiency; solution and powder are light sensitive and must be wrapped in opaque material

Norepinephrine (Levarterenol, Levophed)

Indication	Hypotension
Dosage	1–8 μg/min IV; start at 1–8 μg/min, then titrate to desired effect
	Customary mix: 4 mg in 250 ml of 5% D/W or NSS
Effect	Alpha- > β-adrenergic agonist
Onset	Rapid
Duration	1–2 minutes following discontinuation
Clearance	Monoamine oxidase/catechol O-methyltransferase metabolism
Comments	May cause hypertension, dysrhythmias, myocardial ischemia, increased uterine contractility, constricted microcirculation, or CNS stimulation

Octreotide (Sandostatin)

Indication	1. Upper GI tract bleeding, acute variceal hemorrhage
	2. Control of symptoms in patients with metastatic carcinoid and vasoactive intestinal peptide–secreting tumors; pancreatic tumors, gastrinoma, secretory diarrhea
	3. Off-label uses include AIDS-associated secretory diarrhea, cryptosporidiosis, Cushing's syndrome, insulinomas, small-bowel fistulas, postgastrectomy dumping syndrome, chemotherapy-induced diarrhea, graft-versus-host disease–induced diarrhea, Zollinger-Ellison syndrome

Dosage
1. Adults:
   IV bolus: 25–50 μg followed by continuous IV infusion of 25–50 μg/h
2, 3. Adults:
   SQ: initial 50 μg 1–2 times/d, and titrate dose based on patient tolerance and response
   Carcinoid: 100–600 μg/d in 2–4 divided doses
   VIPomas: 200–300 μg/d in 2–4 divided doses
   Diarrhea: IV, initial 50–100 μg every 8 hours; increase by 100 μg/dose at 48-hour intervals; maximum dose 500 μg every 8 hours
   Pediatric: 1–10 μg/kg every 12 hours beginning at the low end of the range and increasing by 0.3 μg/kg/dose at 3-day intervals

Effect
Somatostatin analogue that suppresses release of serotonin, gastrin, vasoactive intestinal peptide, insulin, glucagon, and secretin

Onset
IV: minutes

Duration
6–12 hours

Clearance
Hepatic and renal (32% eliminated unchanged); decreased in renal failure

Comments
May cause nausea, decreased gastrointestinal motility, transient hyperglycemia; duration of therapy should be no longer than 72 hours due to lack of efficacy beyond this time

Omeprazole (Prilosec)

Indications
Gastric acid hypersecretion or gastritis, gastroesophageal reflux

Dosage
20–40 mg PO daily

Effect
Inhibition of H^+ secretion by irreversibly binding H^+/K^+-ATPase

Onset
1 hour

Duration
>24 hours

Clearance
Extensive hepatic metabolism; 72%–80% renal elimination, 18%–23% fecal elimination

Comments
Increases secretion of gastrin; more rapid healing of gastric ulcer than with histamine-2 blockers; effective in ulcers resistant to histamine-2–blocker therapy; inhibits some cytochrome P-450 enzymes

Ondansetron hydrochloride (Zofran)

Indications
Prevention and treatment of perioperative nausea, vomiting

Dosage	Adult:
	IV: Perioperative 4 mg undiluted over
	>30 seconds
	PO: 8 mg
	Pediatric: 4 mg PO
Effect	Selective serotinin 5-HT$_3$–receptor
	antagonist
Onset	30 minutes
Duration	4–8 hours
Clearance	95% hepatic, 5% renal excretion
Comments	Used in much higher doses for
	chemotherapy-induced nausea; mild side
	effects: headache, reversible transaminase
	elevation

Oxytocin (Pitocin)

Indications	1. Postpartum hemorrhage, uterine atony
	2. Augmentation of labor
Dosage	1. IV infusion at rate necessary to control
	atony (e.g., 0.02–0.04 unit/min)
	2. Labor induction: 0.0005–0.002 unit/min
	Customary mix: 10–40 units in 1,000 ml
	of crystalloid
Effect	Reduced postpartum blood loss by contraction
	of uterine smooth muscle; renal, coronary, and
	cerebral vasodilation
Onset	Immediate
Duration	1 hour
Clearance	Tissue metabolism; renal elimination
Comments	May cause uterine tetany and rupture, fetal
	distress, or anaphylaxis; IV bolus can cause
	hypotension, tachycardia, dysrhythmia

Pentamidine (Pentam)

Indications	1. Prevention and treatment of pneumonia
	caused by *Pneumocystis carinii*
Dosage	1. Adult and pediatric: 4 mg/kg/d IM or IV
	for 14 days
	2. Pediatric: inhalation of 300 mg every
	3–4 weeks via nebulizer
	Adult: inhalation of 300 mg every 4 weeks
	via nebulizer

Effect	Antiprotozoal
Duration	Terminal half-life is 6.4–9.4 hours; may be prolonged in patients with severe renal impairment
Clearance	33%–66% excreted unchanged in urine
Comments	Concomitant use of nephrotoxic drugs may increase risk of nephrotoxicity

Phenobarbital

Indications	1. Sedative/hypnotic 2. Anticonvulsant
Dosage	1. Adult and pediatric: 1–3 mg/kg PO 2. Adult, infant, and pediatric: Loading dose: 10–20 mg/kg, additional 5-mg/kg doses every 15–30 minutes for contol of status epilepticus, maximum 30 mg/kg Maintenance dose: 3–5 mg/kg/d PO, IV in divided doses
Onset	5 minutes, allow 60–90 minutes for full sedative effect
Duration	10–12 hours; half-life may be >100 hours
Clearance	Hepatic metabolism: 25%–50% renal elimination unchanged
Comments	May cause hypotension; multiple-drug interactions through induction of hepatic enzyme systems; therapeutic anticonvulsant concentration 15–40 μg/ml at trough (just before next dose)

Phenoxybenzamine (Dibenzyline)

Indication	Preoperative preparation for pheochromocytoma resection
Dosage	10–40 mg/d PO titrated (start at 10 mg/d and increase dose by 10 mg/d every 4 days prn)
Effect	Nonselective noncompetitive α-adrenergic antagonist
Onset	Hours
Duration	3–4 days
Clearance	Hepatic metabolism; renal/biliary excretion
Comments	May cause orthostatic hypotension (which may be refractory to norepinephrine), reflex tachycardia; nasal congestion expected

Phentolamine (Regitine)

Indications	1. Hypertension from catecholamine excess as in pheochromocytoma 2. Extravasation of α-agonist
Dosage	1. 1–5 mg IV prn for hypertension 2. 5–10 mg in 10 ml of NS SQ into affected area within 12 hours
Effect	Nonselective, competitive α-adrenergic antagonist
Onset	Minutes
Duration	Half-life 19 minutes
Clearance	Unknown metabolism; 10% renal elimination unmetabolized
Comments	May cause hypotension, reflex tachycardia, cerebrovascular spasm, dysrhythmias, stimulation of gastrointestinal tract, or hypoglycemia

Phenylephrine (Neo-Synephrine)

Indication	Hypotension
Dosage	IV: infusion initially at 10 μg/min, then titrated to response IV bolus: 40–100 μg/dose Customary mix: 10–30 mg in 250 ml of 5% D/W or NSS
Effect	α-adrenergic agonist
Onset	Rapid
Duration	5–20 minutes
Clearance	Hepatic metabolism; renal elimination
Comments	May cause hypertension, reflex bradycardia, constricted microcirculation, uterine contraction, or uterine vasoconstriction

Phenytoin (diphenylhydantoin, Dilantin) (see Chapter 29 for treatment of seizures)

Indications	1. Seizures, seizure prophylaxis 2. Digoxin-induced dysrhythmias 3. Refractory ventricular tachycardia

Dosage	1. Seizures IV: Loading dose: Neonates: 15–20 mg/kg in a single or divided dose Infants, children, and adults: 15–18 mg/kg in a single or divided dose Maintenance dose (usually starts 12 hours after the loading dose): Neonates: initial 5 mg/kg/d in two divided doses; usual 5–8 mg/kg/d in two to three divided doses Infants and children: initial 5 mg/kg/d in two to three divided doses; usual doses: 0.5–3 years: 8–10 mg/kg/d 4–6 years: 7.5–9 mg/kg/d 7–9 years: 7–8 mg/kg/d 10–16 years: 6–7 mg/kg/d Adults: 300 mg/d or 4–6 mg/kg/d in two to three divided doses PO: Loading dose: 15–20 mg/kg; based on phenytoin serum concentrations and recent dosing history; administer PO loading dose in three divided doses given every 2–4 hours Maintenance dose: same as daily IV maintenance dose listed above 2, 3. Arrhythmias: Children and adults: Loading dose: IV 1.25 mg/kg every 5 minutes, may repeat up to total loading dose 15 mg/kg Children: Maintenance dose: PO, IV, 5–10 mg/kg/d in two to three divided doses Adults: Loading dose, PO 250 mg four times a day for 1 day, 250 mg twice daily for 2 days Maintenance dose: 300–400 mg/d in divided doses one to four times a day
Effect	Anticonvulsant effect via membrane stabilization; antidysrhythmic effects similar to those of quinidine or procainamide
Onset	3–5 minutes
Duration	Dose dependent; half-life is dose dependent in therapeutic range
Clearance	Hepatic metabolism; renal elimination (enhanced by alkaline urine)
Comments	May cause nystagmus, diplopia, ataxia, drowsiness, gingival hyperplasia, gastrointestinal upset, hyperglycemia, or hepatic microsomal enzyme induction; IV bolus may cause bradycardia, hypotension, respiratory arrest, cardiac arrest, CNS

depression; tissue irritant; crosses placenta; significant interpatient variation, from 7.5 to 20.0 μg/ml, in the dose needed to achieve therapeutic concentration; determination of unbound phenytoin levels may help in patients with renal failure or hypoalbuminemia; divide daily dose into three doses when using suspension, chewable tablets, or non–extended-release preparations; extended-release preparations may be dosed in adults every 12 or 24 hours if patient is not receiving concomitant enzyme-inducing drugs and apparent half-life is sufficiently long

Phosphorus (Phospho-Soda; Neutra-Phos; potassium phosphate; sodium phosphate)

Indications	1. Treatment and prevention of hypophosphatemia
	2. Short-term treatment of constipation
	3. Evacuation of the colon for rectal and bowel exams
Dosage	1. Mild to moderate hypophosphatemia: Children <4 years: PO: 250 mg three to four times a day Children >4 years and adults: PO: 250–500 mg three times a day for 3 days IV: 0.08–0.15 mmol/kg over 6 hours Moderate to severe hypophosphatemia: IV: Children <4 years: 0.15–0.3 mmol/kg over 6 hours Children >4 years and adults: 0.15–0.25 mmol/kg over 6–12 hours
	2. Laxative [Fleet(R) Phospho(R)-Soda]: PO: Children 5–9 years: 5 ml as a single dose Children 10–12 years: 10 ml as a single dose Children >12 years and adults: 20–30 ml as a single dose
	3. Colonoscopy prep regimen [Fleet(R) Phospho(R)-Soda]: PO: Adults: 45 ml diluted to 90 ml with water the evening prior to the examination and repeat the dose again the following morning
Effect	Electrolyte replacement
Onset	Cathartic: 3–6 hours
Clearance	80% of dose reabsorbed by the kidneys

Comments	Infuse doses of IV phosphate over a 4- to 6-hour period; risks of rapid IV infusion include hypocalcemia, hypotension, muscular irritability, calcium deposits, renal function deterioration, and hyperkalemia; orders for IV phosphate preparations should be written in mmol (1 mmol = 31 mg); use with caution in patients with cardiac disease and renal insufficiency; do not give with magnesium- and aluminum-containing antacids or sucralfate, which can bind with phosphate

Physostigmine (Antilirium)

Indications	Postoperative delirium, tricyclic antidepressant overdose, reversal of CNS effects of anticholinergic drugs
Dosage	0.5–2.0 mg IV every 15 min prn
Effect	Inhibition of cholinesterase, central and peripheral cholinergic effects
Onset	Rapid
Duration	30–60 minutes
Clearance	Cholinesterase metabolism
Comments	May cause bradycardia, tremor, convulsions, hallucinations, psychiatric, or CNS depression, mild ganglionic blockade, or cholinergic crisis; crosses blood–brain barrier; antagonized by atropine; contains sulfite

Potassium (KCl)

Indication	Hypokalemia, digoxin toxicity
Dosage	Adult: 20 mEq of KCl administered IV over 30–60 minutes Usual infusion 10 mEq/h Pediatric: 0.02 mEq/kg/min Customary mix: 20 mEq in 1,000 ml of NSS
Effect	To correct severe hypokalemia
Onset	Immediate
Duration	Variable
Clearance	Renal
Comments	Bolus administration may cause cardiac arrest; not to exceed a maximum single dose of 40 mEq in adults; serum potassium levels should be checked prior to repeat administration; a central venous line is preferable for administration

Procainamide (Pronestyl)

Indications	Atrial and ventricular dysrhythmias
Dosage	Loading dose: 10–50 mg/min IV until toxicity or desired effect occurs, up to 12 mg/kg; stop if $\geq$50% QRS widening, or if PR lengthening occurs Maintenance dose: 2 mg/kg/h
Effect	Class IA antiarrhythmic; blocks sodium channels
Onset	Immediate
Duration	Half-life 2.5–4.5 hours, depending on acetylator phenotype
Clearance	25% hepatic conversion to active metabolite N-acetylprocainamide, a class III antiarrhythmic; renal elimination (50%–60% unchanged)
Comments	May cause increased ventricular response in atrial tachydysrhythmias unless predigitalized, asystole (with AV block), myocardial depression, CNS excitement, blood dyscrasia, lupus syndrome with positive antinuclear antibody test, or liver damage; IV administration can cause hypotension from vasodilation, decrease load by one-third in congestive heart failure or shock; therapeutic concentration is 4–8 mg/L;

Prochlorperazine (Compazine)

Indications	Nausea and vomiting
Dosage	5–10 mg/dose IV ($\leq$40 mg/d); 5–10 mg IM q2–4h prn; 25 mg per rectum q12h prn
Effect	Central (δ_2) antagonist with neuroleptic and antiemetic effects; also antimuscarinic and antihistaminic effects
Onset	Rapid
Duration	3–4 hours
Clearance	Hepatic metabolism; renal/biliary elimination
Comments	May cause hypotension (especially when given IV), extrapyramidal reactions, neuroleptic malignant syndrome, leukopenia, or cholestatic jaundice; contains sulfites; caution in liver disease; less sedating than chlorpromazine

Promethazine (Phenergan)

Indications	Allergies, anaphylaxis, nausea and vomiting, sedation

Dosage	12.5–50.0 mg IV q4–6h prn
Effect	Antagonist of H-1, δ-1, and muscarinic receptors; antiemetic, and sedative
Onset	3–5 minutes
Duration	2–4 hours
Clearance	Hepatic metabolism; renal elimination
Comments	May cause mild hypotension or mild anticholinergic effects; crosses placenta; may interfere with blood grouping; extrapyramidal effects rare; contains sulfite; intraarterial injection can cause limb gangrene ("purple glove")

Propofol (Diprivan)

Indications	Short-term sedation during mechanical ventilation
Dosage	Starting dose: 25–75 mg/h Maintenance dose: titrate by 25-mg increments every 15 minutes until desired response is achieved up to a maximum of 200–300 mg/h Bolus dose: 10–50 mg
Effect	General anesthetic and sedation in patients with mechanical ventilation
Onset	Rapid
Duration	10 minutes
Clearance	Cytochrome P-4502B6 (CYP2B6) with a high metabolic clearance that ranges from 1.6 to 3.4 L/min in healthy 70-kg adults, suggesting extrahepatic metabolism
Comments	Side effects include hypotension vomiting, rash, pain at the site of injection; IV bolus doses are associated with histamine release; use with caution in patients with documented egg allergy Sulfite warnings: Baxter propofol injectable emulsion contains sodium metabisulfite; the overall prevalence of sulfite sensitivity in the general population is unknown, is probably low, and is seen more frequently in asthmatics; in our collective experience at Massachusetts General Hospital, this sulfite in propofol has not caused any untoward event, although sulfites have been reported to trigger allergic-type reactions including anaphylaxis and status asthmaticus. There are NO preservatives in either brand of propofol, vial and ampoules are for single use only; propofol is diluted in 10% fat emulsion; propofol should not be administered in the same IV line as other medications; admixed containers and tubing must be changed every 6 hours and unused drug discarded; infusion directly from bottles should be changed every 12 hours

Propranolol (Inderal)

Indications	Hypertension, atrial and ventricular dysrhythmias, myocardial ischemia/infarction, hypertension, thyrotoxicosis, hypertrophic cardiomyopathy, migraine headache
Dosage	Adult: Test dose of 0.25–0.5 mg IV, then titrate ≤1 mg/min to effect PO: 10–40 mg q6–8 h, increased prn Pediatric: 0.05–0.1 mg/kg IV over 10 minutes
Effect	Nonspecific β-adrenergic blockade
Onset	IV: 2 minutes PO: 30 minutes
Duration	IV: 1–6 hours PO: 6 hours
Clearance	Hepatic metabolism; renal elimination
Comments	May cause bradycardia, AV dissociation, and hypoglycemia; bronchospasm, congestive heart failure, and drowsiness can occur with low doses; crosses placenta and blood–brain barrier; abrupt withdrawal can precipitate rebound angina

Prostaglandin E1 (Alprostadil, Prostin VR)

Indications	Pulmonary vasodilator, maintenance of patent ductus arteriosus
Dosage	Starting dose: 0.05–0.1 μg/kg/min Customary mix: 500 μg/250 ml of NSS or 5% D/W
Effect	Prostaglandin E1 will cause vasodilation, inhibition of platelet aggregation, vascular smooth muscle relaxation, and uterine and intestinal smooth muscle stimulation
Onset	Immediate
Duration	60 minutes
Clearance	Pulmonary metabolism; renal elimination
Comments	May cause hypotension, apnea, flushing, and bradycardia

Protamine

Indication	Reversal of the effects of heparin.
Dosage	1 mg/100 units of heparin activity IV at ≤5 mg/min

Effect	Polybasic compound forms complex with polyacidic heparin
Onset	30 seconds–1 minute
Duration	2 hours (dependent on body temperature)
Clearance	Fate of heparin/protamine complex is unknown
Comments	May cause myocardial depression and peripheral vasodilation with sudden hypotension or bradycardia; may cause severe pulmonary hypertension, particularly in the setting of cardiopulmonary bypass; the protamine/heparin complex is antigenically active; transient reversal of heparin may be followed by rebound heparinization; can cause anticoagulation if given in excess relative to amount of circulating heparin (controversial); monitor response with partial thromboplastin time or activated clotting time

Quinidine gluconate (Quinaglute)

Indications	Atrial and ventricular dysrhythmias
Dosage	For acute dysrhythmias: 800 mg IV in 50 ml of 5% D/W, giving 300–750 mg at ≤16 mg/min (≤1 ml/min); stop IV infusion if dysrhythmia is gone or toxicity occurs (25%–50% QRS widening, heart rate >120 beats/min, or loss of P waves); therapeutic concentration is 3–6 mg/L
Effect	Class IA antiarrhythmic; blocks Na channels
Onset	IV: 4–6 minutes
Duration	PO: 6–12 hours
Clearance	Hepatic metabolism; renal elimination (10%–50% unchanged)
Comments	May cause hypotension (from vasodilation and negative inotropic effects), increased ventricular response in atrial tachydysrhythmias, AV block, QT prolongation, congestive heart failure, mild anticholinergic effects, increase in serum digoxin level, cinchonism, or gastrointestinal upset; hemolysis in glucose-6-phosphate dehydrogenase–deficient patients; may potentiate action of oral anticoagulants

Ranitidine (Zantac)

Indications	Duodenal and gastric ulcers, reduction of gastric volume, raising gastric pH, esophageal reflux

Dosage	IV: 50–100 mg q6–8h; bleeding ulcers, 12.5 mg/h PO: 150–300 mg q12h
Effect	Histamine H_2-receptor antagonist; inhibits basal, nocturnal, and stimulated gastric acid secretion
Onset	IV: rapid PO: 1–3 hours
Duration	IV: 6–8 hours PO: 12 hours
Clearance	70% renal elimination unchanged
Comments	Doses should be reduced by 50% with renal failure

Scopolamine (Hyoscine)

Indications	Antisialagogue; amnesia, sedation, antiemetic, anti–motion sickness
Dosage	0.3–0.6 mg IV/IM; 1.5-mg patch
Effect	Peripheral and central cholinergic (muscarinic) antagonism
Onset	Rapid
Duration	Variable
Clearance	Hepatic metabolism; renal elimination
Comments	Excessive CNS depression can be reversed by physostigmine; may cause excitement or delirium, transient tachycardia, hyperthermia, urinary retention; crosses blood–brain barrier and placenta

Streptokinase (Kabikinase, Streptase)

Indications	1. Thrombolytic agent used in treatment of recent severe or massive DVT, pulmonary emboli 2. Myocardial infarction 3. Occluded arteriovenous cannulas
Dosage	Adult: 1. Thromboses: 250,000 units IV over 30 minutes, then 100,000 units/h for 24–72 hours 2. Myocardial infarction: 1.5 million units IV over 1 hour; if hypotension develops, decrease infusion rate by 50%; standard concentration is 1.5 million units/250 ml

3. Cannula occlusion: 250,000 units into cannula, clamp for 2 hours, then aspirate contents and flush with normal saline.

Pediatric: Safety and efficacy not established; limited studies have used 3,500–4,000 units/kg over 30 minutes followed by 1,000–1,500 units/kg/h

Effect   Thrombolytic agent

Onset   Activation of plasminogen occurs almost immediately

Duration   Fibrinolytic effects last only a few hours, whereas anticoagulant effects can persist for 12–24 hours

Clearance   Eliminated by circulating antibodies and via the reticuloendothelial system

Comments   Best results are realized if used within 5–6 hours of myocardial infarction; has been demonstrated to be effective up to 12 hours after coronary artery occlusion and onset of symptoms; give aspirin (160 mg) at the start of streptokinase infusion; begin heparin therapy (800–1,000 units/h) at the end of streptokinase infusion; avoid intramuscular injections and vascular punctures at noncompressible sites before, during, and after therapy; contraindicated with recent administration of streptokinase (antibodies to streptokinase remain for 3–6 months after initial dose), recent streptococcal infection, active internal bleeding, recent cerebrovascular accident (within 2 months), or intracranial or intraspinal surgery; relatively contraindicated following major surgery within the last 10 days, gastrointestinal bleeding, recent trauma, or severe hypertension

Terbutaline (Brethine, Bricanyl)

Indications
1. Bronchospasm
2. Tocolysis (inhibition of premature labor)

Dosage
1. Adult: 0.25 mg SQ; repeat in 15 minutes prn (use <0.5 mg/4h); 2.5–5.0 mg PO q6h prn (<15.0 mg/d)
   Pediatric: 3.5–5.0 μg/kg SQ
2. 10 μg/min IV infusion; titrate to a maximum dose of 80 μg/min

Effect   Beta$_2$-selective adrenergic agonist

Onset   SQ: <15 minutes
PO: <30 minutes

Duration	SQ: 1.5–4 hours
	PO 4–8 hours
Clearance	Hepatic metabolism; renal elimination
Comments	May cause dysrhythmias, pulmonary edema, hypertension, hypokalemia, or CNS excitement

Thiamine (vitamin B_1; Betalin)

Indications	Treatment of thiamine deficiency including beriberi, Wernicke's encephalopathy syndrome, peripheral neuritis associated with pellagra, and pregnancy
Dosage	Adult:
	Non–critically ill thiamine deficiency: 5–50 mg/d orally for 1 month
	Beriberi: 5–50 mg IM three times a day for 2 weeks, then switch to 5–50 mg orally every day for 1 month
	Severe deficiency: 50–100 mg IM or slow IV over 5 minutes repeated daily until oral therapy can be substituted; 300 mg maximum 24-hour dose
	Recommended daily allowance: 1.4 mg (male patient); 1 mg (female patient)
	Pediatric:
	Non–critically ill thiamine deficiency: 10–50 mg/d orally in divided doses for 2 weeks followed by 5–10 mg/d for 1 month
	Beriberi: 10–25 mg/d IM for 2 weeks, then 5–10 mg orally every day for 1 month
	Recommended daily allowance for infants and children: 0.3–1.4 mg
Effect	Vitamin supplement
Clearance	Eliminated unchanged in urine, and as pyrimidine after body storage sites become saturated
Comments	Single vitamin B_1 deficiency is rare, suspect multiple vitamin deficiencies; the IV route of administration is not recommended because of the risk of anaphylaxis

Thiosulfate, sodium

Indication	Cyanide toxicity, cisplatin-induced nephrotoxicity.

Dosage	Adult: 50 ml of a 25% solution IV over 10 minutes; may repeat with 50% of initial dose if signs of cyanide toxicity recur Pediatric: 7–10 g/m^2 (about 250 mg/kg) (maximum $\leq$12.5 g)
Effect	Facilitates conversion of cyanide to less toxic thiocyanate by rhodanese
Clearance	Renal elimination
Comments	Give after amyl nitrite and sodium nitrite

Tissue plasminogen activator
(recombinant; tPA, alteplase, Activase)

Indications	1.	Lysis of thrombi in coronary arteries in hemodynamically unstable patients with acute myocardial infarction
	2.	Management of acute massive pulmonary embolism in adults
	3.	Acute embolic stroke
Dosage	1.	Loading dose: 15 mg (30 ml of the infusion) IV over 1 minute followed by 0.75 mg/kg (not to exceed 50 mg) given over 30 minutes Maintenance infusion: start immediately after loading dose; 0.5 mg/kg up to 35 mg/h for 1 hour, total dose not to exceed 100 mg
	2.	100 mg continuous infusion over 2 hours
	3.	Total dose of 0.9 mg/kg (maximum 90 mg), administer 10% as a bolus and the remainder over 60 minutes
Effect		Tissue plasminogen activator
Onset		Rapid
Duration		80% cleared within 10 minutes of discontinuing infusion
Clearance		Rapid hepatic clearance.
Comments		Aspirin (325 mg) should be given at the initiation of therapy; heparin should be started (1,000 units/h) by continuous infusion 1 hour from the initiation of alteplase; doses above 150 mg have been associated with an increased incidence of intracranial hemorrhage; use within 6 hours of coronary occlusion for best results; contraindicated with active internal bleeding, history of hemorrhagic stroke, intracranial neoplasm, aneurysm, or recent (within 2 months) intracranial or intraspinal surgery or trauma;

should be used with caution in patients who have received chest compressions and patients who are receiving heparin, warfarin, or antiplatelet drugs

Tromethamine (Tris buffer; Tham)

Indications	Metabolic acidosis
Dosage	Adult and pediatric: dose depends on buffer base deficit; tromethamine ml of 0.3 M solution = Body weight (kg) × Base deficit (mEq/L) × 1.1 Pediatric: maximum recommended pediatric dose is 33–40 ml/kg/d or 500 mg/kg/dose
Effect	Organic proton acceptor (buffer)
Onset	Rapid
Duration	Hours
Clearance	Rapidly eliminated by kidneys (>75% in 3 hours)
Comments	Use with caution in patients with renal impairment or chronic respiratory acidosis

Vasopressin (antidiuretic hormone, Pitressin)

Indications	1. Diabetes insipidus
	2. Gastrointestinal bleeding
	3. Vasopressor agmentation in hypotension
	4. Shock-refractory ventricular fibrillation/pulseless ventricular tachycardia
Dosage	1. IM/SQ: 5–10 units q8–12h; IV: 2.4–10 units/hour as required based on serum electrolytes, osmolality, and urine specific gravity
	2. 0.1–0.4 unit/min
	3. 0.01–0.04 unit/min
	4. 40 units IV push × 1
Effect	Synthetic posterior pituitary hormone that increases urine osmolality and decreases urine volume; smooth muscle contraction; constriction in splanchnic, coronary, muscle, and skin vasculature
Onset	Immediate
Duration	2–8 hours
Clearance	Hepatic and renal metabolism; renal elimination

Comments   May cause oliguria, water intoxication,
                       pulmonary edema; hypertension, dysrhythmias,
                       myocardial ischemia; abdominal cramps (from
                       increased peristalsis); anaphylaxis; contraction
                       of gallbladder, urinary bladder, or uterus; vertigo,
                       or nausea; patients with coronary artery disease
                       are often treated with concurrent nitroglycerin

Verapamil (Isoptin, Calan)

Indications   Supraventricular tachycardia, atrial fibrillation
                       or flutter, Lown-Ganong-Levine syndrome
Dosage   Adult:
                       Loading dose: 2.5–10.0 mg (75–150 μg/kg) IV at a
                       rate of 1 mg/min; may repeat 2.5–5 mg every 10
                       minutes, not to exceed 20 mg
                       Maintenance dose: 5–20 mg/h as titrated to
                       patient response.
                       Pediatric:
                       0–1 years: 0.1–0.2 mg/kg IV
                       1–15 years: 0.1–0.3 mg/kg IV; repeat once if no
                       response in 30 minutes
Effect   Blockade of slow calcium channels in heart;
                       prolongation of PR interval with negative
                       inotropy and chronotropy; systemic and coronary
                       vasodilation
Onset   PO: 1–2 hours
                       IV: 1–5 minutes
Duration   PO: 8–24 hours
                       IV: 10 minutes–2 hours
Clearance   Hepatic metabolism; renal elimination
Comments   May cause severe bradycardia, AV block
                       (especially with concomitant β-blockade),
                       excessive hypotension, or congestive heart
                       failure; may increase ventricular response to
                       atrial fibrillation or flutter in patients with
                       accessory tracts; active metabolite has 20%
                       antihypertensive effect

Vitamin K/Phytonadione
(AquaMEPHYTON)

Indications   Deficiency of vitamin K–dependent clotting
                       factors; reversal of warfarin effect

Dosage	IV: 1–5 mg at ≤1 mg/min
	SQ/PO: 2.5–5 mg
	If 8 hours after IV/SQ dose, prothrombin time is not improved, repeat dose prn
Effect	Promotion of synthesis of clotting factors II, VII, IX, and X
Onset	PO: 6–12 hours
	IV: 1–2 hours
Duration	
Clearance	Hepatic metabolism
Comments	If the International Normalized Ratio (INR) is above the therapeutic range but below 5 and rapid reversal is not indicated, omit the next dose or two of warfarin sodium and resume therapy at a lower maintenance dose when the INR returns to the therapeutic range
	If the INR is >5 and <9 **or** rapid reversal is required, vitamin K 0.5–1 mg IV or vitamin K 1–2.5 mg SQ or PO may be administered; if there is a high thrombotic risk, the option to withhold warfarin for two or more doses may be preferred
	If the INR is >9 and <20, vitamin K 2.5 mg IV or 5 mg SQ may be administered.
	If the INR is >20, administration of fresh-frozen plasma is indicated along with vitamin K 2.5 mg IV or 5 mg SQ
	IV vitamin K is associated with a small risk of severe allergic reaction; when administered IV, the rate should not exceed 1 mg/min; reversal of anticoagulation by any means (vitamin K or fresh-frozen plasma) is associated with a risk of thrombosis depending on the patient's underlying need for anticoagulation.

Warfarin (Coumadin, Panwarfin)

Indication	Anticoagulation
Dosage	For patients restarting warfarin, resume warfarin therapy at the patient's maintenance dose
	Initiation:
	Patients ≥80 years old, or patients <80 years old who are <60 kg in weight: 2.5 mg
	Patients <80 years old and >60 kg in weight: 5.0 mg
	Large loading doses (≥10 mg/d) should not be used
	Monitor the International Normalized Ratio (INR) frequently during the first week of warfarin therapy to assure safe and efficient anticoagulation to target INR 2.5 (range 2.0–3.0)

Effect	Interferes with utilization of vitamin K by the liver and inhibits synthesis of factors II, VII, IX, and X
Onset	12–72 hours
Duration	2–5 days
Clearance	Hepatic metabolism; renal elimination
Comments	May be potentiated by ethanol, antibiotics, chloral hydrate, cimetidine, dextran, D-thyroxine, diazoxide, ethacrynic acid, glucagon, methyldopa, monoamine oxidase inhibitors, phenytoin, prolonged use of narcotics, quinidine, sulfonamides, congestive heart failure, hyperthermia, liver disease, malabsorption, and so on; may be antagonized by barbiturates, chlordiazepoxide, haloperidol, oral contraceptives, hypothyroidism, hyperlipidemia; crosses the placenta

AV, atrioventricular; CNS, central nervous system; DVT, deep venous thrombosis; D/W, dextrose in water; ECG, electrocardiogram; IM, intramuscularly; IV, intravenously; NS, normal saline solution; PE, pulmonary embolism; PO, orally; prn, as needed or indicated; q, every (e.g., q12h signifies "every 12 hours"); RBC, red blood cells; SL, sublingually; SQ, subcutaneously.

Table A1-1. Common intravenous antimicrobial agents (See Chapter 11)

Drug	Usual Adult IV Dose[a]	Usual Dose Interval[b]	Comments
Amikacin	300 mg	q8h	Aminoglycoside. Dose adjustment required for renal impairment.
Amphotericin B	Initial dose: 0.25 mg/kg administered over 6 h; dose should be gradually increased, ranging up to 1 mg/kg/d or 1.5 mg/kg on alternate days	q1–2d	Broad-spectrum antifungal. Initial test dose: 1 mg infused over 30 min–1 h. Do not exceed 1.5 mg/kg/d. Because of the high nephrotoxic potential, other nephrotoxic drugs should be avoided.
Amphotericin lipid complex	3–5 mg/kg/d administered over 6 h	Daily	Broad-spectrum antifungal reserved for: Nephrotoxicity to amphotericin with a serum creatinine increase by ≥1.5 mg/dl over baseline despite adequate hydration Initial therapy of fungal infection in patients with preexisting renal disease: baseline serum creatinine ≥2.5 mg/dl Systemic reactions to amphotericin persisting for >3–5 days despite acetaminophen, meperidine, diphenhydramine, and/or corticosteroids Progression of documented fungal disease (by clinical, radiographic, or histopathologic assessment) despite a minimum total course of standard amphotericin B of 500 mg or 7 mg/kg.

Liposomal amphotericin	3–5 mg/kg/d administered over 6 h	Daily	Same as above.
Ampicillin	1 g	q4h	Penicillin. Combined with sulbactam is Unasyn.[1]
Ampicillin– sulbactam (2:1)	3 g	q6h	Not effective against *Pseudomonas*.
Azithromycin	500 mg–1 g	Daily	Macrolide for atypical pneumonia and in with a third-generation cephalosporin for community-acquired pneumonia. Effective against *Legionella*.
Aztreonam	1 g	q8h	Can be used for patients allergic to penicillins or cephalosporins.
Caspofungin	70 mg load, 50 mg daily	Daily	Broad-spectrum antifungal agent particularly effective against fluconazole-resistant *Candida*. Dose must be reduced or interval extended in the presences of severe hepatic insufficiency. May increase the concentrations of other drugs metabolized by the CYP3A4 pathway. Coadministration with phenytoin, carbamazepine, and long-acting barbiturates requires 70 mg daily of caspofungin.
Cefazolin	1 g	q4–8h	First-generation cephalosporin. Adjust dose in renal disease.[c] Use caution in patients allergic to penicillin.[d]
Cefepime	1–2 g	q12h	Fourth-generation cephalosporin. Preferred for *Pseudomonas aeruginosa* infections and neutropenic patients with fever.[c,d]
Cefotetan	1–2 g	q12h	Second-generation cephalosporin. Possible disulfiram-like reaction.[c,d]

(continued)

Table A1-1. *Continued*

Drug	Usual Adult IV Dose[a]	Usual Dose Interval[b]	Comments
Ceftazidime	1 g	q8h	Third-generation cephalosporin.[c,d]
Ceftriaxone	1 g	q24h	Second-generation cephalosporin. Preferred for empiric coverage for bacterial meningitis at higher doses.[c,d]
Chloramphenicol	50–100 mg/kg	q6h	Considered a second-line antibiotic with limited usefulness secondary to an association with aplastic anemia.
Ciprofloxacin	400 mg	q12h	Quinolone. Good absorption via oral route (500 mg q12h). Effective against *Pseudomonas*.
Clindamycin	600 mg	q8h	Associated with *Clostridium difficile* colitis.
Daptomycin	4 mg/kg IV	Daily	Adjust dose for renal insufficiency: Creatine clearance <30 mL/min: 4 mg/kg IV every 48 h. Hemodialysis: 4 mg/kg IV once every 48 h after hemodialysis.
Doxycycline	100 mg	q12h	Rare hepatotoxicity, pseudotumor cerebri, and benign intracranial hypertension have been reported.
Erythromycin	0.5–1 g	q6h	Macrolide. Bacteriostatic. Gastritis with PO route. Venous irritation.
Fluconazole	200–400 mg	q24h	Broad-spectrum antifungal. Well absorbed orally. Dose adjustments required in renal and hepatic insufficiency.
Gentamicin	60–120 mg (3–5 mg/kg/d)	q8–12h over 15–20 min	Aminoglycoside. Decrease dose in renal failure. Renal and ototoxicity. Precipitates with heparin. May prolong neuromuscular blockade.

Imipenem-cilastatin	500 mg	q6h	Carbapenem. Preferred for multiple-drug resistant gram-negative bacterial infections.[c,d]
Levofloxacin	500 mg	Daily	Quinolone. L-isomer of ofloxacin. Well absorbed orally. Dose adjustments required in moderate to severe renal insufficiency.
Linezolid	600 mg	q12	Also available orally with equal efficacy. Anemia, thrombocytopenia, and leukopenia can occur. Will resolve with discontinuation of the drug.
Meropenem	0.5–1 g	q8h	Carbapenem.[c,d] See Imipenem
Metronidazole	500 mg	q8h	Possible acute toxic psychosis; disulfiram-like reaction with convulsions, leukopenia.
Nafcillin	1.5 g	q4h	Preferred for antistaphylococcal coverage.[c,d] May induce interstitial nephritis.
Penicillin G[1]	500,000–2,000,000 U	q4h	Hypersensitivity is common.[c,d]
Piperacillin	4 g	q6h	Usually combined with aminoglycoside for treatment of Pseudomonas.[c,d]
Piperacillin–tazobactam (8:1)	3.375 g	q4–6h	Tazobactam expands activity to include β-lactamase–producing strains of Staphylococcus aureus, Haemophilus influenzae, Enterobacteriaceae, Pseudomonas, Klebsiella, Citrobacter,
	4.5 g	q8h	Serratia, Bacteroides, and other gram-negative anaerobes.[c,d]
Ticarcillin	3 g	q4h	Antipseudomonal penicillin of choice.[c,d]
Ticarcillin-clavulanic acid (30:1)	3.1 g	q4h	Clavulanic acid expands activity to include β-lactamase–producing strains of S. aureus, H. influenzae, Enterobacteriaceae, Pseudomonas, Klebsiella, Citrobacter, and Serratia.[c,d]

(continued)

Table A1-1. Continued

Drug	Usual Adult IV Dose[a]	Usual Dose Interval[b]	Comments
Trimethoprim/ sulfamethoxazole	8–10 mg/kg/d (based on trimethoprim component)	q6–12h	Allergic reactions common. Interferes with secretion of creatinine and potassium; values may increase.
Tobramycin	60–120 mg (3–5 mg/ kg/d over 15–20 min)	q8h	Aminoglycoside. See gentamicin.
Vancomycin	500 mg–1 g over 60 min	q12h	Preferred for oxacillin-resistant staphylococcal infections and patients with penicillin allergy. Decrease dose in renal disease. Histamine release ("red man"), renal damage, deafness. May precipitate with other medications.
Voriconazole	Load: 6 mg/kg IV q12h for two doses Maintenance: 4 mg/kg IV q12h	q12h	Broad-spectrum antifungal. Monitor liver function tests. May increase the concentrations of other drugs metabolized by the CYP3A4 pathway. Coadministration with phenytoin, carbamazepine, and long-acting barbiturates will decrease plasma voriconazole concentrations. Voriconazole increases the plasma concentrations of sirolimus, efavirenz, rifabutin, and ergot alkaloids.

See also Chapter 11.

IV, intravenously; PO, orally; q, every (e.g., q12h signifies "every 12 hours").

[a]Adult doses are those usually given to healthy 70-kg patients and may vary with the patient's condition or concomitant drug intake. Older or debilitated patients may require smaller doses.

[b]Dose adjustments may be required in patients with renal impairment, hepatic dysfunction, and altered volume status.

[c]All β-lactams in high concentrations will cause seizures and should be dosed based on the creatinine clearance.

[d]From 5% to 10% of penicillin-allergic patients will react to cephalosporins and carbapenems.

Table A1-2. Narcotic comparision chart

Drug	Adult Dose[a] (mg)	Pediatric Dose[a] (mg/kg)	Duration of Action (h)	Conversion Factor	Metabolism	Comments
Codeine					Hepatic to morphine	
Parenteral	15–60	0.5–1	4	0.08		Avoid IV route due to large histamine release and cardiovascular effects
Oral	15–60	0.5–1		0.05		
Fentanyl					Hepatic	
Parenteral	0.050–0.10	0.001–0.002	0.5–2	100		Rapid IV injection can result in skeletal muscle and chest wall rigidity
Transdermal patch				100		25, 50, 75, or 100 $\mu g/h$
Hydromorphone (Dilaudid)					Hepatic; eliminated in urine, principally as glucuronide conjugates	Pediatric use not well established
Parenteral	1–2	0.015–0.05	4	0.67		
Oral	2–4	0.03–0.08		1.33		

(continued)

Table A1-2. *Continued*

Drug	Adult Dose^a (mg)	Pediatric Dose^a (mg/kg)	Duration of Action (h)	Conversion Factor	Metabolism	Comments
Meperidine (Demerol) Parenteral	50–150	1–1.5	3–4	0.1	Hepatic; normeperidine (active metabolite) is dependent on renal function and can accumulate with high doses or in patients with decreased renal function	Use with caution in patients with hepatic or renal failure, seizure disorders, or receiving high doses; fluoxetine and other serotonin-uptake inhibitors greatly potentiate the effects of meperidine; normeperidine (CNS stimulant) may accumulate and precipitate twitching, tremor, or seizures; **contraindicated with concurrent use of MAO inhibitors**
Oral **Methadone**	50–150	1–1.5	6–8, increases	0.03		Not recommended Phenytoin, pentazocine, and rifampin may

					Metabolism	
Parenteral	2–10	0.1		1.3	Metabolism is 4 times greater after oral administration than after parenteral administration	increase the metabolism of methadone and may precipitate withdrawal; increased toxicity: CNS depressants, phenothiazines, tricyclic antidepressants, and MAO inhibitors may potentiate the adverse effects of methadone
Oral	2–10	0.1–0.2	to 22–48 with repeated doses	0.7		
Morphine						
Parenteral	5–10	0.1–0.2	3–5	1	In the liver via glucuronide conjugation; excreted unchanged in urine	Histamine release; may cause hypotension in patients with acute myocardial infarction
Oral[b]	10–30	0.2–0.5		0.33		
Oxycodone (Percocet, Roxicet)						
Oral	5	0.05–0.15	4	0.33	Hepatic	

See also Chapter 6.

CNS, central nervous system; IV, intravenous; MAO, monoamine oxidase.

[a]These doses (oral, intramuscular) are recommended starting doses for acute pain. Optimal doses for each patient are determined by titration, and the maximal dose is limited by adverse effects. For single starting intravenous doses, use *half* the intramuscular dose listed. Any oral or parenteral analgesic may be converted into its intramuscular morphine equivalent by multiplying the dose by the conversion factor.

[b]Controversy exists concerning the actual conversion factor (3:1 ratio).

Table A1-3. Comparison of benzodiazepines

Drug	Adult Dose Range (mg/d)	Time to Peak Plasma Level (h)	Half-life (h)	Active Metabolites
Long acting				
Chlordiazepoxide (Librium)	15–100	1–4	5–30	Desmethylchlordiazepoxide Demoxepam N-Desmethyldiazepam
Clonazepam (Klonapin)	1.5–12	1–4	30–40	None
Diazepam (Valium)	6–40	0.5–2	20–80	N-Desmethyldiazepam N-Methyloxazepam (temaxepam) Oxazepam
Flurazepam (Dalmane)	15–60	2–6	40–114	N-Desalkylflurazepam
Short acting				
Alprazolam (Xanax)	0.75–4	1–2	12–15	None
Lorazepam (Ativan)	2–6	2–4	10–20	75% is converted to the glucuronide derivative (12-h half-life), which can accumulate in prolonged dosing
Midazolam (Versed)	2.5–30	0.25–1	1–4	Alpha-Hydroxymidazolam
Oxazepam (Serax)	30–120	2–4	5–16	None

See also Chapter 6.

Laboratory Values for Blood

Richard M. Pino

Chemistry

Adrenocorticotropic hormone	6–76 pg/ml
Albumin	3.1–4.3 g/dl
Alkaline phosphatase	
Male	45–115 U/L
Female	30–100 U/L
Ammonia, plasma	12–48 μmol/L
Amylase, serum	53–123 U/L
Anion gap (AG):	
$[Na] + [K] - [HCO_3] - [Cl]$	5–15 mmol/L
Corrected AG = $AG_{calculated}$ +	
$0.25(Albumin_{normal} - Albumin_{measured})$	
Arterial blood gas tensions and pH	
Po_2	80–100 mm Hg
Pco_2	35–45 mm Hg
pH	7.35–7.45
ALT (alanine aminotransferase [SGPT])	
Male	10–55 U/L
Female	7–30 U/L
AST (aspartate aminotransferase [SGOT])	
Male	10–40 U/L
Female	9–25 U/L
Bicarbonate (Total CO_2)	22–26 mmol/L
Bilirubin, direct	≤0.4 mg/dl
Bilirubin, total	≤1.0 mg/dl
Blood urea nitrogen (BUN)	8–25 mg/dl
Calcium	8.5–10.5 mg/dl
Calcium, ionized	1.14–1.30 mmol/L
Carbon monoxide (CO)	<5% total hemoglobin
Chloride	100–108 mmol/L
Cholesterol	
Desirable	<200 mg/dl
Borderline	200–239 mg/dl
High	>239 mg/dl
Cortisol	
Baseline	10–25 mcg/dl
After corticotropin stimulation	>9 μg/dl
Creatine phosphokinase (CPK)	
Male	60–400 U/L
Female	40–150 U/L
Creatinine	0.6–1.5 mg/dl
Digoxin	0.9–2.0 ng/ml
Ethanol (intoxication)	>1,000 mg/L
Globulin	2.6–4.1 g/dl
Glucose (fasting)	70–110 mg/dl

(continued)

Laboratory Values *Continued*

Haptoglobin	16–199 mg/dl
Iron, serum	30–160 μg/dl
Lactate dehydrogenase (LDH)	110–210 U/L
Lactic acid, plasma	0.5–2.2 mmol/L
Lipase, serum	3–19 U/dl
Magnesium	1.4–2.0 mEq/L
Methemoglobin	0.4%–1.5% total hemoglobin
Osmolality	280–296 mOsm/kg
Phenytoin (serum)	5–20 μg/ml
Phenytoin (calculated free phenytoin)	[Free] = [Serum]/(0.2 × Albumin) + 0.1
Phosphorus	2.6–4.5 mg/dl
Potassium	3.5–5.0 mmol/L
Protein, total	6.0–8.0 g/dl
Sodium	135–145 mmol/L
Thyroid function tests	
Thyroid hormone–binding index	0.77–1.23
Triiodothyronine	60–181 ng/dl
Thyroxine	4.5–10.9 μg/dl
Thyroid-stimulating hormone	0.5–5.0 μU/ml
Total iron-binding capacity (TIBC)	228–428 μg/dl
Triglycerides (fasting)	40–150 mg/dl
Troponin T	<0.1 ng/dl
Uric acid	
Male	3.6–8.5 mg/dl
Female	2.3–6.6 mg/dl
Venous blood gas tensions, mixed	
Po_2	50 mm Hg
Pco_2	40–50 mm Hg
pH	7.32–7.42

Hematology and coagulation values

Activated protein C resistance (screening assay for factor V Leiden)	Normal >2.0
D-dimer	0.0–0.5 μg/ml
Erythrocyte count (RBC)	
Male	4.5–5.3×10^6/mm^3
Female	4.1–5.1×10^6/mm^3
Erythrocyte sedimentation rate (ESR)	
Male	1–17 mm/h
Female	1–25 mm/h
Ferritin, serum	20–300 ng/ml
Fibrin split products (FSP)	0–2.5 μg/ml
Fibrinogen	175–400 mg/dl
Hematocrit	
Male	37%–49%
Female	36%–46%
Hemoglobin	
Male	13–18 g/dl
Female	12–16 g/dl
Heparin assay (anti-Xa activity)	<0.05 IU/ml

(continued)

Laboratory Values *Continued*

Leukocyte count (WBC)	$4.5–11.0 \times 10^3/mm^3$
Neutrophils	45%–75%
Bands	0%–5%
Lymphocytes	16%–46%
Monocytes	4%–11%
Eosinophils	0%–8%
Basophils	0%–3%
Mean corpuscular hemoglobin (MCH)	25–35 pg/cell
Mean corpuscular volume (MCV)	78–100 μm^3
Partial thromboplastin time, activated (aPTT)	22.1–34.1 sec
Platelet count	$150–350 \times 10^3/mm^3$
Prothrombin time (PT)	11.2–13.2 sec
Reticulocyte count	0.5%–2.5%

SELECTED REFERENCES

Kratz A, Lewandrowski B. Case records of the Massachusetts General Hospital. Weekly clinicopathological exercises. Normal reference laboratory values. *N Engl J Med* 1998;339:1063–1072.

Massachusetts General Hospital Lab Handbook 2001 Edition. Available at http://www.massgeneral.org/labmed/adm/handbook/handbook.pdf.

Subject Index

Page numbers followed by f denotes figure; those followed by t denote tables.